Hearing in Children

Sixth Edition

Hearing in Children

Sixth Edition

Jerry L. Northern, PhD

With Significant Contributions From
Deborah Hayes, PhD

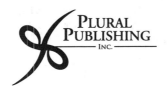
PLURAL
PUBLISHING
INC.

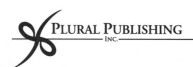

PLURAL PUBLISHING
INC.

5521 Ruffin Road
San Diego, CA 92123

e-mail: info@pluralpublishing.com
Website: http://www.pluralpublishing.com

Typeset in 10½/13 Minion Pro by Flanagan's Publishing Services, Inc.
Printed in the United States of America by McNaughton & Gunn, Inc.

NOTICE TO THE READER
Care has been taken to confirm the accuracy of the indications, procedures, drug dosages, and diagnosis and remediation protocols presented in this book and to ensure that they conform to the practices of the general medical and health services communities. However, the authors, editors, and publisher are not responsible for errors or omissions or for any consequences from application of the information in this book and make no warranty, expressed or implied, with respect to the currency, completeness, or accuracy of the contents of the publication. The diagnostic and remediation protocols and the medications described do not necessarily have specific approval by the Food and Drug administration for use in the disorders and/or diseases and dosages for which they are recommended. Application of this information in a particular situation remains the professional responsibility of the practitioner. Because standards of practice and usage change, it is the responsibility of the practitioner to keep abreast of revised recommendations, dosages, and procedures.

Library of Congress Cataloging-in-Publication Data

Northern, Jerry L., author.
  Hearing in children / Jerry L. Northern, Marion P. Downs ; with significant contributions from Deborah Hayes. — Sixth edition.
       p. ; cm.
  Includes bibliographical references and index.
  ISBN-13: 978-1-59756-392-5 (alk. paper)
  ISBN-10: 1-59756-392-7 (alk. paper)
  I. Downs, Marion P., author. II. Hayes, Deborah, contributor. III. Title.
  [DNLM: 1. Hearing Disorders. 2. Child. 3. Early Diagnosis. 4. Early Intervention (Education)
5. Hearing Tests—methods. 6. Infant. WV 271]
  RF290
  617.80083—dc23
                                                                2013047459

Contents

Foreword		*ix*
Preface		*xi*
Acknowledgments		*xiii*

1 Hearing and Hearing Loss in Children — 1
Hearing Loss in Children—A Hidden Disability — 2
How We Hear — 7
The Nature of Hearing Loss — 20
Demographics of Childhood Hearing Loss — 25
Acoustics of Speech — 30
Team Management of Children with Hearing Loss — 45
Audiologists with Specialty Training in Pediatric Hearing Loss — 47

2 Early Development — 51
Basic Principles of Genetic Inheritance — 52
Inheritance of Genetic Disorders — 63
Abnormalities Related to Gene/Environment Interaction — 67
Prenatal Development — 70
Fetal Development — 77
Development of Ears, Face and Palate — 80
The Nursery Environment — 90
Disorders of the Infant Respiratory System — 96
Disorders of the Cardiovascular System — 99
Disorders of the Central Nervous System — 100
Congenital Infections — 100
Genetic Counseling — 109

3 Auditory and Speech-Language Development — 113
Neuroplasticity — 114
Prenatal Hearing — 118
Neonatal Hearing Development — 121
Development of Oral Communication — 127
Questionnaires for Parents — 132
Studies of Speech Development — 136
Optimal Periods — 143
Listening — 148
Auditory Processing in Children — 151

4 Medical Aspects — 163
Medical Assessment of Newborn Infants — 164

Medical Conditions of the External Ear   166
Otitis Media   173
Medical Disorders and Sensorineural Hearing Loss   189
Childhood Infections Associated With Hearing Loss   199
Cleft Palate   203
Down Syndrome   204
Autism Spectrum Disorder (ASD)   205
Auditory Neuropathy Spectrum Disorder (ANSD)   206

5 Early Intervention   211
Early Intervention Services   211
Implementation of Early Intervention   212
Federal Mandates   215
Cornerstones of Early Intervention   216
Optimal Early Intervention Strategies   221
Family-Centered Services   223
Breaking the News to Parents   228
The Audiologist's Self-Understanding   233
Intervention Strategies for the Child With Otitis Media   239
Telepractice and Teleaudiology   242
Hearing Dogs   244

6 Behavioral Hearing Tests   247
The Audiologist and the Child   249
The Case History   255
Reinforcement Theory   268
Visual Reinforcement Audiometry (VRA): 6 Months to 2 Years of Age   271
Conditioned Play Audiometry With Children Ages 2 to 4 Years   277
Pediatric Speech Audiometry   283
Speech Perception Testing   286
Hearing Testing of the Older Child (5 Years and Older)   294
Evaluating Hearing of Difficult-to-Test Children   295
Functional Hearing Loss in Children   305

7 Physiologic Hearing Tests   309
Managing Toddlers for Physiologic Hearing Tests   310
Acoustic Immittance Measures   315
Clinical Applications of the Immittance Battery With Children   331
Otoacoustic Emissions   337
Evoked Auditory Responses   345
Auditory Brainstem Evoked Responses (ABR)   347
Auditory Middle-Latency Evoked Response (MLR)   355
Late Auditory Evoked Potentials (AEPs)   357
Auditory Steady-State Response (ASSR)   359

Electrocochleography   363
Sedation   365
Vestibular Evaluation in Children   367
Summary of Physiologic Auditory Testing   368

8   Hearing Screening   **373**
Principles of Screening   374
Genetic Screening   382
History of Newborn Hearing Screening   385
Universal Newborn Hearing Screening   390
Hearing Screening: Birth Through 6 Months   399
Hearing Screening: Infants and Toddlers (7 Months to 3 Years)   405
Hearing Screening: Preschool Children (3 to 5 Years)   409
Hearing Screening: School-Age Children (5 to 18 Years)   410
Screening for Middle Ear Disorders   415
Hearing Screening of the Developmentally Delayed Child   418
Screening Follow-Up Issues   419

9   Amplification   **423**
Pediatric Hearing Aid Fittings   426
The Hearing Aid   428
Hearing Aids for Children   431
The Pediatric Hearing Aid Fitting Process   438
Probe Microphone Measurements   439
Prescriptive Fitting Methods   452
Binaural Hearing Aids   456
Frequency Response   458
Hearing Aid Output   460
The Earmold and Sound Channel   462
Monitoring Children's Hearing Aids   464
Pediatric Cochlear Implants   464

10 Education   **483**
The Educational Audiologist   484
Individuals with Disabilities Education Act (IDEA)   487
Educational Goals for the Child With Hearing Loss   490
Current Status of Education   499
Challenges in Teaching Deaf and Hearing-Impaired Students   502
Implementing the Individualized Educational Plan (IEP)   505
Educational Methodologies   507
Mainstream Education   520
Classroom Acoustics   524
Personal FM Systems   527
Parent Education   530

Appendix A. Pediatric Hearing Disorders   535

Appendix B. Guidelines for Identification and Management of Infants   585
and Young Children with Auditory Neuropathy Spectrum Disorder

References   607
Author Index   663
Subject Index   673

Foreword

Pediatric audiology came quietly into being in the early 1940s, spurred by dedicated educators of the hard-of-hearing and deaf who studied auditory behaviors of normal-hearing children and applied those comparisons to their students with hearing loss. These educators were Lord and Lady Ewing in England who developed the earliest behavioral techniques for testing the hearing of very young children. Today many thousands of individuals with hearing loss are enjoying more successful lives as a result of having been identified early in life.

Today we look back to this period of time when the potential of early infant development was finally recognized. Out of an era of mechanistic behaviorism advocated by B.F. Skinner, there gradually grew an understanding of the latent and hidden capabilities of the newborn human infant—capabilities that needed to be stimulated and nurtured in certain ways at certain times to reach full maturity. Foremost in fostering this understanding were individuals such as Chomsky, Piaget, Lennenberg, Apgar, Spock, and Brazelton, and their many, many students. The thoughts, works, and contributions of these clinicians/scientists have extended the purview of the developing infant to other related professionals while recognizing the important roles played by the parent, caregiver, and family.

Nearly all health and education professions have a stake somehow in the human newborn infant; hardly a specialty exists that does not claim a part of this emergent individual. Pediatric audiologists may focus their attentions on the hearing mechanism of the infant, but hearing does not exist in a vacuum; it is part of a complicated, interrelated, living, breathing, thinking child that sustains the auditory response and, in turn, is modified by it. The skills and knowledge that are most interrelated with hearing are linguistics and speech. Both develop in the normal infant through the passive act of listening, albeit in different ways. Normal development and production of speech is dependent on the presence of normal hearing. Most children with normal hearing develop appropriate speech production skills during their early childhood years. For children with hearing loss, speech production intelligibility is directly proportional to the degree of the loss. In other words, the better the hearing, the better is the child's speech.

This is not so for language. Language skills of children with hearing loss appear to be fairly equally affected by almost any degree of significant hearing loss. We have now confirmed that the only factor that significantly affects language abilities in young children with hearing loss and deafness is the time of intervention. In other words, once again, we see that the earlier the intervention, the better the child's language skills.

All children with hearing loss, even those with mild and moderate hearing losses, will show delay in receptive and expressive language. For this reason, all children with hearing loss must be identified early enough in the earliest months of life to enable successful early intervention. The highly technical advancements in hearing aids and cochlear implants provide access to the auditory world even for babies with profound sensory deafness. Early identification followed by early interventions takes advantage of these infants' young brains to help them become fully functional, hearing individuals.

Many thousands of individuals with hearing loss are enjoying more successful lives as a result of having been identified early in life by audiologists. Make no mistake: our goal is for all! Not just the child with parents who can afford testing and monitoring. Not just those children who happen to fall into a category that places them at risk for hearing loss or profound deafness. Not just the infants that happen to be in the right place at the right time to be screened and evaluated. We are talking about all children with hearing loss. They are all entitled to be touched by the hands of pediatric audiologists using the best in modern technology to accurately and promptly diagnosis and manage these babies with hearing loss. There is too much at stake to miss any of these youngsters.

The field of medicine gives us an interesting analog: it has been said that "medicine is unique among the sciences in that it strives incessantly to defeat the object of its own invention." This object, of course, is disease, and there is a parallel in audiology. Since our beginnings in the mid-1940s, we have measured, described, researched, cataloged, analyzed, and synthesized the entity of hearing loss exhaustively. Now,

having defined it completely, we must busy ourselves with preventing the devastation of its effects on children. Such prevention can only be accomplished by early detection of the condition and by proper provision of early intervention, appropriate therapy, and purposeful education. Armed with our new depth of knowledge, we can assuredly enhance and enrich the lives of children with hearing loss and their families.

These observations challenge us to utilize the particular skills that we acquire during our education and training. Our unique knowledge of the interrelated aspects of hearing, speech, and language is an important contribution to understanding the wonder of communication development in infants. The audiologist's goal is to identify hearing problems and to understand the accompanying auditory disorders—an especially challenging task in infants and young children. To this end, we must constantly hone our skills and technologies. Our ultimate goal is that all infants and young children with hearing loss will achieve their full potentials and attain the best future possible as happy, successful, and productive adults.

—Marion P. Downs, DHS, DS
Professor Emerita, University of
Colorado School of Medicine
Denver, Colorado

Preface

I begin by stating that I had no intention of ever writing a sixth edition of *Hearing in Children*. More than a decade had passed since the fifth edition was published in 2002, and I had no desire to undertake such a huge task again. Although my career as an audiologist had taken several unforeseen turns during this time period, my interest in pediatric audiology has never waned. I had given occasional thought to a rewrite and update of the fifth edition, but the necessary time needed for the project was never readily available, and the looming magnitude of the project simply overwhelmed me. I was also well aware of the tremendous growth and advancements in the pediatric audiology arena that would demand a complete overhaul of every topic to make the sixth edition useful and pertinent. Obviously, an update and rewrite would require a huge commitment from me, when, in fact, I had retirement on my mind.

During the years that passed since 2002, many of my academic colleagues who teach pediatric audiology pointed out to me that the fifth edition was outdated, and that they were finding it necessary to supplement the text with outside readings. Many of them urged me to write a new edition of *Hearing in Children* as the book had served them well as a class textbook for so many years. Further, the audiology graduate student populations were studying at an advanced level, and they needed a pediatric audiology textbook that would meet their needs for current knowledge of technologies and the special clinical applications to provide the highest standard of hearing services appropriate for pediatric patients.

I must admit to having several false starts at writing a sixth edition during the past few years, but my time and interests were continually drawn to other projects demanded by my employment and family, making it far too easy for me to procrastinate. I was also well aware of the availability of several new outstanding pediatric audiology textbooks challenging the unique solid position *Hearing in Children* had held for 40 years.

During the long interim since 2002, I have had an active speaking schedule around the United States as well as numerous international speaking engagements. As I traveled and spoke to such a wide divergence of audience, I became keenly aware of the enormous impact that our text, *Hearing in Children*, has had since its inception in 1974 on the worldwide training of audiologists, which hopefully has translated into improved hearing care for uncounted numbers of infants and children. The fact that foreign language translations of the previous editions in Spanish, Portuguese, and Japanese brought our world of pediatric audiology to students and professionals on every continent has provided great satisfaction to us, and now spoke loudly to me for the need and value of a new edition.

But it was the convergence of several factors that made me realize that now was the time to commit to the arduous task of a new sixth edition of *Hearing in Children*. First, my good friend and esteemed colleague, Deborah Hayes of Children's Hospital Colorado, and outstanding pediatric audiologist in her own right, was relentless with her encouragement for me to move forward, and she even went so far as to offer to help me—an offer I obviously couldn't refuse! Then, I experienced unexpected overwhelming responses during a multicity speaking tour in India whereby students and professionals turned out in amazing numbers to express their fondness and appreciation for our previous five editions of *Hearing in Children*. Finally, nearer home, I received not-so-subtle convincing support from my dear wife, Deborah, who desperately needed to get me out from underfoot and would not accept my continued floundering toward retirement. From all of these reasons, I found myself with eager and renewed enthusiasm to get on with the important work of producing a new sixth edition of *Hearing in Children*.

—Jerry L. Northern, PhD
Professor Emeritus, University of
Colorado School of Medicine
Denver, Colorado

Acknowledgments

First Edition. A book of this magnitude cannot be assembled and written without the help of many other people. We pay special tribute to and thank five of our colleagues and good friends who gave graciously of their valuable time and personal material for our benefit: La Vonne Bergstrom, MD; Isamu Sando, MD; Janet M. Stewart, MD; Marlin Weaver, MD; and Winfield McChord, Jr., MS. Many others responded to our needs, willingly and unselfishly, to provide requested information at a moment's notice: Carol Amon, MA; Owen Black, MD; Carol Cox, MA; Kathleen O. Foust, MA; William K. Frankenberg, MD; Aram Glorig, MD; W. G. Hemenway, MD; Brian Hersch, MD; Mrs. Page T. Jenkins; Pat Tesauro, MA; Darrel Teter, PhD; and Harold Weber, MA. Connie H. Knight, MA, audiologist at the Georgia Retardation Center, Atlanta, was our research associate and gathered much of the material presented in the "Index of Selected Birth Defect Syndromes." Sharon Mraz was our editorial assistant. Patricia Jenkins Thompson, MA, diligently proofread and critiqued our efforts. Y. Oishi, MD, served as our primary photographer; Miriam Eliachar illustrated the chapter pictures and embryology figures; and Anita McGuire typed the entire manuscript. We also acknowledge the cooperation of the publishing staff at Williams & Wilkins, especially William R. Hensyl, who encouraged us to write this textbook. Finally, we extend our appreciation and thanks to our spouses, families, children, and friends, who will long remember (as will we!) this period during which we were too busy, too preoccupied, or too tired—our Year of the Book, 1973.

Second Edition. Once again numerous colleagues came to our aid to provide advice, share materials, and labor in the libraries to help prepare the second edition of *Hearing in Children.* We express our warmest thanks to Jeff Adams, Marlin Cohrs, Roni Halpern, Donna Lutz, Winfield McChord, Deborah Smith, Steven Staller, Darrel Teter, Harold Weber, and Janet Zarnoch. We are particularly grateful for the contributions of Mrs. Kathleen Bryant, speech pathologist at the University of Colorado Medical Center. Patsy Tormey, our helpful secretary, typed the manuscript and quietly tolerated our many revisions. Ruby Richardson at Williams & Wilkins nudged us gently, but firmly, throughout this revision. Finally, we appreciate the helpful comments and critique provided by our professional friends who took time to respond to a lengthy questionnaire regarding the first edition. Their guidance and suggestions greatly influenced the second edition of *Hearing in Children.*

Third Edition. We are grateful to a new cadre of friends, students, and associates who responded to our requests for help with the third edition. We thank David Asher, James R. Curran, Sandra Abbott Gabbard, Marianne Geisler, Christine Gerhardt, Katherine Pike Gerkin, Kathryn Grose, Deanie Johnson, Deborah Kinder, Sharon A. Mitchell, Patrick Sullivan, MD, and Ann Wilson. Patsy Tormey-Meredith typed the manuscripts again, but this time during maternity leave. We were delighted to work again with William R. Hensyl, of Williams & Wilkins, who was the original perpetrator of *Hearing in Children.*

Fourth Edition. We are indebted to many of our colleagues for their supportive efforts. Especially helpful through their review, critical commentary, and useful suggestions were Julia M. Davis, Sandy Friel-Patti, Judith S. Gravel, M. Suzanne Hasenstab, Deborah Hayes, John and Claire Jacobson, Susan Jerger, Robert W. Keith, and Laszlo Stein. We thank them for their time and effort. Once again, we are most thankful to our ever-dependable secretary/friend Patsy Tormey-Meredith, for bearing with us again in typing (and retyping) the manuscript. A special thanks is extended to the University Hospital audiology staff for their patience, understanding, and support during the many months spent preparing this new edition.

Fifth Edition. One of the great pleasures in working in the field of audiology has been the close association with colleagues who have stepped forward once again to help with this new edition. I especially acknowledge the contributions of three anonymous reviewers who made many worthwhile suggestions for improvements in this new edition. I also pay special thanks to Harvey Dillon, Kiara Ebinger, Sandra Abbott Gabbard, Parker Haberly, Robert Keith, Patsy Meredith, H. Gus Mueller, and Laszlo Stein, for generously helping and providing materials. Miriam Eliachar, from Jerusalem, willingly created a number of new illustrations in her signature style. I am especially grateful to my esteemed colleague, Deborah Hayes of the Denver Children's Hospital, for her review and comments for each revised chapter and her responsiveness to my requests that were always on a moment's notice. I certainly could not forget to acknowledge the support from my closest colleague for more than 35 years, Marion Downs, who serves as the highest role model for all of us who work with children

with hearing disabilities. Most importantly, a huge thanks and a lot of love to my wife, Deborah, who encouraged and supported me daily and was so understanding of my time and energy commitment throughout the process of rewriting this fifth edition of *Hearing in Children.*

Sixth Edition. I could never have imagined in my wildest dreams that there would be six editions of *Hearing in Children.* I am forever indebted to my colleague and dear friend, Marion Downs, who introduced me to the world of pediatric audiology and then constantly raised questions about every aspect of children's hearing. We didn't have all the answers, but we set out as kindred professional spirits to write a much-needed textbook, way back in 1972, about the hearing and hearing disorders of infants and young children. We realized that we worked in a unique medical center environment, with an amazing group of dedicated medical specialists devoted to helping children with birth defects, who were especially knowledgeable and skillful in the diagnosis and management of children with congenital hearing loss. We jumped at the opportunity to share this knowledge with other audiologists, and audiology students, to improve the overall provision of hearing services for pediatric patients. Working together in a busy audiology clinic, and writing that first edition of *Hearing in Children,* was an unforgettable and enjoyable period of our lives. And, now, six editions and 40 years later, it is overwhelming to look back and realize how many people have been involved in helping to produce various editions of this textbook. I am so very grateful for the encouragement and help provided from many colleagues around the globe for this sixth edition. First and foremost, I extend my appreciation and gratitude to Deborah Hayes of the Children's Hospital Colorado for her support and guidance throughout this long-term project, including the provision of many of her own materials for inclusion in this update. Quite frankly, this book would not have been completed without Dr. Hayes' involvement, contributions and encouragement. I also want to express my appreciation to the Colorado Children's Hospital, Department of Audiology, Speech Pathology and Learning Services staff and clinic families for their help with many of the photographs, taken by Tia Brayman, lead photographer of the CCH Creative Services Department. My appreciation is extended to another good friend, William J. Keith of Auckland, New Zealand, who was very helpful in providing materials about auditory processing in children. Closer to home, my daughter Amy Northern Hardie, director-teacher of the Spokane, Washington, Hearing Oral Program of Excellence (HOPE Preschool for Hearing-Impaired Children) stimulated discussions, provided me with access and photographs, and otherwise kept me moving forward by constantly questioning my progress. The field of pediatric audiology has changed so much over the past decade that I could not have completed this new edition without the help of many experts from various aspects of identification, intervention, and management of children with hearing loss. I am pleased to acknowledge the contributions of Jan Berger, Gini Moore Campbell, Barry Freeman, Erica Friedland, Sandra Gabbard, Jason Galster, Parker Haberly, James "Jay" Hall, III, Valarie Hernandez, Lisa Hunter, Cheryl DeConde Johnson, Robert W. Keith, Lina Kubli, Judith Marlowe, Ryan McCreery, H. Gustav Mueller, Suzzane Purdy, Georgine Ray, Richard Seewald, Shelby Rindahl, Anu Sharma, Dori Segar, Brad Stach, The Colorado Hearing Foundation, Elizabeth Thilo, and Vicki Thompson. And, once again, my loving wife, Deborah, played an important role in this project through her unfaltering encouragement, support, and her willingness to put aside and delay more favorable diversions to allow me to work on this seemingly-never-ending research and writing task. To all, I express my sincere thanks and appreciation.

A Note from Marion P. Downs: *I am immensely grateful to Jerry Northern for letting my name continue as coauthor of these recent and new editions. I have contributed only a few meager paragraphs since that first edition, and the entire burden has been his to update, revise, and rewrite most of the revisions and new editions of* Hearing in Children. *It has been a prodigious effort on his part because even as we write, technology is overtaking us and making many words obsolete. I congratulate him and thank him for continuing our cherished volumes with such fortitude.*

This final edition of Hearing in Children *is dedicated to the legendary Dr. Marion P. Downs who contributed more than 60 years of her career to bring the world of pediatric audiology from its very basic beginnings to today's unlimited promise for all children with hearing loss. As my office colleague and close friend throughout those many years, she continues to inspire us as she serves as our role model even as she reaches her centennial year of life. Marion Downs has changed the world for countless children, families, and professionals; we are grateful for her wisdom, guidance, and immeasurable contributions to the wide arena of pediatric audiology. We have all benefited from her devoted efforts to better our lives.*

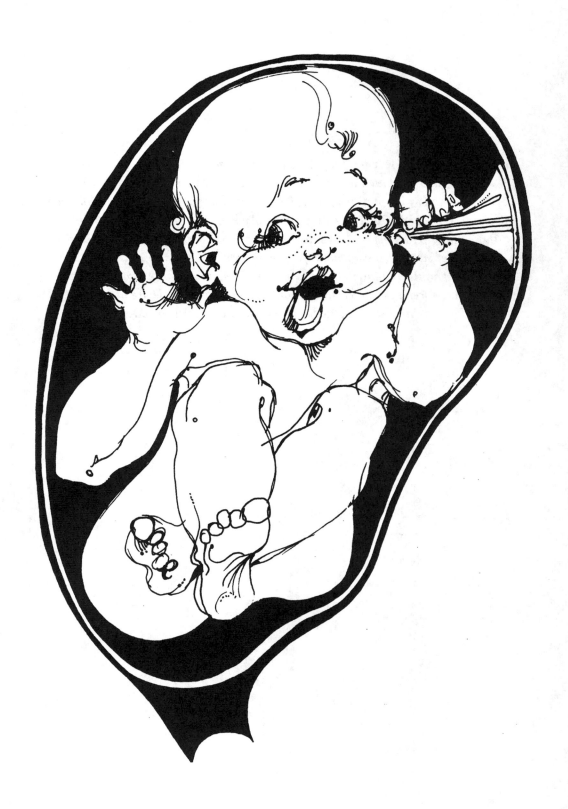

CHAPTER 1

Hearing and Hearing Loss in Children

Long ago the function of hearing became the building block on which our intricate human communication system was constructed. If predawn humans had not inherited an ear, they might have resorted to signing with their fingers or scratching marks on the sand to share their thoughts. The result would have been an awkward method of communication that could have slowed, for millennia, our "progress." For good or bad, we have developed the ear and the vocal mechanism as the media through which language is customarily learned and communicated. An illustration of the interdependence of the ear and speech is found in the direct relationship between the frequencies that make speech intelligible and the differential sensitivity of the human ear. Human ears hear best at precisely those frequencies at which humans formulate speech. The question of which of these factors came first is an ontogenic mystery that no one has solved.

The structure of language is unique to *Homo sapiens*, although experimenters have demonstrated that signed symbols and other visual language forms can be taught to chimpanzees, and experimenters believe that the beginnings of true, rudimentary language are evidenced in these primates (Savage-Rumbaugh et al., 1998). Other investigators insist that the conceptual system learned by these primates is not linguistic; that is, primates do not "think in words" but instead use a signalization system that is far removed from the higher symbolization and syntax of human language (Churchland,

1997; Johnson, 1995). Nevertheless, neither group would question that between the laboriously learned signal responses of the chimpanzee and the first voluntary sentence of the 18-month-old baby lies "a whole day of creation" (Langer, 1957).

The human baby appears to be born with "preexistent knowledge" of language, what Chomsky (1966, 1995) calls a "language organ"—specialized neural wiring that exists only in humans awaiting auditory experience with a symbol-based communication system (either oral or sign language) to trigger it into performing. It follows that language can be termed a *biobehavioral* function. These structures are dependent on auditory stimulation for their emergence in the normally developing child. Thus, there exists a crucial interdependence between language development and the ability to hear.

Both the appearance of language and the development of hearing are time-locked functions. The determining periods for hearing development begin very early. The infant is born with billions of neurons with trillions of connections that, in the case of the auditory cortex, await auditory stimulation to strengthen them (Chugani, 1997). Obviously, for the acoustic speech stimulation to affect the infant's neuronal development, the speech spectrum must be audible. Audibility, or the ability to hear, is vital in the process of normal speech and oral language development. Even in the presence of significant hearing loss, a child with hearing problems who is identified early in life and enrolled in an appropriate intervention

1

program has the opportunity to hear, learn, and develop similar speech and language skills as children with normal hearing.

Some years ago, Kuhl (1988) found through brain wave measurements that an infant's "auditory brain map" is completely formed by 12 months of age. However, even earlier than 12 months—at 6 months of age—the infant has learned all the basic sounds of his or her native language. Almost from birth, infants are sensitized to the subtle auditory cues of their linguistic community (Carney, 1999). Researchers determined that by 8 months of age a Japanese infant is able to distinguish all the sounds that are made in every known language; however, the Japanese adult is not able to make these distinctions. The perceptions for differentiating them have been eliminated in the cortical pathways and are lost almost irretrievably. A baby who is deprived of appropriate language stimulation during the first two or three years of life will have difficulties reaching his or her optimal potential language function, whether the deprivation is from lack of hearing or from lack of high-quality language experience.

The importance of early hearing to language is demonstrated by the story of the deaf-blind Helen Keller, whose remarkable achievement in mastering language skills has become legend. Her proficiency in language can be understood when one realizes that she acquired both deafness and blindness from meningitis in 1882 at 19 months of age (Wepman, 1987). Helen Keller is an example of Lenneberg's (1967) apt description: "It seems as if even a short exposure to language, a brief moment during which the curtain has been lifted and oral communication established, is sufficient to give a child some foundation on which much later language may be based." Helen Keller gave us insight into the importance of hearing to everyday life when she said, "I am just as deaf as I am blind. The problems of deafness are deeper and much more complex, if not more important, than those of blindness. Deafness is a much worse misfortune, for it means the loss of the most vital stimulus—the sound of the voice that brings language, sets thought astir, and keeps us in the intellectual company of man."

It is the importance of oral communication that makes us so uniquely "human." Of course, we can write, draw, and read as well as use gestures and sign language to communicate ideas. Most commonly, however, we choose to talk, we listen, and we "think" using language and speech. It is for these reasons that it is urgent to attack and resolve promptly the hearing problems of children, with all the skill, knowledge, and insights of which we are capable. The prevention of hearing loss in children protects the right of children to their essential humanity, which lies in optimal language function (Figure 1–1).

HEARING LOSS IN CHILDREN— A HIDDEN DISABILITY

Hearing loss in children is a silent, developmental, hidden disability. Hearing loss is a hidden problem because children, especially infants and toddlers, cannot tell us that they are not hearing normally. Nearly all their parents have normal hearing with little or no knowledge about hearing loss in children. Hearing loss is indeed a serious problem for children because, if undetected and untreated, it may cause delayed speech and language development, social and emotional problems, and ultimate academic failures. Undiscovered hearing loss in children may carry difficulties and social problems clear into adulthood. However, it is totally unnecessary for a child to suffer

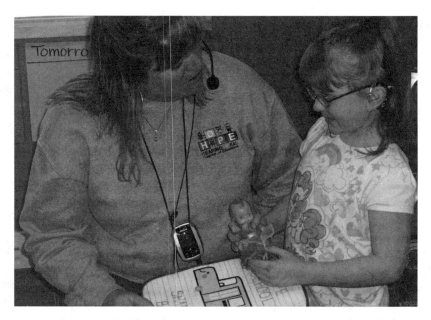

Figure 1–1. Even in the presence of significant hearing loss, a child with hearing loss that is identified early in life and enrolled in an appropriate intervention program has the opportunity to hear, learn, and develop similar speech and language skills as children with normal hearing. Photo courtesy of Spokane H.O.P.E. Preschool.

these debilitating consequences. By detecting hearing loss as early as possible, even as early as during the newborn period, effective treatment, which significantly reduces the handicap of hearing loss, can be applied. All too often, however, identification of a child's hearing loss is delayed because parents are unaware that any child, even a newborn infant, can undergo an accurate hearing test. Fortunately, the implementation of newborn hearing screening has resulted in the fact that 97% of newborns in the United States receive simple hearing screening procedures to help identify the presence of hearing loss prior to discharge from their birthing hospital. Unfortunately, many pediatrician and family practice medical office evaluations may not include the simple hearing screening procedures that could identify those children who develop hearing loss early in life.

The magnitude of problems of hearing loss in children is reflected in the following facts:

- Hearing loss is the most common birth defect in America.
- Of every 1,000 births, two to three children are born with congenital, significant, permanent, bilateral hearing loss.
- Three additional children in 1,000 will acquire deafness in early childhood or by school age (Cunningham & Cox, 2003).
- Thirty-three infants each day (or approximately 12,000 per year) in the United States are born with permanent hearing loss (http://www.infanthearing.org).
- Infants who spend time in the intensive care nursery during the

newborn period are at a higher risk for hearing loss with at least one in 50 showing significant hearing loss (Simmons, 1982).

- Some infants are born with normal hearing but for a variety of reasons may develop progressive hearing loss that occurs gradually during preschool and early school years.
- It is estimated that 90% of very young children's knowledge is attributed to "incidental reception" of sounds around them. Thus, learning is hindered with even the slightest hearing loss.
- Seventeen of every 1,000 children under the age of 18 have hearing loss (NIDCD, 2010).
- There is less than one-half the number of children with severe to profound hearing loss today than two decades ago. But, conversely, there are now more than 10 times the numbers of children with mild to moderate hearing impairments.
- Middle ear infection is the most common infectious disease of childhood and the most common cause of pediatric temporary hearing loss. An estimated five million school days are missed every year due to otitis media.
- Nearly all children will develop some period of hearing loss related to ear infections during the period from birth through 10 years of age.
- Ten to 15% of children who receive hearing screening at school fail because they cannot hear within normal limits.

In 1989, the U.S. federal government undertook a commitment to reduce the harmful effects of childhood hearing loss. In a statement released by the U.S. Public Health Service at that time, the former Surgeon General, C. Everett Koop, MD, emphasized his belief that early identification of hearing problems in children is essential. His remarks, albeit edited somewhat here, are still vibrant 25 years later:

Deafness in infants is a serious concern because it interferes with the development of language—that which sets humans apart from all other living things. The longer a child's deafness goes undiscovered, the worse the outcome is likely to be. Language remediation, which is what specialists call the process of teaching hearing-impaired children to communicate, must begin as early as possible, because language develops so rapidly in the first few months of life. For example, by 6 weeks, a normally hearing infant is more attracted to human speech than to any other sound. A 6-month-old baby already has an ability to analyze language—to break it down into its parts—to put those parts back together again and to store language in its brain and retrieve it. By 18 months, most children are producing simple sentences.

Fortunately, many of the negative results of deafness in babies can be prevented or substantially lessened. Many research studies have demonstrated that early intervention with hearing-impaired children results in improved language development, increased academic success and increased lifetime earnings. Early intervention actually saves money, since hearing-impaired children who receive early help require less costly special education services later. If it is to be effective, early intervention with deaf children should begin before the child's first birthday.

To do a much better job of early identification and early intervention, and to reduce the unnecessary suffering, poor educational performance and lack of productivity that so often accompany deafness, three groups of people must work together:

Parents *are in the best position to identify their child's hearing difficulties. We need to do a better job of making parents aware of normal developmental milestones in speech and language, the danger signals suggesting the presence of hearing loss in their child, and of the sources of help that are available to them.*

Physicians *need to become more responsive to parents' concerns about their child's hearing. Too often, those concerns are brushed aside or ignored. Yet, a recent study found that parents of hearing-impaired children knew about their baby's hearing loss an average of 7 months before it was diagnosed and that almost half of them were given poor advice, such as "don't worry about it" or "wait until the child starts school," when they told their doctors about their concerns.*

State agencies *are helping by sponsoring, initiating and conducting newborn hearing screening and early intervention programs. Studies suggest that such programs can identify up to 95% of infants who are born with various degrees of hearing impairments.*

Many others can help too, of course, from older brothers and sisters to grandparents and babysitters. We in the federal government are committed to doing our part. The 1986 Education of the Deaf Act, which authorized the creation of the Commission on the Education of the Deaf, was a first step. At the National Institutes of Health, a new research institute, the National Institute of Deafness and Communication Disorders (NIDCD) has been authorized and is now in formation. I am optimistic. I

foresee a time in this country, in the near future, in fact, when no child reaches his or her first birthday with an undetected hearing impairment.

Due to incredible innovations in testing equipment over the years, the hearing of newborn infants can be tested at any age with a high degree of accuracy by specially trained audiologists. Using advanced technologies, audiologists can accurately identify even mild degrees of hearing loss in infants during the first day of life. In children with a developmental age of 6 months or older, hearing can be assessed by traditional behavioral procedures that permit identification of any degree of hearing loss with accuracy. Once hearing loss is identified, medical management and/or audiologic intervention can be initiated immediately. At the first sign of hearing loss, children, even newborns, should receive a formal audiologic evaluation by a professional audiologist.

It is well documented by research that adequate hearing is a critical requirement for the development of speech and language. The child with normal hearing typically develops speech in a predictable pattern; young children with hearing loss usually learn in the same developmental way if they have a strong auditory foundation and have access to listening to speech (Caleffe-Schenck & Baker, 2011). Speech and language, in turn, are the cornerstones of communication and learning. Children with hearing difficulties are at high risk for communication disorders and concurrent educational delays. The earlier a hearing loss occurs in a child's life, the more difficulties the child will demonstrate in speech and language development. Significant early hearing loss in a child will cause developmental delay in both receptive and expressive communication skills. The associated language deficit may cause learning difficulties resulting in educational delays and reduced academic achievement. The overall communication difficulties experienced by the child with hearing loss often lead to problematic family and social issues, increased stress and frustration, and poor self-confidence.

On the other hand, the earlier intervention is started in children with hearing loss, the better prognosis the child will have for appropriate development. Early intervention is the process of providing services, education, and support to young children who are deemed to have an established condition, those who are evaluated and deemed to have a diagnosed physical or mental condition, an existing delay, or children who are at risk of developing a delay or special need that may affect their development or impede their education.

There are a number of specific effects on development that can be identified in children with early significant hearing loss (ASHA, 2011a):

- Vocabulary develops more slowly in children who have hearing loss. These children have little difficulty with concrete words that easily can be matched to objects: family names; specific nouns such as desk, cat, and car; colors; and numbers. They are likely to have more difficulty with abstract words such as *before* and *after, over* and *under*; concepts such as dreams and imagination and jealousy; and differentiating between items that are similar and/or different. Another area of difficulty is proper utilization of words such as *the, a, an, are, have, has,* and so forth.
- Children with significant hearing loss understand and express shorter and simpler sentences than children who develop with normal hearing.

Children with hearing loss are more likely to have difficulties with understanding and writing complex sentences. They may not be able to hear word endings such as –s or –ed, which leads to unfortunate and embarrassing misunderstandings of speech, and delay in the proper use of verb tense, pluralization, and possessives as well as nonagreement of subjects and verbs in the same sentence.

- Children with hearing loss often cannot hear soft speech sounds such as /s/, /f/, /t/, and /k/, and therefore may not include them in their speech. With significant hearing loss, the vocal quality of these children may be compromised in terms of prosody, inflection, and rate, making their speech difficult for others to understand. The problem may be that without adequate amplification, the child with hearing loss may not hear his or her own voice as the child speaks, thereby making it difficult for the child to monitor and correct his or her own expressive speech and language as it occurs.
- With the difficulties described above, logically it would be expected that children with significant hearing loss are more likely to have difficulties in all areas of academic achievement, especially reading and mathematical skills. Even children with mild to moderate hearing loss achieve one to four grade levels lower than their normal hearing peers, unless proper intervention and amplification are applied. Children with more severe hearing loss may fall even further behind their peers and achieve skills no higher than third- or fourth-grade level unless appropriate educational

intervention occurs as soon as the hearing loss is identified.

- Children with hearing loss often report feeling alone, without friends, left out of social circles at home and at school, and may be generally unhappy with daily life.

But the good news is that with early identification of the hearing loss in a young child, with appropriate management including early amplification and intervention, appropriate education activities and learning experiences that are enhanced through family activities, speech and language development can be encouraged, promoted, and guided to support the child's cognitive development. Many of today's young children with hearing loss successfully reach the equivalent education levels as their normal hearing peers and compete equally with them in all areas of education and achievements. The prognosis and opportunities for today's children with hearing loss truly are unlimited.

Perhaps the most poignant synopsis of the tremendous advances made over the past two decades were best expressed by former Surgeon General C. Everett Koop, MD, who started the national early identification and intervention initiative:

I set a goal that by the year 2000 all infants with permanent hearing loss would be identified before 12 months of age. Although it was an ambitious goal, and many people thought it was unrealistic, I was optimistic and confident that it could be achieved. Since that time, we have seen remarkable progress. Universal newborn hearing-screening programs are now functioning throughout the United States. With assistance from the federal government, every state has established an Early Hearing Detection and Inter-vention (EHDI) program as a part of its public health system. In some areas with the most effective EHDI programs, most infants and young children who are deaf or hard-of-hearing are being identified at less than 3 months of age. And, research is documenting what we always believed to be the case: deaf or hard-of-hearing children who are identified early and given appropriate educational and health care services develop better language and achieve better in school. I believe it is only a matter of time until we document that such children also grow up to have better jobs and are able to participate more fully and effectively in our communities. The seeds we planted in the 1980s are beginning to bear fruit and will continue to do so. (Koop, 2010)

HOW WE HEAR

Although we generally give little thought to it, there is no doubt that hearing is a critical sense for us. We depend on it for our safety, our education, our communications, and our social interactions. The intricate actions and interactions of the hearing process have fascinated us for more than a century. And fortunately, during these past few years, the micro and macro means by which we perceive and understand complex sounds surely are being revealed and understood by the contributions of researchers working in a wide variety of specialty areas including medical engineering, biomechanics, bioacoustics, and biochemistry, to name just a few. The complex microscopic structures and their interacting anatomy and neural connection mechanisms involved in hearing have long challenged scientists. This complex sensory system has presented research challenges because of its intricacies coupled with the fact that the main structure embedding the hearing and balance mechanisms is smaller in size than an adult's smallest fingernail, and the sensory end organs are totally embedded in the hardest bone of the body, the temporal bone of the skull. The traditional and simplified cross-sectional diagram of the human hearing system is shown in Figure 1–2.

We hear sounds through two basic physiologic pathways. The traditional auditory pathway for hearing is known as the *air conduction route*, through which sound waves enter the external ear, and pass down the ear canal to cause vibration of the tympanic membrane (Figure 1–3A). In the simplest to understand explanation, the tiny microscopic vibrations of the tympanic membrane transmit energy to the cochlea of the inner ear by the three small bones located in the middle ear. Thus, the vibrations of the tympanic membrane are transmitted across the middle ear space by the malleus, incus, and stapes. As the footplate of the third small bone (the stapes) vibrates, wave eddies are created within the fluids within the inner ear. Vibrations in the inner ear fluid create pressure changes in the numerous micro-hairs protruding from the hair cell sensory cells. The bending of the stereocilia at the top of the hair cells causes significant chemical and electrical changes within the sensory cells that in turn stimulate neural impulses that travel upward to specific centers in the brain, creating the sensation we recognize as "hearing."

Not so well recognized is the second route for hearing known as the *bone conduction pathway* (Figure 1–3B). Because the inner ear is encased within the bones of the skull, vibrations carried through the

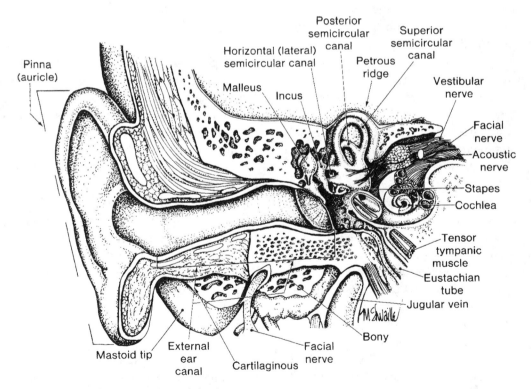

Figure 1–2. Cross-section of the human ear.

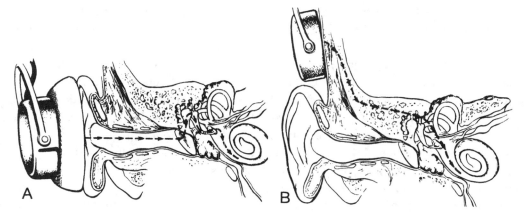

Figure 1–3. The two pathways of human hearing. **A–B.** Broken arrows show the routes of the air-conduction hearing pathway and the bone-conduction hearing pathway.

skull, mandible, and jaw (and even through the throat) cause the fluids to move within the inner ear. Thus, vibrations of the skull are transmitted directly to the inner ear, effectively bypassing the external and middle portions of the ear. These bone-conducted vibrations stimulate the sensory cells of the inner ear in the same way as sound waves passing through the air conduction pathway, again resulting in the neural phenomenon we recognize as "hearing." Audiologists determine thresholds by air conduction signals through insert earphones and/or bone-conducted signals presented through a small, specialized vibration transducer pressed against the mastoid portion of the skull's temporal bone behind the pinna.

Sounds transmitted by air-conducted vibrations and bone-conducted vibrations are perceived as precisely the same sound. When a person hears his or her own voice from a tape or video recording, the typical response is that our voice sounds "totally strange." Our recorded voice sounds "natural" to others because they always listen to our voice by air-conducted sound waves through their own hearing systems. For the individual listening to his or her recorded voice, however, the sounds are strange

because we are accustomed to hearing our own voices mostly by bone conduction as we speak. For the audiologist performing hearing evaluations, it is the comparison of air-conducted and bone-conducted sounds during the hearing test that provides the differential determination of the general type of a hearing problem.

The organ of hearing must process sounds that range from the soft rustle of leaves in the wind to the thunderous roar of a departing jet airplane. To understand the process of hearing, one must include consideration of the nature of sound, the structure and function of the auditory system, and the basic perceptions that result when a sound is present. As described by Yost (2007), the process of hearing involves a complex network and intricate coordination of neural coding, auditory processing, and cortical integration which lead to an appropriate response to sound.

The Nature of Sound

Psychologists and physicists describe sound very differently. This difference was emphasized in the early 1700s when philosophers loved to debate the question of whether a falling tree makes noise if no one is available to hear the sound. The psychologist views sound as a personal quality of sensory perception. The physicist views sound as a propagating disturbance in the air initiated by a vibrating source. The physicist studies the generation, transmission, reception, and modification of sound waves as the science of acoustics. The psychologist studies the human reaction to sound waves that we know as "hearing." There is important information contained within both points of view which needs to be acknowledged to understand how we hear and communicate.

Sound waves in the air follow the physical rules of wave motion, much like the ripples created when a pebble is tossed in a pond. The vibrations produce wave motion. Sound waves are vibrating air particles set into motion by an energy source, bumping each other to create repetitive waves. These sound waves are measured in terms of frequency and intensity.

Frequency is a physical parameter of sound defined as the number of vibrations per second. The vibrating movements of an object alternately increase *(compression)* and decrease *(rarefaction)* the density of surrounding air molecules, creating waves like those seen when a stone is dropped into a quiet pool of water. Thus, the pattern of movement of the vibrator is imprinted on the air in the form of waves. The number of complete cycles of waves that pass a given point in 1 second is the frequency of the sound. The sound of a single frequency is known as a *pure tone*. The fewer the cycles per second, the lower is the frequency; as more cycles per second pass the given point, the higher is the frequency measurement. Frequency was historically expressed as cycles per second (cps) and is now known by the internationally agreed upon term, hertz (Hz). A young child's hearing encom-

passes the frequencies from 20 to 20,000 Hz. Unfortunately, the ability to hear higher frequencies decrease with age. Adults seldom hear sounds above 8000 Hz, and we tend to lose our high-frequency hearing as we age.

The frequency of a sound determines the *pitch* of a tone. Pitch is the psychological perception of the frequency of a stimulus. As frequency is increased, the pitch of the sound also increases. A tuning fork produces a specific vibratory pattern determined by its mass and length that is a single pure tone frequency. Pure tones rarely exist in nature; instead, most sounds are complex because they consist of a spectrum of frequencies that differ in intensity and frequency. Although the middle C note on the musical scale is 256 Hz, the actual musical sound carries additional frequency harmonics related to the resonance of the instrument. The output pitch range of human speech is a broad range of frequencies from approximately 500 to 3500 Hz, which is nearly identical to the optimal frequency sensitivity of our hearing mechanism.

Intensity describes the physical measurement of the strength or magnitude of a sound. Intensity is determined by the force applied to the moving air molecules; greater forces cause larger sound waves. The psychological correlate of intensity is "loudness." The dynamic range of intensity in the human ability to hear is remarkable. The ratio of intensity of the faintest audible sound to the most intolerable sound is approximately 1 to 10,000,000. To manage numbers with such a huge dynamic range, we use a logarithmic notation system with the unit of measure known as the *decibel* (dB), defined as one-tenth of a bel and named for Alexander Graham Bell. The decibel is a logarithmic unit that indicates the ratio of a physical quantity (usually power or intensity) relative to a specified or implied reference level. A ratio in decibels is 10 times the logarithm to base 10 of the ratio of two power quantities. The decibel is used for a wide variety of measurements in science and engineering, most prominently in acoustics, electronics, and even in astronomy. In electronics, the gains of amplifiers, attenuation of signals, and signal-to-noise ratios are often expressed in decibels. The decibel confers a number of advantages, such as the ability to conveniently represent very large or small numbers, and the ability to carry out multiplication of ratios by simple addition and subtraction.

The decibel (dB) is an arbitrary unit that expresses the ratio of a measured power or pressure to a specified reference value. Because it is not an absolute measure, it has no meaning unless the reference value is identified. In audiology, we use several reference bases for the dB including dB HL (hearing level) which is a biologic scale based on normal hearing values; dB SL (sensation level) which uses the patient's speech reception threshold as a base; and dB SPL (sound pressure level), a purely physical measure. In audiology measurements, the reference level for the decibel shown on audiograms is the biologic normal hearing baseline, or 0 dB HL. Because of the logarithmic nature of the decibel scale, every 10-dB increase represents a 10-fold multiplication of sound. Thus, 50 dB is 10 times more intense than 40 dB; 100 dB is a million times more intense than 40 dB. Furthermore, the 10-dB difference between 110 and 120 dB is much greater than the 10-dB difference between 40 and 50 dB.

Audiologists and acoustic engineers measure environmental sound in dB SPL. Sound pressure or acoustic pressure is the local pressure deviation from the ambient (average or equilibrium) atmospheric pressure caused by a sound wave. Sound pressure in air can be measured using a microphone, and in water using a hydrophone. The unit

for sound pressure p is the pascal (symbol: Pa). The usual physical reference value for sound pressure is 20 microPascals (symbol: daPa), and the value is referred to as dB SPL. Sound pressure level (SPL) or sound level is a logarithmic measure of the effective sound pressure of a sound relative to a reference value. It is measured in decibels (dB) above a standard reference level. The commonly used "zero" reference sound pressure in air is 20 μPa RMS, which is approximately the threshold of human hearing at 1000 Hz.

Speech patterns in English vary considerably based on intensity, frequency, and duration. The speech sounds of greatest intensity (central vowel sounds) are also typically low in frequency, while the weakest sounds (unvoiced fricatives such as /f/ and /s/) are typically composed of higher frequencies. The overall intensity of conversational speech normally varies within a dynamic range of about 30 dB from the quietest consonant (the unvoiced /th/ sound) to the loudest vowel (aw). The intensity of speech sounds also vary dependent on whether or not the word is stressed or unstressed. For conversational speech, the average pressure level of the voice from 5 feet away is approximately 60 dB SPL, while the loudest adult speech can easily generate levels greater than 110 dB SPL.

Audiologists evaluate hearing by presenting single-frequency tones (known as "pure tones") to patients at varying intensities to establish auditory thresholds across a frequency range, typically from 250 to 8000 Hz. For psychology purposes, threshold is defined as the minimum effective stimulus that is capable of evoking a response. In audiometry, however, hearing thresholds are defined as the minimum intensity of a pure tone or speech signal at which the patient responds correctly approximately 50% of the time. As "hearing thresholds" are identified at the various test frequencies, it is marked on a special chart known as an audiogram. However, inasmuch as the data plotted on the audiogram are based on normal speech and normal hearing, audiologists have long recognized that the audiogram underestimates problems of hearing due to distortions contributed by sensorineural damage and dysfunction as well as from environmental factors such as reverberation and competing noise (Chial, 1998). The frequency and intensity of general English sounds during conversational speech are plotted on an audiogram and compared with common environmental sounds in Figure 1–4. The diagrammatic audiogram shown in Figure 1–4 has proven useful in counseling parents about the audibility of speech in regard to their child's hearing loss.

Our Amazing Hearing System

The majesty of creation is abundantly evident in the structure and function of the human hearing mechanism. The human hearing mechanism is a product of evolution, originating as a simple extension of a pressure-sensing organ in primitive sea animals, and developing in a highly complex sensory system in mammals (Lipscomb, 1996). Great strides have been made in recent years toward a more thorough understanding of how the auditory system translates physical acoustic energy into neural impulses that are interpreted by the brain. However, the truth is that many questions remain to be answered concerning the precise biologic, mechanical, and neurochemical relationships that operate at all levels within the auditory system. The reader interested in more detail about otologic anatomy and physiology is referred to traditional references such as Schuknecht (1993), Nadol and McKenna (2004), Guly (2007), and more recent resource materials

including Yost (2007), McFarland (2008), and Fuller, Pimente, and Peregoy (2011).

Although far too simple a description, the basic anatomical structure of the ear is most easily understood if the ear is discussed in three major sections: the outer ear, the middle ear, and the inner ear. The discussion below is necessarily an overview and does not reflect the detail and intricate workings of our hearing mechanism. These three components of the hearing mechanism work together in a complex manner to let us hear and appreciate a wide diversity of sounds. With normal hearing we can easily identify and discriminate among more than 400,000 individual sounds. It is still almost beyond our understanding that the ear performs in such an amazing manner. We can hear everything from the softness of leaves rustling in the wind to the powerful sounds of the space shuttle liftoff. We can make the fine distinction between music played by a violin and a cello in the midst of an orchestral performance while listening to the whisper of our companion. We are able to shut out the hub-bub of a noisy cocktail party with a band playing while listening to a single speaker's voice. Even during sleep, our hearing and brain function to wake us in the event of an unusual event or let us sleep soundly through noisy traffic. Yet our hearing wakes us with the gentle sound of a door opening down the hall. The ear is obviously a master of multitasking!

The Outer Ear

Human ears, the characteristic, and sometimes prominent, flaps of skin and cartilage on the sides of our head, at first glance, are not much to appreciate. Perhaps valued most of the time for decorating with a wide variety of jewelry, human ears do not seem to do much. The outer ear consists of the external ear (pinna) and the ear canal that

Audiogram of Familiar Sounds

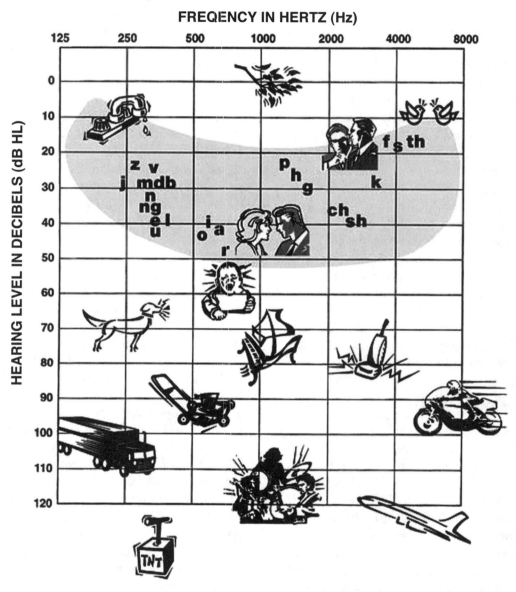

Figure 1–4. Frequency spectrum of familiar sounds plotted on a standard audiogram. Shaded area represents the "speech banana" that contains most of the sound elements of spoken speech.

collects and funnels air vibrations to the tympanic membrane. The outer ear and external ear canal help us localize sound and provide resonance to the sounds we hear. Functionally, the ear canal resonates at the frequencies most important for us to understand speech (between 2000 and 4000 Hz). This resonance amplifies the peaks and troughs of air pressure that make up sound waves, so that the peak pressure at the eardrum is approximately double the pressure at the open end of the ear canal. The ear canal contains modified sweat glands that secrete wax (cerumen) that actually serve to clean the ear canal. It has been suggested that an individual's pinnae could be a better and more unique identification mark in human beings than fingerprints, as no two outer ears are exactly alike. There are some key identification points on the outer ear that do not change throughout life. In fact, the outer ears do not contribute much to our auditory sensitivity, per se, as individuals without pinnae have been shown to have hearing within normal limits.

The Middle Ear

The middle ear includes the tympanic membrane (eardrum) and a small air-space cavity that contains the three smallest bones of the body known as the malleus, the incus, and the stapes (commonly known as the hammer, anvil, and stirrup). The three ossicles are suspended in the middle ear space by seven ligaments and two small muscles, (a) the tensor tympani attached to the malleus, and (b) the stapedial muscle attached to the posterior crus of the stapes. The three ossicles form a system of levers linked together to further amplify the force of sound vibrations picked up by the tympanic membrane. Working together, the middle ear ossicles nearly triple the force of the vibrations they carry to the inner ear. The tiny, but powerful, stapes bone passes the amplified vibrations directly to the cochlea portion of the inner ear. In brief, the middle ear is a mechanical system that serves as a transformer and impedance matching mechanism to convert low-pressure, high-amplitude airborne vibrations into low-amplitude, higher pressure fluid vibrations directed to the inner ear. Working together, the outer and middle ear mechanisms increase amplification by 180 times before the sound waves set the fluids of the inner ear in motion. Even with such powerful amplification, the transmitting mechanisms actually vibrate much less than the diameter of a hydrogen molecule; a vibration so small it is imperceptible to the human eye.

The Inner Ear

The inner ear contains two major divisions: (a) the cochlea or hearing mechanism and (b) the structures of the balance or vestibular mechanisms. The fluid-filled cochlea is the "hearing" portion of the inner ear and contains thousands of sensory cells that operate in a complex, highly developed, and intricate manner to stimulate an extremely complex neural network passing through brainstem neural centers to the cortex of the brain. The cochlea converts mechanical energy received from the middle ear into hydraulic pressure and electrical energy that imparts movement through minute vibrations to the cochlear duct and the organ of Corti, which contains thousands of sensory structures known as hair cells. The entire hearing and vestibular components of the inner ear are so tiny that they contain only a drop of specialized fluids (perilymph: a fluid almost identical to spinal fluid; and endolymph: a fluid similar to that found within cells) to fill the ducts and spaces.

The organ of Corti is basically a frequency analyzer, with the highest pitches monitored from the base of the coil of the cochlea and the intermediate and higher pitches tonotopically organized toward the tip or apex. The organ of Corti is a papillary structure resting on the basilar membrane within the scala media (cochlear duct) containing hair cell sensory structures and supporting elements. The hair cells are attached to a cuticular surface at their tops, and their bases are in contact with the dendritic processes of the neurons of the spiral ganglion. Technically, the hair cells convert the mechanical fluid vibration into electromechanical feedback and electrochemical events, which in turn promote synaptic transmission between the hair cells and the neurons of the auditory portion of the eighth nerve (Ryan & Dallos, 1996; Yost, 2007). The spiral-shaped organ of Corti contains two types of sensory cells, inner and outer hair cells, topped by several rows of stereocilia (Figure 1–5).

There are some 40 stereocilia extending from the top surface of each of the 3,500 inner hair cells and about 150 stereocilia extending from the 12,000 outer hair cells. The inner hair cells, which are shaped like a flask, are completely surrounded by specialized supporting cells except for their hair-bearing tops. The outer hair cells are arranged in three (at the base) to five (at the apex) parallel rows (Table 1–1). The outer hair cells are rectangular, shaped like elongated cylinders, and in contact with

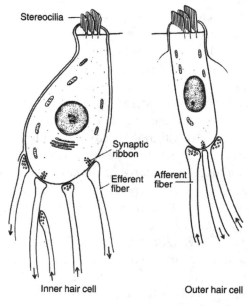

Figure 1–5. Diagrammatic representation of inner and outer hair cells found in the inner ear within the organ of Corti.

Table 1–1. Comparison of Inner and Outer Hair Cells

Inner hair cells	Outer hair cells
3,500	12,500
Flask shape	Cylinder shape
Single row	3–5 rows
"C"-shaped stereocilia	"V"-shaped stereocilia
Surrounded by support cells	Attached at top and bottom
Afferent innervation	Multiple innervation
One neuron—one cell	One neuron—multiple cell

supporting cells only at their very tops and bottoms. The approximately 15,500 hair cells rest on supporting cells that, in turn, rest on the basilar membrane and extend into a third cochlear duct filled with endolymph fluid that is known as the scala media or cochlear duct. This third duct is interposed between the scala vestibuli and scala tympani throughout the entire 2.5 turns of the cochlea.

Thus, with the arrival of a vibratory stimulus to the cochlea, transduction of the mechanical traveling wave into a neural activity begins with the deflection of the outer hair cell's stereocilia rows. The tips of the tallest outer hair cell stereocilia are embedded within the tectorial membrane, where it appears that the inner hair cells do not touch the tectorial membrane. The stereocilia of the outer hair cells are displaced directly by the combined displacement of the tectorial and the basilar membranes. With the vibration of the basilar membrane, a shearing force is produced with an accompanying displacement of the stereocilia; this results because the tectorial membrane does not move to the same degree as the hair cells (Noback, Strominger, & Demarest, 1996).

Ryan and Dallos (1996) demonstrated that the selective destruction of outer hair cells resulted in a loss of threshold sensitivity in the cochlea of approximately 40 to 50 dB accompanied by compromised or eliminated frequency selectivity. Examination of the hair cell innervation patterns has led to the conclusion that outer hair cells amplify signals that are subsequently processed by inner hair cells (Dallos, 2008). Van Tasell (1993) concluded that hearing loss of cochlear origin, with air-conduction thresholds less than 60 dB HL, is consistent with damage to the outer hair cells, whereas hearing losses greater than 60 dB HL are likely to involve widespread destruction

of inner hair cells and disruption of their afferent function, in addition to the loss of outer hair cell function. This absolute loss in inner hair cell function, if extensive, can produce greatly degraded speech recognition and auditory discrimination abilities.

The peripheral neurons of the cochlear nerve are distributed to hair cells from beneath the basilar membrane and its supporting shelf, the osseous spiral lamina. The fluid motion of the scala tympani due to its physical properties of width, length, thickness, mass, and elasticity displaces the basilar membrane in a traveling wave pattern, producing torsion on the hair-like processes of the cell and creating a mechanical-chemical change resulting in peripheral nerve-ending stimulation.

The scala vestibuli and scala tympani (filled with perilymph, a fluid with a low potassium ion concentration) surround the third duct, the scala media or cochlear duct (a chamber filled with endolymph, a fluid with a high potassium ion concentration). The mechanical-chemical process occurs as sound vibrations travel along the basilar membrane causing activation of the hair cells by opening transducer channels in the stereocilia. These channels allow an influx of calcium and potassium ions, which cause the hair cells to depolarize, initiating signals in the auditory nerve. The resultant electrical potentials in the eighth nerve dendrites initiate impulses that are transmitted to the central nervous system via the higher auditory neural pathways. Through this intricate and complex system, the external vibratory energy in the ear canal, and transmitted by the tympanic membrane, is ultimately transformed into neural impulses dispatched as a coded version of the original sound (including information about frequencies, intensities, timbre, etc.) to the brain. These neuroelectrical signals pass up the auditory nerves to be processed in various brainstem neural stations and forwarded upward to be interpreted by auditory brain centers in the temporal lobe.

The Auditory Nerve

The nerve fibers that innervate the hair cells have their cell bodies in the bipolar spiral ganglion located in Rosenthal's canal. Axons from the spiral ganglion cells join in the modiolus and collect as the auditory, or cochlear, branch of the eighth (VIII) cranial nerve. The auditory nerve is composed of two main sets of fibers: one group of fibers for auditory stimuli and a set of fibers for the vestibular system. Outside the cochlea, the vestibular portion of the VIIIth nerve ascends from the semicircular canals, utricle, and saccule joins the cochlear portion of the VIIIth nerve. The two portions of the eighth nerve come together like a rope and pass through the internal auditory meatus toward the brainstem. The structure of the auditory nerve is orderly, with fibers from the apical quarter of the cochlea forming the core of the nerve. Around the core, nerve fibers from the apex of the cochlea twist one way, while the fibers from the middle turn of the cochlea twist the opposite way. Fifty percent of the nerve fibers from the cochlea come from the basal coil and represent sensory elements that respond to frequencies higher than 2000 Hz.

Research by Spoendlin (1967, 1969) demonstrated that the vast majority (90%) of the afferent neurons innervate the inner hair cells, whereas only some 10% of the fibers come from the outer hair cells. Each outer hair cell is innervated by several different neurons, and each neuron innervates a large number of outer hair cells. The inner hair cells are innervated by a large number of different neurons, but each neuron innervates only one inner hair cell. Most of the information transmitted to the brain originates from the inner hair cells, not the outer hair cells (Ryan & Dallos, 1996).

Although the cochlea is stimulated by hydromechanical pressures, the electrical neural impulses leave the cochlea via the afferent neurons that join together to form the acoustic division of the eighth cranial nerve. The VIIIth nerve divides into acoustic and vestibular branches before it reaches the brainstem. The acoustic nerve enters the brainstem at the level of the pons. The auditory portion then divides into dorsal and ventral branches that go to corresponding nuclei in the brainstem wherein the second-order afferent auditory neuron cell bodies are located.

The fibers in the VIIIth nerve are "tuned" to certain frequencies. That is, certain fibers are more responsive to certain stimulating frequencies. This fact is shown by inserting microelectrodes into single nerve fibers, determining the threshold for the action potential "spike" of that nerve fiber for a variety of frequencies, and then plotting the response area for that particular fiber. The threshold sensitivity of a fiber increases gradually and is most sensitive at its "tuned" frequency. The tuned frequency is used to name the fiber (e.g., 7000 Hz fiber). Individual inner hair cells also show characteristic responses to tuned frequencies.

Brainstem Pathways

The brainstem auditory pathway can be seen in Figure 1–6. It is important to realize that although first-order neurons from the cochlea reach the brainstem in the cochlear nuclei, most of the activity that ultimately reaches the cortex is by way of fourth-order neurons. This seemingly too complex system seldom breaks down because of alternate

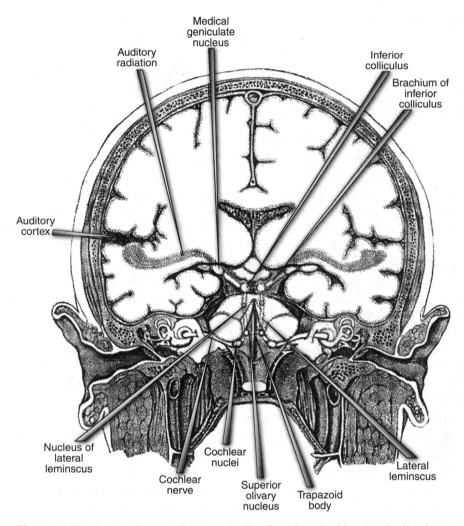

Figure 1–6. Ascending auditory pathway. Reprinted with permission from *The human brain: An introduction to its functional anatomy* (4th ed.), by J. Nolte, 1988, St. Louis, MO: CV Mosby.

paths to the cerebral cortex (Thompson, 1983).

Two pairs of cochlear nuclei exist, a dorsal and a ventral cochlear nucleus on each side of the medulla; they are referred to collectively as the cochlear nuclei of the medulla. Although some of the neurons of the cochlear nuclei ascend to higher nuclei on the same side of the system, most cross over to the opposite side in the trapezoid body. Auditory units in the cochlear nuclei are also tuned to specific frequencies as noted previously with the auditory nerve fibers. Inhibitory units have also been reported in the cochlear nuclei, which under certain circumstances actually inhibit response rather than excite the unit under examination. Thus, a particular frequency stimulus may excite certain neurons of the auditory system while inhibiting other units from firing. What starts out in the cochlea as the excitation of the relatively large group of hair cells is narrowed down to a smaller group of neurons through this process of inhibition. The number of discharges from a single cochlear nucleus unit is related to the intensity of the acoustic stimulus.

The principal terminations of second-order afferent auditory neurons are in the nuclei of the trapezoid body and superior olivary body. The superior olive is the first structure in the medulla that receives fibers from both ears, and it may play a role in the localization of sound. From here, neurons originate that course upward in the loosely compacted neurons of the lateral lemniscus to another principal relay station, the inferior colliculus. Collaterals of second- and third-order neurons are given off to the reticular formation that provides an indirect, diffuse, sensory pathway to the cerebral cortex. The reticular formation is closely related to arousal and attention during sleep and may be responsible for the fact that a crying baby may wake only the mother but no one else in the family, or that a person may sleep soundly through a barrage of noise but wake suddenly on hearing a soft familiar voice.

The auditory cortex is, of course, responsible for the fine discrimination necessary in the understanding of speech. The "tuning" function of the higher auditory centers, including the inferior colliculus, the medial geniculate body, and the auditory cortex, has been summarized by Ryan and Dallos (1996); some units at higher levels in the auditory system are frequency specific, and some are not. An estimated cell count of each of the levels in the afferent auditory pathway is presented in Table 1–2.

Attempts to map the cortical responses to auditory stimuli have identified the temporal lobe as the responsive area, sometimes further localized as Brodmann's areas 41 and 42. The primary cortex (area 41) area in the temporal lobe has at least five tonotopic

Table 1–2. Afferent Auditory Pathways Count and Estimated Cell at Each Level

Cochlear nuclei	8,800
Superior olivary complex	34,000
Nuclei of lateral lemniscus	38,000
Inferior colliculus	392,000
Medial geniculate body	364,000
Auditory cortex	10,000,000

frequency projections that are the reverse of each other. Kryter and Ades (1943) established a very important fact with significant clinical implication by showing cortical lesions have no appreciable effect on the absolute thresholds of pure tone stimuli. This is true even when extensive bilateral cortical lesions are made. Thus, the ability to respond to simple pure tones is not dependent on the cerebral cortex. These same investigators reported that removal of the inferior colliculi created an approximate 15-dB loss in pure tone sensitivity; destruction of the entire auditory system from the midbrain to the cortex created a pure tone hearing loss of about 40 dB. It may be concluded that the most important aspect of auditory sensitivity to pure tones is due to intact neurons below the inferior colliculi, and a nearly normal audiogram may be obtained with a loss of 75% of the neurons of the auditory nerve. Unilateral lesions of the ascending auditory pathways above the level of the cochlear nuclei produce only minor impairments because of the strong bilaterality of the pathway. Bilateral lesions of the central auditory pathways are relatively uncommon because tracts and nuclei of the system are redundant and widely separated.

In addition to the afferent (ascending) auditory pathways to the cortex, a separate system of neurons provides an efferent (descending) pathway from the cortex to the cochlea. Of particular interest is the olivocochlear bundle, which consists of: (a) lateral olivocochlear neurons that project ipsilaterally and terminate on the peripheral processes of afferent fibers beneath the inner hair cells, and (b) medial olivocochlear neurons that project contralaterally and terminate primarily beneath the outer hair cells (Figure 1–7). The medial olivocochlear pathway is associated with interaction between the two ears at the level of the brainstem and most likely has a role in suppression of otoacoustic emissions (Hood & Berlin, 1996).

THE NATURE OF HEARING LOSS

Hearing loss can result from a wide spectrum of causes including inherited or congenital problems, infections, diseases, or traumatic situations that affect different portions of the ear and hearing mechanism. Audiologists traditionally describe hearing loss in three categories as conductive hearing loss, sensorineural hearing loss, or mixed hearing loss, which is a combination of the two major categories. However, considerable success has been achieved

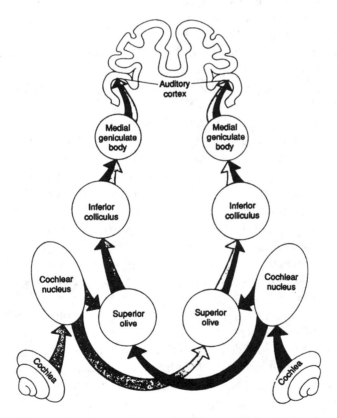

Figure 1–7. A diagrammatic scheme of the ascending auditory pathway. Reprinted with permission from *Fundamentals of hearing: An introduction* (5th ed.), by W. A. Yost, 2007, San Diego, CA: Academic Press.

through newer measurement technologies that differentiate between sensory and neural hearing deficits. Thus, audiologists are commonly able to discern between hearing loss caused by damage to the sensory elements of the cochlea versus neural damage in the auditory pathways leading to more specific descriptions of sensorineural hearing loss as either "sensory" or "neural." It is not uncommon for a conductive component to the hearing loss to be concurrent with a permanent-type sensorineural hearing loss, with the resultant hearing problem described as a mixed hearing loss. When auditory dysfunction is present in light of normal or near-normal peripheral hearing (i.e., normal hearing levels with no conductive or sensorineural hearing loss), the auditory dysfunction may be described as a central auditory processing (CAP) disorder.

Conductive Hearing Loss

Conductive hearing loss is the most common cause of hearing problems in children often resulting from ongoing ear infections. The "conductive" component of the problem describes the blockage of sounds from reaching the sensory cells of the inner ear and may often be a temporary condition. Although conductive hearing loss has a wide range of etiologies, the actual hearing loss is created by interference of any sort in the transmission of sound from the external auditory canal to the inner ear. Although the inner ear may function normally in persons with conductive hearing loss, the sound vibration is unable to stimulate the cochlea via the normal air conduction pathway because of blockage in the ear canal, tympanic membrane, or middle ear. Conductive hearing loss is usually mild to moderate in degree, may occur in one or

both ears at the same time, and may resolve spontaneously over time without treatment. However, conductive hearing loss may also persist in many patients leading to the necessity of minor medical or surgical treatment to clear up disease and return the hearing to normal limits. More significant conductive hearing loss may be associated with facial or skull malformations that require significant surgical intervention to correct.

A conductive component to the hearing problem may be present along with permanent sensorineural-type hearing loss. In these patients, the bone conduction threshold values represent "better hearing" than the air conduction threshold measures. Eliminating the conductive component through treatment or spontaneous recovery will result in the improvement of the hearing loss to the levels of permanent hearing loss (Stach, 2008). The most common causes of conductive hearing loss are sterile fluid in the middle ear; ear infections of the ear canal, the middle ear, or both; or foreign objects in the ear canal (i.e., pop beads, broken crayons, insects, etc.) that inadvertently find their way into the ear canal and must be removed. Earwax found in the ear canal can be pushed deeper through personal cleaning efforts and should be cleaned out only by someone with proper experience and safe instruments. Public health officials warn against the use of cotton swabs, sometimes known as Q-tips, as a dangerous procedure that deposits shreds of cotton fibers in the ear canal and may actually result in causing more significant problems. These situations lead to the familiar adage cautioning to "stick nothing in your ear smaller than your elbow."

Conductive hearing losses are the most common type of hearing loss found in children, usually resulting from transient ear infections known technically as "otitis media." Conductive hearing loss can also occur when the ear canal or middle ear air conduction pathway is totally blocked (occluded) with wax or some other physical obstruction, producing a maximal 60 dB HL conductive hearing loss. Conductive-type hearing loss is often found in individuals with craniofacial malformations that might include malformation of the middle ear structures. Although most conductive hearing losses caused by otitis media resolve spontaneously, more severe cases require medical or surgical treatment to return the hearing to normal levels.

Sensorineural Hearing Loss

The term *sensorineural* has long been used to describe permanent hearing loss caused by damage to the cochlear hair cells or auditory nerve fibers leading to the brain. Until recent years, audiologists could not accurately differentiate between sensorineural hearing loss due to hair cell dysfunction and auditory nerve dysfunction, so it proved easier to lump the two causes together under one term. Traditionally, damage to the sensory hair cells was not easily differentiated from damage to the auditory nerve system and pathways, so the resultant hearing loss was simply described as sensorineural. Sensorineural hearing losses were almost universally assumed to involve the hair cells of the cochlea with, or without, accompanying loss of auditory nerve fibers (Sininger, 2008). However, current audiometric testing techniques, such as otoacoustic emissions, electrocochleography, and auditory evoked potentials, can provide an objective means to differentiate between sensory and neural hearing loss (see Chapter 7).

For individuals with sensorineural hearing losses, the air and bone conduction auditory thresholds should be, theoretically, equal or at least within ±5dB. Sensorineural hearing losses are not likely to be identified during routine medical otoscopic examination as the external auditory canal and tympanic membrane typically appear normal. Accordingly, it requires an audiometric evaluation with air conduction and bone conduction threshold testing to establish an accurate diagnosis of the sensorineural hearing loss. Sensorineural hearing loss may be caused by a wide variety of etiologies including bacterial and viral infections; genetic or familial inheritance; disease processes involving the otic capsule, auditory nerve, or membranous labyrinth; metabolic disorders; excessive noise exposure; or toxic pharmacological agents. Sensorineural hearing loss is nearly always permanent and irreversible.

Mixed Hearing Loss

When both a sensorineural and a conductive loss are present, the result is termed a mixed hearing loss. The audiogram (Figure 1–8) shows abnormal bone conduction thresholds that are closer to normal hearing levels than the air conduction thresholds. This audiometric threshold configuration with a separation between the air and bone conduction thresholds is termed the *air–bone gap*. The air conduction and bone conduction threshold differences generally disappear when the conductive portion of the hearing loss is ameliorated. The sensorineural part of the mixed hearing loss will typically improve to the level of the previously established bone conduction threshold level. In mixed hearing loss, the hearing levels are not likely to return to normal limits due to the presence of sensorineural hearing impairment.

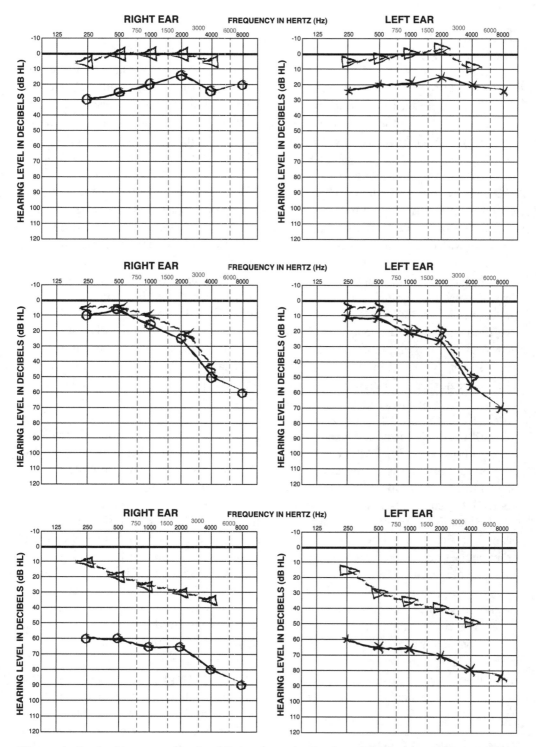

Figure 1–8. Audiograms showing bilateral conductive hearing loss *(top),* bilateral sensorineural hearing loss *(center),* and bilateral mixed-type hearing loss *(bottom).*

Central Auditory Processing Disorder

Central auditory processing disorders (CAPDs) refer to difficulties in the processing of auditory information in the central nervous system. This problem was described by Jerger and Musiek (2000) as a deficit in the processing of information that is specific to the auditory modality. This deficit is a problem that is likely to be exacerbated in unfavorable acoustic environments as in situations with competing noise background. CAPD may be associated with difficulties in listening, speech understanding, language development, and learning. Childhood central auditory disorders can be classified into two groups: those with identifiable neuropathology and those of unknown etiologies that present as communication disorders. The vast majority of children whose conditions are diagnosed as central auditory disorders show communication disorder symptoms with normal hearing and no observable neuropathology (Stach, 1998). This type of auditory dysfunction is not usually accompanied by a decrease in auditory thresholds but tends to manifest itself in varying degrees as a decrease in auditory comprehension. For example, the child may have a normal audiogram but be unable to comprehend complex speech, which in turn, may lead to learning disabilities. Approximately 30% of all students diagnosed with learning disabilities have histories of chronic middle ear problems and conductive hearing loss (Upfold, 1988). The diagnosis and treatment of central auditory dysfunction are controversial and complex and are discussed more fully in Chapter 6.

Degree and Severity of Hearing Loss

An important consideration in any hearing loss is its degree of impairment. The common terms used to identify the degree of hearing loss are mild, moderate, severe, profound, and anacusis (total hearing loss). Sometimes, borderline categories of hearing impairment are described with a combination of terms, such as moderately severe hearing loss. The person-first phrase "children with hearing loss" is used in this text to describe children with all degrees of decreased hearing from mild hearing loss to profound deafness. More specifically, children with hearing losses in the mild, moderate, and severe categories are likely to be described as hard-of-hearing. Children with hearing losses in the profound category are more likely to be classified as deaf. The historical differences between children who were generally categorized as hard-of-hearing and those children who were profoundly deaf were significant. In terms of prognosis of educational attainment, clarity of speech, language development, and reading skills, and general adjustment to the "hearing world," the children who were hard-of-hearing had much better chance of success than the children who were profoundly deaf. In today's climate, however, the lines between children who are hard-of-hearing and children who are deaf has become blurred. Early identification of babies with hearing loss followed with early intervention strategies and the early application of advanced amplification technologies has set aside the degree of hearing loss, per se, as a major deterrent to the prognosis of the child with hearing loss.

Additional consideration regarding the severity of hearing loss is related to whether one ear (unilateral) or two ears (bilateral) are affected. The child with a unilateral mild hearing loss or complete loss of hearing in one ear with normal hearing in the other may function adequately in some situations and falter in other situations, particularly in noisy background environments or when auditory localization is required. The child with unilateral hearing loss will fail the school screening test, however, and presents special testing and management challenges to the audiologist. Considerable research with the child who shows mild bilateral or unilateral hearing loss has shown that these children often need supplementary educational support and may benefit from amplification (Gravel, Fischer, & Chase, 2009; Tharpe, Sladen, Dodd-Murphy, & Boney, 2009).

A complete description of a child's hearing loss should include whether it is unilateral or bilateral, the degree of auditory impairment, and the type of loss (conductive, sensorineural, or mixed). The cause of the hearing loss should also be included when known and a brief summary of the audiometric evaluation should be provided. Sample descriptions of hearing loss are "unilateral, severe sensory (or neural) hearing loss due to ototoxic medications" and "bilateral, moderate conductive hearing loss due to middle ear fluid."

DEMOGRAPHICS OF CHILDHOOD HEARING LOSS

The federal government has funded a number of attempts to determine the demographics of hearing loss in children in the United States over the past 50 years (Blanchfield, Feldman, Dunbar, & Gardner, 2001). However, accurate determination of the national incidence and prevalence of hearing loss in children continues to be an ongoing challenge. The incidence and prevalence results are dependent on numerous complex and interactive variables such as the research sampling technique (i.e., collection of data from testing the hearing of a large random sample of children versus the subjective questionnaire approach, whereby the parents are asked if their child has difficulty with hearing). Results between studies have been difficult to compare as each of the sampling projects used different age groups as well as different definitions of what decibel level cutoff constitutes a hearing loss in their pediatric sample.

The growing national population in the United States over this period of years makes it difficult to determine absolute numbers for the incidence and prevalence of hearing loss in our children. Over the years, improvements in the medical treatment of correctable hearing loss have no doubt influenced the demographic numbers. And, finally, the choice and power of the statistical analysis of the data have influenced the final demographic estimates of childhood hearing loss in each of the studies. However, it is important that we continue this process of trying to correctly identify the numbers of children with hearing loss in the United States because of the important implications for our public health services and appropriate funding sources. The demographic studies described below illustrate some of the study variables that make it difficult to compare hearing survey results among national research efforts.

Early federal projects to establish the national prevalence of hearing loss in children were reported by Hull, Mielke, Timmons, and Williford (1971), Kessner, Snow, and Singer (1974), Leske (1981), Delgado, Johnson, Roy, and Trevino (1990), and Ries (1994). The Hispanic Health and Nutrition Examination Survey of 1990 included a comparative analysis of hearing in African American, Hispanic American, and non-Hispanic white children. The results showed a significantly higher prevalence of hearing loss in Cuban American and Puerto Rican children relative to the three ethnic study groups (Lee, Gomez-Marion, & Lee, 1996, 1998).

One of the most comprehensive attempts to establish the numbers of children with hearing loss in the United States was undertaken by the National Health and Nutrition Examination Surveys (NHANES II: 1976–1980 and NHANES III: 1988–1994). These surveys attempted to examine children's hearing, ages 6 to 19, through objective audiometric examinations and questionnaires. The sample sizes were 7,119 in NHANES II and 6,166 in NHANES III. Prevalence rates for combinations of better and worse ear hearing levels were generally similar in these two nationally representative surveys. High-frequency hearing loss was more prevalent than low-frequency hearing loss (12.7% versus 7.1%), and 4.9% of children had combined high- and low-frequency hearing loss. Most of the hearing loss noted was unilateral and of mild degree (Niskar et al., 1998).

Audiometric measurements were obtained for the NHANES studies making it possible to estimate the number of children with hearing loss with differing degrees of hearing loss. These estimates have subsequently been adjusted for the growth in the U.S. population of children to provide prevalence data calculated for 2005:

- The prevalence of profound bilateral hearing loss was 0.75 and 0.57 in NHANES II and NHANES III, respectively. Because the number of U.S. children, 6 to 19 years old, increased to 57.5 million in 2005, applying these two prevalence rates to the 2005 population yielded estimates of 43,000 and 33,000 with profound bilateral hearing loss.
- The prevalence of moderate hearing loss (30 to 45 dB) in the better ear was 2.37 and 1.66 in NHANES II and NHANES III. Adjusting for the 2005 population increase, the estimates were 136,000 and 96,000.
- The prevalence of mild hearing loss (15 to 30 dB) was 1.37% and 1.38%

in NHANES II and III, and adjusted for the 2005 population increase, the estimates were similar at 791,000 with mild hearing loss in the better hearing ear.
- The prevalence of children with severe unilateral hearing loss, adjusted for the 2005 population increase, was estimated at 30,000 and 16,000.
- Thus, with the exception of children with profound bilateral hearing loss, the total estimate in 2005 was 903,000 (NHANES II) to 957,000 (NHANES III) children with mild, moderate, or severe hearing loss between the ages of 6 to 19 years.

The estimates above are for children with hearing loss in both ears; however, some children have normal hearing in their better ear while having significant hearing loss in their other (worse) hearing ear. The prevalence of "unilateral" mild, moderate, or severe hearing loss in the worse ear and normal hearing in the better ear was 4.9% and 5.7% in NHANES II and NHANES III. Adjusting for the 2005 population increase, the estimates are 2.8 and 3.0 million children in the United States with mild, moderate, or severe unilateral hearing loss in their worse hearing ear. By this point in your reading, you should be gaining an appreciation of the difficulties in determining the incidence and prevalence of pediatric hearing loss in the United States.

Obviously it was a more difficult task for the NHANES group to determine the incidence of hearing loss in children younger than five years. In 2005, 25 million children were younger than 5 years of age. Because nationally representative hearing examination data were lacking for children in this age range, incidence statistics derived from states with newborn hearing screening programs were used as a surrogate. Through statistical approximations, the estimate was 26,310 children in the United States in 2005 with hearing loss since birth. After adjusting for other known medical etiologies of acquired early childhood hearing loss, the overall total estimate was rounded up to be at least 30,000 children with significant hearing loss below 6 years of age. Other studies have shown wide variance in the prevalence of newborns with congenital hearing loss in the United States. The overall estimates have been estimated to be between one and six per 1,000 newborns (American Academy of Pediatrics, 1999; Cunningham & Cox, 2003; Hayes & Northern, 1994). Most children with congenital hearing are identifiable by newborn screening. However, some congenital hearing loss may not become evident until later in childhood.

Each year the NHIS uses interview survey techniques to ask parents or caregivers about the hearing of their children. In another attempt to estimate the national prevalence of childhood hearing loss, parents and caregivers were asked: Which statement best describes your child's hearing (without a hearing aid)? (a) good, (b) little trouble, (c) lot of trouble, or (d) deaf. Since 1997, 12,000 to 15,000 children have been sampled annually. The statistical mean prevalence of "deaf" is 0.81 per 1,000, corresponding to 67,000 children reported as deaf. The mean prevalence of a "lot of trouble" hearing is 3.1 per 1,000, corresponding to 260,000 children with a "lot of trouble" hearing. The mean prevalence of a "little trouble" hearing is 2.9%, corresponding to 2.5 million children with a "little trouble" hearing. These governmental pediatric hearing surveys can be reviewed at the following websites: http://www.cdc.gov/nchs/nhis.htm; http://www.cdc.gov/nchs/nhanes; and http://www.cdc.gov/ncbddd/ehdi/

The national prevalence of hearing loss in children under the age of 18, as determined through a large-scale consumer survey conducted by the Better Hearing Institute in the MarkeTrak VII study, was estimated to be approximately 1.67% (Kochkin, 2005; Kochkin, Luxford, Northern, Mason, & Tharpe, 2007). Shargorodsky, Curhan, Curhan, and Eavey (2010) reported a change in the prevalence of hearing loss in U.S. adolescents through cross-sectional analyses of U.S. demographic and audiometric data from NHANES studies of 1988 to 1994 and 2005 to 2006. The prevalence of hearing loss in teenagers 12 to 19 years increased significantly from 14.9% in 1988 to 1994 to 19.5% in 2005 to 2006 in teenagers. In 2005 to 2006, hearing loss was more commonly unilateral (prevalence, 14.0%) and involved the high frequencies (prevalence, 16.4%). Individuals from families below the federal poverty threshold (prevalence, 23.6%) had significantly higher odds of hearing loss than those above the threshold (prevalence, 18.4%).

As you can see, the question of how many children in the United States have hearing loss requires a complex answer that incorporates many variables, the most important of which is what hearing level constitutes hearing loss in our children? Although our data and estimates become more accurate with each survey, the costs and administrative effort involved in answering the question is huge.

Defining Pediatric Hearing Loss

It is first necessary to ask if there is a definition for hearing loss in children. At what point does hearing in children cease to be normal and become abnormal? At what decibel hearing levels does "hard-of-hearing" or "deafness" begin? The problem is that no one has adequately defined the parameters of a pediatric hearing handicap, or established an agreed upon "standard" definition of normal hearing in children, or determined the best method of securing the necessary data for such definition. The true and accurate definition of a handicapping hearing loss in any given child lies in the entire diagnostic process, which includes not only hearing tests but requires measurements of a child's receptive and expressive language, vocalization and speech levels, and behavioral functioning evaluations. Such diagnostic evaluations are best conducted by establishing a team of professionals from other disciplines, including speech-language pathologists, to help determine if the child is sufficiently language delayed to warrant educational intervention.

The foregoing concepts can be used in proposing a realistic definition of hearing loss in children: *A significant hearing loss in a child is any degree of hearing that reduces the intelligibility of speech to a degree inadequate for accurate interpretation or as to interfere with learning.* Such a definition recognizes that it may not be possible to place specific measure on what precisely handicaps a child's ability to learn. Too many variables are present in the learning process of children: amount of parental stimulation, quality of parental stimulation, innate intelligence, age of onset of hearing loss, personality factors, health conditions, and socioeconomic status. These variables may so affect the learning abilities of children that a 15 dB HL loss may be a significant hindrance in hearing for one child, whereas a 20 dB HL loss will not be much of a problem for another child.

Minimal Hearing Loss in Children

There have been few studies that have attempted to establish normative data for normal hearing in children. The majority of available data about the hearing status of school-aged children are based solely on the results of hearing screening examinations. These studies are somewhat suspect because of deficient testing conditions and protocols, and thus cannot be used to establish absolute normative levels for hearing in children. Haapaniemi (1996) reported a scientific study of more than 1,000 school-aged children in Finland. The Finnish study found that hearing levels in children had a tendency to improve with age up to 10 years (i.e., the mean threshold average for 10-year-olds was 3 dB better than in children of 7 years of age). Mean hearing thresholds were 0.4 dB to 1.2 dB better in girls than in boys. This finding raises the question, do hearing levels really improve with age in childhood or is this improvement the result of better attention to the hearing test procedure and motivation to respond correctly?

The American Academy of Otolaryngology's *Guide for the Evaluation of Hearing Handicap* gives directions to agencies for rating the percentage of hearing loss in compensation cases involving adults. It must be noted that this rating schedule was never intended for use with children. The important point to consider in their hearing handicap formula is that only hearing loss averages greater than 25 dB are considered to be "handicapping" for compensation rating. This "low-fence" value of 25 dB has been used for many years to evaluate the hearing of adults, with the inherent assumption, apparently, that adults do not experience communication difficulties until their hearing impairment exceeds an average of 25 dB between 500 and 3000 Hz. Most audiologists realize that in real-life situations with environmental noise, the traditional low-fence of 25 dB does not adequately represent the "true" hearing handicap. Is it possible that modern times are producing background noises so loud that they make hearing of speech increasingly difficult? And how realistic is it to apply this adult "low-fence" value to children's hearing needs? Davis, Elfenbein, Schum, and Bentler (1986) reported that hearing loss of any degree appears to affect the psycho-educational development of children adversely, leading to the conclusion that even minimal hearing loss places children at risk for language and learning problems.

Bess, Dodd-Murphy, and Parker (1998) conducted a study of school-aged children in Nashville, Tennessee, to determine the prevalence of minimal sensorineural hearing loss and to assess the relationship of the minimal loss to educational performance and functional status. Minimal hearing loss was defined as 20 dB HL or greater in the speech frequencies or a high-frequency loss of 20 to 40 dB at 1000, 2000, and 4000 Hz. They sampled 1,218 children from the third, sixth, and ninth grades and concluded that children with minimal sensorineural hearing loss experienced more difficulty than normal-hearing children on a series of educational and functional test measures. In fact, 31% of children with minimal sensorineural hearing loss had failed at least one grade. Edwards (1991, 1996) suggested that hearing aids might serve some of these children well and that other management intervention strategy, such as enhancement of listening skills, auditory programming, and modification of the listening environment, might be helpful as well. Fitzpatrick, Durieux-Smith, and Whittingham (2010) conducted a retrospective chart review of a large group of children with mild bilateral or unilateral hearing loss in a Canadian pediatric clinic to document amplification practices. They identified parental uncertainty related to clinical amplification recommendations, as well as considerable delay between confirmation of the hearing loss and the ultimate fitting of hearing aids. In review, they found inconsistent practice patterns from audiologists who recommended amplification in 60.1% of children with mild bilateral hearing loss and 26.1% of those with unilateral hearing loss. An important point in the study was the finding that although more than 90% of the sample received a recommendation for amplification, chart documentation revealed that less than two thirds of the children consistently used their amplification devices.

Dobie & Berlin (1979) undertook to find out what kind of speech perception problems such a child with a mild 20 dB HL hearing loss would have in language learning situations. They recorded speech samples through correcting filters as a "normal hearing" example and then attenuated the samples by 20 dB to simulate how a person with a 20 dB HL conductive hearing loss would perceive the material. Their results demonstrated that the treated utterances revealed that: (a) there was a potential loss of transitional information, especially plural endings and related final position fricatives; and (b) brief utterances or high-frequency information could either be distorted or degraded if signal-to-noise conditions were less than satisfactory. Dobie and Berlin reasoned that on the basis of their findings, a child with a 20 dB HL hearing loss might be handicapped acoustically in the following ways:

- Morphologic markers might be lost or sporadically misunderstood. For example, "Where are Jack's gloves to be placed?" might be perceived as "Where Jack glove be place?"
- Very short words that are often elided in connected speech (see "are" and "to" above) will lose considerable loudness because of the critical

relationship between intensity, duration, and loudness.

- Inflections or markers carrying subtle nuances, such as questioning and related intonation contouring, can at the very best be expected to come through inconsistently.

It must be acknowledged that children have a more critical need for hearing during their developmental and school years than do adults for understanding everyday speech. Children are unable to "fill in the blanks" when listening to conversation when a sample of the speech is not heard clearly. Accordingly, we believe strongly that 15 dB HL should be considered the lower limit of normal hearing for children and that impairment increases with each decibel of hearing loss greater than 15 dB HL.

Some may question why a 15 dB HL hearing loss may result in speech and language delays. The reasons lie in the nature of speech sounds, with the major amount of speech energy residing in the voiced vowels and voiced consonants. The unvoiced consonants /s, p, t, k, th, f, sh/ contain so little energy that they often fall below even normal hearing thresholds in average rapid conversation. However, it is important to note that frequencies above 3000 Hz contribute approximately 25% to audibility of speech. The frequency of the fricative /s/ sound may be between 6300 and 8300 Hz depending on the speaker's voice fundamentals (Stelmachowicz, Lewis, Choi, & Hoover, 2007). The phoneme /s/ is one of the most frequently occurring sounds in the English language and carries significant linguistic and grammatical cues such as passive voice, plurality, possession, and verb tense. Persons with normal hearing in their childhood development learn to use listening strategies for understanding speech based on their experiences using the context of the speech material for comprehension (i.e., their brain fills in the missing sounds). However, infants, toddlers, and young children who are just learning and building speech and language relationships need to hear *all* the sounds clearly to implant the perceptions solidly in their developing brains.

ACOUSTICS OF SPEECH

The sounds of the English language can be basically classified as vowels or consonants. Vowel sounds carry the most vocal energy (intensity) in speech, whereas the higher frequency consonant sounds contribute to the intelligibility of speech. The relative importance of speech frequency bands for the understanding of spoken language is shown in Figure 1–9. Spoken language is further characterized by its *prosody*—described in terms of pitch and loudness, duration of spoken elements, as well as vocal stress and temporal patterns.

Vowels are the first sounds learned by children as they attempt to formulate words. Children with normal hearing usually develop all of their vowel sounds by the ages of 24 to 36 months. Vowels are characterized by periodicity produced by vocal fold vibration. Vowel quality is determined by energy in several frequency regions, called *formants,* whose center frequency depends on the shape of the vocal tract. The first three formants are the most important for correct recognition of English vowels. The frequency response of the first formant, F_1, is about 250 to 1000 Hz; the second formant, F_2, is found in the frequency region between 1000 and 2000 Hz; and the third formant, F_3, occurs between 2000 and 3000 Hz. Vowels are usually more intense and of relatively longer duration than consonants and tend to be of lower frequency, but both vowels and consonants contain harmonic cues that extend into the higher frequencies (Figure 1–9).

However, general American English speech sounds can also be described in more specific detail by the way they are produced. In traditional articulatory phonetics, the main divisions are: (a) voicing, related to vocal fold vibration (e.g., voiced or voiceless); (b) place, related to articulators used to constrict the vocal tract (e.g., tongue or

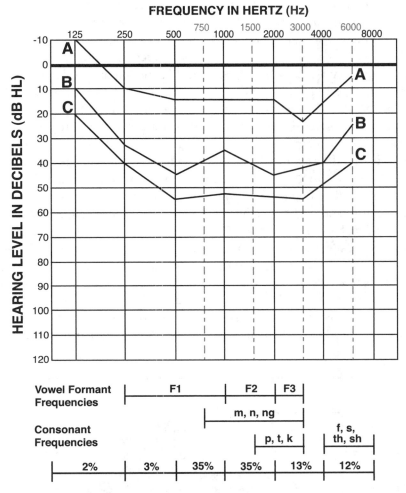

Figure 1–9. The area between curves A and B represents 80% of normal conversational speech levels. As hearing thresholds fall below curve B, difficulty understanding speech or even isolated words spoken in quiet surroundings are expected. Conversational speech exceeds curve A 90% of the time, speech exceeds curve B only 50% of the time, and curve C merely 10% of the time. With permission from "Yet another audiogram," by M. Chial, 1998, *ASHA Hearing and Hearing Disorders: Research and Diagnostics Newsletter, 2,* pp. 2–3.

lips); and (c) manner, related to degree of nasal, oral, or pharyngeal cavity construction (e.g., plosives, fricatives, nasals). Thus, /b/ in the word *be* is a voiced bilabial plosive. In contrast, acoustic phonetics identifies speech sounds in terms of acoustic parameters—frequency composition, relative intensities, and changes in duration. Human vocal cords convert only a fraction of the energy of the air stream flowing from the lungs into the acoustic energy required for speech.

Fricative consonants (i.e., /f/, /z/) are characterized by aperiodic noise and may be voiced or voiceless. Fricatives are classified in voiced-unvoiced cognate pairs. Each member of the pair is articulated in the same way and has similar acoustic characteristics except for the presence or absence of voicing. The frequency regions differentiate consonant pair, that is, the /zh, sh/ pair has energy between 2500 and 4500 Hz, whereas the /z, s/ pair has energy in the frequency region of 3500 through 8000 Hz. The /h/, /f/, and /a/ have less energy than the rest of the fricatives.

Stop consonants, also known as plosives or occlusives, are produced when air pressure is built up to the point of complete closure in the vocal tract and is then released abruptly, causing a burst of air. A silent period followed by a burst of air is distinctive in plosives and identifies them as different from other consonants. The unvoiced stop consonants are characterized by an aspiration period before the onset of the succeeding voiced vowels. The voiced stop consonants are characterized by the burst of air immediately preceding the onset of the succeeding vowel. Acoustic cues for differentiation among the various plosives are the frequency of the released burst and the second formants transitions. That is, changes in the center frequency of energy in the burst of /b/ and /p/ are relatively low frequency, those changes of /d/ and /t/ are relatively high frequency, and those changes in the center frequency burst of /k/ vary with the adjacent vowel. The relative contribution of the consonant frequencies to the understanding of speech is shown by the fact that nearly 70% of word recognition is determined by speech energy between 500 and 2000 Hz. An additional 25% of word recognition energy occurs by energy falling above 2000 Hz as shown in Figure 1–10.

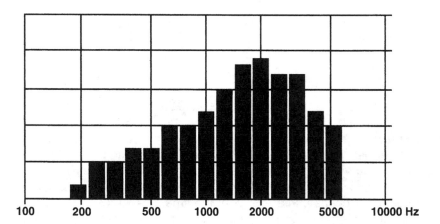

Figure 1–10. Graph showing the relative importance of individual speech bands for speech intelligibility. (American National Standards Institute. *Specifications for audiometers.* ANSI S36-1969. New York, NY: Author.)

The concentrations of acoustic energy in speech sounds (formants) make each speech sound somewhat different than other similar sounds. Many sounds look precisely alike on the lips to children with hearing loss, as the difference between similar sounds may just be whether or not the sound is voiced or unvoiced. Voicing places the vocal folds into vibration, permitting the child with profound deafness to actually feel the sound on the throat. Most sounds are grouped in pairs where one sound is voiced and the other sound is unvoiced (i.e., b/p, t/d, etc.). Hearing speech sounds is much more effective for children with hearing loss to learn speech and language than depending on speech reading.

Caleffe-Schenck and Baker (2011) provided a classification summary for the sounds of speech as follows.

Manner of place tells us how a sound is made:

- Plosives and stops: a release of built-up pressure occurs with plosives; the pressure is not released for stops: p/b, t/d, k/g.
- Fricatives: a point of constriction causes friction in the breath stream that creates a sound: h, f/v, s/z, sh/zh.
- Nasals: the breath stream goes mainly through the nose: m, n, ng.
- Semivowels: these are produced like vowels except there is greater constriction: w, y.
- Liquids: the tongue diverts the breath stream in the mouth: l, r.
- Affricatives: a stop is released with a fricative: ch, j.

Place of production is where in the mouth the sound is made:

- Bilabial: two lips: p, b, m, w;
- Labiodental: bottom lip and teeth: f, v;
- Linguadental: tongue and teeth: th;
- Alveolar: ridge on hard palate behind the inner teeth: t, d, s, z, n, l, r;
- Palatal: hard palate: sh, zh, y, ch, j;
- Velar: back of soft palate: k, g, ng; and
- Glottal: back of mouth: h.

Supersegmental patterns in speech refer to the duration, intensity, and pitch that give us our personal qualities of speech. A suprasegmental is a vocal effect that extends over more than one sound segment in an utterance. Suprasegmentals allow us to vary the meaning of our messages without changing the words. We do this by putting stress on different words by conveying emotion in what we say. Children learn at a very early stage if the speaker is angry or happy simply from the person's volume and intonation. So even if the listener cannot understand all the words, the listener can usually determine the emotion of the message. Without appropriate use of suprasegmentals, the voice can sound flat or mono-pitched, such as traditional "deaf speech" from a profoundly deaf individual, which can affect communication and socialization. With appropriate use of hearing aids and cochlear implants, children with profound hearing loss can develop the rich suprasegmental speech of persons with normal hearing (CASTLE Staff, 2011).

Variation in Acoustic Parameters of Speech Sounds

Skinner (1978) suggested that infants would recognize speech sounds with relative ease if they were not spoken in rapid succession and if the acoustic features were constant. However, speech-sound acoustic cues vary: (a) each time an individual speaker produces a speech sound, (b) from speaker to speaker, and (c) with changes in phonetic context as they are modified by adjacent speech sounds and stress patterns. Most children and adults recognize the ambiguous, sometimes even distorted, acoustic cues provided in everyday conversation with remarkable ease. Although there are multiple acoustic cues for recognizing speech sounds, other cues include the general speech situation or context, previous experience and expectations, and most importantly, knowledge of the language. Speech recognition depends partially on the acoustic signal and partially on the listener's language experience. Through extensive listening experiences, the infant learns where the boundaries of speech sounds and words occur in connected speech. The process is called segmentation. In different listening environments over time, the average intensity of speech varies between 20 and 60 dB HL, with an average of approximately 40 dB HL (Figure 1–11).

A good loud shout is about 75 dB HL; but for the soft whisper, the average intensity level may drop 10 to 20 dB below normal speech levels. The human vocal range constitutes a 700:1 ratio of intensities between the weakest and strongest speech sounds made while speaking at a normal conversational level (Fletcher, 1953). Ordinary background noise varies between approximately 35 and 68 dB SPL. For normal-hearing adults, the situation in which noise is 5 to 10 dB below the level of speech (known as the signal-to-noise ratio and abbreviated as S/N) does not create difficulty in listening, because the listener can fill in missing

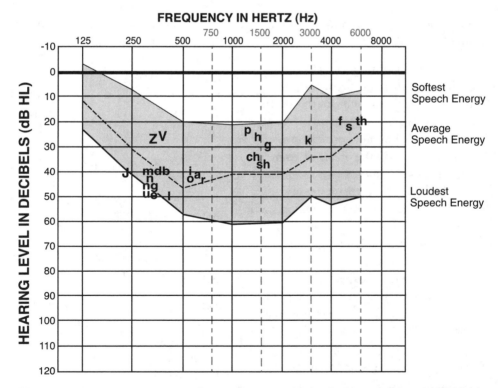

Figure 1–11. Average range of speech energy in decibel hearing level (dB HL) is shown in audiogram form, with the average range of softest and loudest speech energy in conversation.

acoustic cues. In contrast, the linguistically unsophisticated infant cannot fill in the missing acoustic details, and the speech energy needs to be some 30 dB louder than the background masking noise.

Connected speech carries suprasegmental information, which depends on the rhythm of speech and consists of stress and intonation patterns as well as duration characteristics. Stressed speech sounds or words are longer in duration, more intense, and higher in fundamental frequency than unstressed speech sounds. Change in the fundamental frequency of voiced sounds contributes to intonation that helps the listener identify sentence type. There is little definitive information about the specific role of suprasegmental parameters, but within broad limits they can be specified for various grammatical configurations.

Effect of Hearing Loss on Speech and Language

Hearing loss does not cause one specific kind of communication problem. The effects of a hearing loss depend on its severity, configuration, duration, and stability as well as the age of the person at onset. In the child with hearing loss, the extent and type of early training; the type and timing of amplification; visual, emotional, and intellectual factors; and cultural and family support also influence language development. Age at identification and intervention are especially important factors in language development. A child who sustains significant hearing loss after acquiring language (3 or 4 years of age) will have a less severe linguistic deficit than the child whose hearing loss is present at birth or develops within the first few months of life.

Children with hearing losses have limited opportunities to "overhear" information from various input sources, which leads to impoverished experiences with negative consequences for language rules formation, world knowledge, and vocabulary development (Carney & Moeller, 1998). Children love to listen in on conversations and no doubt this incidental hearing forms an important part of their learning new words. Dunn and Shatz (1989) showed that 2- and 3-year-olds monitor third-party conversations demonstrated by the children joining the conversation in appropriate topic interludes. An interesting study by Akhtar, Jipson, and Callanan (2001) confirmed that 2-year-olds learn novel words through overhearing. Moller (2010) reported a series of studies conducted at Boys Town National Research Hospital, Omaha, Nebraska, to learn more specifically how children listen in on adult conversations to identify behaviors that might lead to future word, speech, and language development.

Adults know the language they are listening to in the sense of its phonemes, its words, and its grammar. They have subtly learned what phoneme sequences make up meaningful words and how the rules of grammar and semantics determine word order. The major effect of a hearing loss is the loss of audibility for some or all of the important acoustic speech cues. Persons with hearing loss typically complain of an inability to understand speech, especially in the presence of background noises. Conversation may be loud enough for them, but they cannot understand the words because the hearing loss distorts the acoustic signal and interferes with auditory processing. Carney (1999) wisely cautioned audiologists against assuming linearity of a hearing loss. That is, hearing loss does not progress in an orderly fashion, and each 10 dB of additional hearing loss does not cause the same decrease in auditory function, regardless of the degree of hearing loss.

Skinner (1978) listed a number of detrimental general principles of "acoustic liabilities" to a child's language learning when a hearing loss exists:

- *Lack of Constancy of Auditory Clues When Acoustic Information Fluctuates.* When a child does not hear speech sounds in the same way from one time to another, there is confusion in abstracting the meanings of words due to inconsistent categorization of speech sounds.
- *Confusion of Acoustic Parameters in Rapid Speech.* Even the normal-hearing child suffers from variations of speech occurring among speakers and even in the same speaker. Frequency, duration, and intensity vary as a result of differences among speakers of different ages, genders, and personality types. The child with hearing loss will be confused in language learning as a result.
- *Confusion in Segmentation and Prosody.* The child with hearing loss may miss linguistic boundaries such as plurals, tenses, intonation, and stress patterns. These factors are requisite to meaningful interpretation of speech.
- *Masking of Ambient Noise.* Children with hearing loss who are in classroom settings need a signal-to-noise ratio of at least +15 dB; that is, the speech signal must be 15 dB louder than the background noise for learning to take place (Crandell, 1991; Crandell & Smaldino, 1995; Crandell, Smaldino, & Flexer, 2005). Unfortunately, it is rare in our modern, open, school classrooms for this preferred listening ratio to be present. Public school classrooms typically have signal-to-noise ratios that range between +7 and −5 dB (Finitzo-Hieber, 1988; Markides, 1986). Negative value S/N ratios indicate that the background noise is actually louder than the speaker's voice. Obviously, a child with even a minimal hearing loss is significantly handicapped under such poor listening situations.
- *Breakdown of Early Ability to Perceive Speech Sounds.* The infant begins to learn to discriminate speech sounds almost immediately after birth. Studies have shown that at between 1 and 4 months of age an infant can discriminate between most of the English speech sound pairs. By 6 months of age, the infant recognizes many of the speech sounds of language and is making ongoing cataloging of speech sounds. If the sounds of speech are not perceived early, due to the presence of a hearing loss, learning can be impeded.
- *Breakdown in Early Perceptions of Meanings.* During ordinary speech, the normal listener often misses some unstressed or elided words or sounds but is able to fill in by understanding the context of the message. However, when a hearing loss causes a young child to miss many of these soft or inaudible sounds, there is confusion in word naming, difficulty in developing classes of objects, and misunderstanding of multiple meanings.
- *Faulty Abstraction of Grammatical Rules.* When short words are soft or elided, as they often are, it becomes more difficult for a hearing-impaired child to identify the relationships between words and to understand word order.

- *Subtle Stress Patterns Missing.*
  The emotional content of speech,
  its rhythm, and its intonation
  are communicated through the
  low frequencies. When there is
  low-frequency hearing loss, the
  emotional content of speech is
  confused—another condition that
  impairs the learning of speech
  and language.

Effects of Hearing Loss

It is common practice to simplify hearing
losses into terms such as mild, moderate,
severe, and profound for ease of general
description. However, this categorization
by degree is potentially misleading and,
perhaps, an unfortunate practice. Yet, these
terms are in common use although there is
no agreed upon standard agreement as to
the definitive criteria for each category. For
example, a child labeled with "mild" hearing loss is likely to be considered to have
only "minimal" dysfunction—a descriptor
that parents, teachers, and physicians may
interpret to mean that no significant hearing problem exists. Yet, research by Wohlner
(cited by Matkin, 1984) found that young
children categorized with "mild" bilateral
sensorineural hearing loss showed delay in
development of at least 2 years in expressive
oral language by the age of 7 years. Children in the study with "moderate" hearing
impairment at age 7 scored below the norms
for normal-hearing 4-year-olds.

Of course, undetected hearing loss of
any degree can have a significant impact on
speech, language, cognitive, and psychosocial development. We not only need to be
concerned with children with moderate to
profound hearing loss, the "minimal hearing loss" group also needs our attention. The
impact of bilateral mild and unilateral hear-

ing loss on the development of children has
only recently been recognized by educators
and health care providers. Many children
are being identified with unilateral hearing loss from birth, and early bilateral mild
hearing loss that previously had not been
detected prior to school hearing screening. It is no longer reasonable to accept that
children with mild and unilateral hearing
losses are not at risk for speech and language delays, academic failure, and poor
self-esteem. These children, in fact, have
difficulties with speech and language development resulting in lower scores in school
achievement and more behavioral problems
than their peers with normal hearing (Eichwald & Gabbard, 2008).

Mild Hearing Loss (15 to 30 dB)

As we have repeatedly pointed out in this
chapter, a 15 to 30 dB hearing loss will have
a significant effect on communication, language learning, and educational achievement. Vowel sounds are heard clearly, but
voiceless consonants may be missed. In
children with this degree of hearing loss,
auditory learning dysfunction may result
in inattention, classroom behavior problems, and possible mild language delay and
speech problems. This child with "mild" loss
hears only the louder, voiced speech sounds.
The short, unstressed words and less intense
speech sounds (such as voiceless stops and
fricatives) are inaudible. The acoustic cues
of speech that are audible may be perceived
differently by a child with a 15 to 30 dB conductive loss than by another child with a 15
to 30 dB sensorineural hearing loss.

Moderate Hearing Loss
(31 to 50 dB HL)

These children miss most conversational
speech sounds, but they typically respond

well to educational activities with the help of hearing aid amplification. Children with moderate hearing loss may demonstrate behavioral problems, inattention, language delay, speech problems, and learning problems. These children may have difficulty learning abstraction in the meaning of words and the grammatical rules of language because they do not hear some of the speech sounds. With this degree of hearing loss, vowels are heard better than consonants. Short, unstressed words such as prepositions and relational words, as well as word endings (–s, –ed), are particularly difficult to hear. This reduction of cues and information may lead to confusion among speech sounds and word meanings, limited vocabulary, difficulty with multiple meanings of words, difficulty in developing object classes, confusion of grammatical rules, errors in word placement in sentences, and omission of articles, conjunctions, and prepositions. Omission and distortion of consonants typically characterize the speech articulation of the individual with moderate hearing loss. Strangers may have difficulty understanding the speech of a child with moderate hearing loss.

Severe Hearing Loss (50 to 70 dB HL)

Language and speech will not develop spontaneously in children with severe hearing loss. With early intervention, use of appropriately fitted hearing aids, and special education, these children may function very well. Without amplification, children with severe hearing loss cannot hear sounds or normal conversation. They can hear their own vocalizations, albeit distorted, some very loud environmental sounds, and only the most intense conversational speech when spoken loudly at close range. With the use of hearing aids, they can discern vowel sounds and differences in manner of consonant articulation. This degree of hearing loss generally results in significant language problems, speech problems, and associated educational problems.

Profound Hearing Loss (71 dB HL or Greater)

Children with profound hearing loss learn language and speech only with intensive special education supplemented through powerful hearing aids or cochlear implants. Their success in life is greatly improved with early identification and early treatment of their hearing loss problem. Without some means of amplification, children with profound hearing loss are generally unable to hear or understand sounds. With appropriately fitted amplification, they will hear the rhythm patterns of speech, their own vocalizations, and environmental sounds. Profound hearing loss may result in severe language delay, speech problems, and possible related learning dysfunction. Boothroyd (1993) suggested three additional subcategories to describe those children with more than profound hearing losses: (a) those children with considerable residual hearing with thresholds between 90 and 100 dB HL; (b) those with limited residual hearing between 101 and 120 dB HL; and (c) those children with no measurable hearing or auditory thresholds of 121 dB HL or greater.

The speech of children with profound hearing loss may be characterized with voice, articulation, resonance, and prosody problems and require extensive speech therapy. Their vocal pitch is frequently higher than that of normal-hearing people, and the prosodic features of intonation and stress are missing, giving their voices a monotone quality. The speech of children with profound deafness may be characterized with: (a) slow temporal patterning, (b) inefficient use of the breath stream, (c) prolongation of vowels, (d) distortion of vowels, (e) abnormal rhythm, (f) excessive nasality, and (g) addition of an undifferentiated neutral vowel between abutting consonants. The articulation of children with severe to profound hearing loss has been observed to have excessive mandibular movement, lack of tongue movement, posterior tongue positioning, voiced-voiceless confusions for consonants, problems with coarticulation, substitution of visible sounds for those sounds that are difficult to see, better articulation for initial speech sounds than for medial or final speech sounds, stop/plosive confusion, and the intrusion of an undifferentiated neutral vowel between abutting consonants. Studies of speech intelligibility indicate that, at best, naive listeners understand 20% to 25% of the deaf speech produced by young children with profound deafness (Table 1–3). Deaf children use concrete rather than abstract words and concepts with poor syntactic constructions limited by their lack of exposure to natural language.

Hereditary Deafness

Hereditary deafness is a fairly common disease entity, occurring with between one and three children in 1,000 live births. The terms *hereditary deafness* and *congenital deafness* are often interchanged to describe children with profound, irreversible, bilateral sensorineural hearing loss that is present at birth. Hereditary deafness may be related to any condition including anatomic malformations of the outer, middle, or inner ear, in utero infection, birth trauma, and genetic causes. In studying a child with apparent congenital severe deafness, the audiologist must be aware of possible late onset exogenous, or outside, factors that can cause childhood deafness.

Hereditary hearing impairment may be categorized in a variety of ways including: (a) by type of inheritance (single-gene, chromosomal, multifactorial); (b) by time of onset (congenital, acquired, early onset, late onset); (c) by degree of hearing loss (mild through profound); or (d) by affected structures (external ear, middle ear, inner ear, neural), and associated with other abnormalities (syndrome delineation).

A high percentage of congenital deafness is hereditary: about 40% of profound childhood deafness is autosomal recessive in origin; 10% dominant transmission; and 3% due to a sex-linked gene. Current research has shown that genetics is responsible for hearing loss among 50% to 60% of children with hearing loss, whereas infections during pregnancy in the mother, or other environmental causes, and complications after birth are responsible in about 30% of hearing-impaired infants. The marriage of two deaf persons gives a slightly increased risk of deafness in their children because there is a small chance that two such persons would be affected by the same genetic deafness. Should the same recessive gene be carried by two normal-hearing parents, theoretically one fourth of their offspring would be affected and one half of the children would be carriers. However, if the same recessive type of hereditary deafness overtly affects both parents, they are homozygous for the trait; therefore, all of their children will be affected and will also be capable of passing the trait on to some of their offspring.

Hereditary hearing loss is often associated with congenital craniofacial anomalies such as malformations of the external ear and canal, cleft lip and palate, ear tags, and other head and facial dysmorphic features. Hayes (1994) described results of auditory

Table 1–3. Handicapping Effects of Hearing Loss in Children

Average hearing level (500–2000 Hz)	Description	Possible condition	What can be heard without amplification	Handicapping effects (if not treated in first year of life)	Probable needs
0–15 dB	Normal range	Conductive hearing losses	All speech sounds	None	None
15–25 dB	Slight hearing loss	Conductive hearing losses, some sensorineural hearing losses	Vowel sounds heard clearly; may miss unvoiced consonants sounds	Mild auditory dysfunction in language learning	Consideration of need for hearing aid; speech reading, auditory training, speech therapy, preferential seating
25–30 dB	Mild hearing loss	Conductive or sensorineural hearing loss	Only some speech sounds, the louder voiced sounds	Auditory learning dysfunction, mild language retardation, mild speech problems, inattention	Hearing aid, speech reading, auditory training, speech therapy
30–50 dB	Moderate hearing loss	Conductive hearing loss from chronic middle ear disorders; sensorineural hearing losses	Almost no speech sounds at normal conversational level	Speech problems, language retardation, learning dysfunction, inattention	All of the above plus consideration of special classroom situation
50–70 dB	Severe hearing loss	Sensorineural or mixed losses due to a combination of middle ear disease and sensorineural involvement	No speech sounds at normal conversational level	Severe speech problems, language retardation, learning dysfunction, inattention	All of the above plus probable assignment to special classes
70+ dB	Profound hearing loss	Sensorineural or mixed losses due to a combination of middle ear disease and sensorineural involvement	No speech or other sounds	Severe speech problems, language retardation, learning dysfunction, inattention	All of the above, plus possible cochlear implant and long-term educational support

evaluation of 145 infants with craniofacial anomalies and found that 50% evidenced hearing loss. The presence and degree of hearing loss associated with craniofacial anomalies varied by the specific anomaly. Some syndromic disorders may manifest progressive-type hearing loss, so that although normal hearing may be noted on the initial visit, these children require regular reevaluation. The verification of hearing loss is the realm of the audiologist who can substantiate accurately the progression of hearing loss in such children.

Economic Burden of Hearing Loss and Deafness

A major concern that has a significant effect on parents when they learn that their child has significant hearing loss is worry about immediate and future potential financial stress. Although no specific amount of money can be identified that will apply to every hearing-impaired or deaf child, at least some consideration and estimates can be given to a number of possible factors that should be included to make the child's daily living optimal for communication and education purposes. This information may be used for parents' financial planning, or for advising agencies, or it may be helpful as a baseline in medical-legal cases as the result of inadvertent hearing loss resulting from an accident or as an iatrogenic misadventure from medical treatment.

It is a thought-provoking exercise to consider the economic burden created by childhood deafness. A number of general areas should be considered, including routine medical and audiologic expenses over the lifetime of the child as well as special educational and vocational expenses that are above and beyond those expenses incurred by parents of children with normal hearing.

The child with hearing loss may require any number of special living expenses for assistive listening devices and other supportive accessories to meet ordinary daily life circumstances. Finally, there is the question of potential loss of income borne by every individual with profound deafness over the course of his or her adult working life due to the inability to obtain employment of full and equal status with the average, normal-hearing adult. In addition to the specific expenditures that can be estimated, consideration must include a number of intangible costs of deafness that affect the persons with hearing loss from childhood and throughout their adult lives.

Although statistics to determine the precise economic penalty of hearing loss and deafness are not readily available, it is possible that not every child with hearing impairment will need all the services or supplies described below. However, there is no doubt that our cursory overview reveals a potentially enormous financial obligation to be shared among the child's parents, state and federal social service agencies, and the individual with hearing loss. Shown below are examples of possible or necessary, financial responsibilities associated with childhood deafness and the estimated recurring costs over a lifetime. Be aware that these expenses begin at the time of the first identification of the child with hearing loss that likely occurs early in life and will extend through the individual's life expectancy of approximately 75 years.

Medical and Audiologic Expenses

The child with hearing loss can count on numerous visits to clinical offices and medical facilities throughout life. Otolaryngology and pediatric consultations are needed approximately twice each year until 16 years of age and then annual evaluations throughout adult life; audiologic services are required on a quarterly basis through age 6 and then semiannual hearing evaluations through age 13; annual hearing monitoring is needed until age 18 and as needed throughout adult life. Technology tools and assistive devices are undergoing constant improvement so there will be visits for hearing aids, personal FM auditory systems, cochlear implant tuning and upgrades, assistive listening devices, battery replacements, maintenance, and insurance based on utilization of binaural amplification devices. Most amplification devices if used daily, need to be replaced every 4 to 5 years throughout life.

Education and Training Expenses

Education and training expenses might include parent-infant program training; speech, language, and auditory therapy during preschool years; private school placement, with special educational tutoring services as needed through age 18; computer-assisted learning systems; attendance at Gallaudet University, the National Technical Institute for the Deaf, or any regular college or community adult education program, perhaps with interpreter services needed along with special electronic media needs to keep up with lectures and course requirements.

Special Living Expenses

Special living expenses begin at the time of early identification of the child's hearing loss and continue throughout adulthood. Parents with hearing loss and a new baby with hearing loss may need a baby-cry amplifier or home video monitoring system; special home signaling devices might include lighting doorbells, video telephone systems, special smoke and fire alarms, vibrating or super-loud alarm clock, wristwatch, cell phone with texting or face-to-face capability, computers and notebooks with visual conference abilities, and upgrades for all these devices as needed and replacements throughout life; social media paraphernalia; special interpreter fees as needed for daily living; telecaption system for televisions; captioned films, videos, and DVDs for entertainment, educational, and recreational purposes; and of course, hearing dog services throughout life including provisions for pet food, shelter, transportation, and veterinarian care.

Lifetime Loss of Income Considerations

Based on a work life expectancy of 50 years and a comparison of the average annual salary with the fact that employed deaf adults earn 30% less annually than normal-hearing persons (Schein & Delk, 1974), it can be further noted that unemployment of deaf adults is more than twice the U.S. national unemployment figure, and (as reported by Internal Revenue Service statistics) more than 20% of deaf adults report no income.

Additional Intangible Costs of Hearing Loss and Deafness

The price of hearing loss and deafness is not limited to economic costs. One must also take into consideration the deep wounds of emotional trauma to the parents and family of the child with hearing loss. Many have compared the parents' realization of deafness in their child to an actual death inasmuch as the parents have "lost" the normal child they had expected for 9 months. Many parents go through a denial phase during which they may go from clinic to clinic, searching for a diagnosis and cure that will allow their child to be normal; an anger phase during which they may lash out at clinicians and doctors and try to place blame; a mourning phase during which they experience sadness and depression over the deafness; and finally an acceptance phase that allows them to become active participants in the child's habilitation process. Other intangibles comprise a never-ending recital of problems that only begin with the initial documentation of the child's hearing loss.

According to information provided on the Centers for Disease Control and Prevention (CDC) website, the annual educational cost for a child with significant hearing loss (i.e., greater than 40 dB HL) was estimated at $115,600 as of 2007. In addition, the total lifetime costs associated with childhood hearing loss, direct medical costs, such as doctor visits, prescription drugs, and inpatient medical stays, will account for about 6% of total living expenses; direct non-medical expenses such as home modifications and special education support, make up 30% of lifetime expenses; and indirect costs to include the value of lost wages when a person cannot work or is limited in the amount or type of work that he or she can do, will make up 63% of lifetime expenses. The CDC points out that these estimates do not include other expenses such as medical outpatient visits, sign language interpreters, and family out-of-pocket expenses.

Breakdown of Normal Family Communications

Beyond the financial burden, parents are denied the pleasure of being understood easily by their child and perhaps of hearing their own child speak normally. Without substantial training and assistive hearing devices in place, their child does not come when they call, does not obey their verbal commands, can neither be praised nor reprimanded orally, and cannot play the kinds of games the rest of the family plays—all these things present difficulties for the parents of a child with severe to profound hearing loss. Other children in the family are deprived of the attention of their parents, who must spend a great deal of time in coping with the needs of the deaf child. The extra time required to teach that child the basic elements of living, as well as communicating, is taken away from the other siblings who may suffer from this deprivation. The child with hearing loss suffers as well, for jealousy and anger can arise from siblings and cause significant undesirable family upheaval.

Problems in School

The child with significant hearing loss is isolated from peers in every educational system circumstance. As the mainstreamed child in normal-hearing classes, he or she may stand aside while the other children play games involving rapid verbal commands. In the classroom, he or she requires special attention and help that set him or her apart from fellow student peers. Studies have shown that although a deaf child may learn well in a mainstreamed environment, he or she may be scarred by the psychological feeling of inferiority and poor self-image (Davis et al., 1986). In a special school for the deaf, he or she is among deaf peers but is only able to communicate fully with them if signing is the mode of communication. The economic cost of special education in the United States for the 1999–2000 school years to deliver special programs for children who were deaf or hard-of-hearing was $625 million.

Language learning is always impaired to some degree in the deaf child. The average language level of the young deaf adult has been shown to be often equivalent to the third- or fourth-grade level. This fact has accounted for the poorer earning power of the deaf. It also deprives them of one of the great joys of life: an appreciation of humor that relies on verbal play or on an understanding of some daily usages. For example, a deaf child takes expressions such as "put your best foot forward" absolutely literally unless additional explanation is provided. And possibly, speech defects associated with hearing loss and deafness seriously diminish the social relations of the deaf child with normal-hearing peers. Nothing makes a child an outcast more than "funny speech," and children are notoriously cruel to a child with any deviations from the norm.

Problems in Adulthood

The lower income of the deaf necessitates a more modest lifestyle than is possible for their peers, consigning them to a lower level of living than their potential abilities would have allowed them. When it comes to marriage, the choices of the deaf are narrowed. If the deaf person has been led by his or her family and educational environment to expect to find a hearing mate, he or she may be doomed to disappointment.

One of the most devastating problems facing the deaf is dealing with the demands of the "hearing establishment." Society is organized around hearing people, and major adjustments have to be made for the deaf to confront everyday problems. Hopefully, hearing aids and cochlear implants help the adult who is fortunate enough to utilize these hearing devices. However, for adults who communicate through sign language, significant problems exist in daily living in our hearing world. Imagine the difficulties of a person who is deaf and signing, trying to explain a tax problem to the Internal Revenue Service agent. Interpreters must be scheduled in advance to accompany the deaf individual in court and legal matters. Going to the doctor to explain a medical problem may require special vocabulary that is yet unfamiliar to the person with deafness. Consider the difficulty of getting out of a burning public building in time without hearing the fire alarm, or trying to mobilize the authorities to help find a child lost in the mall.

The choice of a career is reportedly limited for some individuals with profound deafness, although successful auditory-oriented persons with severe to profound hearing loss are more likely to succeed in adult careers. Recognized graduate professions such as medicine, allied health professions, as well as careers in law, dentistry, and so forth, may be difficult (but certainly not impossible) for some persons with hearing loss to successfully complete and graduate. Many occupations are limited or closed to persons with profound hearing loss if the position requires extensive verbal communication or difficult hearing situations. However, in spite of hearing limitations, the use of amplification and cochlear implants has elevated the opportunities for persons with hearing loss and deafness in many ways not previously possible. It is to the everlasting credit of the human spirit that individuals with hearing loss are able to rise above their hearing problems and lead normal, productive, and happy lives. For those individuals who choose to be a part of the deaf community, they can count on a cohesive, supportive, and close group whose members are generally as active and content as their normal-hearing peers.

TEAM MANAGEMENT OF CHILDREN WITH HEARING LOSS

Due to the complex nature of hearing loss in children, and the fact that the hearing function is not an isolated phenomenon, it is imperative that a team of professionals work together to diagnose and manage each individual case. Emphasizing the value of the team approach in no way minimizes the audiologist's contribution. The role of the audiologist in decisions concerning diagnosis and management is vital and necessary. The audiologist contributes essential information on the degree of loss, auditory behavior and development, and auditory functioning of the child and provides familiarity with educational methods in decisions on school placements. The clinical insight and observation of the experienced pediatric audiologist contribute a much-needed element to the decisions that will be made by the family and team: How does the child relate to others? Is eye contact good? Is the behavior even minimally distractible? Does there seem to be perseveration of auditory behavior? What is the vocal quality and how does the child use his or her voice? How do parent and child relate to each other? These are the questions that can be answered more through the audiologist's experienced observations than through calibrated measurements.

Once the audiologist has specified the degree of hearing loss that exists and has delineated the status of the auditory development of the child, a standard protocol of examinations is indicated. Any of these studies, if made in isolation, will furnish only a fragment of the total picture of the child and his or her needs. When these fragments are brought together in a team conference, the picture becomes a whole.

The team together makes a diagnosis of the etiology, extent, and degree of the problem and decides on the proper management for the child.

After the initial thorough evaluation, it is customary to follow the young child every 3 to 6 months to complete the diagnostic process. The family and their child with hearing loss will likely be well-acquainted with their pediatrician and audiologist for sure, and maybe other members of the deafness team, by the time the child transitions into school at 5 or 6 years of age. During these early years, the team will work to identify other possible associated anomalies, health, or education problems. The pediatrician or family practitioner will continue presence as the medical home for the child with hearing loss for several years until the child approaches adulthood. The medical home physician will assess the overall development of the child and even provide for genetic counseling to the family and the child with hearing loss.

The audiologist contributes diagnostic audiometry, evaluates possible vestibular involvement when necessary, evaluates the relationship of the child's functioning to the degree of hearing loss, and pursues hearing aids or cochlear implants for the child. The speech-language pathologist provides a baseline speech and language evaluation that will be used throughout the child's developing years. During the diagnostic workup, the social worker helps determine where parents are in their process of accepting the problems of their child. How can they be helped to an acceptance of the problem? What can be done to best nurture the child? The team may decide at any given point to bring in a psychologist for counseling. The ophthalmologist evaluates associated eye abnormalities and vision acuity as well as examines for retinitis pigmentosa with electroretinography to rule out Usher's syndrome. A renal consultant should be involved in cases such as hereditary chronic nephritis or Alport's syndrome. Cardiologists and neurologists are called in as indicated, and it is found that in such complex cases as Hunter-Hurler syndrome that the entire roster of a hospital's specialists may be involved.

Routine regular medical examinations should be performed for the child with hearing impairment until the child is at least 10 years of age. An otolaryngologic examination should be obtained at least annually and more frequently if warranted. An erroneous assumption is that after a child has sustained a hearing loss, nothing more can happen to their hearing. Not only is this belief incorrect with the onset of middle ear infections, but there may be progressive sensorineural hearing loss accompanied by increased susceptibility to other ear diseases, to noise-induced loss, or to ototoxicity. Therefore, it is imperative that the auditory thresholds of the child with hearing loss be monitored frequently. The importance of every decibel of residual hearing that the child possesses may be in exponential ratio to each decibel of hearing loss. Routine audiologic monitoring of the hearing loss pays dividends in information on changes in hearing that are pertinent for the child's habilitation program. A more extensive otologic and physical examination may be recommended when deterioration of the auditory threshold or the speech discrimination is found.

During the first two years, the child with hearing loss should be seen every 3 to 6 months for periodic reassessment of the hearing loss, review of medical conditions, and progress in education for the reasons listed below:

- Repeat audiometry will become more accurate as the child matures; routine reevaluation of hearing may reveal progression of hearing loss or identification of previously unsuspected opposite ear involvement; changes in the child's hearing may reveal the need to adjust hearing aids or re-tune the cochlear implant.
- Individual case history review by the team members may reveal overlooked historical items such as early history of disease or previously unnoted or unmentioned symptoms.
- Physical examination may reveal physical findings or newly developed symptoms, such as thyroid problems, renal problems, and night blindness.
- Repeat family history may show suppressed information or false-positive items. An incorrect initial diagnosis may be corrected by reevaluation.
- Progressive concomitant disease may be identified by follow-up evaluations.
- New information, new scientific knowledge, and new technology may become available with application to benefit to the child.
- Speech and language evaluations are given to monitor the performance of the child in the particular program in which he or she has been entered. If at any point it is obvious that the child is not making reasonable progress in the system, consideration can be given to evaluating a change of educational program.
- Psychosocial reevaluation and monitoring are extremely useful to determine whether any help should be given to the family in psychological or social matters.

In the hearing team's function as an objective advocate for the child (apart from the methodology of the program the child is in), it may be necessary to arbitrate between the family and the system. If the parents believe that the school system has mismanaged the child's placement, it may be necessary for the team to represent the family at a hearing called to evaluate the disagreement. Federal law mandates hearings that the parents can request whenever they believe a change is indicated (see Chapter 10). When college age is reached, the team may be called on to support the special interests of the student in obtaining a specific type of education. It should be evident that the work of a child's hearing team will continue until the patient is fully achieving and completely comfortable in the environment that has been chosen.

AUDIOLOGISTS WITH SPECIALTY TRAINING IN PEDIATRIC HEARING LOSS

There may be no more challenging audiology task than conducting hearing evaluations and intervention services to pediatric patients. Unlike adults with hearing impairment who generally present with similar hearing problems, every child is so uniquely different. However, it is recognized that not every audiologist wants to deal with the challenge of working with these oft-times difficult young patients. It is often stated that, "children are not just small adults; they must be tested, fitted, and managed in a total different manner than adults." The specialty focus of working with pediatric patients requires clinicians to seek training beyond the core courses related to the field of audiology. The pediatric-oriented audiologist must, first and foremost, have a strong calling and love for working with children; second, they must have an exceptional

knowledge base, masterful clinical skills, and sufficient clinical experience to meet the special needs of these young patients.

Scollie and Seewald (2002) pointed out numerous differences between working with pediatric patients and the audiology procedures used with adults. With pediatric patients, the audiologist often has to work with less-than-complete audiometric information. Thus, judgments must necessarily come from estimates of auditory thresholds obtained through electrophysiological measures, real ear measurements of growing and changing ear canal volumes and resonances, and confronting the issue of hearing fluctuations due to transient middle ear fluid situations. And, needless to say, many of the infants, toddlers, and young children are less than cooperative with the audiologic processes, and the children may be unable to contribute reliable behavioral responses. The audiologist who specializes in pediatric patients must be skillful at quickly determining the best way to gain the child's cooperation, and skillful enough to complete the hearing evaluation while keeping the child interested and on task.

Pediatric audiology is a dynamic and rapidly changing specialty area of audiology practice. Where we used to provide confirmation for parents who suspected their 2- or 3-year-old child might have hearing loss, pediatric audiologists routinely diagnose the hearing loss during the first month after the child's birth followed by completion of the hearing aid fitting process by the time the infant is 6 months of age. This has created entirely different challenges for the pediatric audiologist in regard to early identification and early intervention for infants diagnosed with hearing loss. Counseling is now more important than ever as the surprised and shocked parents learn of their baby's hearing loss. Parental counseling by the pediatric audiologist requires tact and empathy without understating the child's hearing problem. Fortunately, during the past decade, there have been new technological developments along with advanced testing and fitting protocols to help overcome pediatric hearing loss challenges.

The American Academy of Audiology (AAA) has recently instituted a program to identify those audiologists who are especially qualified and skilled at evaluating and managing children with hearing loss. Obtaining the AAA Specialty Certification in Pediatrics ensures that the audiologist has demonstrated a high level of knowledge in all areas of pediatric audiology and that the audiologist has a significant background of experience in working with children (i.e., at least 2 years and direct contact and case management with 600 pediatric patients) who have hearing loss. A certification is not a guarantee of any particular skill or competency, but an audiologist holding this certification has demonstrated the ability to pass a rigorous written examination in pediatric audiology that covers core audiology knowledge as well as pertinent federal and state law pediatric hearing issues, normal and abnormal child development, screening and assessment procedures, counseling, communication enhancement technologies as well as habilitation/rehabilitation strategies, and educational support systems and programs.

It goes without question that every child with hearing loss deserves the best hearing solution possible. This requires the highest standards of care developed from evidence-based practices whenever possible and a methodical system of careful analysis of the child's hearing loss and the child's hearing and communication needs within his or her family and educational environments. Taking all of that information and data into consideration, the next steps require thoughtful analysis of the pediatric patient's hearing threshold configurations, individual ear acoustics, and determination of prescriptive hearing aid fitting targets, as well as the selection, programming, and fitting of appropriate technology features in personal amplification devices. The final audiology solution for each child must be determined by auditory performance through standardized outcome and verification measures. And, in fact, a "final solution" may not apply to many pediatric patients who require ongoing evaluation and monitoring for many years as they approach adulthood.

Each pediatric patient provides an opportunity for the audiologist to have a unique intervening and positive factor in people's lives. Although the responsibilities of the audiologist working with young children are huge, the diagnostic and treatment outcomes will likely have significant intervening influence (hopefully successful and positive) for the family and the ultimate educational progress and lifetime achievements of the child. It is critical that pediatric audiologists be fully cognizant that the decisions they make and counseling they provide may have life-changing ramifications for their patients.

In addition to the fact that pediatric patients are often cute and fun to work with, they each present a unique and different challenge to the audiologist. Although working with older adults often results in management of similar hearing loss and similar hearing complaints, each child seems to display a totally different hearing loss presentation requiring individual management requirements. That is to say, every child (and the child's parent or caretaker) is completely different from the last pediatric patient. Audiologists who work with pediatric patients tend to have a strong sense of calling to provide personalized services to their small patients and their families along with a professional attachment that grows through the years as they see their patients for follow-up evaluations. In return, pediatric audiologists gain considerable self-fulfillment and satisfaction from utilizing their unique expertise to benefit children and their families.

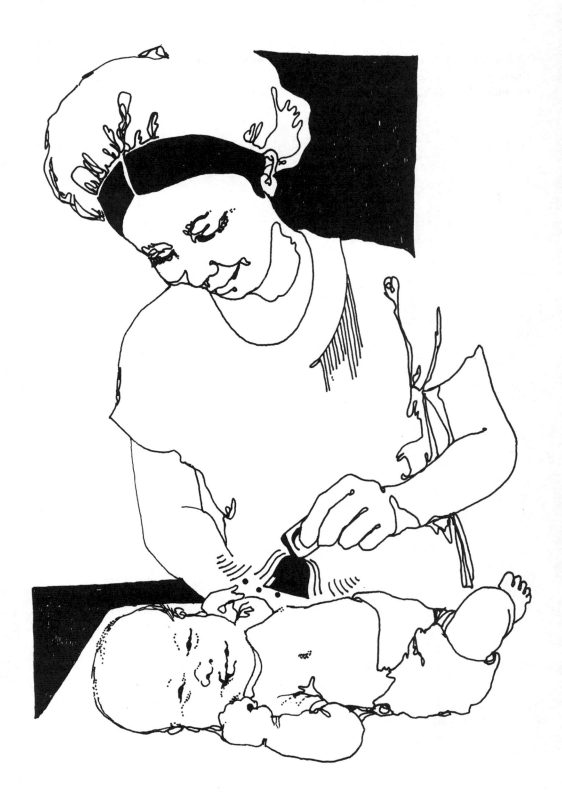

CHAPTER 2

Early Development

There are few events in life that surpass the birth of a new baby. The mystery and beauty of the origins of life have been well documented in books, videos, and the Internet, and yet, with each new birth, we continue to be awestruck. The time leading up to the normal birthing process is generally 266 days (38 weeks) from conception to birth, although it should be noted that only about 5% of births occur on the actual due date. Parents typically develop growing anticipation as the delivery time draws near. And, the satisfaction of taking the new baby home is an emotion that remains strong throughout life. Birthing is a miraculous event that produces an amazing 97% of normal births in spite of the complexities of prenatal development.

However, the fact is that about 3%, or one in every 33 babies born in the United States, is born with a birth defect (NICHD, 2012). Prematurity and low birth weights are identified as the primary causes of birth defects. Many different factors may be associated with the development of birth defects, such as genetic and chromosomal aberrations, *in utero* exposure to viruses or bacteria, uncontrolled maternal diabetes, maternal cigarette smoke, maternal use of drugs and alcohol during pregnancy, and prenatal exposure to chemicals. All of these factors may influence normal infant growth or development, resulting in different types of birth defects. From the audiologist's point of view, each of these factors can result in an infant being born with hearing impairment as a single isolated defect or an associated symptom to other birth defects. It is important that

audiologists have a full understanding of the numerous processes involved in the earliest embryonic and fetal development of organ systems in the newborn.

The embryologic development of the ear is of more than academic interest to the clinician. An understanding of embryologic relationships helps confirm a diagnosis and suggests the need for early hearing assessments. If one is aware of the timetable of prenatal development and the association of the various organs and structures with each other, the suspicion of deafness and its subsequent diagnosis and treatment become easier. The origination and major changes in the development of the ear and the hearing system take place in the mother's womb as the baby becomes a progressively more complex structure over time. Several processes occur concurrently to produce the final structure, including enlargements, constrictions, and foldings, which are further modified by evaginations and invaginations. However, development of the auditory structure does not cease, and is not totally complete, at the time of birth.

Knowledge of the origins of auditory structures (known as *phylogeny*) can be of diagnostic significance to the clinician. For example, when an infant presents with a congenital skin disorder, the clinician considers the fact that the skin and the otocyst (the primitive cochlear structure) both originate from ectoderm. It may then be logical to suspect that anomalies of the cochlear structures may have occurred contiguously with the skin disorder and that a search for severe sensorineural deafness is in order. Similarly, the timing of development of the various organ systems guides the clinician to suspect that a hearing loss may have occurred at the same time that other systems were affected. A noxious influence on the fetus at 2 months of gestation may result in a malformation of the pinna developing at that time. The pinna malformation, however, does not necessarily imply malformation of the ossicles of the middle ear. Although, as you will see later in this chapter, the ossicles of the middle ear partially share the same time clock as the pinna in embryologic development, the basic origins of the structures are different; on the other hand, an insult to one may well result in a related insult to the other.

Principles such as these allow clinicians to look for the occult symptom of hearing loss whenever an overt embryologic-related symptom becomes evident. The prognosis for auditory function can then be evaluated with consideration of what is known regarding the origin of the structures in question and the expected auditory pathology (Jones, 2011).

BASIC PRINCIPLES OF GENETIC INHERITANCE

Humans take great pride in identifying distinguishing traits from one generation to the next. We enjoy speculating on the resemblance of children to their parents and grandparents. With such observations begins the appreciation of genetics. Genetics and the study of hereditary disorders are among the most rapidly evolving disciplines among the medical sciences. There is probably some genetic component in almost all disease conditions, but the extent of the genetic component likely varies. To provide competent services to infants and their families, audiologists need an elementary understanding of the basic genetics, cyto-

genetics and molecular genetics, the inheritance of hereditary disorders, specific disorders associated with genetic disease, and the process of genetic evaluations. Tremendous strides have been made in understanding the genetics of deafness during the past two decades. In 2002, about 200 syndromes associated with deafness had been typed with genetic origins; by 2006, investigators had identified the genetic identity of about 300 syndromes; in 2012 at least 400 genetic-based syndromes were described that are likely to include permanent hearing loss. It should be obvious that the study of clinical genetics is important as it allows investigators and clinicians to understand genetic transmission and to ultimately prevent and treat inherited conditions in the future.

It is important to distinguish among the many terms used in describing pediatric hearing loss. *Congenital* means present at birth; "congenital" does not make any implications regarding the etiology of the condition. Infants born with hearing loss, regardless of the cause, have congenital hearing loss. *Heredity* means inherited, or "passed down" from previous generations through DNA, genes, or chromosomes; *hereditary* implies chromosome or gene control of the condition in question. *Genetic* means caused by a gene; *genetic* may also be considered a special subset of hereditary. *Familial* means the symptom or sign is present in several related family members; however, the term *familial* does not in any way imply etiology.

Although hereditary disease can become apparent at any point in an individual's life span, genetic and chromosomal abnormalities and associated congenital malformations are especially important in pediatric specialties. The relative contribution of these disorders to infant mortality rate has increased as the prevalence of infectious childhood disease has decreased. In the pre-antibiotic era, most infant mortality was attributable to infectious disease; today, in developed countries, most infant mortality is attributable to genetic disorders and congenital malformations. Of recognized pregnancies that end in spontaneous abortion, 50% to 60% have detectable chromosomal anomalies. It is estimated that 2% of all newborns demonstrate chromosomal or single-gene disorders. These abnormalities produce significant neonatal mortality and morbidity. Infants with genetic anomalies who survive into childhood require substantially greater health and educational care than nonaffected children.

DNA

Cells are the fundamental working units of every living system. All the instructions needed to direct their activities are contained within the chemical DNA (deoxyribonucleic acid). DNA is the base unit of heredity, "the code of life," or the molecular "letters" of inheritance. DNA from all organisms is made up of the same chemical and physical components. The DNA sequence is the particular side-by-side arrangement of bases along the DNA strand. This order spells out the exact instructions required to create a particular organism with its own unique traits. When changes or errors occur in this ordered sequence of the genetic code, disease may result. DNA is a nucleic acid consisting of four nitrogen-containing bases attached to a sugar-phosphate polymer and arranged on intertwining strands, the well-known "double-helix." The four bases, adenine (A), guanine (G), cytosine (C), and thymine (T), occur in predictable pairs on complementary strands such that A on one strand always pairs with T on its complementary strand, and G on one strand always pairs with C on its complementary strand. One set of complementary bases, <AT> and <CG> is a base pair. There are three billion base pairs of DNA that tell the body how to grow and

build and how to repair itself. Because bases occur in these invariant pairs, one strand of DNA contains all the information necessary to construct its complementary pair.

DNA stores and encodes a vast amount of information based on the sequence of base pairs. For segment N bases long, there are N^4 possible base-pair sequences. The base-pair arrangement of DNA encodes the complete genetic information of an organism; it is called the organism's genome. Genomes vary widely in size: the smallest known genome for a free-living organism (a bacterium) contains about 600,000 DNA base pairs, while human and mouse genomes have some three billion.

Accurate replication and transmission of the genetic code are ensured by the base-pair coding and double-helix structure of DNA. Figure 2–1 shows the double-helix structure of DNA (upper half of figure) and replication (lower half of figure). During replication, the double helix unwinds and separates into two single strands with their associated bases. Each strand serves as the template for a new, complementary strand. For example, the unwound DNA strand at the bottom right of Figure 2–1 with bases <ATCACT> will direct synthesis of a strand with complementary bases <TAGTGA>. After replication, two "daughter" double helixes will result; each daughter will contain one original parent strand and one newly synthesized complementary strand. In addition, if a base on one strand is lost or damaged, it can be replaced using the complementary strand to direct its repair.

Genes

Genes are the fundamental physical and functional units of heredity. Genes are sequences of DNA that direct protein synthesis. A gene may contain several hundreds or even thousands of base pairs of DNA.

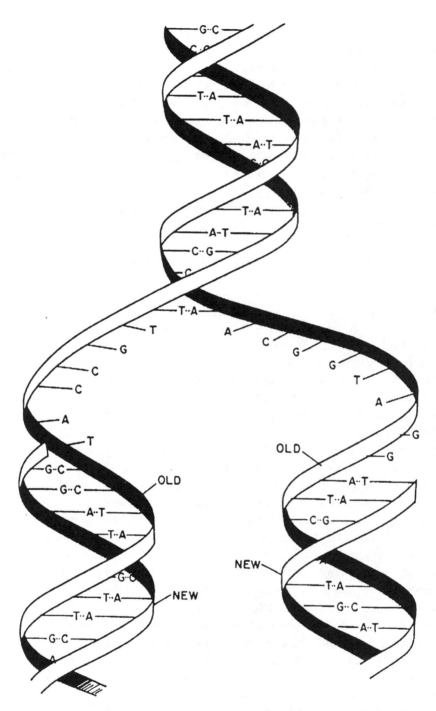

Figure 2–1. DNA, showing base-pair arrangement on intertwining sugar phosphate strands creating the double-helix structure of DNA. As the double helix unwinds and separates into single strings, each strand serves as a template for reproducing the complementary strand. With permission from *Clinical genetics and genetic counseling*, 2nd ed., by T. E. Kelly, 1986, Chicago, IL: Year Book Medical.

Genes are the main working parts of DNA; they instruct the body to perform specific functions. A mutation in even a single base pair may result in inaccurate synthesis of an essential protein and lead to genetic disease. Approximately 60% of hearing loss is estimated to be due to mutations in genes. This can be further broken down into syndromic hearing loss, estimated at about 30% of genetic hearing loss, and nonsyndromic hearing loss comprises the remaining 70% of hereditary hearing loss (Avraham, 2011).

Humans have about 20,000 genes. Genes are ordered in a linear fashion on uniquely identifiable structures known as chromosomes, contained in the nucleus of all cells. Genes, by themselves, do not directly make us who we are. Instead, the genes produce proteins that are dispatched throughout the body to execute the genetic will; if the genes are the blueprints, the proteins are the working parts (*Time,* May 20, 2013). Because genes occur at a specific locus on a chromosome, in many cases it is possible to identify the precise gene responsible for a specific genetic disorder (Keats, 1996). For example, researchers have determined that individuals with neurofibromatosis type II (bilateral acoustic neuromas) demonstrate an abnormal gene on chromosome 22; individuals with Waardenburg's syndrome demonstrate an abnormal sequence of DNA on chromosome 2; and individuals with Huntington's disease have an abnormal prolongation or repetition of a particular DNA sequence on the tip of chromosome 4.

Chromosomes

Chromosomes are long segments of DNA containing hundreds of genes. They are observed by light microscopy in nucleated cells undergoing active cell division. Chromosomes are categorized by their distinctive sizes and shapes. Prior to cell division, the chromatids separate, and one chromatid contributes a complete copy of DNA to each daughter cell. Chromosomes manifest this appearance during only one phase of active cell division. During other phases of the cell cycle (growth and protein synthesis), chromosomes are uncondensed, single, elongated strands. Figure 2–2 is a diagrammatic representation of a chromosome during one phase of cell division. At this stage, the DNA has condensed and doubled; the chromosome appears as two longitudinal rods, called chromatids, joined at a single point called the centromere. The chromatids each contain one complete copy of the

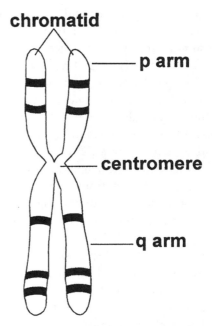

Figure 2–2. A chromosome during cell division. DNA has condensed and doubled. The two longitudinal halves of the chromosome are called chromatids, each of which contains a complete copy of DNA. The chromatids are joined at the centromere that divides the chromatids into unequal arms, the short (p) arm and the longer (q) arm.

DNA. The centromere divides each chromatid into unequal length, or arms; the short arms above the centromere are called the *p* arms (from the French, petite) and the long arms below the centromere are called the *q* arms. Deletion or duplication in the *p* or *q* arm of a given chromosome results in a specific pattern of birth defect.

Each species has a characteristic number of distinctly identifiable chromosomes known as the karyotype. The human karyotype consists of 46 chromosomes (23 distinct chromosome pairs). Of these, 44 chromosomes occur in 22 homologous pairs (autosomes) with one member of each pair containing the same genetic information. Autosomes are identical in both genders of the species; these chromosomes contain genes that code for and regulate somatic cell development. The 23rd pair of chromosomes differs in the two genders (sex chromosomes). The sex chromosomes determine gender and regulate some aspects of sexual development and function. Normal human females have two X chromosomes (XX); normal human males have one X and one Y chromosome (XY). One chromosome of each autosome pair and one sex chromosome are derived from each parent.

In contrast to somatic cell nuclei with their complement of 46 chromosomes (diploid number or 2N), mature sex cells, or gametes (ova and sperm) contain 23 chromosomes (haploid number or IN). Upon fertilization of the ovum by a sperm, a single cell, the zygote, containing the diploid number of chromosomes (46) is formed. This single cell, with equal genetic contributions from the mother and the father, contains the code necessary to develop into a unique human individual.

The principal functions of DNA, genes, and chromosomes are: (a) to provide the template for protein synthesis, and (b) to direct accurate replication and transmission of the genetic code to the next genera-tion. Protein synthesis is necessary for biologic function, and accurate replication and transmission are necessary for preservation of the species.

Protein Synthesis

The genetic code, DNA, directs synthesis of proteins. Proteins regulate cell growth and differentiation, inheritance of characteristics, and response to the environment. Errors in protein synthesis related to errors in DNA result in significant morbidity and mortality. Proteins are composed of amino acids, organic compounds extracted from ingested proteins, or produced by the body in small quantities. The DNA code specifies the sequence of amino acids that make up a specific protein. Twenty amino acids are commonly found in proteins of the human body. A distinct set of three DNA base pairs, called a triplet or codon, codes for a specific amino acid. A gene may contain hundreds of triplets that specify the amino acid sequence of a single protein. For example, insulin, a protein necessary for sugar metabolism, consists of 51 amino acids coded by a sequence of approximately 1,430 base pairs of DNA.

Protein synthesis is accomplished by a complex process in which a second form of nucleic acid, ribonucleic acid, or RNA, decodes and translates the DNA sequence into the constituent amino acids. This multistage process involves generation of an RNA molecule from the DNA template in the cell nucleus, transmission of this information from the cell nucleus to specific cellular bodies (ribosomes), translation of the code into the intended protein, and some intrinsic signaling mechanism to both initiate and terminate the process.

Most genes consist of protein-coding segments, exons, interrupted by a nonprotein coding segment, known as an intron.

An intron is any nucleotide sequence within a gene that is removed by RNA splicing to generate the final mature RNA product of a gene. The term *intron* refers to both the DNA sequence within a gene and the corresponding sequence in RNA transcripts. Sequences that are joined together in the final mature RNA after RNA splicing are *exons*. Introns are found in the genes of most organisms and many viruses and can be located in a wide range of genes, including those that generate proteins, ribosomal RNA, and transfer RNA. When proteins are generated from intron-containing genes, RNA splicing takes place as part of the RNA processing pathway that follows transcription and precedes translation. Introns are sometimes called *intervening sequences*, the term *intervening sequence* can refer to any of several families of internal nucleic acid sequences that are not present in the final gene product.

During protein synthesis, RNA initially decodes the entire gene sequence, including introns. These segments are eventually spliced out of the genetic code before the final production of a protein. If splicing is inaccurate because of base-pair derangement, then no protein or an abnormal protein may be produced. All nucleated cells have an identical genome, but only about 1% of the total genome is active in any given cell at any given time. Areas of DNA adjacent to specific protein-coding segments appear to influence decoding and synthesis of proteins. If these adjacent segments mutate, gene regulation of protein synthesis may fail.

Cell Division: Replication and Transmission of Genetic Information

Cell division is the process through which species grow and reproduce. It can result in exact replication of genetic material of the parent cell, mitosis, or reshuffling of and reduction in genetic material, meiosis. Mitosis results in preservation of the diploid number of chromosomes in somatic cells (in humans, 46). Meiosis results in reduction of chromosomes to the haploid number in gametes (in humans, 23).

Mitosis

Mitosis occurs in somatic cells and results in two genetically identical diploid daughter cells from a single diploid parent cell. Mitosis allows a single-celled fertilized egg (zygote) to develop into a complete human being, blood and skin cells to replace dead or dying cells, and the organism to expand in size and grow.

The cycle of cell function and duplication through mitosis occurs in continuous stages. When cells are engaged in their normal, specific functions, and when they are not dividing, they are in interphase. During interphase, chromosomes are active but invisible; they are an unformed granularity in the cell nucleus. As shown in Figure 2–3, during this stage DNA replication results in duplication of chromosomes before cell division actually begins. Mitosis is the process of cell division that segregates this double DNA into two identical daughter cells.

As the parent cell enters into active cell division, the previously invisible chromosomes become visible by light microscopy. The DNA has already doubled, the membrane surrounding the cell nucleus begins to disappear, and two distinct small bodies, the centrioles, appear and migrate to opposite poles of the cell. Eventually, the cell's nuclear membrane completely disappears and the duplicated chromosomes line up side-by-side on the cell's central spindle or equator.

Next, the chromosomes separate longitudinally at the centromere, and one chromatid

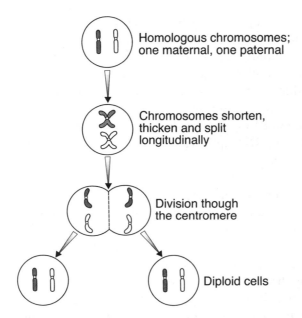

Homologous chromosomes; one maternal, one paternal

Chromosomes shorten, thicken and split longitudinally

Division though the centromere

Diploid cells

Figure 2–3. Mitosis. Mitosis is the process through which a single somatic cell replicates to produce two daughter cells. Each identical daughter cell contains two complete sets of chromosomes.

of each chromosome pair migrates to the centrioles at opposite poles of the cell. In this manner, each pole receives a set of chromosomes identical to the original, nondividing cell prior to DNA duplication. In the final phase of mitosis, the original parent cell divides into two identical daughter cells. The new daughter cells contain the diploid number of chromosomes that cluster at the poles of the two new cells. The chromosomes lose their distinct form and the process begins anew.

Meiosis

In a process similar to mitosis but with important differences, meiosis occurs in sex cells and results in reduction of a single diploid germ cell into four haploid gametes. As shown in Figure 2–4, the important differences during meiosis are *crossing over*, or recombination of genetic material from the chromatids on a chromosome pair, and reduction in chromosome number from 46 to 23. Crossing over permits genetic material from the two parents to be shuffled into virtually infinite combinations. On the average, 30 to 40 crossing overs (one or two per chromosome) occur during meiotic division. Reduction in chromosome number results in a haploid germ cell that, when joined with the haploid germ cell from the parent of the opposite sex, produces a zygote with the species-specific diploid complement of chromosomes.

Meiosis occurs in two divisional processes: Between the first and second meiotic division, genetic material is not duplicated. Crossing over and recombination of genetic information occur early in the first divisional process. During the process, chromosomal rearrangements that produce

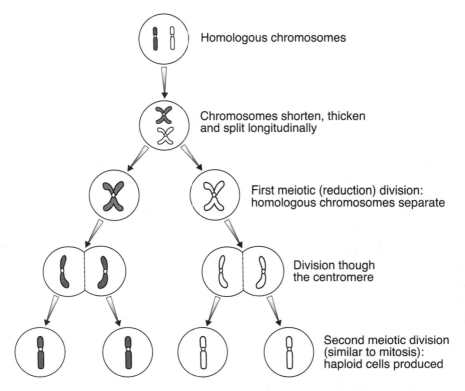

Homologous chromosomes

Chromosomes shorten, thicken and split longitudinally

First meiotic (reduction) division: homologous chromosomes separate

Division though the centromere

Second meiotic division (similar to mitosis): haploid cells produced

Figure 2–4. Meiosis is the process that produces germ cells. The recombination or *crossing over* of genetic material during meiosis produces genetic differences in germ cells. During the crossover process, chromosomal rearrangements may arise which produce congenital anomalies.

congenital abnormalities may occur. Reduction of genetic information into the haploid germ cell is the terminal meiotic event. During this process, errors in chromosomal separation and migration (chromosomal nondisjunctions) may also produce congenital anomalies.

Gametogenesis

In human males, the process of meiosis begins at puberty. The entire process takes approximately 65 days and results in four sperm cells with the haploid number of chromosomes from each original male germ cell (spermatogonia). In human females, early germ cells in the first meiotic divisional process are present at birth and remain suspended in this stage until sexual maturity. At sexual maturity, a germ cell that has completed the first meiotic division (oocyte) is extruded each month. As it travels through the fallopian tube to the uterus, this cell undergoes the second meiotic division. In females, only one potentially fertile cell, the ovum, results from meiosis. After the first meiotic division, a major portion of cytoplasm goes to one daughter cell; the other daughter cell (polar body) contains 23 chromosomes but insignificant cytoplasm. The polar body is eventually discarded. Similarly, after the second meiotic division, another unequal division of cytoplasm occurs, and an ovum and another polar body develop. This polar body is also discarded.

Cytogenetics

Cytogenetics is the specialized area of laboratory medicine involving the study of normal and abnormal chromosomes and their relationship to human development and disease. In medical practice, the study of human chromosomes is important because changes in the human chromosome number and structure can lead to birth defects, anomalies, hearing impairment, and deafness. To evaluate chromosomes, cytogeneticists must obtain body cells capable of growth and rapid division. White blood cells are easily acquired and suitable for chromosome analysis. Generally, a sample of peripheral blood is drawn and centrifuged to separate out white blood cells. These cells

are placed in a tissue culture medium, and cell division is stimulated by the addition of a chemical agent. After a 3-day incubation period, cell division is chemically arrested, the cell membrane is disintegrated, and the intact chromosomes are released. These chromosomes are fixed, mounted on slides, and stained. The prepared chromosomes are now ready for analysis. A variety of techniques are used for chromosome staining.

An international recognized system of human chromosome classification was formulated in the early 1970s. The human karyotype layout is known as the "Denver System," so called because it was formulated at a meeting of cytologists in Denver, Colorado. Figures 2–5 and 2–6 show normal human chromosome arranged in this

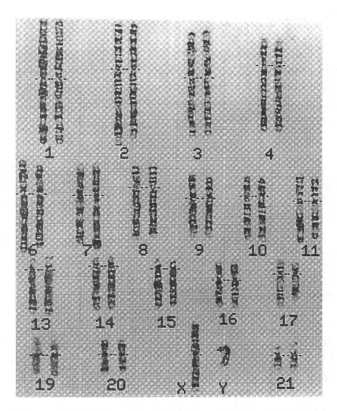

Figure 2–5. The normal human male karyotype with normal chromosomes (46, XY). There are 22 pairs of autosomes arranged by size and one pair of sex chromosomes, XY.

classification system. Figure 2–5 shows the normal male karyotype (46, XY); Figure 2–6 shows the normal female karyotype (46, XX). The 22 autosomes are arranged according to length with the longest chromosome numbered one and the shortest numbered 22. The sex chromosomes are displayed following chromosome 22.

Recently, techniques developed for recombinant DNA research are being applied to examine chromosomes. Termed *molecular cytogenetics*, these techniques permit examination of specific regions of individual chromosomes. One technique, fluorescence in situ hybridization (FISH), allows detection of chromosomal aberrations through fluorescing DNA probes (segments of DNA that are labeled by radioisotopes and contain a specific DNA code). DNA probes will bind to complementary DNA if it is present in the sample. Molecular cytogenetics is a rapidly growing subspecialty of cytogenetics.

Molecular Genetics

Molecular genetics refers to study of the structure and function of genes through analysis of DNA. The highly sophisticated techniques used in molecular genetics have been developed primarily in the past three decades. These techniques permit detailed examination of the genetic code in both normal and abnormal genes. Molecular genetics has revolutionized understanding

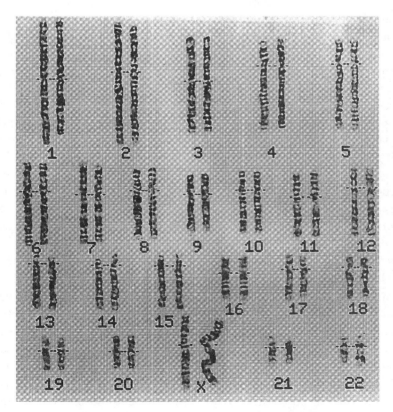

Figure 2–6. The normal human female karyotype with normal chromosomes (46, XX). There are 22 pairs of autosomes arranged by size and one pair of sex chromosomes, XX.

of human genetic disease, its inheritance, its diagnosis, and its treatment.

Because single genes cannot be seen directly, other methods are needed to visualize and analyze DNA. Some techniques of molecular genetic analysis include restriction endonucleases that yield restriction fragments of DNA, Southern blots, DNA probes, and polymerase chain reactions (PCRs). These techniques are applied to DNA isolated from blood or tissue cells.

Polymerase chain reaction (PCR) permits selective amplification of a specific fragment of DNA. A fragment of interest (e.g., a segment thought to contain the DNA code for a specific hereditary disease) is isolated and bound to single-stranded complements of DNA. Under treatment with certain enzymes, these strands will double. Multiple cycles of enzyme treatment will amplify the target DNA sequence exponentially. DNA from relatively poor quality samples, for example, saliva swabs or single embryonic cells, can be amplified quickly for molecular analysis. DNA probes can then be added to the sample to identify and label specific sections of code.

Molecular genetic analysis may be useful for assessing the probability of genetic disease in families at risk, especially if the locus of the genetic defect is known. Through these techniques, scientists have identified the DNA abnormality in more than 125 conditions including adult polycystic kidney disease, neurofibromatosis type I and type II, hemophilia A, Usher syndrome type II, Fragile X syndrome, Treacher Collins syndrome, and Waardenburg's syndrome.

Many conditions may be diagnosed at an early stage in fetal development through ultrasonographic imaging, cytogenetic or DNA analysis of fetal cells, or biochemical analysis of maternal serum. Prenatal diagnostic tests provide definitive information about the genetic information about the fetus, measuring the exact number of chromosomes and genetic makeup of the fetus, including whether or not the fetus has Down syndrome or other genetic abnormalities.

Techniques for prenatal diagnosis range from indirect, noninvasive imaging by sophisticated ultrasonography to direct sampling of fetal skin or blood. Cytogenetic and molecular genetic techniques applied to fetal cells permit diagnosis of some congenital abnormalities that can be accurately detected through a variety of prenatal diagnostic techniques include neural tube defects, chromosomal disorders, structural malformations, and severe hermatological and metabolic disorders. Techniques are available to assess genetic characteristics of material germ cells (ova) before fertilizations and very early embryos (e.g., within 1 week after conception before implantation).

Ultrasonography is a sensitive and relatively risk-free approach to prenatal diagnosis. The fetus is imaged in utero by reflection of very high frequency energy (e.g., 2.0 Megahertz) delivered across the mother's abdominal wall. Experienced ultrasonographers can detect major central nervous system abnormalities (e.g., anencephaly, myelomeningocele, hydrocephalus), skeletal abnormalities (e.g., osteogenesis imperfect and severe neonatal bone dysplasia), and internal abnormalities (e.g., severe congenital heart defects, renal agenesis, and fetal abdominal wall defects).

Cytogenetic or molecular genetic analysis can be applied to fetal blood or tissue cells. As described previously, cytogenetic analysis is useful for diagnosis of chromosomal abnormalities (changes in chromosome number or alterations in chromosome structure); molecular genetic analysis is useful when the location of an abnormal gene on a specific chromosome is generally known.

Fetal cells for analysis can be obtained by several invasive procedures. The most common procedure, amniocentesis, entails removal of a small amount of amniotic fluid, the fluid that surrounds the fetus, in mid-gestation. It is typically performed under local anesthetic as an outpatient procedure. Under visualization by ultrasonographic scanning, a hollow needle is guided into the uterus through the mother's abdominal and uterine wall. A small (e.g., 20 mL) sample of amniotic fluid is withdrawn for analysis. Amniotic fluid contains maternal serum and fetal cells, including skin cells and cells from the epithelial layer that lines the gastrointestinal, respiratory, and urinary tracts. Both the fluid and the fetal cells can be analyzed for fetal defects. For example, amniotic fluid can be investigated for the presence of teratogenic agents such as rubella virus or specific proteins associated with neural tube defects. Viable cells obtained through amniocentesis can be cultured for cytologic, biochemical, or molecular genetic analysis. Amniocentesis is typically performed at about 15 to 16 weeks following the last menstrual period. Because of recent advances in ultrasonographic scanning, amniocentesis may be performed earlier in pregnancy. This procedure is reported to have a 95% accuracy rate. The results typically are available in 2 to 3 weeks. The associated risk of miscarriage is between 1 in 200 and 1 in 400.

Fetal cells may also be obtained by chorionic villus sampling (CVS). The chorionic villus is a fetal component of the placenta. A sample of placental tissue is obtained by passing a plastic tube through the vagina and cervix or by inserting a needle through the abdomen. Results are usually known in 2 to 3 weeks. CVS may be performed either transabdominally or transcervically as early as 9 weeks (although it is typically conducted between 10 and 14 weeks) following the last menstrual period. The risk of miscarriage associated with CVS is approximately 1 in 100 to 1 in 200.

A newer procedure allows mothers-to-be to undergo a simple blood test to determine as early as 10 weeks into the pregnancy whether or not the Down syndrome chromosome abnormality exists. The test called MaterniT21 requires only a blood sample in order to detect the Trisomy 21 chromosome with 99% accuracy. The current cost of MaterniT21 will be about the same as amniocentesis.

INHERITANCE OF GENETIC DISORDERS

Over the past decade one of the most dramatic changes in the evaluation of children with hearing loss has been the ability to offer diagnostic genetic testing. Since the first nonsyndromic deafness gene discovery in 1988, the variety of genes and the proteins they encode is astounding (Avraham, 2011). Since that first deafness gene discovery, genetic counseling has become an important clinical contribution to the overall management of deafness in children. Genetics counselors have developed specific predictive relationships that can help assure parents about the possibilities of their future offspring having normal hearing or being hearing impaired. Along with genetic testing of the parents and their children, a careful family history of the inheritance of the trait in question results in a graph known as a family pedigree. The family pedigree format provides a simple, universal method for recording the relevant family medical history and for illustrating familial inheritance of traits and disease.

Inherited disorders may result from a variety of factors including single-gene and chromosomal abnormalities. Other means of inheritance have also been identified that do not follow classically described single gene or chromosomal mechanisms. These mechanisms, *nontraditional inheritance*, reveal that genetic inheritance is much more complex than previously understood. All of these mechanisms, single-gene, chromosomal abnormalities, and nontraditional inheritance, can be modeled by constructing a family pedigree.

Single-Gene Defects

Single-gene defects are those that follow patterns of inheritance predicted by Mendel's famous garden pea experiments. A single-gene defect may be the result of abnormal gene or genes on one of the 22 pairs of autosomes (autosomal gene defect) or an abnormal gene on one of the sex chromosomes (X-linked defect). Recall that upon fertilization of the ovum by a sperm, each parent contributes one copy (allele) of each autosomal gene to the offspring. If the two alleles on the matched chromosome pair are identical, the individual is homozygous for the trait produced by that gene. If the two alleles are different, the individual is heterozygous for the trait. From his extraordinary study of garden pea generation, Mendel deduced several principles of genetic transmission including inheritance of recessive and dominant characteristics.

Autosomal Dominant Disorders

Autosomal dominant disorders are due to an abnormality of a gene located on one of the 22 autosome pairs (chromosome numbers 1 to 22). A disorder is dominant if one of the alleles produces the defect. In this case, the abnormal gene on one of the autosome pairs "overrides" the normal gene on its matched pair. Dominant disorders, therefore, represent a heterozygous effect. Examples of autosomal dominant disorders

include Treacher Collins syndrome, Apert syndrome, and Crouzon syndrome.

The rule of inheritance of autosomal dominant includes: (a) one affected parent, (b) both males and females are affected and transmit the disorder to their offspring, (c) 50% risk for offspring to inherit the disorder from an affected parent, and (d) nonaffected offspring cannot transmit the disorder (no carrier state). A negative family history does not preclude the presence of an autosomal dominant disorder. Reasons for a negative family history include: (a) new mutation in the affected individual, (b) undiagnosed mild expression of the disorder in the parent, (c) inaccurately identified paternity, or (d) nontraditional inheritance through germ cell abnormality in one parent (gonadal mosaicism). Figure 2–7 shows a family pedigree associated with an idealized example of autosomal dominant inheritance.

An individual may inherit two copies of an abnormal autosomal dominant gene. In this relatively unusual case, the individual is homozygous for a dominant effect. For some autosomal dominant characteristics such as achondroplasia, this "double-dose" of the abnormal gene results in very severe or lethal disease. Homozygosity for dominant characteristics can occur when the prevalence of the defective gene in the general population is relatively high and its effect is relatively mild or when affected individuals preferentially marry (e.g., deaf marrying deaf).

Among the factors that may complicate diagnosis of autosomal dominant disorders is lack of penetrance and variable expression of the disorder. Lack of penetrance refers to the proportion of individuals known to carry the gene who fail to demonstrate the trait. Theoretically, all individuals who are heterozygous for an autosomal dominant trait should demonstrate the trait. In reality, a proportion of individuals known to carry the gene do not demonstrate the trait. These cases are typically detected by a family pedigree in which an unaffected individual is detected who is the offspring of an affected parent and the parent of affected offspring. This "skipped generation" is the result of a variety of mechanisms including subclinical presence of the disease, late onset, or absence of other obligatory genetic or environmental interactions in the skipped generation.

Variability in expression refers to the degree to which the disorder is manifest in the affected individual. Some autosomal dominant disorders are expressed with little variability; most demonstrate a range of expression. Individuals with Waardenburg's syndrome, a genetic syndrome including sensorineural hearing loss, characteristic facial features, hair and skin pigmentary changes, ocular findings, and other symptoms, exhibit striking variability in expression of this disorder. Hearing sensitivity, for example, may range from normal to profound deafness; pigmentary changes may include none to marked areas of depigmentation. Lack of both penetrance and variability in expression presents dilemmas in the genetic evaluation. Lack of penetrance may complicate unambiguous identification of an autosomal dominant disorder; variability in expression may mislead parents into underestimating the severity of the genetic condition.

Autosomal Recessive Disorders

Autosomal recessive disorders are due to abnormalities of both alleles of a given gene. Affected individuals are thus homozygous for the effect. For an individual to exhibit an autosomal recessive disorder, the person must inherit identical abnormal genes from each parent. Typically, the parent is heterozygous for the disorder, and because two abnormal genes must be present for the disorder to be expressed, the parent is an unaffected carrier. Examples of autosomal

recessive disorder include phenylketonuria (PKU), cystic fibrosis, and Tay-Sachs disease.

The rule of inheritance of autosomal recessive transmission includes: (a) unaffected parents, both of whom are heterozygous for the trait; (b) both males and females are affected; (c) 25% of offspring of two carrier parents are affected (homozygous); and (d) two-thirds of unaffected offspring of heterozygous parents (carriers) are also heterozygous (carriers). Figure 2–8 shows a family pedigree associated with idealized autosomal recessive inheritance.

In autosomal recessive disorders, variability in expression is less pronounced than in autosomal dominant disorders. An important factor influencing successful diagnosis of an autosomal recessive condition is often lack of a positive family history. In some rare autosomal recessive disorders, consanguinity (marriage/mating of close relatives) may be a factor. The risk of inheritance of abnormal traits in consanguineous marriages is related to the proportion of shared genes. Table 2–1 summarizes the degree of family relationship and proportion of shared genes; as you can see, the higher the proportion of shared genes, the greater is the risk of inheritance of abnormal traits.

X-Linked Disorders

X-linked disorders are caused by an abnormal gene or genes on the X sex chromosome. Most X-linked disorders are recessive. In these cases, females are unaffected because they have two X chromosomes with at least one normal gene. If a female is heterozygous for the defect, 50% of her male offspring will be affected (each male offspring will inherit one X chromosome; those who inherit the X chromosome with the abnormal gene will exhibit the disorder). Female offspring of the same heterozygous mother will have a 50% chance of being

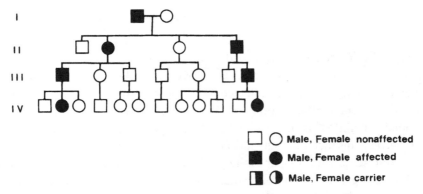

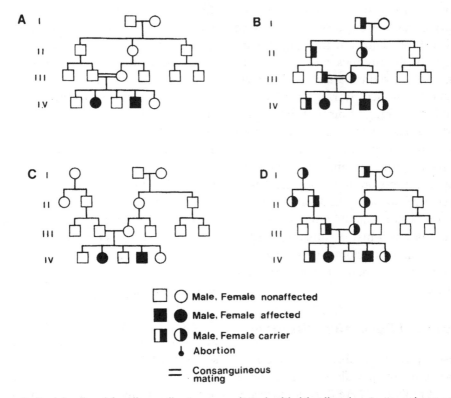

Figure 2–7. Idealized family pedigree associated with an idealized example of autosomal dominant inheritance. Notice the vertical transmission and that affected individuals appear in every generation. On average, the trait is transmitted to 50% of offspring. Unaffected individuals do not transmit the trait. Used with permission from *Developmental pathology of the embryo and fetus,* by J. E. Dimmick and D. K. Kalousek, Eds., 1992, p. 114, Philadelphia, PA: Lippincott.

Figure 2–8. Idealized family pedigree associated with idealized autosomal recessive inheritance. Notice the horizontal distribution of affected individuals. Carriers are present among parents, siblings, offspring, and other relatives. On average, 25% of the offspring of two carriers will be affected, and 50% will be carriers. **A** and **C** do not show carrier status, whereas **B** and **D** indicate carriers. **A–B.** A family with consanguinity and the inheritance of the abnormal gene from the common ancestor, the grandfather. Used with permission from *Developmental pathology of the embryo and fetus,* by J. E. Dimmick and D. K. Kalousek, Eds., 1992, p. 114, Philadelphia, PA: Lippincott.

Table 2–1. Degree of Family Relationships and Proportion of Shared Genes

Degree	Proportion of shared genes
First	One-half
Siblings	
Dizygotic twins	
Parents	
Children	
Second	One-fourth
Half-siblings	
Uncles, aunts	
Nephews, nieces	
Third	One-eighth
First cousins	
Half-uncles, aunts	
Half-nephews, nieces	

a carrier for the trait. An example of an X-linked inheritance includes hemophilia. The rule of inheritance for X-linked disorders includes: (a) inheritance through the material line, (b) no male-to-male (father-to-son) inheritance, (c) 50% male offspring of a carrier female affected, (d) 50% of a female offspring of a carrier female are also carriers, and (e) absence or milder form of the disorder in the carrier female.

ABNORMALITIES RELATED TO GENE/ENVIRONMENT INTERACTION

Many common congenital anomalies do not exhibit classic Mendelian inheritance and are not associated with a chromosomal abnormality. Although the exact causes of these anomalies remain largely unknown, it is believed that birth defects such as con-genital heart defects, cleft lip and palate, and neural tube defects are inherited through the interaction of multiple genes with environmental influences (multifactorial inheritance). Similar to single-gene defects, multifactorial disorders often cluster in families. Unlike single-gene defects, which exhibit predictable patterns of familial inheritance, these disorders demonstrate no predictable pattern of family inheritance.

Risk for multifactorial inheritance is often described by the liability model with a threshold effect. By this model, all individuals in a population are at risk (liable) for a specific disorder, but only individuals who exceed an imaginary threshold will exhibit the disorder. For example, consider a case in which there are seven conditions that influence development of a defect: three gene pairs (six alleles) and one environmental condition (e.g., prenatal nutrition). An individual may exhibit normal function with as many as four unfavorable conditions (e.g., three abnormal alleles and inadequate prenatal nutrition). If five unfavorable conditions exist (e.g., four abnormal alleles and inadequate prenatal nutrition), the individual will exhibit the disorder; the imaginary threshold has been exceeded. Recurrence risk for multifactorial disorders cannot be predicted by mathematical rules based on population studies. Factors influencing risk include number of family members affected, degree of relatedness to those affected (e.g., first-degree versus second-degree relatives), severity of the disorder, and frequency of the disorder in specific populations (e.g., neural tube defects are more prevalent in Irish and English populations).

Chromosomal Abnormalities

Two basic defects result in chromosomal abnormalities: changes in chromosome number termed *chromosomal nondisjunctions* and changes in chromosome structure known as *chromosomal rearrangements*. To understand the result of changes in chromosome number, recall that the human karyotype contains 46 chromosomes, 22 autosomal pairs, and one sex pair. During meiosis, the diploid cell with its 46 chromosomes replicates and reduces into four haploid cells with 23 chromosomes each. Nondisjunction, or failure of chromosomes to separate during this process, results in development of at least one gamete with 24 chromosomes and one gamete with 22 chromosomes. The other two gametes may either be normal haploid cells with 23 chromosomes, or abnormal with 24 and 22 chromosomes, respectively, depending on when nondisjunction occurred. If one of these abnormal gametes fertilizes or is fertilized, the resulting zygote will have trisomy (2N + 1 chromosomes) or monosomy (2N − 1 chromosomes). Trisomy 21 (three copies of the 21st chromosome) causes Down syndrome, a common birth defect occurring with an overall frequency of 1 in 600 live births. Figure 2–9 shows a human karyotype with an extra copy of chromosome 21 (trisomy 21 also known as Down syndrome). Few monosomies are compatible with life; monosomy of the X chromosome results in Turner syndrome. Changes in chromosome number typically result in marked physical abnormalities including dysmorphism (unusual appearance), congenital malformations, and mental retar-

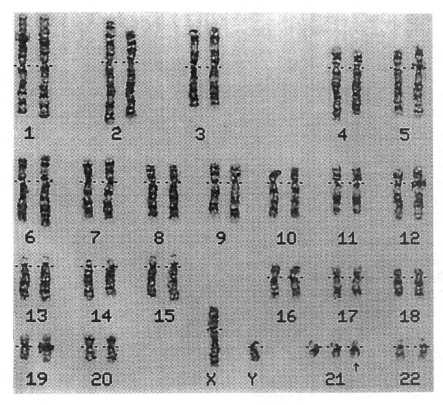

Figure 2–9. Karyotype of a male infant with trisomy 21 (Down syndrome). Note the presence of an extra copy of the 21st chromosome.

dation. Changes in chromosome structure, chromosomal rearrangements, are relatively common. Depending on the location of the abnormality, there may be little or no effect, or a severe disorder. The major types of chromosome rearrangements are deletions, duplications, inversions, and translocations. These chromosomal rearrangements occur during the crossing-over phase of meiosis.

Deletions occur when a portion of the chromosome is missing. Deletions may occur at the ends of long (q–) or short arms (p–), or as an interstitial deletion. Interstitial deletions result when the chromosome breaks in two locations and the distal portion reattaches to the remaining chromosome fragment. Genes located on the deleted portion of the chromosome are missing. Because a portion of the genetic code is lost in chromosome deletions, individuals with this chromosomal abnormality are often severely affected.

Duplications occur when a segment of a chromosome occurs more than the normal number of times within a given chromosome. The process of duplication results in extra copies of specific genes on the chromosome which may or may not result in noticeable characteristics. Some individuals with Cornelia de Lange syndrome have been identified with duplication in a segment of the long arm (*q*) of chromosome 3.

Inversions occur when a portion of a chromosome is rearranged in reverse order. When this occurs, the chromosome breaks in two locations, and the portion of the chromosome intermediary to the break rotates 180 degrees and reattaches.

Translocations occur when one segment of a chromosome transfers to another chromosome following breakage. During translocation, all genetic information may be transferred unaltered (balance translocation) or genetic information may be added or lost (unbalanced translocation). Persons with balanced translocations appear normal but are at risk for transmitting unbalanced translocations to their offspring. Persons with unbalanced translocations may demonstrate specific disorders.

Mitochondrial Inheritance

Nontraditional inheritance is a recent concept that explains genetic inheritance by mechanisms other than Mendelian principles or chromosomal abnormalities. One example of nontraditional inheritance is mitochondrial inheritance. Mitochondria are small spherical bodies found in the cytoplasm of cells. They are the principal energy source for the cell. Mitochondria are believed to have evolved from microorganisms that formed a symbiotic relationship with the progenitors of animal cells many millennia ago. Because these bodies evolved from separate biologic material, they contain their own DNA which replicates independently of nuclear DNA.

Similar to nuclear DNA, mutation of mitochondrial DNA can produce inherited disorders. Typically, these disorders affect muscle and nervous tissue. Several specific disorders associated with mitochondrial DNA mutation have been identified associated with hearing loss (Elverland & Torbergsen, 1991; Hutchin & Cortopassi, 1995). In most cases, onset of dysfunction associated with mitochondrial inheritance is similar to autosomal dominant inheritance with two important differences. First, in mitochondrial inheritance, 100% of offspring are affected rather than the 50% in highly penetrant autosomal dominant inheritance. Second, traits inherited through mitochondrial DNA are never transmitted through a male. Although males and females are affected at equal rates, males do not transmit mitochondria to future generations.

PRENATAL DEVELOPMENT

During the 38 weeks between fertilization of an ovum by a sperm and the birth of a human baby, a remarkable and highly intricate sequence of development results in a unique human individual. Knowledge of the developmental sequence, the critical periods of development, and the conditions that affect development will aid in understanding congenital birth defects, including deafness. Human prenatal development is defined in three stages: (a) pre-embryonic development encompassing the period from fertilization through 3 weeks; (b) embryonic development from 4 through 8 weeks; and (c) fetal development from 9 weeks through term.

The 40 weeks of a normal pregnancy (gestation) encompasses the time span from the first day of the mother's last menstrual period (LMP) until birth. Although few women can be certain of when they conceived, most women can remember the date of their LMP. For this reason, physicians use the LMP to date the pregnancy. Of course, in most cases, the ovum was not fertilized by the sperm until about 2 weeks after the LMP. A *term pregnancy* is 40 weeks or 10 lunar months after the LMP (or approximately 9 months). Premature birth is any birth that occurs before the completion of the 37th week.

Pre-embryonic Stage

The pre-embryonic stage consists of the first 2 to 3 weeks following fertilization. The female gamete, or ovum, is fertilized by the male gamete, or sperm, in the fallopian tube near the ovary. Fertilization of the ovum creates a diploid cell called a *zygote* with 22 autosomes and one sex chromosome from each parent (46 chromosomes in total). At the moment of fertilization, the genetic characteristics of the future individual are determined; this unique human's genetic code is encoded within this single cell.

The zygote increases in size by mitosis, the cell division process that results in genetically identical cells. At about day 3, a solid ball of approximately 12 to 16 cells reaches the uterus. This cell mass evolves into a blastocyst, a structure with three distinct components: (a) an inner cell mass, or embryoblast, that develops into the embryo; (b) a large, central fluid-filled cavity into which the embryoblast projects; and (c) a thin outer layer of cells that encloses the embryoblast and central cavity and contributes to formation of the placenta. Between the sixth and seventh day following fertilization, the blastocyst superficially implants into the wall of the uterus. It is estimated that approximately 45% of fertilized ova fail to develop and implant, or abort shortly after implantation.

During the second week of development, the blastocyst becomes firmly implanted. Maternal blood supply to the embryoblast is established and nourishes the embryoblast prior to development of the placenta. The embryoblast differentiates into a flattened, circular embryonic disk with two layers. By the end of the second week, a slight thickening indicates the future cranial region of the embryo, and the location of the future mouth.

During the third week of development, rapid proliferation and growth result in evolution of the bilaminar embryonic disk into a trilaminar disk. This phenomenon, termed *gastrulation*, is one of the most important events in prenatal development. It marks the beginning of rapid development of the embryo. The three superimposed cellular plates, known as *germ cell layers*, are established during this process. The germ layers, ectoderm, mesoderm, and endoderm, will eventually give rise to all fetal organs and tissues.

The primary germ layers and their derivations, tissue and organ systems, are reviewed in Table 2–2. Ectoderm gives rise to skin, hair, and nails; sensory epithelia of the ear, eye, and nose; teeth enamel; the mammary glands; pituitary gland; and subcutaneous glands. Organ systems derived from ectoderm include the central and peripheral nervous systems. Mesoderm gives rise to cartilage, bone, connective tissues, and striated and smooth muscles. Organ systems that develop from mesoderm include the heart, kidneys, gonads, and spleen. Endoderm gives rise to epithelial lining of the digestive and respiratory tracts including the eustachian tube and tympanic cavity, the thyroid and parathyroid glands, and the thymus. Organ systems associated with endoderm include the liver and pancreas.

During this important third week of development, the notochord (the structure that evolves into the bony axial skeleton, vertebral column, ribs, sternum, and skull) develops. The notochord induces development of the primitive nervous system. The primitive ectoderm layer, overlying the notochord, thickens to form the neural plate. The neural plate ultimately develops into the central nervous system. It invaginates to form the neural groove at about day 18 with edges (neural folds) that approach each other and fuse to form an enclosed

Table 2–2. Derivatives of the Three Primary Germ Layers: Ectoderm, Mesoderm, and Endoderm

Germ layer	Tissues	Organ systems

Ectoderm	Epidermis (skin)
	  Hair
	  Nail
	Sensory epithelia
	Lens
	  Inner ear
	  Olfactory
	Teeth enamel
	Mammary glands
	Pituitary gland
	Subcutaneous glands
		Central nervous system
		  Brain
		  Spinal cord
		  Autonomic ganglia
		  Meninges
		Peripheral nervous system

Mesoderm	Cartilage Bone Connective tissues Striated and smooth muscles	Heart Kidneys Gonads Spleen

Endoderm	Epithelia membranes that line:
	  Digestive and respiratory systems
	  Eustachian tube and middle ear cavity
	Thyroid and parathyroid glands
	Thymus
		Liver
		Pancreas

neural tube (Figure 2–10). As the neural folds join, neuro-ectodermal cells lying lateral to the folds separate into cells that will evolve into spinal ganglia and ganglia of the autonomic nervous system. Fusion of the neural tube begins in the middle of the embryo and progresses to the cranial and caudal end. By the end of the fourth week of development, closure of the neural tube is complete. Disruption in fusion of the neural folds and incomplete closure of the neural tube result in severe congenital abnormalities of the brain and spinal cord.

The primitive cardiovascular system also begins to form during the third week of human development. This important organ system is the first system to become functional in the embryo (from the Greek word meaning "to swell"). The heart begins to develop at the end of the third week; during the same period, primitive blood is forming. The primitive heart has only one atrium and one ventricle. It begins to beat by the 22nd day.

In summary, during the first 3 weeks following fertilization, the single, diploid cell (zygote) resulting from the union of the ovum and the sperm rapidly evolves from a dividing cell mass into an embryo with well-defined cell layers and the primitive beginnings of major organ systems. The first week of development is characterized by rapid mitosis of the zygote into a ball of identical cells. Upon entering the uterus, this cell mass develops into a blastocyst with structures that ultimately evolve into the embryo. By the end of the first week, the blastocyst is superficially implanted into the uterine wall. The second week of development is marked by differentiation of the inner cell mass of the blastocyst into a bilaminar disc. A localized thickening in this bilaminar disc marks the position of the future mouth. Finally, rapid cell proliferation and differentiation during the third week of development generate a trilaminar embryonic disc with three well-defined germ layers. Precursors to the axial skeleton (notochord) and central nervous system (neural plate, groove and tube) arise, and a primitive cardiovascular system is developing. Although the first 3 weeks of development are traditionally viewed as the pre-embryonic period, events in the fourth week signal rapid development of the embryo and early development of the inner ear (Figure 2–11).

Embryonic Development

The embryonic period of development continues from about the beginning of the

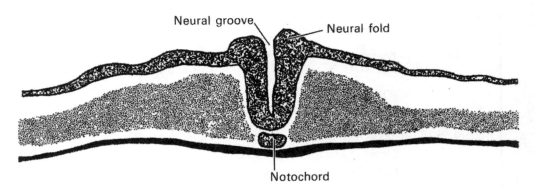

Figure 2–10. Ectodermal evagination and fusion of the neural tube. Modified from *Developmental anatomy,* by L. B. Arey, 1940, Philadelphia, PA: W. B. Saunders.

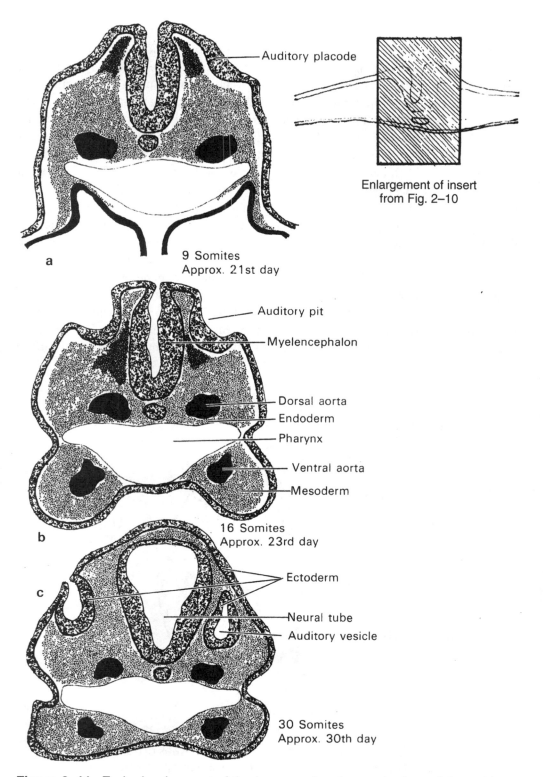

Figure 2–11. Early development of the inner ear in a human embryo. Adapted from *Developmental anatomy,* by L. B. Arey, 1940, Philadelphia, PA: W. B. Saunders.

fourth week through the end of the eighth week following fertilization. During this period, all major organ systems begin and undergo critical development, and the embryo achieves a human-like appearance. This period of development is crucial: exposure to teratogens (drugs, infections, or toxins that cause birth defects) during this period results in either death of the developing embryo or major congenital anomalies affecting multiple organ systems. Early in the embryonic period, the flat trilaminar embryonic disk folds into a more cylindrical appearing embryo. Brisk growth of the embryo, especially of its central nervous system, and differences in relative growth rate of the sides of the embryo versus its long axis are responsible for development

of the characteristic C-shaped appearance of the embryo at the end of the fourth week.

Major events during the fourth week include appearance of structures destined to become principal components of the face and ear. Figure 2–12 shows a representation of an embryo at this time. By the end of this week, four pairs of branchial (from the Greek *branchia* for gill; at this stage the embryo resembles a fish at a similar stage of development) or pharyngeal arches are discernible. The first, or mandibular arch, which is visible early in the fourth week, will evolve into the mandible (lower jaw), the maxilla (upper jaw), and other structures of the face. Otic pits, which will develop into the sensory structure of the inner ear, are visible as thickenings on the lateral surface

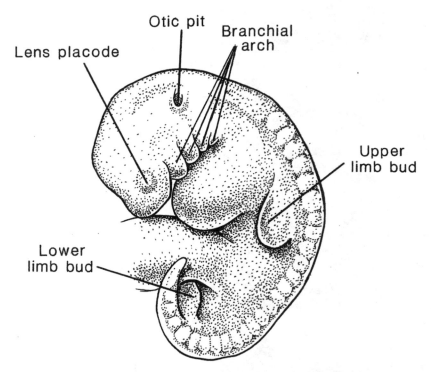

Figure 2–12. An embryo at the end of the fourth week of development. The lens placodes will develop into the eye, the otic pit will become the inner ear, and the branchial arches will contribute to development of the ear and face. Both upper and lower limb buds are apparent.

of the head. Lens placodes that will develop into the lenses of the eyes, are also apparent on the lateral surface of the head. Earlier in the fourth week, upper limb buds appear; by the end of the fourth week, lower limb buds are also visible.

Major external features apparent during the fifth week of development include enlargement of the head and differentiation of structures in the limbs. Head growth is secondary to increase in brain size. On the upper limbs, hand plates develop and elbows become evident. On the lower limbs, foot plates appear. The major features of the face develop primarily during the fifth through eighth weeks.

During the sixth week, structures important to future development of the external ear emerge. Several small swellings (auricular hillocks) develop around the groove between the first and second branchial arches; these auricular hillocks will eventually fuse and form the external ear. The first branchial groove will deepen to become the external auditory meatus. The eye is especially apparent during the sixth week because it has become pigmented. Both the upper and lower limbs continue to differentiate. In the upper limbs, both elbow and wrist regions can be observed, and condensation of mesenchymal tissue in the hand plates (digital rays) marks the beginnings of future fingers. In a 6-week-old embryo, increases in head size are substantial relative to increase in trunk size.

A major external feature of the seventh week is further differentiation of the limbs. On the upper limbs, notches between the digital rays early mark the future fingers and thumb. Lower limb development parallels upper limb development but lags by a day or two.

The eighth week marks the final week of embryonic development. As shown in Figure 2–13, by the end of this week, the embryo has a distinctly human appearance. Differentiation of the limbs produces clearly recognizable structures with distinct joints, fingers, and toes. The head remains disproportionately large; it comprises one half the length of the embryo. Facial features are clearly distinguishable with well-formed eyes, nose, and mouth. The ears remain low-set but show both external auditory canals and auricles.

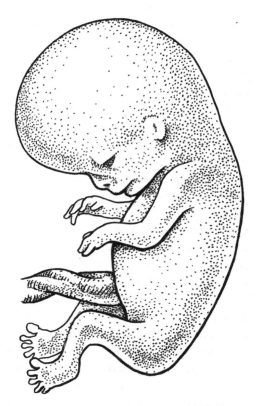

Figure 2–13. An embryo at the end of the eighth week of development. The embryo has a distinctly human-like appearance. Well-formed extremities with distinct joints, fingers, and toes are clearly recognizable, and the face has well-formed eyes, nose, and mouth. The ears are low-set but show both external auditory meati and auricles.

Organogenesis

The embryonic period is critical for differentiation and development of the major organ systems. As described previously, the nervous system initiates development during the third week (pre-embryonic period). The central nervous system (brain and spinal cord) arise from the neural tube; the peripheral nervous system evolves from the neural crest. The neural tube closes by the fourth week of development; failure of the neural tube to close results in severe congenital malformations of the brain, most commonly anencephaly.

The cardiovascular system, which also begins to develop during the pre-embryonic period, continues to evolve during the embryonic period. During the fourth week, for example, differentiation of the primitive heart into two ventricles begins; by about the end of the seventh week, communication between the two ventricles is eliminated with closure of the intraventricular foramen. Incomplete closure into two ventricles results in the most common congenital heart defect, ventricular septal defect. The critical period for development of the heart is encompassed within the embryonic period.

The respiratory system begins to develop during the fourth week with formation of the precursor to the trachea and larynx, the laryngotracheal tube. This structure arises from the primitive pharynx that will develop into the esophagus. Incomplete separation of the laryngotracheal tube from the primitive pharynx results in tracheoesophageal fistula, a congenital abnormality that occurs in about 1 in 2,500 births.

During weeks five through eight, important structures of the respiratory system evolve from rapid development of the laryngotracheal tube. The bronchi emerge and lung development ensues. It is not until well into the fetal period (weeks 9 through 38), however, that the critical interface between the respiratory and circulatory systems develops.

The primitive gut also begins to develop during the fourth week. The foregut consists of the esophagus, stomach, liver, and pancreas; it communicates through the stomodeum (future mouth) with the amniotic cavity. The midgut consists of the small intestines, ascending colon, and substantial portions of the transverse colon. During the embryonic period, portions of the midgut develop in the umbilical cord because the mass of the developing liver and kidneys limits space in the abdominal cavity.

The hindgut consists of portions of the colon, the rectum, and the cloaca (Latin for "drain" or "sewer"); the embryologic common terminus of the urologic, reproductive, and intestinal systems). Initially, the rectum is isolated from the exterior by an anal membrane that breaks down by the beginning of the eighth week of development. Failure of normal development of the hindgut results in a variety of congenital malformations including persistent cloaca, imperforate anus, anal stenosis or atresia, and anorectal agenesis.

The urinary system, consisting of the kidneys, ureters, bladder, and urethra, begins to develop in the early embryonic period. The kidney appears in the fifth week and begins to produce urine at about the 11th week of development.

A baby's gender is determined at the moment of fertilization based on the presence of an X or Y chromosome in the sperm. Without chromosomal analysis, however, male and female embryos cannot be distinguished before about the seventh week when the gonads (testes or ovaries) begin to develop. The exterior genitalia do not become distinctly male or female until the fetal period.

In summary, during the embryonic period, the three germ layers differentiate into the major tissue and organ systems. By the end of the eighth week, all major organ systems have become established, at least in a primitive state. During this period of rapid differentiation, major congenital anomalies may arise from exposure to teratogens, or from genetic or chromosomal abnormalities.

FETAL DEVELOPMENT

The interval from approximately nine weeks to birth represents the period of fetal development. During this period, the human-appearing *fetus* (Latin for offspring) undergoes rapid growth of body structures, and growth and differentiation of tissues and major organ systems. Because major organ systems were established during the embryonic period, the fetus is less susceptible to death or major deformity from teratogens, although these agents may interfere with growth and normal functional development.

At the beginning of the ninth week of development, a major external characteristic of the fetus is its relative head size. At this time, the head constitutes almost one-half of the length of the fetus as measured from crown to rump. However, during the ninth week, acceleration in growth of the body alters the relationship of head size to body length. By the end of the 12th week, overall fetal length has more than doubled primarily due to growth in body length. Lower limb growth continues to lag behind upper limb growth. By the end of the 12th week, the upper limbs have almost achieved their final relative length (length relative to body length), but the lower limbs remain somewhat shorter than their final relative length.

During the 13th through 16th weeks of development, growth is brisk. Similar to the previous three weeks, growth in body length outpaces growth in head size; by the end of the 16th week, the head-to-body ratio is relatively small compared to a 12-week-old fetus. The external ears become repositioned through growth of the head and lie closer to their final birth position.

During the next three weeks of fetal development, weeks 17 through 20, the rate of growth slows. The very thin fetal skin becomes protected by a mixture of fatty secretions and dead skin cells (vernix caseosa). In addition, a fine, downy-like hair (lanugo) covers the body of the fetus. Eyebrows as well as head hair become apparent on a 20-week-old fetus. Fetal movements (quickening) become noticeable to the mother.

During weeks 21 through 25 of development, the fetus gains substantial weight. Blood in peripheral vessels is visible giving the fetal skin a pink-to-red appearance. At about 24 weeks, gas-exchange sites (alveoli) in the fetal lungs are apparent and begin to produce surfactant, a substance necessary to maintain alveolar patency at birth.

During weeks 26 through 29, further development of the lungs and alveoli improves the fetus's chance of extrauterine survival. Head hair and lanugo are well developed, and the fetus has developed substantial subcutaneous fat resulting in smoother skin appearance. The fetus may rotate into a head-down orientation in the uterus due to uterine shape and relative weight of the fetal head.

And during the final 9 to 10 weeks of gestation, the fetus is preparing for extrauterine life by rapid development of the respiratory system, and by adding subcutaneous fat. Prior to approximately 24 weeks of development, the fetus is incapable of survival outside the womb due to immaturity of the respiratory system. After approximately 25 weeks of intrauterine development, the fetus may survive in an extrauterine environment with sophisticated medical care available in the neonatal intensive care unit.

In summary, the fetal period, from approximately 9 weeks after fertilization until birth, is characterized by rapid body growth and completion of organ system differentiation. As shown in Figure 2–14 the relative size of the fetus decreases from almost one-half fetal crown-to-rump length at 8 weeks to one-quarter fetal length at 38 weeks. In addition to growth in body length, the fetus gains substantial weight during this period, much of it in the form of subcutaneous fat. Fetuses less than 30 weeks appear thin with wrinkled skin; fetuses close to term appear relatively plump with smooth skin. Although changes during the fetal period are less dramatic than changes during the embryonic period, they are essential for preparing the infant for independent, extrauterine survival.

Fetal Respiratory System

The purpose of respiration is to introduce oxygen to blood hemoglobin molecules for circulation to all body tissues. At the tissue level, oxygen is exchanged with carbon dioxide and transported back to the lungs for elimination. Oxygen/carbon dioxide gas exchange occurs in mature lungs in the alveoli. In the developing fetus, gas exchange occurs in the placenta; compromise of maternal-fetal circulation results in fetal distress due to decreased oxygenation to the developing tissues and organ systems. At birth, the infant must rapidly convert from a placental-based oxygenation system to a lung-based oxygenation system.

Prior to about 24 to 25 weeks, the fetal respiratory system is not sufficiently mature to support extrauterine life. The fetal lungs exhibit no functional gas exchange mechanisms to oxygenate blood. From approximately 24 through 28 weeks, the oxygen/carbon dioxide gas exchange system of capillary surrounded alveoli begins to develop, and gas exchange sites form. Infants born at 24 weeks of development may survive if the lungs can be expanded, respiration sus-

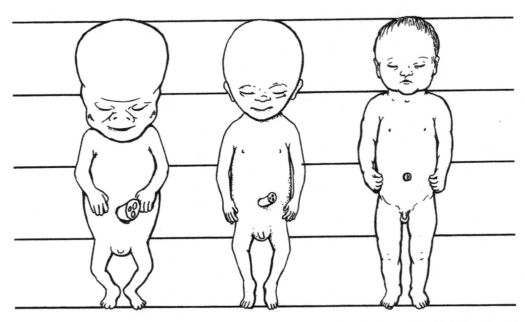

Figure 2–14. Representation of a fetus at about 8, 16, and 38 weeks. Relative head size of the fetus decreases from approximately one-half length to one-quarter length at 38 weeks.

tained, and gas exchange maintained. From 29 through 35 weeks, mature, vascularized gas exchange sites form. Babies born during this period have adequate anatomy to support gas exchange but may develop alveoli collapse and compromised gas exchange. From 36 weeks through term, there is a marked expansion of gas exchange surface area and production of surfactant, a surface tension reducing biocompound that prevents alveoli collapse at expiration.

Fetal Circulatory System

Blood circulation in fetal life is markedly different from blood circulation after birth. Because blood is oxygenated by placental-based mechanisms in the fetus, a fetal circulatory pattern is developed which shunts blood away from the dormant fetal lungs (fetal circulatory pattern). In the newborn infant, blood is oxygenated by gas exchange in the lungs; the fetal pattern of circulation must rapidly change to shunt blood into the now active lungs (extrauterine circulatory pattern).

In the adult, the heart acts as a simple double pump; the first pump is the right chambers of the heart, responsible for delivering poorly oxygenated blood to the lungs. Following gas exchange in the lungs, the well-oxygenated blood is returned to the second pump of the heart, the left atrium and ventricle. From these chambers, the oxygen-rich blood is pumped through the aorta for distribution to all parts of the body. Oxygen is exchanged with carbon dioxide at the tissue level in the body, and the oxygen-depleted blood is returned to the right atrium of the heart to begin the cycle anew.

Fetal circulation is actually a more complex circulatory pattern. It is often described in two parallel circuits that interact in the right atrium. In one circuit, blood from the placenta flows into the fetus through the umbilical vein. About one half of this blood enters the fetus's liver, and the other half flows directly into the inferior vena cava. In the inferior vena cava, the well-oxygenated blood mixes with less well-oxygenated blood returning from the fetus's gastrointestinal tract, lower extremities, and liver. This mixture enters the right atrium where more than half of it flows through the foramen ovale, an opening that closes shortly after birth, into the left atrium. Blood in the left atrium flows into the left ventricle where it is pumped into the ascending aorta to perfuse the heart and brain.

In a second circuit, blood from the fetus's head and upper extremities enters the right atrium via the superior vena cava. This poorly oxygenated blood mixes with blood from the inferior vena cava which did not flow through the foramen ovale. Blood in the right atrium is now a mixture of blood from the superior vena cava (returning head and upper extremity circulation) and blood from the inferior vena cava (umbilical vein and returning gastrointestinal tract, lower extremity, and liver circulation). This mixture flows into the right ventricle where it is pumped into the pulmonary artery. Although a small amount of blood circulates into the fluid-filled fetal lungs, the majority is shunted through the ductus arteriosus (a second fetal circulatory opening that closes shortly after birth) into the descending aorta. The blood in this circulatory pattern is less well-oxygenated than the blood in the ascending aortic circulation; it perfuses the trunk and lower extremities and returns, via the umbilical arteries to the placenta for reoxygenation.

At birth, circulation must rapidly convert from this fetal pattern to the extrauterine pattern. This is accomplished by the complex interactions of clamping the umbilical cord and expanding the lungs with air. The resulting changes to pulmonary vascular resistance and oxygen tension result in closure of the foramen ovale and constriction of the ductus arteriosus. Closure of these fetal circulatory pathways and decreased pulmonary artery pressure results in blood flow to the lungs.

Teratogens and the Developing Fetus

In addition to disorders related to genetic and chromosomal factors, the developing fetus is vulnerable to injury from environmental factors such as infection, drugs, radiation, and mechanical compromise. Any environmental agent, substance, organism, or process (such as a virus, a drug, or radiation) that causes malformation of an embryo or fetus is called a teratogen. In general, teratogens result in malformations and anomalies of specific organ systems when the fetus is undergoing rapid differentiation (for most organ systems during the third through the eighth week of development).

Three factors influence the possible teratogenicity of an agent: (a) critical period of human development, (b) concentration of the exposure or dosage, and (c) maternal-fetal and teratogen interaction. Exposure of the embryo to teratogens during periods of rapid tissue and organ differentiation typically results in major congenital anomaly of the organ system under development. For humans, the critical period of development generally occurs between the third and eighth week for most organ systems and extends through the 16th week for the central nervous system. Exposure to teratogens prior to the third week may result in early death and spontaneous abortion of the pre-embryo but does not cause congenital anomalies because cell differentiation has not occurred. Prior to implantation into the uterus (during the second week post fertilization), the pre-embryonic cell mass is not susceptible to teratogens.

The dosage or concentration of the teratogen is a factor contributing to the development of congenital anomalies. Because of the complex interaction between the dosage or concentration of exposure and maternal and fetal reactions to that exposure, a specific dose threshold cannot be established for most teratogens. For this reason, pregnant women are advised to avoid any exposure to potentially teratogenic agents prior to and during pregnancy (e.g., eliminate consumption of alcohol and smoking prior to and during pregnancy).

Finally, animal studies have shown that there are genetic differences in response to teratogens. In humans, not all embryos that are exposed to a specific teratogen develop major congenital anomalies. It appears, therefore, that the genetic characteristics of the embryo influence whether a teratogen will affect its development. Familiar teratogen agents include infectious diseases such as rubella, cytomegalovirus, toxoplasmosis, and syphilis. Drugs such as alcohol, cocaine, thalidomide, nicotine, and other agents in cigarette smoke, as well as environmental chemicals such as mercury and lead, are also potential teratogens.

DEVELOPMENT OF EARS, FACE, AND PALATE

For professionals interested in human communication, knowledge of prenatal development of the ears, face, and palate is especially important. Major congenital anomalies such as aural atresia or cleft lip and palate typically result in speech and language delays that affect the infant's overall development. The major features of the ears, face, and palate emerge and differentiate primarily during the fourth through eighth week of development (the embryonic period). Formation of the external structures of the head and neck depends largely on development of the branchial structures: development of the face, including the eyes, nose, lip, mouth, and palate, requires contributions from both branchial and other embryonic structures.

The Branchial Structures

Most congenital malformations of the head and neck arise from abnormalities of the branchial structures. The branchial structures include: (a) the branchial arches, numbered one through four in a crania-to-caudal sequence; (b) the pharyngeal pouches, outpocketings of the primitive foregut (pharynx) which arise internally and balloon out between the branchial arches; (c) the branchial grooves that separate the branchial arches externally; and (d) the branchial membranes that develop from the approximation of pharyngeal pouch and branchial groove epithelia.

The branchial arches emerge early in the embryonic period during the fourth week following fertilization. They appear as surface elevations on the head and neck area of the embryo lateral to the developing pharynx. The first and second branchial arches appear at about day 24, and the four most apparent arches are visible by about day 28. The branchial arches are composed of mesenchyme derived from embryonic mesoderm, covered externally with ectoderm and lined internally with endoderm. All three tissue layers are important in transformation of the branchial arches into their ultimate structures.

The branchial arches include arteries, cartilage, muscle, and nerve tissues. These components develop into structures associated with the head, neck, face, and ear. For example, the cartilage of the first branchial arch (Meckel's cartilage) contributes to formation of two middle ear ossicles, the malleus and the incus. Similarly, the cartilage of the second arch (Reichert's cartilage) evolves into the stapes. Table 2–3 summarizes the structures derived from branchial arch components.

Table 2–3. Structures Derived from Components of the Branchial Arches

Arch	Nerve	Muscles	Bone and Cartilage
Mandibular (First)	Trigeminal (Vth cranial)	Tensor tympani Tensor veli palatini Muscles of mastication	Malleus Incus
Hyoid (Second)	Facial (VIIth cranial)	Stapedius stylohyoid Muscles of expression	Stapes Styloid process Upper part of hyoid bone
Third	Glossopharyngeal (IXth cranial)	Stylopharyngeus	Portions of hyoid bone
Fourth	Superior laryngeal branch of the vagus (Xth cranial)	Cricothyroid Levator veli palatini Muscles of the larynx and pharynx	Cartilages: Thyroid Aryteniod Cricoid Corniculate Cuneiform

The first branchial arch (mandibular) is especially important in head and face development. Derivatives from this structure include the mandible (lower jaw), maxilla (upper jaw), zygomatic bone (cheekbone), and squamous portion of the temporal bone. The second branchial arch (hyoid) contributes to development of the hyoid bone (suspension for the larynx). The third branchial arch also contributes to development of the hyoid bone. The fourth branchial arch contributes to formation of the larynx.

The four pharyngeal pouches separate the branchial arches internally: the four branchial grooves separate the branchial arches externally. Of these, only the first branchial groove persists into a permanent structure. The first branchial groove involutes into the external auditory meatus (ear canal). Swellings of the mesenchymal tissue (auricular hillocks) on the first and second branchial arch around the first branchial groove evolve into the external ear. Auricular hillocks are clearly apparent on embryos of 5 to 6 weeks of development. The other three branchial grooves transform during embryonic development into a sinus that becomes obliterated as the neck develops.

The branchial membranes appear where the branchial grooves approximate the pharyngeal pouches. Approximation of the ectoderm of the grooves with the endoderm of the pouches induces formation of mesenchyme. Only the mesenchyme of the first groove/pouch persists into an adult structure: it becomes the middle layer of the tympanic membrane.

The pharyngeal pouches are outpocketings of the primitive foregut or pharynx. The pharynx will evolve into the digestive tract of the fetus; the pharyngeal pouches will contribute to structures important in head, face, and ear development. Four functional pharyngeal pouches balloon out internally into the space between the branchial arches (e.g., the first pharyngeal pouch occupies the space between the first and second branchial arch). The first pharyngeal pouch evolves into the tubotympanic recess including the middle ear cavity, the mastoid antrum, and the eustachian tube. The second, third, and fourth pharyngeal pouches contribute to the development of the lymphoid system, the parathyroid, and thymus gland.

Development of the Ear

Formation and evolution of the branchial arch apparatus during the fourth through eighth weeks are signal events in development of the external and middle ear. As described above, these structures are important for development of the auricle, the external auditory meatus, the tympanic membrane, the middle ear cavity and eustachian tube, and the ossicles. The inner ear develops simultaneously with the external and middle ear but arises from different embryonic tissue. It is often normal in the presence of congenital malformation of the external and/or middle ear.

The External Ear

Development of the external ear is initiated by formation of the branchial arches during the fourth week. Of the four identifiable arches, the first (mandibular) and second (hyoid) arches are critical to development of the external ear. The auricle develops from swellings that arise around the first branchial arch during the fifth week as shown in Figure 2–15. These irregular enlargements, auricular hillocks, grow and fuse into a recognizable external ear by about the eighth week. Scanning electron microscopic examination of human embryos has confirmed the contributions of each hillock

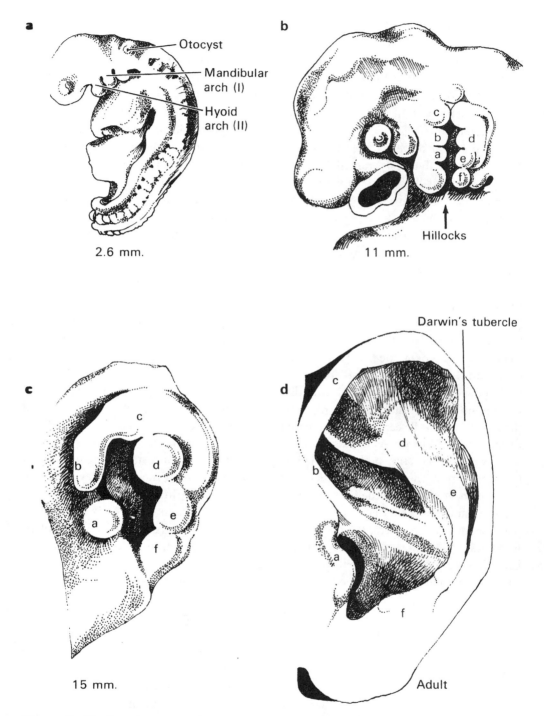

Figure 2–15. Development of the auricle from approximately the third week to adult stage. Modified with persmission from *An atlas of human anatomy,* 2nd ed., by B. J. Anson,1963, Philadelphia, PA: W. B. Saunders.

to the structures of the auricle. In general, the auricular hillocks associated with the first branchial arch contribute to formation of the tragus; auricular hillocks associated with the second branchial arch contribute to the formation of all other structures of the external ear.

The external auditory meatus (EAM) develops from the first branchial groove beginning about the fourth to fifth week. The ectoderm-lined groove deepens toward the endoderm-lined first pharyngeal pouch; approximation of these two tissue layers induces formation of a third tissue layer, the mesoderm. Eventually, the tympanic membrane arises from tissue derived from the ectoderm of the first branchial arch (outer, radial fiber layer), the mesoderm (middle, fibrous layer). Through the 20th week of development, the EAM is occluded by a solid tissue plug, the meatal plug. The EAM opens during the 21st week with disintegration of the meatal plug. By this time, the inner and middle ear structures are well formed. The EAM opens during the 21st week with disintegration of the meatal plug, thereby forming a canal. The innermost layer of meatal plug epithelium becomes the squamous epithelial layer of the tympanic membrane. At birth, the floor of the EAM has no bony portion. In the infant, the EAM is short and straight, with the tympanic membrane lying at the medial end in an oblique or almost horizontal position, making it very difficult to visualize with otoscopy.

The Middle Ear

The middle ear cavity and eustachian tube develop from the endoderm-lined first pharyngeal pouch (the internal separation of the first and second branchial arches). As this pouch expands, it gradually encompasses the developing middle ear ossicles and their attachments. Development of the tympanic cavity begins at about 5 weeks and is virtually complete by the 30th week. The mastoid antrum arises from expansion of the middle ear cavity during late fetal development.

Cartilaginous derivatives of the first and second branchial arch contribute to development of the middle ear ossicles. Meckel's cartilage, associated with the first arch, gives rise to the head and neck of the malleus and the body and short arm of the incus. Riechert's cartilage, associated with the second arch, contributes to the manubrium of the malleus, the long arm of the incus, and the head, neck, and crura of the stapes.

The branchial arches contain primitive blood vessels termed *aortic arch arteries*. The stapes develops around the artery associated with the second branchial arch, the stapedial artery. The distinctive stirrup-like appearance of the stapes results from embryonic molding of the ossicle around this artery. By 8½ weeks, the incus and malleus have attained complete cartilaginous form similar to that in an adult. The malleus, incus, and stapes begin to ossify about the fourth month of development. These are the first bones to attain adult size in the human body; early in the sixth month growth of the ossicles is complete. The auricle, EAM, and middle ear space will continue to grow during the first decade of life until the child is 9 to 10 years of age.

The Inner Ear

The inner ear sensory structures are derived from ectoderm tissue thickenings on the lateral surface of the head (Kelley et al., 2005). These thickenings, the otic placodes, become apparent about the fourth week. Shortly thereafter each otic placodes invaginates to form an otic pit. The edges of the otic pit approximate and eventually fuse to form an otic vesicle (otocyst). The otic vesicle pinches off from the surface ecto-derm to become a closed ectodermal lined cavity and migrates internally.

Figure 2–16 shows development of the membranous labyrinth from the otocyst during weeks 5 through 11. During this period, the otocyst rapidly differentiates through a series of folds, evaginations, and elongations into the vestibular and cochlear portion of the membranous labyrinth. Initially, the otocyst lengthens more rapidly than it widens to form two pouches, a large, triangular pouch that will evolve into the vestibular membranous labyrinth and a slender, flattened pouch that will evolve into the cochlear membranous labyrinth. A tubular extension appears that becomes the endolymphatic duct. By the sixth week,

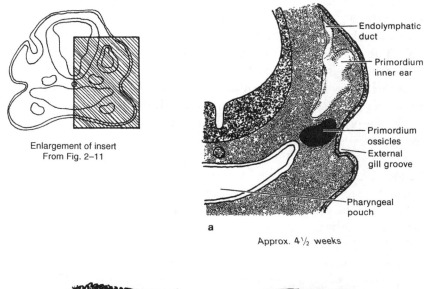

Enlargement of insert
From Fig. 2–11

— Endolymphatic duct

— Primordium inner ear

— Primordium ossicles
— External gill groove

— Pharyngeal pouch

a

Approx. 4½ weeks

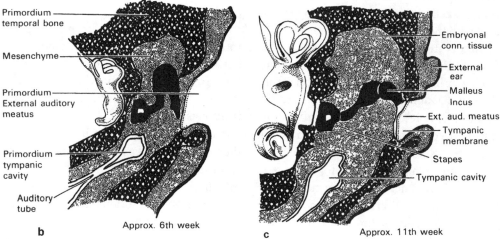

Primordium temporal bone

Mesenchyme

Primordium External auditory meatus

Primordium tympanic cavity

Auditory tube

b
Approx. 6th week

— Embryonal conn. tissue

— External ear
— Malleus Incus
— Ext. aud. meatus
— Tympanic membrane
— Stapes
— Tympanic cavity

c
Approx. 11th week

Figure 2–16. Development of the inner and middle portions of the auditory mechanism. Adapted from *Human embryology,* 3rd ed., by B. M. Patten, 1968, New York, NY: McGraw-Hill.

the cochlear pouch begins to coil. By the eighth week, 1.5 coils are apparent; by 9 weeks, the full 2.5 coils of the cochlea are complete. The membranous cochlea continues to grow through 16 weeks when the length of the cochlear duct approximates the adult length of 33 to 37 millimeters. Mesenchyme surrounding the otic vesicle forms the cartilaginous otic capsule. This capsule eventually ossifies to form the bony labyrinth.

From the seventh through the 20th weeks, the sensory structures of the inner ear are developing from cells within the membranous labyrinth. As the membranous labyrinth attains its ultimate structure, six sensory structures develop and differentiate: the three ampullae of the semicircular canals, the maculae of the saccule and utricle, and the organ of Corti. By about the 11th or 12th week, incompletely differentiated hair cells are apparent. Inner hair cells can be identified throughout the cochlear duct, but outer hair cells are observed only in the basal half of the cochlea. Differentiated hair cells are visible by the 16th week, and by 17 weeks the full number of adult hair cells is apparent in the cochlea of the developing fetus. Supporting cells in the organ of Corti (Dieter's cells, Hensen's cells) develop in parallel with the sensory structures.

Innervation of the cochlea progresses from the seventh through about the 20th week. During the period, ganglion cells from the spiral ganglion start to grow toward the membranous labyrinth. Shortly after coiling of the cochlea is complete (ninth week), nerve fibers enter the developing sensory epithelium. Synaptic endings for both afferent and efferent nerve fibers form when the hair cells begin differentiating in the 11th week. By 20 weeks, mature synaptic patterns are achieved on the inner hair cells; synaptic patterns on the outer hair cells continue to evolve. The fetus acquires rudimentary functional hearing around the 20th week. By about 34 weeks, the cochlea has achieved its final size and structure, and growth and development are complete. A summary of the embryologic development of the ear is shown in Figure 2–17 and Table 2–4.

Development of the Face

The face includes the mouth, chin, jaws, lips, nose, cheeks, eyes, and forehead. The mouth evolves from a slight depression in the surface ectoderm of the embryo early in the fourth week of development. This depression, the stomodeum, is separated from the primitive pharynx by a membrane which ruptures on about day 24 and permits communication between the primitive digestive system and the amniotic cavity. The other structures of the face arise from prominences or swellings surrounding the stomodeum. Five prominences are apparent early in the fourth week; facial development occurs primarily during the fourth through eighth weeks. The five prominences are the single, midline, frontonasal prominence, and the paired maxillary and mandibular prominences.

The single frontonasal prominence surrounds the forebrain and accommodates the optic vesicles. These structures are projections from the forebrain which will evolve into the eyes. The frontal portion of the frontonasal prominence will become the forehead, and the portion intermediary to the frontal portion and the stomodeum will contribute to development of the nose. The maxillary and mandibular prominences arise from the first branchial arches. These structures contribute to development of the upper and lower jaws, the upper and lower cheeks, the upper and lower lips, and the chin.

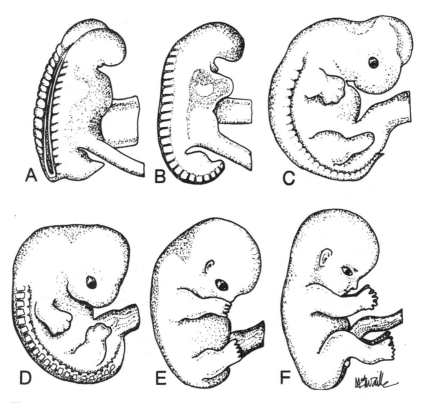

Figure 2–17. Human life and hearing develop together. **A.** The neural tube, the heart and the brain begin to develop at 3 weeks concurrently with the auditory pit and tubotympanic recess. **B.** In the 4-week-old embryo, limbs begin to appear and the otocyst develops. **C.** The embryo is only one-third inch in length at the fifth week when the auditory meatus begins to form. **D.** At 6 weeks, eyes, semicircular canals, and external ear hillocks develop. **E.** Embryonic seventh week includes initial formation of teeth, muscles, genitals, external ear, and cochlea. **F.** Now nearly 1 inch long, at 8 weeks the embryo becomes a fetus and the middle ear and ossicles and tympanic membrane begin to form.

The palate begins development during the fifth week and completes the process during the 12th week. The critical period of palatal development encompasses the sixth through ninth weeks of development. The palate arises from two structures. The primary palate is a wedge-shaped mass of mesenchyme formed midline between the two maxillary prominences (segments of the first branchial arches). The primary palate contributes to formation of a small portion of the hard palate. The secondary palate evolves into both the hard and soft palates. It arises from lateral mesenchymal projections from the internal segments of the maxillary prominences. These projections elongate on each side of the midline and fuse to form the complete palate.

Table 2–4. Embryology Summary of the Ear

Fetal week	Inner ear	Middle ear	External ear
Third	Auditory placode; auditory pit	Tubotympanic recess begins to develop	—
Fourth	Auditory vesicle (otocyst); vestibular-cochlear division	—	Tissue thickenings begin to form
Fifth	—	—	Primary auditory meatus begins
Sixth	Utricle and saccule present; semicircular canals begin	—	Six hillocks evident; cartilage begins to form
Seventh	One cochlear coil present; sensory cells in utricle and saccule	—	Auricles move dorsolaterally
Eighth	Ductus reunions present; sensory cells in semicircular canals	Incus and malleus present in cartilage; lower half of tympanic cavity formed	Outer cartilaginous one-third of external canal formed
Ninth	—	Three tissue layers at tympanic membrane are present	—
11th	2.5 cochlear coils present; nerve VIII attaches to cochlear duct	—	—
12th	Sensory cells in cochlea; membranous labyrinth complete; otic capsule begins to ossify	—	—
15th	—	Cartilaginous stapes formed	—
16th	—	Ossification of malleus and incus begins	—
18th	—	Stapes begins to ossify	—
20th	Maturation of inner ear; inner ear adult size	—	Auricle is adult shape but continues to grow until age 9
21st	—	Meatal plug disintergrates exposing tympanic membrane	—
30th	—	Pneumatization of tympanum	External auditory canal continues to mature until age 7

Table 2–4. *continued*

Fetal week	Inner ear	Middle ear	External ear
32nd	—	Malleus and incus complete ossification	—
34th	—	Mastoid air cells develop	—
35th	—	Antrum is pneumatized	—
37th	—	Epitympanum is pneumatized; stapes continues to develop until adulthood; tympanic membrane changes relative position during first 2 years of life	—

Developmental Anomalies of the Ears, Face, and Palate

Not unexpectedly, developmental anomalies of the first branchial arch result in a complex range of anomalies affecting the external and middle ear, face, and palate. Although developing simultaneously with the external and middle ear, the inner ear is unaffected because it originates from different embryonic tissue (ectoderm).

First arch syndrome (for first branchial arch) describes a constellation of defects including aural atresia, microtia, and developmental anomalies of the middle ear ossicles, mandible, maxilla, eyes, and palate. It is believed to result from disruption in normal cell migration patterns during the fourth week of development. Mandibulofacial dysostosis (Treacher Collins syndrome) includes malar hypoplasia (underdevelopment of the zygomatic bone); abnormalities of the external, middle, and inner ear; and defects of the lower eyelids. Pierre Robin sequence, a constellation of abnormalities secondary to the primary defect of mandibular hypoplasia (small lower jaw) includes cleft palate and defects of the external ear. Both mandibulofacial dysostosis and Robin sequence represent disorders within the spectrum of first arch syndrome.

During the period from 4 to about 10 weeks of development, the embryo/fetus is especially vulnerable to anomalies of inner ear development. Exposure to teratogens, for example, the rubella virus, during this critical period may result in disruption of the normal developmental sequence and congenital deafness. Genetic effects are also capable of disrupting inner ear development during this period; at least one form of congenital deafness of genetic origin, Mondini aplasia, originates from arrest in development of the inner ear during about the seventh to eighth week. This disorder is characterized by 1.5 turns of the bony cochlea rather than the normal 2.5 turns. Mondini aplasia is also associated with several syndromic anomalies as well as exposure to teratogens (e.g., cytomegalovirus). Regardless of the etiology of the Mondini defect, its presence suggests developmental effects during the seventh week to eighth week.

Isolated cleft lip and palate are relatively common birth defects. Approximately 1 in 700 children born have a cleft lip or cleft palate or both. Cleft lip almost always refers to fissure in the upper lip; cleft of the lower lip is exceedingly rare. Cleft lip may be unilateral or bilateral; both unilateral and bilateral forms result when processes within the maxillary prominence (derived from the first branchial arch) fail to fuse with medial nasal prominences. Cleft palate results from failure in fusion of either the primary (intramaxillary mesenchyme) or the secondary (lateral maxillary mesenchyme) palate, or both. A cleft palate may involve only the uvula or both the hard and soft palates.

Cleft lip and palate typically result from multifactorial inheritance. Both genetic and nongenetic effects influence embryologic development of cleft lip and palate. Single gene defects and chromosomal anomalies may also result in cleft lip and palate. For example, infants with an extra copy of chromosome 13 (trisomy 13) commonly exhibit cleft lip and palate. Teratogenic agents are also implicated in cleft lip and palate.

THE NURSERY ENVIRONMENT

The Neonatal or Newborn Intensive Care Unit (NICU)—also called a Special Care Nursery, intensive care nursery (ICN), and special care baby unit (SCBU)—is an intensive care unit specializing in the care of ill or premature newborn infants. The NICU is typically directed by neonatologists and staffed by nurses, nurse practitioners, pharmacists, physician assistants, resident physicians, and respiratory therapists. NICUs concentrate on treating very small, premature, or congenitally ill babies. Some of these babies may be from higher order multiple births, but most are still single babies born too early. Premature maternal labor, and how to prevent it, remain a perplexing problem for doctors even though medical advancements allow doctors to save low birth weight babies.

Besides prematurity and extreme low birth weight, common diseases cared for in a NICU include perinatal asphyxia, major birth defects, sepsis, neonatal jaundice, and infant respiratory distress syndrome due to immaturity of the lungs. An infant may spend a day of observation in a NICU or may spend many months there. Neonatology and NICUs have greatly increased the survival of very low birth weight and extremely premature infants. In the era before NICUs, infants of birth weight less than 1,400 grams (3 pounds at about 30 weeks' gestation) rarely survived. Today, infants of 500 grams at 26 weeks have a fair chance of survival. Overall survival rates, for all gestational ages lumped together, are roughly 70%.

The NICU environment provides challenges as well as benefits. Stressors for the infants can include continual light, a high level of noise, separation from their mothers, reduced physical contact, painful procedures, and interference with the opportunity to breastfeed. The NICU can be stressful for the staff as well. The critical pressures of the NICU environment contribute to increased stress for the tiny patients, their parents, and the medical staff.

Medical care around the time of birth is known as perinatal care and is generally organized into three levels depending on the complexity of services needed by the mother and her infant. Perinatal care programs are usually coordinated jointly by medical and nursing directors for obstetrics and pediatric services. Most community hospitals offer Perinatal level I services; higher levels of services, levels II and III, may be available only in larger institutions affiliated with teaching facilities as described in Table 2–5.

Perinatal level I care represents routine post-delivery care of the mother and infant. Mothers and babies in this setting require no unusual medical or nursing services. In hospitals with level I nurseries, babies with an uneventful prenatal and birth experience receive complete physical assessment and initial observation, care, and management. On discharge, usually within 24 hours of birth, parents assume responsibility for ongoing observation, care, and management of their babies. Services not necessary for routine care of an infant must be coordinated within the very short length of stay in the level I nursery. In most institutions, parents have the option of "rooming-in" or nursery infant care. Infants who room-in receive care in the same hospital room where the mother is receiving postpartum care; infants who receive nursery care are housed in the nursery except for feedings and other care delivered in the mother's room. The nursery is typically an open room with unobstructed line of sight of babies in Plexiglas-sided bassinets. The testing of hearing in this environment may be complicated by excessive noise levels.

Table 2–5. Characteristics of Levels I, II, and III Perinatal Care

Level I
Management and care of uncomplicated patients
Normal pregnancy, labor, delivery
Identify at-risk patients and prepare for transport
Emergency management/stabilization of unexpected complications
Prepare patients for transport
Level II
Provide all services of a level I facility
Management and care of selected high-risk patients (e.g., premature infants >32 weeks)
Identify high-risk patients requiring care beyond level II capability (e.g., premature infants <32 weeks)
Initiate and receive transport
Level III
Provide all services of a level II facility
Management and care of all high-risk patients
Long-term care of high-risk infants
Coordination of transport services
Outcome evaluation of regional services

Perinatal level II care is provided to mothers and infants who are at risk for complications due to premature delivery, small size/low birth weight, unusual conditions of labor or delivery, or other medical events. Infants who receive level II care require monitoring for development of complications associated with their underlying conditions. In these units, babies receive more interventions and treatments than babies in a level I nursery. Infants who develop respiratory or other complications may receive continuing care in the level II nursery, or they may be transferred to a level III nursery depending on the severity of their illness. Length of stay in a level II nursery ranges from 24 hours for infants who are under observation to several weeks for babies receiving uncomplicated treatment for prematurity or other general conditions. Babies who receive level II care are housed in nursery units that permit optimum observation and care of these higher risk infants. Level II nurseries access more technology than level I nurseries and include capability for isolation of infants with potentially infectious conditions. Cardiopulmonary monitoring and other electronic technology are common in level II nurseries and may affect hearing testing. Similar to level I nurseries, excessive noise is frequently encountered in this environment.

Perinatal level III perinatal care is provided to mothers and infants at high risk for morbidity and mortality due to conditions of pregnancy, labor, or delivery. This level of care may be organized on a regional basis; that is, one site in a geographic region is designed to provide level III perinatal care. Connected to regional level I and level II programs by telephone and transport services, the regional level III program provides rapid access to mothers laboring prematurely and to unstable newborns who require complex medical care. Medical and nursing personnel in level III settings are highly specialized in maternal and neonatal diseases and their complications. These professionals are trained to provide emergency medical care to every patient they receive.

Level III nurseries are typically designated as newborn intensive care units (NICUs). In these units, services are highly individualized to the unique needs of the newborn's complex medical condition. Nursing staff-to-infant ratios may exceed one-to-one in the care of unstable infants with complicated medical conditions. Physicians who specialize in newborn intensive care medicine (neonatologists) are present 24 hours a day to admit incoming transports, and respond to medical emergencies of patients under care. Length of stay in level III nurseries may range from 24 hours to many months for babies with severe complications from their underlying condition or its treatment. The physical environment of the level III nursery is intense with electronic equipment surrounding each bassinet in close proximity to facilitate nursing care. Several professionals may surround a single infant, and monitors and other audible alarms are frequently activated. The level III nursery is one of the most challenging environments for accurate hearing testing.

In recent years, a fourth level of perinatal medical care is available in only a few highly specialized medical centers. The level IV NICU is the highest level of neonatal care. Although there is no official definition for a level IV NICU, some states and hospital systems use this designation for NICUs that care for babies with the highest needs. A level IV NICU can provide care for babies at the lowest ages of viability; necessary mechanical ventilation, including high-frequency ventilation. A wide variety of intrauterine surgeries may be conducted in the level IV NICU. The term *quaternary care* is used to refer to care required of patients who receive organ transplants. Newborn infants who receive organ transplants may be placed in a special maternal fetal nursery to receive this highly technical support for weeks or months following transplantation.

Technology in the NICU

The history of the NICU is intimately related to technological achievements in respiratory and other biomedical instrumentation. The development and use of the neonatal positive pressure respirator in the 1970s provided one of the earliest breakthroughs in the management of premature infants and infants with respiratory distress syndrome. It has been followed by a host of complicated technology specific to monitoring and treating premature and critically ill newborns.

The basic premise of the NICU is to rescue newborns from life-threatening medical emergencies in the face of uncertain medical or developmental outcomes. The considerable resources of the NICU are directed at managing medical crises and perilous events in the earliest days and weeks of life. Care in the NICU is complicated by unavoidable uncertainty. Prognosis for very low birth weight babies or infants with severe congenital disorders is often unknown and unpredictably affected by the very treatment necessary to sustain life. Until a situation is deemed final and hopeless, no effort may be spared in sustaining life. In the not-uncommon moment of crisis, professionals and parents may be thrown into immediate actions in the efforts to save an infant's life. The pediatric audiologist may spend time in the NICU screening the hearing of infants and should appreciate the advanced tech-

nologies described below in common use to aid these at-risk babies.

To detect potentially damaging episodes of bradycardia (slow heart rate) and apnea (periodic cessation of breathing), babies in the NICU are continuously monitored for heart rate and respiration. CR monitors are passive devices; they monitor but do not alter the infant's state. Infants are monitored by electrodes attached on either side of the chest (active electrodes) and abdomen or leg (ground). The active electrodes detect the electrophysiologic signal that stimulates cardiac muscle contraction (heartbeat) and chest expansion (respiration). These signals are displayed on the monitor oscilloscope and an electronic counter. Nursing staff sets the limits of the acceptable range for heart rate and respiration for individual babies. Any deviation from this range of 15 seconds or longer results in an alerting audible alarm.

Pulse oximetry, or pulse ox, is a noninvasive test that measures how much oxygen is in the blood, known as the blood-oxygen saturation level. Infants with heart problems may have low blood oxygen levels, and therefore, the pulse ox test can help identify babies that may have critical congenital heart disease (CCHD). The monitor consists of a light-emitting probe attached to a distal extremity (typically a finger or toe) which measures the arterial hemoglobin oxygen saturation. Oxygen saturation is calculated from the light absorption characteristics of the blood flow as it passes through the skin beneath the probe. If oxygen saturation drops below a preset limit, an audible alarm triggers. The pulse ox test takes only a couple of minutes and is performed after the baby is 24 hours old and before he or she leaves the newborn nursery.

Neonatal ventilators are one of the most important technologies in the nursery. Premature infants, and some term infants, may suffer progressive respiratory failure from a number of underlying conditions. The purpose of the ventilator is to maintain lung inflation and to deliver a measured flow of oxygen to the baby. Oxygen from a compression tank or wall delivery system is mixed with room air to achieve the required concentration of oxygen. The respirator pump delivers the air and oxygen mixture at a prescribed rate and pressure through a nebulizer and heater system that adds moisture and warms the mixture. An inflow tube delivers the moist, warm oxygen to the infant through a pressure monitoring device that monitors the inflow to the infant. Oxygen may be delivered through an endotracheal tube, a polyethylene tube fed through the infant's mouth into the trachea, and ending below the level of the vocal folds, or through nasal cannula. For infants with specific medical conditions, a continuous airway pressure may be maintained to prevent collapse of the alveoli and reinflation of the lungs with each breath.

Extracorporeal membrane oxygenation (ECMO) is a variant of cardiopulmonary bypass first developed in the 1950s for open heart surgery. By these procedures, blood is removed from the patient and pumped through an oxygenator prior to return to the patient. These systems permit tissue preservation during surgery in which normal heart and lung function is stopped. During the 1980s, this concept was applied to neonatal medicine in the form of ECMO. The essential difference between surgical cardiopulmonary bypass and ECMO is length of time on the bypass machine. In the case of surgery, patients are on bypass for hours; in the case of ECMO, infants are on bypass for periods extending up to several days. A catheter in the infant's right atrium drains deoxygenated blood into a pressure-sensitive reservoir that is connected to the ECMO pump. A servocontrol mechanism, coupled with a pressure-sensitive reservoir, detects blood outflow from and inflow to the infant, and maintains a constant infant blood volume. Deoxygenated blood is returned through the infant's aortic arch. ECMO is an expensive, labor-intensive procedure associated with considerable morbidity and mortality.

For premature or sick infants, nutrition, fluids, and medication may have to be supplied directly into the bloodstream to avoid stressing the immature digestive tract. This is accomplished by insertion of an intravenous (IV) line into a superficial (small, peripheral) or central (larger, major) vein. An infusion pump attached to the IV line regulates the amount of nutrition, fluids, and medications that are delivered to the baby. The IV fluid, usually a glucose/sterile water solution, is hung on a stand attached to the infusion pump. The fluid is gravity-fed into the pump through a calibrated burette. The pump controls rate of fluid dispersement through the IV line. A variety of juncture or membrane-capped joints are interspersed in the line to permit administration of medications. An IV line may be inserted into a small, superficial vein of the arm, leg, or scalp, or into a larger central vein of the arm, leg, scalp, or neck.

One of the factors important to survival of premature infants is appropriate nutrition. Infants less than approximately 34 to 36 weeks gestation do not exhibit neurologically mature swallow, gag, or cough reflex. These babies may not be able to coordinate sucking, swallowing, and breathing in the correct sequence and are at risk for aspiration of formula or breast milk into the lungs. In addition, babies on ventilators may aspirate if fed by mouth. If an infant cannot be fed orally, the baby will receive nutrition via gavage feeding. Feeding is accomplished by positioning a flexible polyethylene tube through the infant's nose or mouth directly into the stomach. A syringe containing a specified amount of breast milk or formula is connected to the tubing. By elevating the syringe above the baby, breast milk or formula flows through the tube into the baby's stomach by gravity. Rate or flow can be controlled by raising or lowering the syringe. During feeding, the infant may be offered a pacifier to stimulate nonnutritive sucking, calm the infant, and promote earlier nipple feeding. Gavage feeding may be scheduled on an intermittent or continuous basis depending on the infant's tolerance for feeding. Infants who cannot be fed orally or by gavage methods due to esophageal anomalies, or who require long-term tube feeding due to significant neurological compromise, will receive gastrostomy placement, surgical insertion of a feeding tube through the abdominal wall directly into the stomach. These infants may require tube feeding for months or even years.

Mild hyperbilirubinemia is a condition that exists in almost all newborn infants. Bilirubin is a toxic by-product of the normal process of red blood cell breakdown. It is normally detoxified in the liver. In the first week of life, however, the liver is not fully effective in conjugating, or detoxifying, bilirubin. Increasing bilirubin levels in the blood lead to hyperbilirubinemia and jaundice. For most infants, the condition is transient and does not require an intervention. For premature infants, or infants with birth trauma or infection, potentially damaging levels of bilirubin may develop. For cases of hyperbilirubinemia that approach but do not exceed the bilirubin level associated with central nervous system damage, infants may receive phototherapy. Under this treatment, infants are exposed to a specific wavelength of light under special lights.

These bililights alter the molecular structure of bilirubin which improves liver detoxification and natural excretion. An infant may receive bililight treatments for periods ranging from a few days to more than a week. Effective phototherapy prevents the need for exchange transfusion that occurs when hyperbilirubinemia reaches levels associated with central nervous system damage.

Any visitor to the NICU is immediately aware of the high noise levels. Originally, hospital nurseries were small rooms with four to eight infants in incubators or cribs with virtually no life-support equipment. However, modern technology has created a much noisier nursery environment with the use of machines for life support, diagnosis, and monitoring of activity. The modern-day NICU is a multitude of sound sources, respirators, and monitors that generate both background sound and alarm signals.

Noise levels in the NICU may be 20 dB higher than in the well-baby nursery, day and night, causing staff aggravation, fatigue, and stresses. Ambient noise levels in ICU have been reported to range between 56 and 77 dBA. This noise is generally low frequency (most energy lower than 250 Hz), persistent, and continuous (Falk & Woods, 1973; Redding, Hargest, & Minsky, 1977). Although prolonged exposure to the noise levels characteristic of intensive care equipment and infant incubators may be harmful to the developing neonate, direct evidence for such insult has not been reported. A number of concerned investigators measured the ambient sound level generated within infant incubators. The SPLs of incubators were found to be greater than 60 dBA (Blennow, Svenningsen, & Almquist, 1974; Douek, Dodson, Banister, Ashcroft, & Humphries, 1976; Falk & Farmer, 1973; League, Parker, Robertson, Valentine, & Powell, 1972). As early as 1974, the American Academy of

Pediatrics Committee on Environmental Hazards took action and recommended that manufacturers of incubators reduce noise levels below 58 dBA.

Although these sound levels are not in excess of acceptable damage risk criteria, it must be remembered that infants in such incubators are usually in poor health, may be undergoing treatment with potentially ototoxic drugs, and are exposed to the noise continuously for several weeks to months. Long, Lucey, and Philip (1980) recorded infants' heart rates, respiratory rates, transcutaneous oxygen tensions, and intracranial pressures during the routine NICU schedule. They found that sudden loud noises caused agitation and crying in the infants, which led to decreases in transcutaneous oxygen tensions and increases in intracranial pressures, as well as increases in heart and respiratory rates.

Bess, Peek, and Chapman (1979) measured incubator noise with different types of life-support equipment when impulse noise was created by health professionals striking the side of the incubator or by opening and closing the doors of the storage unit. The life-support equipment increased the overall noise levels of the incubators by as much as 20 dBA with a predominance of high-frequency energy. Opening and closing the storage unit doors created peak amplitudes of 114 dBA SPL. The impulse signals created by striking the side of the incubator (a common practice of physicians and nurses to forcefully stimulate breathing in apneic infants) ranged from 130 to 140 dBA SPL.

DISORDERS OF THE INFANT RESPIRATORY SYSTEM

Babies are most often admitted to the NICU due to pulmonary immaturity and respiratory illness. The pulmonary and circulatory systems work in tandem to produce adequate oxygenation; both systems are involved when newborn infants develop respiratory dysfunction.

Respiratory Distress Syndrome (RDS)/Hyaline Membrane Disease (HMD)

The terms *respiratory distress syndrome* (RDS) and *hyaline membrane disease* (HMD) are used interchangeably to describe the most common cause of respiratory disease in premature infants. A complex, coordinated cardiorespiratory response must occur at birth to change from a placenta-based to a lung-based gas exchange (oxygenation) system. Upon first breath, all infants must inflate their lungs and increase blood flow into the lungs. Surfactant, a surface-tension reducing component produced in specific lung tissue, is essential to maintain lung expansion. Because the major period of differentiation of the lung cells that produce surfactant is between 24 and 34 weeks' gestation, premature infants are especially vulnerable to RDS. Surfactant allows some air to remain in the lungs upon exhalation and thus prevents collapse of the alveoli. Subsequent breaths will require less effort than the first. In infants with inadequate surfactant production, all air will be expelled upon exhalation and the alveoli will collapse. Subsequent breaths will require as much effort as the first. During the early hours of life, the infant will become progressively fatigued with the effort of breathing. Over time, the baby will be unable to reinflate completely all alveoli with each breath, leading to progressive atelectasis and low lung volumes.

Oxygen/carbon dioxide gas exchange decreases. The infant works harder to obtain progressively less oxygen. Carbon dioxide in the bloodstream increases, and respiratory academia (shift in blood pH to an abnormally acid range) further impedes respiration. As the disease progresses, collapsed alveoli stick together (atelectasis), pulmonary cell death accelerates, and sloughed cells combine with fluid leaking from the capillaries to form thick hyaline membranes. These membranes further impede gas exchange in the lungs.

When premature birth is likely, a mother may receive corticosteroids to accelerate lung maturation in the fetus. If birth can be delayed for days or even hours, severity of RDS may be lessened. After birth, treatment for RDS includes maintaining lung volume delivering oxygen through mechanical ventilation, and instilling a surfactant replacement. To sustain lung expansion, ventilators that supply continuous positive pressures are typically used (continuous positive airway pressure, CPAP; or positive end-expiratory pressure, PEEP). Artificial surfactant, usually extracted from bovine or sheep lung, is instilled through the endotracheal tube into the lungs. Infants are maintained on ventilatory support until they produce sufficient surfactant to sustain lung expansion and adequate gas exchange.

Injury to the respiratory system in infants is not uncommon. Delicate lung tissue may be injured by mechanical ventilation and by oxygen toxicity. A cycle of injury-healing-reinjure of immature lung tissue results in chronic lung disease. Infants with chronic lung disease often require supplemental oxygen during the early years of life. Other respiratory complications include pneumothorax, or air leakage from the lungs into the surrounding chest cavity. Pneumothorax is a life-threatening complication because pressure within the chest cavity compromises lung excursion and cardiac output. Without emergency surgical relief of pressure,

the infant will not survive. The most serious central nervous system (CNS) complication is intracranial hemorrhage, or periventricular or intraventricular hemorrhage (P/IVH). P/IVH is classified by the severity of the bleed which can range from mild to severe. Infants with severe P/IVH typically exhibit serious neurodevelopmental delay. Because infants with RDS receive treatment by invasive procedures such as intubation and suctioning, they are at increased risk of developing infection. Infants who become septic (generalized infection) are typically treated with antibiotics with potentially ototoxic properties.

Persistent Pulmonary Hypertension of the Newborn (PPHN)

PPHN results from complex cardiopulmonary dysfunction shortly after birth. It is diagnosed in infants who maintain a fetal pattern of blood circulation instead of converting to an extrauterine pattern of circulation. For this reason, PPHN is also termed *persistent fetal circulation* (PFC). The blood circulation in the fetus is markedly different than blood circulation after birth. In infants with PPHN, pulmonary vascular resistance remains high (pulmonary hypertension) after birth, and blood flow to the lungs does not increase. PPHN is diagnosed in infants who exhibit pulmonary hypertension, shunting of blood through the fetal cardiovascular channels (foramen ovale, ductus arteriosus or both) away from the lungs, and a structurally normal heart. The syndrome may be without a known cause (idiopathic), or it may be secondary to other disorders such as respiratory distress syndrome (RDS), congenital diaphragmatic hernia, sepsis, or meconium aspiration syndrome (MAS). Infants with PPHN experience inadequate oxygenation leading to diminished cardiac output and further decreased oxygenation. PPHN is often a disorder of late preterm or term infants.

Maintaining adequate oxygenation is the primary goal in caring for infants with PPHN. Treatment is directed at decreasing pulmonary vascular resistance through use of mechanical ventilation to achieve adequate lung inflation and ventilation, and inhaled nitric oxide (iNO), a potent pulmonary vasodilator. In severe cases, extracorporeal membrane oxygenation (ECMO) may be used as a treatment for PPHN. This treatment involves shunting the blood through an oxygenation circuit outside the body (extracorporeal), similar to cardiopulmonary bypass for open heart surgery. Babies are typically maintained on ECMO for durations of 72 hours to 2 weeks, depending on the underlying problem. Mortality from PPHN is high. Prior to ECMO, mortality rates as high as 80% were reported in infants with PPHN. Mortality rates in infants treated by ECMO range from 13% to 33%. For infants who survive, complications include those associated with mechanical ventilation such as chronic lung disease and pneumothorax.

Meconium Aspiration Syndrome (MAS)

MAS is compromise of respiratory function secondary to obstruction of the respiratory tract and lung tissue by aspirated meconium, a blackish-green substance produced in the intestinal tract of fetuses. Meconium is normally passed shortly after birth and represents the newborn infant's first bowel movement. Fetuses who experience hypoxia in utero may pass meconium prior to birth as decreased oxygen causes the anal sphinc-

ter to relax. With ongoing hypoxia, the fetus may exhibit gasping respiratory movements that draw meconium-stained amniotic fluid into the nose, mouth, and oropharynx. MAS results when deeply inspired meconium obstructs the respiratory tract, induces an inflammatory response, and compromises gas exchange in the lungs following birth. Because the greatest quantities of meconium are produced in fetuses age 34 weeks and older, MAS is a disorder of term or late preterm infants. These infants are no longer routinely suctioned unless they are depressed at birth with poor respiratory efforts. In that case the trachea is suctioned before beginning resuscitation with positive pressure ventilation. If the infants are vigorous at birth, no routine tracheal suctioning is performed. These babies may require supplemental oxygen or more vigorous treatment with mechanical ventilation if the pneumonitis is severe or is complicated by PPHN. Infants who require mechanical ventilation are susceptible to mechanical injury to the lung and oxygen toxicity resulting in chronic lung disease.

Bronchopulmonary Dysplasia (BPD)

In the late 1960s, investigators described chronic radiographic changes in lungs of infants who were premature and required mechanical ventilation after birth. BPD is perhaps largely an iatrogenic disease; that is, it is an adverse condition resulting from medical treatment, although the most premature infants are prone to develop it even if they never had significant respiratory distress syndrome in the days immediately after birth. The pulmonary changes observed in BPD reflect the cycle of injury/healing/reinjury of delicate lung tissue in infants who receive supplemental oxygen or mechanical ventilation. Infants with BPD exhibit decreased lung compliance, increased pulmonary airways resistance, and pulmonary edema. Because BPD affects oxygen and carbon dioxide exchange in the lungs, infants with this disorder often require mechanical ventilation and supplemental oxygen for weeks or even months after birth. To manage the complications associated with BPD, infants may receive diuretics and antibiotics with ototoxic properties.

The literature documents associations between respiratory system disorders in premature and term newborns and sensorineural hearing loss. In 1985, Sell, Gaines, Gluckman, & Williams reported long-term neurodevelopmental outcomes of infants with PPHN. In their investigation, more than 50% of infants demonstrated sensorineural hearing loss. Naulty, Weiss, and Herer (1986) followed 11 children with PPHN for 36 months with behavioral audiometry and auditory brainstem evaluations and identified three babies (27%) with bilateral, progressive hearing loss and language delays. All infants required prolonged ventilation and were treated with ototoxic drugs. Hendricks et al. (1988) reported sensorineural hearing loss in 21 of 40 PFC infants, 14 of whom required hearing aids. In their study, the authors reported a high association of delayed onset and progressive sensorineural hearing loss. Conservative management of infants with PPHN may reduce the prevalence of neurologic abnormalities and sensorineural hearing loss (Marron et al., 1992).

Fujikawa, Yang, Waffarn, and Lerner (1997) reported treatment of 28 infants with PPHN with inhaled nitric oxide; none of these infants had significant sensorineural hearing losses. The probability of sensorineural hearing loss in these PPHN infants is high enough that the Joint Committee on Infant Hearing 2007 Guidelines recommended referral of all infants who have been mechanically ventilated for additional audiologic evaluation.

DISORDERS OF THE CARDIOVASCULAR SYSTEM

Congenital heart disease (CHD) is among the most common birth defects affecting as many as 1 in 100 newborns. Some conditions are benign and require no intervention; other conditions are life threatening and require immediate surgical treatment. The heart develops during the first 7 weeks following fertilization. During this critical period, major CHD can arise from genetic and chromosomal abnormalities, infection, and exposure to teratogens, or maternal metabolic or nutritional factors. Newborns with severe CHD may exhibit cyanosis, respiratory distress syndrome (RDS), and congestive heart failure with decreased cardiac output. Congestive heart failure is a clinical syndrome signaling the inability of the heart to meet the metabolic needs of the body. Signs of congestive heart failure include enlarged heart, increased heart rate, generalized malaise, fluid retention and edema, and failure to thrive. CHDs often encountered in the NICU include ventricular septal defect, patent ductus arteriosus, coarticulation of the aorta, tetralogy of Fallot, and hypoplastic left heart syndrome.

Although there is no reported association between hearing impairment and isolated CHD, hearing loss is often present in infants with CHD and other congenital anomalies. Several syndromes have been identified which include cardiac and auditory dysfunction. A sample of such syndromes would include CHARGE association, Jervell and Lange-Nielsen syndrome, as well as Down syndrome and congenital rubella syndrome. Furthermore, medical management of CHD may include use of ototoxic medications such as loop diuretics and aminoglycoside antibiotics. It is therefore important to consider the effects of both the infant's underlying condition and the treatment for that condition as potential etiologies in sensorineural hearing loss.

DISORDERS OF THE CENTRAL NERVOUS SYSTEM

The central nervous system is vulnerable to genetic and teratogenic disorders, as well as iatrogenic effects secondary to treatment for respiratory, cardiovascular, infections, and metabolic dysfunction. The CNS is one of the first major organ systems to initiate development in the embryo, and functional development continues through the early years of childhood because the brain controls all other organ systems and is responsible for all learning. CNS disorders and their related neurologic effects are among the most feared complications of prematurity and neonatal disease. Common CNS medical problems include anencephaly, spina bifida, intracranial hemorrhage, hydrocephalus, hypoxic encephalopathy, and neonatal seizures. Although neurologic dysfunction *per se* does not result in hearing impairment, it may substantially affect central auditory processing and speech and language development. Infants with neurologic dysfunction during the newborn period should be monitored for hearing status and neurodevelopmental effects.

CONGENITAL INFECTIONS

Maternal infections during pregnancy are the cause of a host of congenital malformations and abnormalities. Congenital infections often cause fetal death and miscarriage. Damage to the fetus attributed to congenital viral infections has included congenital malformations such as clubfoot, intrauterine growth retardation, serious damage to the nervous system (including spina bifida), congenital heart disease, and disease of other organs (such as the liver, pancreas, and adrenals). Prenatal and postnatal bacterial and viral infections have long been recognized as causes of hearing loss and deafness.

Widespread vaccine programs in the modernized nations have done much to decrease common childhood infectious diseases such as measles, mumps, diphtheria, tetanus, hepatitis B, meningitis, pertussis, and polio. Children are born with a natural immunity to certain infections. Antibodies pass through the mother's placenta to the fetus before birth, protecting the baby from infection. Breast-fed babies continue to receive antibodies from their mothers' breast milk. However, this natural immunity eventually wears off, usually within the first year of life. In the past, a number of serious childhood diseases reached epidemic proportions claiming thousands of lives, and often leaving children with lasting mental or physical problems including deafness. Vaccines prevent many of these diseases by introducing modified versions of viruses and bacteria into the body, causing the body to produce antibodies. These antibodies remain in the body to identify and fight the virus or bacteria in the future. Immunization with vaccines provides people with lifetime protection to once common diseases.

The damaging effects of congenital infections on the developing fetus were first described more than 70 years ago. N. McAllister Gregg, an ophthalmologist in Australia, recognized the association between congenital cataracts in infants and maternal rubella. His pioneering observation initiated investigation into the potential teratogenicity of fetal exposure to maternal infection. Although the fetus develops within the normally protected environment of the womb, specific microbes can cross the placental membranes and infect the fetus. Infections acquired transplacentally during the first trimester of pregnancy are especially damaging. Because organs systems are undergoing rapid differentiation and growth, infection during this period results in major congenital anomalies and multisystem disease. Because congenital infections are a major consideration in the identification of hearing loss in infants, every infant with history of congenital infection should receive audiologic assessment during the newborn period and routinely thereafter to identify late-onset or progressive sensorineural hearing loss. Congenital infections have been identified as an important risk factor on every register developed by the Joint Committee on Infant Hearing (JCIH) since 1972.

The Centers for Disease Control and Prevention (CDC) repeatedly call attention to the fact that less than 80% of U.S. children are adequately protected by immunization by the time they reach 2 years of age. Vaccination programs have practically eradicated maternal rubella infections in the United States and Canada, but isolated cases of these diseases do appear occasionally due to parents' unfounded fears regarding adverse effects from vaccinations in general. Stein and Boyer (1994) described medical advances in the treatment and prevention of bacterial meningitis due to *Haemophilus influenzae* type b through universal immunization programs and the introduction of cephalosporin antibiotics and corticosteroid treatment of congenital toxoplasmosis. These public health programs represent important progress in the prevention of childhood deafness. Unfortunately, without widespread vaccination programs in developing countries, children with these diseases continue to show a high incidence of significant hearing loss due to infectious diseases.

Congenital Rubella Syndrome (CRS)

Rubella, also called German measles, is a viral infection that results in a mild flu-like illness. The rubella virus has a worldwide distribution, and prior to the introduction of the rubella vaccine, epidemics generally occurred in spring and early summer months in countries with temperate climates. Although congenital rubella syndrome (CRS) was the single most important cause of nongenetic hearing loss in the United States during the 1960s, the disease has been virtually eliminated through successful vaccination programs. According to the CDC, the number of reported cases of congenital rubella syndrome in the United States declined more than 97.4% from 77 new cases in 1970 to a total of 2 cases reported in 1996. However, in countries without a widespread vaccination program, CRS remains an important cause of deafness even in current times (Atkinson, Hamborsky, McIntyre, & Wolfe, 2007; Neighbors & Tannehill-Jones, 2010; Reef, 2006).

Transmission of rubella virus occurs from close contact with infected individuals. Characteristic features of primary rubella infection in adults are rash, malaise, swollen lymph nodes, and joint pain. As many as 10% of patients may be asymptomatic. For this reason, primary rubella infection in a pregnant woman may be undetected. If a primary maternal infection occurs during the first trimester of pregnancy and the virus crosses the placenta, the fetus may develop generalized infection and multiorgan disease. Spontaneous abortion occurs in as many as 20% of cases when maternal rubella occurs in the first eight weeks of pregnancy. In fetuses exposed during the first trimester who survive, the reported incidence of congenital anomalies ranges up to 54%; the incidence of congenital anomalies in fetuses exposed between 13 and 16 weeks' gestation is approximately 17%. For fetuses exposed after 16 weeks' gestation, risk of congenital anomaly is low. The only abnormalities reported in infants infected after the first trimester are deafness and retinopathy.

Infants who are born infected characteristically exhibit lethargy, petechiae (small subdermal hemorrhages; "blueberry muffin" rash), intrauterine growth retardation (IUGR), and enlarged liver and spleen (hepatosplenomegaly). The classic triad for congenital rubella syndrome is sensorineural deafness (58% of patients); eye abnormalities—especially retinopathy, cataract, and microphthalmia (43% of patients), and congenital heart disease—especially patent ductus arteriosus (50% of patients). Cultures for rubella virus may remain positive in infants up to age 1 year, and rubella virus has been recovered from intracellular tissue of children with congenital infections up to age 3 years. Congenital rubella infection is a chronic disease and may result in progressive disability.

Prevention of maternal infection is the most effective treatment for CRS. In the United States, CRS has been virtually eliminated as a major cause of birth defects because of successful vaccination programs initiated in the late 1960s and early 1970s. The characteristic features of CRS are cardiac defects, congenital cataracts, and deafness; other features include mental retardation, glaucoma, and microphthalmia. During the last large-scale rubella epidemic in the United States in 1964, an estimated 10,000 to 20,000 infants were born with hearing loss secondary to congenital rubella infections.

Cytomegalovirus (CMV)

CMV is a member of the herpes family of viruses which includes herpes simplex, Epstein-Barr, and varicella (chickenpox) virus. CMV is endemic throughout the world. CMV causes cytomegalic inclusion disease that is a generalized "herpeslike" viral infection of infants caused by intrauterine or postnatal passage from the mother. Fortunately, CMV is not highly contagious and is harmless to most people who experience a CMV infection with no symptomatology. Although antibodies are established, the virus remains in body cells in an inactive state, making future infection possible for the remainder of the person's life. This inactive virus can be reactivated under certain circumstances, including pregnancy. When the virus is reactivated, it is excreted in body fluids such as urine, saliva, feces, blood, semen, and cervical secretions. Unlike rubella, infection by CMV in any stage of gestation may result in damage to the fetus. The infection may be contracted during the perinatal period with passage down the birth canal where the viral infection shows little pathogenicity and no symptoms in the mother. Like other herpes viruses, exposure to CMV results in a primary infection that then becomes dormant for extended periods of time. Reinfections result in recurrence of CMV. It is the most common viral infection in the human fetus. The incidence of congenital CMV infection is reported to range from 0.3% to 3% of live births. If 1% of all babies born in the United States are infected, then as many as 40,000 infants with congenital CMV infection are born in this country each year (Raynor, 1993).

Cytomegalovirus (CMV) is a leading cause of nongenetic hearing impairment in infants and young children. There may be as many as 6,000 children born in the United States each year who experience sensorineural hearing impairment as a consequence of congenital CMV infection (McCollister, Simpson, Dahle, & Pass, 1996). Sensorineural hearing loss is the most common sequela following congenital CMV infection (Dahle et al., 2000; Fowler & Boppana, 2006; Ross, Gaffney, Green, & Holstrum, 2008). CMV is estimated to be the leading environmental cause of childhood hearing loss, accounting for approximately 15% to 21% of all hearing loss at birth in the United States (Grosse, 2007; Morton & Nance, 2006). In addition, CMV-related hearing losses have been well documented as progressive or late onset, conditions that require more frequent audiologic monitoring of infants and young children who have been diagnosed with congenital CMV infection. Radiographic studies of children with hearing loss and symptomatic CMV have also revealed temporal bone abnormalities including Mondini dysplasia.

CMV is not highly contagious. Transmission occurs through direct contact with infected secretions (urine, blood, semen, vaginal secretions, breast milk, and other bodily fluids). Because CMV is ubiquitous; most people acquire CMV infection at some time in their lives. Although adults with both primary and recurrent CMV infections are usually asymptomatic, some individuals may experience a flu-like illness. Primary CMV infection in a pregnant woman results in congenital CMV infection in the infant in about 30% to 40% of cases. Much less frequently, recurrent infection in the mother results in congenital infection in the fetus. Unlike rubella, infection by CMV in any stage of gestation may result in damage to the fetus. As many as 90% to 95% of infants with congenital CMV infection are asymptomatic at birth. Although most of these infants develop normally with no developmental deficits attributable to their infection, about 5% to 10% of these normal newborns will be identified with sensorineural hearing impairment that is often progressive. Approximately 10% of infants infected from primary maternal disease are symptomatic at birth. These babies demonstrate characteristics similar to those seen in CRS including microcephaly, congenital cataracts, hepatosplenomegaly, and petechiae.

Unfortunately, there is no treatment for congenital CMV. Although congenital infection can be detected at birth through urine, saliva, or blood cultures, screening for congenital CMV infection in U.S. hospitals is not routinely performed. Primary maternal disease is most devastating, and congenital CMV infection occurs in 30% to 40% of infants born to mothers with primary disease. Approximately 15% of these infants will be asymptomatic at birth; of these, as many as 30% will die. Ninety percent of survivors will exhibit neurodevelopmental deficits including deafness, microcephaly, mental retardation, cerebral palsy, and chorioretinitis. The remaining 85% to 90% of infants with congenital CMV acquired during primary maternal disease will be asymptomatic at birth, but as many as 15% of these infants will develop neuro-developmental deficits.

Infants born to mothers with recurrent CMV disease are much less likely to be infected. Only about 1% of recurrent maternal disease results in congenital CMV infection, and 10% or less may result in progressive hearing loss in infants and young children. Research suggests that the hearing impairment may first appear after the newborn period. Identification of hearing loss in asymptomatic infected infants may be delayed because these babies will not be recognized as at risk for progressive hearing loss.

CMV-related hearing losses do not have a unique audiometric configuration, and the loss may be present at birth or occur in the first years of life. Hearing loss from congenital CMV infection can be either unilateral or bilateral and varies from mild to profound. In addition, CMV-related hearing loss may be fluctuating and/or progressive (Littman, Demmoer, Williams, Istas, & Griesser, 1995; Peckham, Stark, Dudgeon, Martin, & Hawkins, 1987; Williamson, Demmler, Percy, & Catlin, 1992). In fact, approximately half of the cases of hearing loss due to congenital CMV infection are late-onset and progressive and, therefore, will not be detected at birth through newborn hearing screening (Fowler et al., 1997).

Harris, Ahlfors, Ivarsson, Lemmark, and Svanberg (1984) reported data from a large-scale prospective study conducted in Sweden. Some 10,328 infants were followed for a 5-year period in which it was shown that 50 (0.5%) had a congenital CMV infection. Of this group, five children had sensorineural hearing loss (four with total deafness and one with mild hearing loss). Hicks et al. (1993) reported the rate of sensorineural hearing loss resulting from congenital CMV infection to be 1.1 per 1,000 live births. Fowler et al. (1997) found that 70% of children with asymptomatic congenital CMV infection also had sensorineural hearing loss characterized by delayed onset and threshold fluctuation. Fowler et al. (1992) found that the risk of acquiring hearing loss from CMV increases substantially if the infection is acquired during pregnancy. Furthermore, the presence of antibodies to CMV in the mother before conception may improve the infant's protection against hearing loss.

Toxoplasmosis

This is a parasitic infection transmitted by pregnant women to their unborn children. Most adults infected with the parasite have no symptoms. However, the infected child with congenital toxoplasmosis typically has chorioretinitis (inflammation of the choroid and retina of the eye), cerebral calcification, severe psychomotor developmental delay, hydrocephalus or microcephaly, and convulsions. Although reports of hearing disorders related to toxoplasmosis are in fact sparse, the congenital infection is so serious that there is no doubt that it may cause hearing loss. Active congenital infection may be fatal in days or weeks or become inactive with residuals of medical problems in varying degrees and combinations. The full impact of the infection may not become evident until some weeks or months after its apparent cessation. Apparently, the later in pregnancy the infection occurs, the less severe the clinical symptoms. Some afflicted newborns appear normal but develop blindness, epilepsy, or mental retardation in later years.

Toxoplasmosis gondii is a single-celled protozoan parasite that is widespread in domestic and wild animals (e.g., dogs, cats, rabbits). *Toxoplasma gondii* infections are found worldwide but are less common in cold climates, hot and arid regions, and at high altitudes. Human infection by *Toxoplasma gondii* occurs following ingestion of toxoplasma cysts in undercooked meat or contaminated raw vegetables or through close contact with domestic animals, typically cats, harboring the infection (Babson, 1980; Robillard & Gersdorff, 1986).

Toxoplasma infection crosses the placenta and infects the fetus in about 40% to 50% of untreated maternal infections. Manifestations of toxoplasmosis infection at birth range from infants who are asymptomatic (approximately 80% to 90% of cases) to infants with severe disease. If untreated, asymptomatic infants will develop retinal disease in about 85% of cases. In fact, visual disease is the most important sequelae of congenital toxoplasmosis (Stagno et al., 1982; Stein & Boyer, 1994). Late development of hearing impairment and mental retardation has also been reported. Clinical features of severe congenital toxoplasmosis at birth include hydrocephalus, infection of retinal tissue, cerebral calcification, and other organ system disease.

Unlike rubella or CMV, acute maternal toxoplasmosis infection can be treated to prevent the parasite from infecting the fetus. Infected infants also receive direct treatment of congenital toxoplasmosis. Infants are treated with antiparasitic medications and vitamin supplements. Treatment appears effective in reducing morbidity associated with congenital toxoplasmosis infection. Neurodevelopmental sequelae of untreated congenital toxoplasmosis include mental retardation, microcephaly, microphthalmia, and hearing loss. The most common disorder is visual defects and blindness. Stein and Boyer (1994) reported that auditory, visual, and central nervous system

sequelae of toxoplasmosis can be virtually eliminated with long-term treatment with antiparasitic drugs. In their study, none of 57 treated children developed sensorineural hearing loss.

Syphilis

Syphilis is a sexually transmitted disease caused by the bacterium *Treponema pallidum*. It is estimated that 1 in 10,000 live-born infants in the United States is infected with congenital syphilis. Although the incidence of syphilis steadily declined through the 1970s, syphilis is now on the increase with more reported cases of the disease now than in the previous two decades. Despite the fact that this disease can be cured with antibiotics if caught early, rising rates of syphilis among pregnant women in the United States have increased the number of infants born with congenital syphilis. Nearly half of all children infected with syphilis while they are in the womb die shortly before or after birth.

Congenital syphilis (also known as congenital lues) may be present in utero and at birth and occurs when a child is born to a mother with secondary syphilis. Untreated syphilis results in a high risk of a bad outcome of pregnancy, including mulberry molars in the fetus. Syphilis can cause miscarriages, premature births, stillbirths, or death of newborn babies. Some infants with congenital syphilis have symptoms at birth, but most develop symptoms later. Untreated babies can have deformities, delays in development, or seizures along with many other problems such as rash, fever, hepatosplenomegaly, anemia, and jaundice. Sores on infected babies are infectious. Rarely, the symptoms of syphilis go unseen in infants so that they develop the symptoms of late-stage syphilis, including damage to their bones, teeth, eyes, ears, and brain. Hearing impairment from congenital syphilis typically is not present at birth. Auditory impairment may not be present at birth, but manifests in later childhood or early teen years with sudden onset, generally bilaterally symmetrical severe-to-profound loss.

Treponema pallidum is a frail organism that does not survive long outside a host organism. It is transmitted through sexual intercourse when the lesions of the infected individual come into intimate contact with minute breaks in the epithelial surfaces of his or her partner. There are several stages of syphilis infection: during the first and second stages (known as early syphilis), viable organisms are present and the individual can transmit the disease through sexual contact as described. During the third, or latent, stage (late syphilis), the individual no longer transmits the disease through sexual contact although the infection can be transmitted to the fetus. The early stage of syphilis in adults usually causes a single, small, painless sore. Sometimes it causes swelling in nearby lymph nodes. If not treated, syphilis usually causes a nonitchy skin rash, often on hands and feet. Many people do not notice symptoms for years. Symptoms can disappear for indeterminate times and then return.

An infected mother in either the early or late stage of syphilis may transmit the infection to her fetus. In early, untreated syphilis, transmission to the fetus occurs in 80% to 90% of cases. Approximately 25% to 30% of infected fetuses die in utero, 25% to 30% die postnatally, and 40% of survivors develop late symptomatic syphilis. Transmission can occur in any stage of pregnancy; untreated maternal infection in the first two trimesters leads to significant fetal morbidity but maternal infection in the third trimester does not always result in fetal infection.

Treatment of primary syphilis with penicillin during pregnancy is highly effective in preventing infection of the fetus. Penicillin is also an effective treatment of congenital syphilis. Approximately 60% of infants with congenital syphilis are asymptomatic at birth. Congenital syphilis is defined as early or late depending on whether clinical signs are present before or after the second year of life. In early congenital syphilis, the infant develops rhinitis (snuffles) and treponemas are present in the nasal discharge. Shortly thereafter, a rash develops that especially affects the palms, soles, perianal, and perioral regions. Skin on the palms and soles is vulnerable to sloughing. Late congenital syphilis manifests after age 2 years with a variety of lesions affecting the bones, connective tissue, and central nervous system. Progressive sensorineural hearing loss is a common finding in late congenital syphilis.

Human Immunodeficiency Virus (HIV)

In 1981, the first cases of acquired immunodeficiency syndrome (AIDS) were recognized. HIV is a retrovirus that is now known to cause AIDS. HIV replicated in the host's immune system, thereby diminishing the host's immune response. HIV infection is often difficult to diagnose in very young children. Infected babies, especially in the first few months of life, often appear normal and may exhibit no telltale signs that would allow a definitive diagnosis of HIV infection. Moreover, all children born to infected mothers have antibodies to HIV, made by the mother's immune system, that cross the placenta to the baby's bloodstream before birth and persist for up to 18 months. Because these maternal antibodies reflect the mother's and not the infant's infection status, the test is not useful in newborns or young infants.

In recent years, investigators have demonstrated the utility of highly accurate blood tests in diagnosing HIV infection in children 6 months of age and younger. One laboratory technique called polymerase chain reaction (PCR) can detect minute quantities of the virus in an infant's blood. Another procedure allows physicians to culture a sample of an infant's blood and test it for the presence of HIV. Currently, PCR assays or HIV culture techniques can identify at birth about one third of infants who are truly HIV infected. With these techniques, approximately 90% of HIV-infected infants are identifiable by 2 months of age, and 95% by 3 months of age. One innovative new approach to both RNA and DNA PCR testing uses dried blood spot specimens, which makes it simpler to gather and store specimens in field settings. Infants with congenital HIV infection are at risk for acquiring hearing loss secondary to other opportunistic infections such as meningitis and otitis media, or ototoxic antibiotic treatment for these infections.

HIV is transmitted through sexual intercourse, infected blood products, infected breast milk, or transplacentally. Typically no symptoms are present at initial infection although some individuals demonstrate a mild flu-like illness. Most infected individuals remain asymptomatic for years after infection. An individual who is HIV positive develops AIDS when he or she exhibits signs of generalized constitutional diseases, opportunistic infections, neurologic disease, secondary cancer, and other systemic effects. AIDS is the end stage of a complex disease process.

The risk of transmission of the HIV from an infected mother to her fetus is estimated to range from 10% to 40%. Early treatment of the infected pregnant woman with antiviral drugs has been shown to reduce transmission of HIV to the fetus. The spectrum of embryopathologic effects of HIV can be significant and include growth retardation, premature birth, low birth weight, and dysmorphic features in infected infants. Researchers have observed two general patterns of illness in HIV-infected children. About 20 percent of children develop serious disease in the first year of life; most of these children die by age 4 years. The remaining 80% of infected children have a slower rate of disease progression, many not developing the most serious symptoms of AIDS until school entry or even adolescence. HIV-infected children frequently have severe candidiasis, a yeast infection that can cause unrelenting diaper rash and infections in the mouth and throat that make eating difficult. Many children with HIV infection do not gain weight or grow normally. HIV-infected children frequently are slow to reach important milestones in motor skills and mental development such as crawling, walking, and speaking. As the disease progresses, many children develop neurologic problems such as difficulty walking, poor school performance, seizures, and other symptoms of HIV encephalopathy.

The most effective treatment for children with HIV is antiretroviral therapy (ARV), which reduces illness and mortality among children living with HIV. In high-income countries, children can be tested soon after birth usually using PCR tests that can detect the genetic material of HIV. Many of the drugs that are conventionally used to treat adults living with HIV are not available in an appropriate form, are unpalatable for children, or are licensed or approved for use in children. Most children on HIV treatment need to take three or more types of ARVs every day for the rest of their lives as this prevents their HIV from becoming resistant to any single drug. ARV treatment for children living with HIV is highly effective at reducing mortality and illness so that children living with HIV can expect to survive well into adulthood.

In some low- and middle-income countries, "dried blood spot" testing has been introduced. This is where a small sample of blood is taken from a child, dropped onto paper, and sent to a laboratory where it can be tested. Because these samples do not need to be refrigerated and are easy to transport, they can potentially be sent miles away to places where PCR testing is available. This means that even children living in resource-poor areas can be tested relatively quickly. However, dried blood spot testing can be expensive, and it can take a long time for test results to return.

Individuals do not die of AIDS, per se, but rather from the opportunistic infections and disease. HIV develops rapidly among infants and children and, without treatment, one third of children infected with HIV will die of AIDS before their first birthday. In 2010, there were 250,000 worldwide AIDS-related deaths in children under 15, most of which could have been prevented through early diagnosis and effective treatment. In many high-income countries, children who were infected with HIV at birth in the 1980s and 1990s are now entering adulthood as a result of access to AVR treatment. However, although the number of children receiving antiretroviral therapy (ART) has increased significantly in recent years, at the end of 2010 only 23% of the 2 million children in need of ART in low- and middle-income countries were receiving it.

TORCH Infections

The TORCH complex is an acronym for a set of perinatal infections (i.e., infections that are passed from a pregnant woman to her fetus). The TORCH infections can lead to severe fetal anomalies or even fetal loss. They are a group of viral, bacterial, and protozoan infections that gain access to the fetal bloodstream transplacentally. TORCH infections are acquired by the embryo or fetus during gestation or by the newborn at delivery. In the acronym, T stands for toxoplasmosis, R for rubella virus, C for cytomegalovirus (CMV), H for herpes simplex virus (HSV), and O for other bacterial infections, especially syphilis, that result in hearing loss (Nahmias, 1974). TORCH infections are often clinically unapparent, and when the infections are identified, their associated signs and symptoms are sometimes nearly indistinguishable. Prognosis for the involved infant is usually grim.

The lack of symptomatology in the pregnant woman makes the diagnosis of TORCH infections very difficult. Even when symptoms are manifest, the diagnosis cannot be confirmed without special laboratory tests. Toxoplasma infections and CMV rarely cause a clinically definable syndrome in the pregnant woman; the rash associated with rubella is not specific enough to differentiate it from other entities. In the case of herpes simplex infections, it is not the readily diagnosable cold sores or fever blisters that are of particular concern, but it is the less discernible genital infections of concern. Some of the TORCH infections, such as toxoplasmosis and syphilis, can be effectively treated with antibiotics if the mother is diagnosed early in her pregnancy. Many of the viral TORCH infections have no effective treatment, but some, notably rubella and varicella zoster, can be prevented by vaccinating the mother prior to pregnancy. If the mother has active herpes simplex (as may be suggested by a Pap test), delivery by Caesarean section can prevent the newborn from contact, and consequent infection, with this virus.

There is no clear-cut pattern in the sensorineural hearing loss attributed to TORCH complex infections. The hearing loss can be progressive and range from mild to profound, and cases of both bilateral and unilateral losses are well documented. Virus excretions may remain active for several years following birth, constituting a contributing factor in the degenerative process. In terms of infant follow-up, it is important to realize that any pattern and degree of hearing loss may occur with the TORCH complex.

GENETIC COUNSELING

Genetic counseling varies with the complexity of the problem but always requires: (a) a careful family, pregnancy, birth, and infancy history to identify factors that might explain the abnormality; (b) a thorough physical examination of the affected individual and other family members; and (c) necessary laboratory work as required. When the evaluation has been completed and the diagnosis reached, the parents return for the actual counseling sessions. Both parents are generally required to attend, and the counseling is done in an unhurried and relaxed atmosphere. They are given the final diagnosis and the risk figures for future pregnancies. When possible, an attempt is made by the genetic counselors to minimize guilt; however, in situations in which one parent is obviously the carrier of the gene causing the defect, it may be better to acknowledge the guilt and help the parent deal with it. In many instances, more than one counseling session is necessary. There is good evidence that parents who seek genetic advice will usually make appropriate and expected decisions about future children. Comprehensive medical histories for all family members are essential to determine the etiology of a disorder, especially if genetic factors are likely to play a role. Family history may demonstrate a clear pattern of inheritance on which recurrence and future risk calculations for family members can be based.

Most geneticists approach their responsibilities as counselors in a supportive and nondirective manner. Ultimately, the family must decide how to respond and act on the information provided through genetic evaluation. Prenatal diagnosis is an important tool in diagnosing and preventing genetic disease for selected couples.

Preferential Marriage. During genetic evaluation and counseling, consideration must be given to the influence of cultural, religious, and ethical traditions on the family's response to, and benefit from, genetic counseling. In some communities, individuals with similar traits and customs frequently marry. Marriage of deaf individuals is not uncommon; it is estimated that as many as 90% of deaf adults marry deaf persons. The probability of bearing hearing or deaf offspring may be of interest to these individuals, their families, or even their children in future planning.

The probability of deaf versus hearing offspring is dependent on the mode of inheritance in the parents. If both partners in a marriage have the same recessive hearing loss, the probability of deaf offspring is 100%. If one parent has a dominant hearing loss and the other a recessive loss, the probability of deaf offspring with dominant inheritance is 50%, and the probability of being a carrier for recessive inheritance is 100%. Of course, the genetic basis and gene locus are rarely known, and precise predictions of probability are obviously limited. Genetic counselors who work with deaf couples should acquire a communication system and style, including sign language proficiency, appropriate to their client base and sensitivity to deaf culture.

Consanguinity. Similar to preferential marriage, consanguinity (marriage between close relatives) represents nonrandom mating and thus nonrandom assortment of genes available to future generations. Consanguinity is more common in other countries where marriage among close family members is encouraged. It is an important fact to note in clinical genetics because the offspring from a consanguineous marriage are at increased risk for autosomal recessive disorders. Because each individual in the population is estimated to carry at least one mutant recessive gene for a serious or lethal abnormality, the likelihood that a couple will transmit two copies of this mutant, recessive gene is increased if they share a common ancestor from whom the gene originated. In general, consanguinity in a family without known genetic disease appears to increase the probability of serious or lethal conditions. In first-degree relationships (incestuous mating, e.g., father-daughter, brother-sister), the risk is marked; in relationships more distant than third degree (e.g., greater than first cousins), the risk is insignificant. In the United States there are legal restrictions on marriage between relatives; all states ban first-degree relationship marriages.

Prenatal Diagnosis and Ethical Dilemmas. The ability to diagnose certain hereditary conditions in utero is an important benefit to families at risk for serious genetic disorders. Through prenatal diagnosis, couples can determine the health of their infant for certain conditions before birth. If the prenatal diagnosis reveals a healthy fetus, the couple is spared many months of anxiety; if prenatal diagnosis reveals an affected fetus, the couple may elect therapeutic abortion. Therapeutic abortion remains an issue of intense moral and ethical debate. For couples who consider abortion to be unjustifiable under any circumstances, prenatal diagnosis may be inappropriate. For couples who believe that abortion is a justifiable choice to prevent serious disease and disability, prenatal diagnosis is appropriate if risk of disease is present. Conditions usually considered necessary to justify prenatal diagnosis include increased risk of hereditary or congenital disorder such as increased maternal age, family history of genetic disease or abnormality, or in utero exposure to viral infection.

Because the procedures are often extremely accurate as a diagnostic test, the option of therapeutic abortion is available to the couple. Preimplantation diagnosis obviates the need for therapeutic abortion of affected fetuses. It may be an acceptable alternative for couples at risk of transmission of a grave genetic condition for whom elective abortion is not an option. Although not routinely available, preimplantation diagnosis represents the current frontier in prevention of genetic disease.

Another area of interest is the ethical issues arising in medicine concerning the prenatal care and treatment of the unborn fetus. Developments in this area over the past 20 years have been recognized in medical and legal circles as bearing immense significance for the practice and ethics of medicine concerning the pregnant woman and her fetus. Advances in medical science in recent years have revolutionized a new era in prenatal care. Scientific procedures now can reveal previously undetectable secrets about the unborn child. Perinatologists not only have the ability to discern fetal abnormalities of an extraordinary variety, but they also have become increasingly successful in correcting many of these defects in utero, albeit raising more issues of morality, ethics, and legality. Again, decisions concerning the appropriateness and willingness to permit prenatal treatment of the unborn fetus depend on the personal beliefs and preferences of the parents.

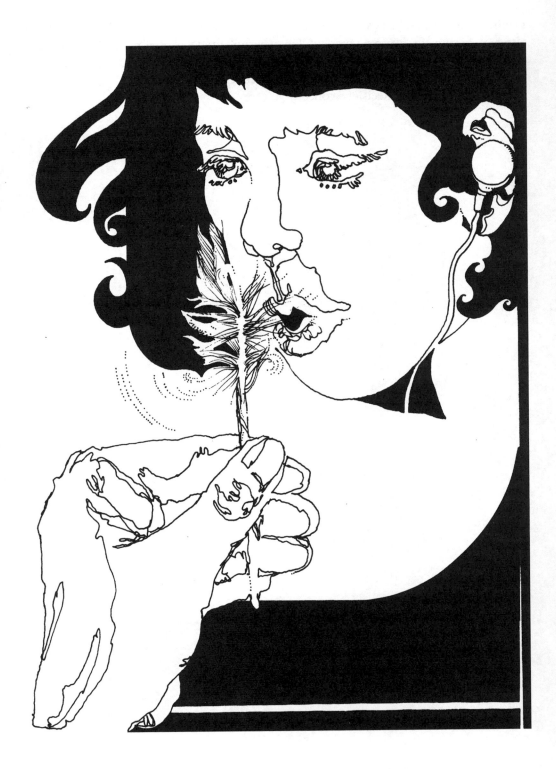

CHAPTER 3

Auditory and Speech-Language Development

One of the most important aspects in any child's development is the acquisition and production of spoken language. Spoken language is the doorway to successful communication and the social interaction that is so important to daily life. Language is the key to the doors by which we express our thoughts, needs, and feelings and by which we receive and comprehend the thoughts, needs, and feelings of others. Although it is language in a child that opens the door to education, the successful acquisition of language is highly dependent on an adequately functioning auditory system. With our success in early identification of infants with hearing loss, and through appropriate interventions, hard-of-hearing and deaf children have new opportunities to achieve higher levels of spoken language, reading abilities, and academic competencies than were available to most children in previous generations (Flexer, 2012).

As adults, we give little thought to the development of speech and language because it comes so naturally and easily to most children. We listen with awe, however, as the child's sounds develop into phonemes, then into words, and finally into sentences complete with appropriate expression and speech patterns. As audiologists we know that the child with hearing loss does not automatically develop speech. The child with hearing loss may be confronted with a life of language difficulties and educational struggles. Language develops so rapidly in the first few months of life that the longer

an infant's hearing loss goes undetected, the worse the outcome is likely to be; thus, we realize the importance of early intervention.

The audiologist has a unique contribution to make to the understanding of how language develops in infants—one that linguists and psychologists cannot offer. That is, the study of the degree to which the acoustic parameters of language learning in the infant are innate, preprogrammed processes and how acoustic factors influence language learning. There is research evidence that there are special biologic predetermined processes of perception for the various acoustic dimensions of speech. For example, we know that the newborn infant responds selectively to the dimensionality of human speech within hours after birth and is especially tuned to the voice of its mother (DeCasper & Fifer, 1980). It appears that the perception of speech signals by infants is mediated in some manner by central neural events, because although infants have had little listening experience by 2 months of age, they can differentiate between voiced stops /b/ and /g/ (Lieberman, 1975).

According to Stark (1996), Jacobson, a well-known linguist of the 1940s, made the claim that the vocal sounds made by infants during their first year of life are completely at random. Jacobson believed that these early infant sounds are made only for "practice" in the manipulation of the oral articulators, because their vocal productions do not resemble the sounds of any known language. Stark, an expert in child language development, pointed out that the International Phonetic Alphabet cannot be used to transcribe the unique sounds made by very young infants. However, in contrast to Jacobson's beliefs of the 1940s, other researchers documented that infants produce similar sounds across all languages. By the early 1970s, scientists noted that the patterns of vocal development in all infants, regardless of nationality, are universal. The milestones of cooing, vocal play, and replicated babbling appear in that general order in all normally developing infants. There is, furthermore, a lawful relationship between sounds that babies make in babbling at the end of the first year of life and those they make in their first attempts at words during the second year.

It is important for us to know that the auditory development and maturation of a normal-hearing baby follow a standard sequence of behaviors from birth to 12 months that is as regular as clockwork. The experiences of sounds and exposure to speech shape the auditory system of infants during their first year of life. Although infants are unable to produce recognizable words until about 12 months of age, they quickly develop a remarkable ability to distinguish auditorily among speech sounds. Newborns quickly learn to recognize words, phrases, vocal intent, rhythm, and names and to perform sophisticated auditory functions long before they produce their own speech.

This chapter discusses the intricate pattern of auditory development in normal-hearing infants and contrasts their auditory, speech, and language development with infants who have significant hearing loss. The studies cited have been selected for their contributions to understanding the auditory aspects of oral speech development. Numerous classic studies, as well as more recent research, that establish the basics of prenatal and neonatal hearing development, the neuroplasticity of the auditory system, and normal speech and language development are reviewed. It is critical that the pediatric specialist audiologist completely understands the normal development of auditory behavior in normal-hearing infants to be able to recognize the similarities and differences in infants with congenital and acquired hearing impairments. The positive result of our efforts is that there is evidence that earlier identification of children with hearing loss, when intervened with timely and appropriate interventions, can result in language, communication, cognitive, and social-emotional skills that are consistent with children's cognitive abilities and chronological age (Moeller, 2000; Yoshinaga-Itano, Sedey, Coulter, & Mehl, 1998; Yoshinaga-Itano et al., 2010). Of course, our ultimate goal in early hearing loss detection and intervention is to optimize language, social, and literacy development for children with hearing loss.

NEUROPLASTICITY

William James, author of *The Principles of Psychology* (1890) was one of the first scientists to suggest that the brain is not a static structure. During the latter part of the 20th century, scientists believed that active brain development was only possible during infancy and early childhood. However, through studies conducted over the past three decades, researchers have gained new insights into the early development of the brain and nervous system. Sophisticated technologies, such as elaborate brain scans and brain mapping, as well as important animal research studies, have helped illuminate the developing brain in greater detail than ever before. One of the most important conclusions from such studies is that the brain development that takes place during the first 12 months of life is more rapid and more extensive than previously realized. Since the late 1950s, one of the major themes in neuroscience is that the brain is not a "rigid" structure but a malleable, "plastic" organ with the capability of reorganizing itself based on sensory and motor input, a phenomenon known as *neuroplasticity*. Through the concepts of plasticity, the brain is a dynamic structure that is changing throughout life and is capable of new learning at any time.

Neuroplasticity refers to the brain's ability to reorganize itself, forming new connections and pathways in response to sensory and motor input, learning new skills, or in creating new memories upon which to build additional behaviors. This process involves orderly increases in the number and density of neurons, dendrites, synapses, and the proteins that are essential to the survival of nerve cells. We now know that the brain is constantly laying down new pathways and rearranging existing routes. Connections between neurons that are inefficient or infrequently used fade away, while those connections that are frequently utilized will be strengthened through a process known as *pruning*. It is likely that the majority of synapses in the brain have the capacity to grow, connect, disconnect, and reconnect to each other in response to environmental experiences of all sorts. Neuroplasticity occurs in each of us every day as we encounter new experiences. It is the brain's ability to act and react in ever changing ways to constantly lay down new pathways for neural communication and to rearrange existing ones, thereby aiding our process of learning.

The brain is an amazing organ in terms of its development, organization, efficiency, and abilities. From early neurogenesis and

the beginning of life, brain cells proliferate rapidly, making connections in a preprogrammed, orderly, and sequential manner (Mundkur, 2005). The growing brain of an embryo, by 6 weeks nearly as big as its entire body, is richly irrigated by a vast system of blood vessels. As each neuron matures, it sends out multiple axons and dendrites to lay out the basic communication routes in the brain. At this embryo stage, the brain produces many more neurons (or nerve cells) than it actually needs. At birth, each neuron in the cerebral cortex has approximately 7,500 synapses. By the time an infant is 2 years old, the number of synapses has doubled and grown to approximately 15,000 synapses per neuron (Gopnik, Meltzoff, & Kuhl, 1999), considerably more than we find in the adult brain. Although plasticity of the brain is maximal during the first 4 years of life, the brain changes throughout life as a function of experiences (i.e., it adapts to its environment) (Tremblay, 2003).

The estimated 15,000 synapses *per neuron* at birth increases with astounding rapidity, growing the total number of synapses at least 20-fold (i.e., from 50 trillion to 1,000 trillion synapses by 2 to 4 years of age) (Chugani, Phelps, & Mazziotta, 1987; Kolb, 1989). Considerable research has been completed to establish critical periods for plasticity, especially for speech and language development, which has confirmed again that the most sensitive period for functional maturation of the auditory system is within the first 2 to 4 years of life. Thus, it is critical that hard-of-hearing and deaf infants are provided with auditory input as early as possible to take advantage of the ongoing neuroplasticity.

Brain mapping studies show that the biochemical patterns noted in a 1-year-old's brain qualitatively resemble those patterns found in the brain of a normal young adult. Brain cell formation is virtually complete before birth, but brain maturation is far from over. The next challenge is the formation of connections among the neurons to form the brain's physical "maps" that allow learning to take place. Research conducted by Tremblay and Kraus (2002) suggests that a series of frequency maps exist in central auditory systems that can be altered due to auditory training or injury to the peripheral hearing system.

However, synaptic pruning, more technically known as apoptosis or programmed cell death, eliminates the weaker synaptic contacts while stronger connections are kept and strengthened (Sarnat & Menkes, 2000). The process of pruning excessive synapses continues actively until approximately age 16 to 18 when it begins to slow down. Experience ultimately determines which connections will be used more (i.e., strengthened) and which will disappear. Many types of brain cells are involved in neuroplastic processes including neurons, glia, and vascular cells. Although plasticity occurs over an individual's lifetime, it appears that different types of plasticity dominate during certain periods of one's life and are less prevalent during other periods (Raff et al., 1993).

As the neurons carry electrical signals along the nervous system, systematic pathways are established through coordinated routes that are used over and over again. The stimulated neurons develop long axons that spin out multiple branches that connect with a vast number of different neurons. Current theory suggests that spontaneous bursts of electrical activity strengthen some of these pathway connections, while other neurons that are not reinforced by electrical activity begin to atrophy and finally disappear. The brain eliminates the excess neurons and connections that are seldom or never used. During early life, the number of neuronal connections explodes, and each of the brain's billions of neurons will forge links to thousands of other neurons. The resultant increase in cortical and brainstem electrical activity, triggered by the new flood of sensory experiences, fine tunes the brain's circuitry and determines which connections will be retained and which connections will be pruned (Chugani, 1993).

Decades of research have shown that substantial changes occur in both the brain's physical structure and functional organization. Cortical implants in animals have been used to study plasticity in both the somatosensory and the auditory systems (Blake, Heiser, Caywood, & Merzenich, 2006; Blake, Strata, Churchland, & Merzenich, 2002; Blake, Strata, Kempter, & Merzenich, 2005; Syka & Merzenich, 2011). Both systems show similar changes with respect to behavior. When a stimulus is cognitively associated with reinforcement, its cortical representation is strengthened and enlarged. These researchers showed that cortical representation can double or even triple in 1 to 2 days when a new sensory or motor behavior is first acquired. Control studies show that these changes are not caused by sensory experience alone; they require learning about the sensory experience and are strongest for the stimuli that are associated with reward.

Among the first systematic circuits laid down by the brain are those that govern the emotions such as contentment, distress, and anger. Although the newborn can feel, see, hear, and smell, these senses operate somewhat dimly and reflexively. Over the first few days, weeks, and months of life, sensory activity stimulates the neuronal connections from the brainstem to the appropriate areas of the cortex. The results of these early sensory experiences are those actions we have come to expect as normal infant development: by 2 months the baby is able to grasp objects, by 4 months the complex actions required to locate a sound in space are initiated, by 6 months a baby can recognize and mimic the vowel sounds that are the precursors to speech formation, and by 12 months we begin to see the results of neural pathways formed to produce the first words that mark the beginning of language expression.

Genetics certainly play a role in establishing an individual's brain plasticity, and the environment exerts heavy influence in maintaining it. For example, the newborn's brain is absolutely flooded each day with new information. When the body receives input through its many different sensory organs, different neurons are responsible for sending that input back to the appropriate part of the brain. Neuroplasticity can work in two directions; it is responsible for creating new connections and frequently deletes old connections that are not used as often. Each neuron acts independently, and learning skills may require large collections of neurons to be active simultaneously to process complex neural information. In response to a new experience or novel information, neuroplasticity allows either an alteration to the structure of already existing connections between neurons, or forms new connections between neurons; the latter leads to an increase in overall synaptic density, while the former merely makes existing pathways more efficient or suitable. In either way, the brain is remolded to take in this new data and, if useful, retain it. Further repetitions of the same information or experience may lead to more modifications in the connections or routing or may actually increase the number of connections that can access the new information (Drubach, 2000).

Scientific study has shown that early brain development is much more vulnerable

to environmental influence than previously suspected. The influence of environment on early development may be long lasting. The prenatal environment and conditions affect not only the number of brain cells and the number of connections among them, but also the way that these connections are "wired." For example, we know that inadequate nutrition before birth and during the first years of life can seriously interfere with brain development. Poor early nutrition may lead to a host of neurologic and behavioral disorders, including learning disabilities and mental retardation. Other detrimental changes in the environment of the embryo, such as drug abuse or viral infection, can wreck the clockwork precision of neural development, resulting in epilepsy, autism, or other serious disorders. Thus, one can understand and appreciate the increased focus that society has given to the importance of proper prenatal care (Carnegie Corporation, 1994).

Knowledge of these facts demands that more attention be focused on the importance of early childhood intervention. At birth the brain is very immature; in fact, the brain is not fully mature for at least 20 years. During this long period of development, the brain is highly dependent on and is modified and shaped by experiences. However, without the experience of auditory stimulation, the brain reorganizes itself to receive input from other senses—primarily vision. This is called *cross-model regeneration,* and it reduces subsequent auditory neural capacity (Flexer, 2012; Sharma, Purdy, & Kelly, 2009; Tremblay, 2003). Therefore, programs and environments that provide enriched activities to stimulate the auditory pathways and various sensory, motor, and language centers will enhance neuroplasticity and bring about changes in the infant brain (Boatman et al., 1999).

There appear to be three major means by which plasticity of the brain occurs known as synaptic, neurogenesis, and functional compensatory plasticity: (a) *Synaptic plasticity* refers to the brain's ability to create new interconnecting neurons through learning and practice. The neurons in a neural pathway communicate with each other at a meeting point, the synapse. Every time new knowledge is acquired (through repeated practice), synaptic communication or transmission is enhanced among implicated neurons. Revisiting the neural circuit and reestablishing neuronal transmission between the implicated neurons at each new attempt enhances the efficiency of synaptic transmission. Communication between the relevant neurons is facilitated, and cognition made it faster. Synaptic plasticity is perhaps the pillar on which the brain's amazing malleability rests. (b) *Neurogenesis* plasticity refers to the birth and proliferation of new neurons in the brain. In recent years the existence of neurogenesis has become scientifically established. Stem cells can divide into two cells, each of which will become a neuron fully equipped with axon and dendrites. Those new neurons will then migrate to distant neurons. (c) *Functional compensatory plasticity* of the brain describes a situation in which a region of the brain demonstrates sensory reassignment. An example of this would be a situation in which one sensory modality (vision for example) is damaged and, in response, another sensory modality (touch for example) contributes inputs into the cortical space previously committed to the damaged modality. In the presence of age-related deficits and decreased synaptic plasticity that accompany aging, the brain manifests its multisource plasticity by reorganizing its neurocognitive networks. Studies show that the brain reaches this functional solution through the activation of alternative neural pathways, which most often activate regions in both hemispheres (Sousa, 2011).

Sininger, Doyle, & Moore (1999) reviewed the experimental evidence to support the notion of auditory system plasticity. Animal experiments show that the developing auditory nerve, brainstem nuclei, and auditory cortex have the capacity to change during normal development and during times of interrupted sensory input. There is also experimental evidence that reintroduction of sensory input after auditory deprivation induces further plastic changes, and deleterious effects may be reversed only during early stages of development. This important research evidence obtained in animal anatomic studies supports the view those critical periods may exist for intervention to ameliorate the experimentally created deficits.

The brain's growth spurts begin to slow around 10 years of age. By the end of adolescence, around age 18, the brain has declined in plasticity but increased in power. These physiologic findings, confirmed by modern neuroscience, show the importance and value of early interventions. Although the adult nervous system continues to lay down new synaptic connections as we learn new ideas and skills, never again will the brain be able to assimilate and master new information so readily as it can during the first 3 years of life.

PRENATAL HEARING

The auditory system in the fetus is under structural development during the first 20 weeks of gestation, followed by the initial neurosensory maturation. Thus, the auditory system becomes functional around 25 weeks' gestation when the ganglion cells of the spiral nucleus in the cochlea connect inner hair cells to the brainstem and temporal lobe of the cortex (Hall, 2000). Elliot and Elliot (1964) confirmed that the human cochlea shows response to sound after the 20th week of gestation.

Johansson, Wedenberg, and Westin (1964) were among the first to attempt to test hearing function in the fetus. Using pure tones presented through a microphone placed on the mother's abdomen, fetal heart rate increase in response to the tones was recorded after the 20th week of gestation. The demonstration of fetal hearing has value in contradicting the theory that the child is born a *tabula rasa* insofar as hearing is concerned. At the time of birth then, the infant has actually been hearing sounds for at least 4 months—fluid-borne sounds, to be sure— but nonetheless, perceiving sounds. The important question is not so much precisely when we first hear sound, but rather what long-term impact hearing loss has on the development of the auditory brain structures.

How early does the infant perceive speech and act on the acoustic environment? To be sure, the developmental response to sound in the fetus is primarily reflexive, including startle, generalized body movement, possible cessation of activity, and the auropalpebral reflex (involuntary eye blink). Nevertheless, there is also research evidence for the existence of preadaptive processes of perception of the acoustic dimensions of speech. Knowing that the fetus is physiologically prepared to respond to sound is important, but the difficult task is determining when the developing fetus begins to "hear." Birnholz and Benacerraf (1983) observed the auropalpebral reflex systematically in 236 intrauterine babies in a study of screening for deafness. Stimuli were presented via vibroacoustic stimuli applied to the maternal abdominal wall directly over the fetal ear, and fetal eye clenching was observed with ultrasonic imaging. Their results, confirmed by Kuczwara, Birnholz, and Klodd (1984), indicated that auropalpebral reflexes consistently occur at approximately 24 to 25 weeks' gestational age in normal fetuses.

At birth the infant is able to discriminate his or her mother's voice and will behave in such a way as to elicit the mother's voice in preference to the voice of another female. DeCasper and Fifer (1980) used a sucking stimulus-response paradigm to demonstrate these capacities with infants shortly after delivery. Earphones were placed over the ears of the supine infant, and a nonnutritive nipple was placed in the infant's mouth. The nipple was connected by way of a pressure transducer to recording equipment that produced either another nonmaternal voice or the mother's voice. For five randomly selected infants, sucking bursts first produced only the mother's voice on the tape for a predetermined interval and then the voice of another infant's mother. For another five infants the conditions were reversed. A preference for the maternal voice was indicated if the infant produced the sucking response more often to his or her own mother's voice than to the nonmaternal voice. The infants soon learned to gain access to their own mother's voice, because specific temporal properties of sucking could be used to produce the recorded maternal voice.

Is there sufficient acoustic exposure in the uterus to permit such a precocious development? Bench (1968) reported that for a 72 dB SPL signal there is the least attenuation of sound going into the uterus at 200 Hz (19 dB), slightly more at 500 Hz (24 dB), more at 1000 Hz (38 dB), and the most at 2000 and 4000 Hz (48 dB). The frequencies below 1000 Hz contained the frequency response of the maternal voice that may be heard by the fetus from the fourth month of gestation.

A later study by Armitage et al. (1980) measured the actual sound level inside the amniotic sac of pregnant ewes by means of hydrophones inside the sac, within the normal fluid environment of the fetus. These investigators found that although sounds from the maternal cardiovascular system were not perceived, the sounds of the mother's eating, drinking, ruminating, breathing, and muscular movements were discernible, as were sounds from outside the mother. They found that the attenuation of sounds measured reached a maximum of 37 dB below 1000 Hz, but it was reduced below and above this frequency. The higher frequencies were attenuated about 20 dB up to 5000 Hz. Human conversations at normal levels outside the sheep could be understood, and raised voices were heard distinctly. If the leap is made from this animal model to the case of the human fetus, then it is likely that the mother's and even the father's voices can be heard by a fetus.

Querleu, Renard, and Crepin (1981) performed intrauterine measures on humans and demonstrated that the fetus could hear the mother's voice and other voices that were perfectly audible but lacking in tone because the high frequencies were absorbed. When there is no fetal distress, the fetus reacts to the sound stimulus by a change in heart rate, often associated with movement. Querleu made additional observations of seven patients during term labor after amniotomy, implanting hydrophones and microphones in the uterine cavity. When external speech was recorded through the uterus, two observers could recognize 64% of the mother's phonemes and 57% of a male's speech.

Apparently a great deal of auditory experience is necessary to produce the abilities of the newborn to prefer the mother's voice to other voices. Before such early discriminations can be made, the infant auditory system has to be preadapted to various acoustic discriminations. Such discriminations have been shown to be present in the newborn, and assuming a normal hearing system and normal CNS, the same capabilities are present in the 4-month-old fetus. The innate discriminations that subserve the preference for the mother's voice require the auditory competencies of discriminating rhythm, intonation, frequency variation, stress (suprasegmental aspects of speech), and phonetic components of speech (linguistic aspects).

Hepper and Shahidullah (1994) attempted to systematically evaluate the development of fetal behavioral responsiveness to pure tone auditory stimuli (100 Hz, 250 Hz, 500 Hz, 1000 Hz, and 3000 Hz) in infants from 19 to 35 weeks of gestational age. Stimuli were presented by a loudspeaker placed on the maternal abdomen and the fetus's response, a movement, was recorded by ultrasound. In their study the fetus initially responded to the 500 Hz tone at 19 weeks' gestational age. The range of frequencies subsequently responded to expanded first to lower frequencies (e.g., 100 Hz and 250 Hz) and then upwards to higher frequencies (e.g., 1000 Hz and 3000 Hz). By 27 weeks' gestational age, 96% of fetuses responded to the 250 and 500 Hz tones but none responded to the 1000 and 3000 Hz tones. Responsiveness to 1000 and 3000 Hz tones was observed in all fetuses at 33 and 35 weeks' gestational age, respectively. For all frequencies there was a large decrease (20 to 30 dB) in the intensity level required to elicit a response as the fetus matured. These researchers concluded that the observed pattern of behavioral responsiveness reflected the prenatal maturation of the auditory system.

In summary, it would appear that there is ample evidence that perceptual learning of the more global, prosodic aspects of language actually commences prior to birth. Studies using the sucking and heart rate paradigms show that exposure to sound in utero resulted in a preference of newborn infants for native-language over foreign-language utterances (Moon, Cooper, & Fifer, 1993), for the mother's voice over another female's voice (DeCasper & Fifer, 1980), and for simple stories the mother read during the last trimester over unfamiliar stories (DeCasper & Spence, 1986). This indicates that the prosodic aspects of human speech, including voice pitch and the stress and intonation characteristics of a particular language and speaker, are transmitted to the fetus and are learnable. According to Doupe and Kulh (1999), these studies on learning during the first year of life indicate that prior to the time that infants learn the meanings of individual words or phrases, they learn to recognize general perceptual characteristics that describe phonemes, words, and phrases that typify their native language. Thus, as a first step toward vocal learning, infants avidly acquire information about the perceptual regularities that describe their native language and commit them to memory in some form. Understanding the nature of this early phonetic learning and the mechanisms underlying it is one of the key issues in human language development.

NEONATAL HEARING DEVELOPMENT

It has long been established that normal-hearing infants and neonates between the ages of 4 and 16 months undergo an orderly maturation and development of predictable auditory response behaviors (Murphy, 1962, 1979). These responses are easily observable and can be elicited with soft acoustic signals or simple noise makers. In the hands of an experienced audiologist, knowledge of the normal auditory behavioral responses may

be used as a preliminary hearing screening method. The normal-hearing, alert infant will respond in the predictable manner in accordance with his or her mental age. These auditory maturation responses are so reliable that in skillful hands, they can serve as an initial orientation for the audiologist as to what to expect in the more formal hearing evaluation. In fact, these auditory development responses are very age specific, depending on the maturation of the infant, as shown in Figure 3–1. In older pediatric patients with developmental delay, for example 3 to 6 years of age, these auditory developmental responses may actually prove to be a good starting technique for screening the hearing of difficult-to-test individuals.

Kearsley, Snider, Richie, Crawford, and Talbot (1962) found that if an unexpected noise of 70 dB SPL reaches maximum intensity within a few milliseconds, a newborn infant closes his or her eyes, startles, and shows an increase in heart rate. If the same sound reaches its maximal intensity in 2 seconds, the infant opens his or her eyes, looks around, and is likely to show a decrease in heart rate. The first reaction is a defensive one; the latter displays interest in the changing environment. This easiest auditory reflex response to elicit and observe is the startle, or Moro, response. All normal-hearing infants younger than 30 months will show an easily observable startle response to a sudden onset stimulus of 65 dB HL or louder. An easy and simple way to observe this response is to present a sudden speech stimulus through the sound-field speakers, with the baby seated quietly on the parent's knees as far forward as possible with minimal support. When a sudden and loud auditory stimulus is presented, such as an intensity controlled speech signal, the normal infant will likely provide an immediate, brisk, reflexive, whole-body response coincident with the presentation of

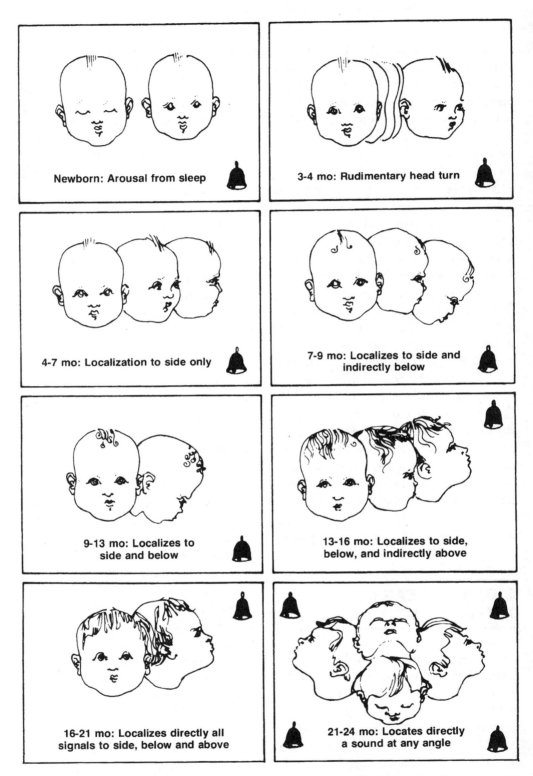

Figure 3–1. Normal infant-neonate maturation of the auditory localization response. (From Bench, 1962; Northern & Downs, 1974.)

the signal. We reserve observation of this startle response as our final presentation of the screening procedure, because the loud stimulus may actually frighten the baby into crying. The parent should be warned quietly beforehand about the presentation of the sudden loud sound as to not jump and startle the child. The Moro response is specific and reliable but is only a screening test and cannot be tied to any specific decibel hearing level (dB HL) threshold value. It is recommended that infants and babies who do not demonstrate an appropriate startle response to sudden, intense auditory signals should be scheduled for additional audiologic evaluation.

Auditory Maturation

Other normal developmental auditory maturation milestones can be used in hearing screening protocols. It has been our experience that at least 95% of normal-hearing babies will demonstrate the following auditory maturation responses when properly administered by an audiologist in a quiet setting with minimal visual distractions. It is best to observe the baby for 30 to 45 seconds before applying the screening noise sources to confirm that the state of the infant or toddler is calm, collected, and comfortable. Babies with severe-to-profound hearing loss, or developmental delay problems, may not show age-appropriate auditory maturation responses, and the Moro response may be limited, absent, or not easily elicited. It behooves the pediatric audiologist to observe and become familiar with normal responses from a large sample of normal-hearing infants before using the techniques with infants and toddlers who are more difficult to test and those who might have hearing losses. The age catego-

ries and boundaries shown below are presented for hearing screening purposes only and are likely to be quite variable among infants. These auditory response behaviors described below should be accepted as "normal" if appropriate and observed within a week or two of the age boundaries described.

We often use these auditory developmental responses to "break the ice" or reduce the suspicions of a timorous child we are seeing for the first time. It makes for a nice opening and meeting with the nervous child to have the child sit on the parent's lap in the sound-treated room while you kneel in front of them, casually holding noise-making toys below and out of the child's eyesight. With a friendly smile and happy greeting to hold the eyes of the child, slowly grasp the noisemaker in one hand, hold it off to the side, and present a soft stimulus sound while observing the child's localization skills. With the older child, we might present the first stimulus at the lower level on each side and look for the more mature localization response that is age appropriate. This auditory screening procedure takes only a few minutes, befriends the child and parent, and provides initial information about the child's hearing status and auditory maturity. Children with unilateral hearing loss will often demonstrate quite different localization behaviors with this protocol. And, now having developed the child's trust, the audiologist will have an easier time placing insert earphones, making immittance measurements, and generally proceeding with the hearing evaluation.

Birth to Four Months of Age

At this early age, babies may turn toward their mother's voice and even smile when they hear a new voice. They may be observed suddenly quieting, or becoming still, at the presentation of a new sound if they are crying or fussing. However, in general, infant auditory responses are limited and largely reflexive. In a very quiet environment one may only see an eye-blink or eye-widening response to soft sounds from noisemakers or other subtle auditory signals, but the tester must be aware that these responses are highly variable and may be late in evolving (i.e., more easily elicited at 6 weeks to 4 months of age rather than near birth). The only reliable behavioral (but reflexive) auditory response at this early age is the Moro startle response or the "surprise" eye-blink to louder sounds. However, the Moro startle response can be observed sometimes while the baby is comfortable in the mother's arms even within weeks of birth. Be patient and cautious in your interpretation because at 3 or 4 months of age, the infant may begin to show a slow head turn toward a sound, but this response is also not yet consistent and still quite variable among infants.

Four to Seven Months of Age

By 4 months of age auditory development is noted as the infant begins to turn his or her head toward the sound source in a more consistent, but still slow and wobbly manner. By 7 months, the infant's neck muscles will be strong enough to permit a stronger and more direct turn on a lateral plane toward the side from which the sound is presented. The head turn may not be a direct localization to sounds presented at lower plane levels. When the stimulus sound is presented at a lower level beneath the eyes of the baby, the response may be initially a turn to the appropriate side of the sound and then a slow search downward for the source.

Seven to Nine Months of Age

Between 7 and 9 months the infant develops the ability to identify the precise location of the sound source with a direct head turn, either on a lateral plane or to a lower level. By this age the localization response is brisk and firm. Sound stimuli presented below the child should draw a direct localization down to the sound source. However, it is likely that the infant will not yet look directly at a sound on a higher plane (i.e., above eye level), as the ability to localize sound above the head is not demonstrated for another month or two. It is a bit remarkable that although the infant can localize sounds to the side or below with briskness and accuracy, they seem unable to localize sounds presented above and over their heads.

Nine to Thirteen Months of Age

Certainly, by 12 to 13 months of age, the normal-hearing infant is able to localize sounds briskly and directly in any plane to the side, above, or below eye level. Usually, by 12 months of age, the curiosity of the child is full blown and one will see quick localizations to appropriately presented auditory stimulus which will be noted by children with bilaterally normal hearing. Full maturation of the child's auditory development has usually been attained by this age.

Thirteen Months and Older

Although it is generally easy for the pediatric audiologist to elicit and observe these nonconditioned localizing auditory responses in this older age group, other factors may influence expected auditory behaviors up through 36 months of age and must be taken into consideration. For example, when a 2- or 3-year-old hears the auditory stimulus sound, the audiologist can actually see the child willfully inhibiting the orienting response. Perhaps the child may suspect that the examiner is making the sound, realizes the expected behavior, and simply rebels against responding. Skill and experience of the audiologist must prevail with these younger children to be sure any responses noted are specific only to the presentation of the auditory stimulus. Of course, for this older age group, reinforced behavioral response techniques such as visual response audiometry or conditioned orientation response audiometry are the required audiologic testing methods (see Chapter 6).

Condon and Sander (1974) as well as Demany, McKenzie, and Vurpillot (1977) demonstrated that neonates move in precise and sustained segments of movements that are synchronous with the articulated structure of speech. Spring and Dale (1977) showed that 1- to 4-month-old babies could discriminate linguistic stress as well as location, fundamental frequency, intensity, and duration. Thus, the entire gamut of suprasegmental aspects of speech is available and understandable to the infant at birth.

Rhythm, intonation, duration, and stress are extremely important to understanding multiple meanings of words as well as the meanings of homophones. Many words and phrases contain multiple meanings that are made clear only by intonation, rhythm, duration, and stress. This fact explains a part of the problem of a deaf child in understanding some of the subtle parameters of irony, satire, scorn, implied anger, or humor that convey the sense of multimeaning words or phrases. "You're tired." and "You're tired?" are two different sentences depending on the intonation of the rising or falling fundamental frequency. Sentences such as, "You drive me up the wall," and "I can't bear

it," make for humorous misconceptions, but it is the kind of thing that is difficult for the concrete-minded, hard-of-hearing or deaf child who has not heard the stress and intonations that made these phrases meaningful.

Eimas, Siqueland, Juscyzk, and Vigorito (1972), Eimas (1975), and Eimas and Tartter (1979) documented evidence that the very young child is also able to discriminate the segmental aspects of speech in a categorical and presumably linguistic manner. In an experiment with 26 one-month-old infants, Eimas used the classic sucking paradigm in discriminating the differences between the voiced stop /b/ and the voiceless stop /p/ combined with the vowel /a/. His results indicated that infants as young as 1 month of age are not only responsive to speech but are able to make fine distinctions between similar speech sounds.

Eisenberg (1970, 1976) demonstrated that newborns, including those with known CNS abnormalities, can discriminate sound on the basis of frequency, intensity, and stimulus-dimensionality. Thus, neuronal mechanisms for processing and discriminating between SPLs are fully mature at birth. She found that the low frequencies tend to have a soothing or inhibiting effect on the infant, while sounds with higher frequencies have the property of occasioning distress rather than inhibiting it. However, signals in the range below 4000 Hz are two or three times more response provoking than those in the very high frequency ranges. It is intriguing to speculate whether speech dimensional signals are more attention-getting because of some preadaptive auditory reactivity or whether the known frequency-dependent sensitivity of the human ear is operating here. That dependency in itself is intriguing; one wonders which came first, the human ear's greater sensitivity to frequencies in the speech range or the peculiar properties of the human larynx and resonators to produce speech in that particular range of frequencies.

The theoretical considerations of the infant's ability to process a segmental unit of speech have occasioned a great deal of speculation. The arguments revolve around the fact that speech is a very complex code; transformation of the acoustic energy signaling speech to the perceptual event may not be a simple conversion mediated by an auditory decoder. Lieberman (1975) states that the acoustic cues for successive phonemes are intermixed in the sound stream to such an extent that definable segments of sound do not correspond to segments at the phoneme level. These studies lead to the inescapable conclusion that the infant enters this world with considerable awareness to the phonologic component of language.

That the infant is able to discriminate the acoustic features of speech means that the infant can segment an almost continuous acoustic input into discrete elements. This ability to process language into discrete elements is a basis for development of full language competence. The infant's ability to do this at the very beginning of language acquisition means that he or she does not have to learn that language is formed by discrete elements. The result is a facilitation of the language acquisition process, and indeed, the ability to break down discrete elementary language may even be requisite to its formation.

Bench (1971) described the relationship between the infant's activity or sleep state and auditory response in terms of the law of initial value: the magnitude of response change is influenced by the state of the infant before stimulation. The lower the initial or prestimulus state, the greater the increase in level of activity on stimulation; the higher the initial state, the greater the decrease in level of activity. Bench measured the heart rate of 10 normal newborn babies for 10 seconds before and after stimulation by a 95 dB SPL broadband noise. The results indicated that the heart rate change to auditory stimulation was dependent on the prestimulus heart rate. The implication of this work for infant audiometry is that any given baby may show an increase or decrease in behavioral activity, or no change at all, depending entirely on the prestimulus state. Exploring the responsiveness of birth to 6-month-old infants to various stimuli, Bench, Collyer, Mentz, et al. (1977) found that infants up to 6 months of age were notably unresponsive to pure tone and narrow-band auditory stimuli. However, broad-spectrum noise elicited better responses in the younger infants (1 week and 6 weeks), and the 6-month-olds responded well to recorded voice stimuli. Moderate-intensity signals were not effective for the month molds. The younger infants were mostly in sleep states when studied, so stimuli of 90 dB SPL were necessary for response.

In addition to responding differently in a passive way to stimulus patterns and intensity, newborns can be active in regulating auditory events in their environment. Butterfield (1968) reported that babies made bursts of contingent sucking responses that controlled the onset and offset of tape-recorded music: classical, popular, and vocal. An instrumental pacifier nipple operated the musical selections. Four 1-day-old infants were used in his study, and all responded consistently over several tests. This study leaves no doubt but that newborn infants are not passive in their hearing function. Their feedback loop operates actively at as early an age as study is possible. The availability of such an auditory function strengthens the idea of early application of hearing aids to hearing-impaired infants who have sufficient residual hearing to benefit from them.

Eisenberg (1976) conducted a classic study based on response observations of newborns. She included as possible overt newborn reactions a listing that included arousal, gross body movements, orienting behavior, turning of head, wide-eyed "what-is-it" look, pupillary dilation, motor reflexes, facial grimaces, displacement of a hand or single digit, crying, or cessation of crying. Eisenberg's studies have important significance to those interested in early auditory behavior of infants. It was she who first described differences in habituation to sound as an index of CNS integrity. Newborn infants with known CNS involvement failed to extinguish their responses to repeated acoustic signals. Normal infants habituated to the repeated stimuli in a short time, a behavior known as *response decrement*. Neonates' sensory habituation to a pure tone was shown by Bridger (1961) using heart rate measures to indicate a startle response to pure tones. All babies who were tested showed a cessation of marked startle to successive stimuli presentations, provided the interval between the stimuli was less than 5 seconds. Bridger also showed that changing the frequency of the pure tone would renew the startle response after habituation to one tone, showing that babies do discriminate between frequencies.

DEVELOPMENT OF ORAL COMMUNICATION

In the most basic terms, communication has two aspects: receptive language and expressive language. Receptive language is what we hear and understand; expressive language is what we say to others. These two facets of language are very different but equally important. Good oral language development, both receptive and expressive, is a good predictor of later ability to read and write well. Receptive language is the ability to listen and understand language. Expressive language is the ability to communicate with others using language.

We recognize a special kind of speech that parents, and most adults, use when they speak to infants termed *parentese*. It has long been observed that adults speak to infants using a unique tone of voice characterized by increased pitch, animated intonation contours, and slower speech rate, and that when given a choice, infants prefer this kind of speech (Fernald, 1985; Fernald & Kuhl, 1987; Grieser & Kuhl, 1988). Of interest is the fact that parentese speech provides infants with greatly exaggerated and overly articulated prototypical samples of the phonetic units of language. When speaking to infants, adults may intuitively produce a signal that aids in speech development with their exaggerated and clear enunciation. This type of speech provides a signal that emphasizes the relevant distinctions and increases the contrast between phonetic instances. Thus, it is possible that these exaggerated but overly clear speech instances along with the great variability characteristic of infant-directed speech may actually promote learning after the normal critical period (Kuhl et al., 1997).

Babies and toddlers develop receptive language skills much earlier than their expressive language skills. At about 4 years old, most children have a speaking vocabulary of about 2,300 words but a receptive language vocabulary of about 8,000 words. Receptive vocabulary plays a big part in listening comprehension and is necessary for understanding directions and for social contact. It is difficult to state with certainty the absolute age of onset and cessation of various stages of speech development during the first year of life. However, there is agreement about the general order of succession of speech development—the onset of cooing, laughter, and reduplicated babbling follows the onset of vocal play and ultimately leads to single-word production. Receptive language development is not necessarily easy to recognize. When the baby responds to the sound of a pleasant voice, we see the beginnings of receptive language. When a baby coos in response to a familiar voice, we see the beginning of expressive language. These are signs that the baby is beginning to understand that communication is important and useful.

Between birth and 3 months, babies learn to turn to mother when she speaks, and they may smile when they hear a new voice or the dog bark. In fact, they seem to recognize familiar voices and may quiet at the onset of a new sound if they are fussing or crying. Between 4 and 6 months, babies become responsive to changes in vocal tone of voice, and to sounds other than speech. For example, they can be fascinated by toys that make sounds, enjoy music and rhythm, and show interest in all sorts of new sounds such as the kitchen sounds, birdsong, children playing, or the noise of machines.

Big changes begin to occur between the ages of 7 and 12 months and are exciting and fun as the baby now obviously listens when spoken to, turns when called by name, and discovers the fun of games like, "peek-a-boo," "I see you," and "pat-a-cake." These babies love to hear music, singing, and out-loud reading. During this period the baby recognizes the names of familiar objects ("Daddy," "car," "eyes," "phone," "key") and responds with a head shake or by facial expression to requests such as, "Give it to Granny" and simple questions, "More juice?"

We need both receptive and expressive language abilities to communicate and both begin to develop at birth. As children grow, their ability to understand and use language grows as well. Toddlers begin to respond to simple requests or questions —"Please get your shoes so we can go outside." "Would you like more juice?" This is when simple word games like "Show me your eye; your ear; your nose" begin to be enjoyable. Toddlers also begin to use one-word sentences—"Doggie!" "Candy!" "No!"—and may even use a few two-word sentences—"More juice!" "Go out!" Preschoolers usually understand most of what is said to them. They can respond to complex requests—"Put on your shoes, get your coat, and wait by the door so that we can go for a drive in the car."—and because of their increased receptive language abilities, they have good comprehension of stories and can answer simple questions about them. Their expressive language is also well developed. Preschoolers can form complex sentences—"We went to the zoo and saw the monkeys swing by their tails, and I had popcorn!" Because preschool children have better developed language abilities, this is often the age when hearing or speech problems begin to be noticeable (http://www. waisman.wisc.edu/birthto3/communica tions.pdf).

Concurrent with the maturation of the auditory function is the development of speech and language and other developmental skills. Certainly, the beginnings of language occur at birth and possibly even before birth. Condon and Sander (1974) showed that the human neonate moves in segments of movements synchronous with the articulated structure of adult speech demonstrated and that the infant is a participant in the rhythm of many repetitious speech structures long before use in communication. These rhythms comprise a prelinguistic activity of the human infant even at birth.

The infant's first use of sounds in a repetitive manner indicates the time at which the auditory feedback loop has become effective. By 2 months the baby is beginning to make certain sounds more than others. The selection of which sounds to repeat seems to depend on the nature of the sound. From 2 to 4 months these sounds are vowel-like. The sequence of use of vowels is presumably from middle (the "schwa" sound) to front and back vowels (Menyuk, 1972). By 5 months the consonant-vowel (CV) sequences begin. The back consonants (velars and glottals) predominate at 5 to 6 months of age, with some of labial (front) consonants noted. At 9 to 10 months, the glottal sounds decrease and the alveolar sounds (middle) are frequently used.

Although the infant is able to differentiate various speech sounds in the first few months of life, production of the sounds does not develop at the same rate. Berko and Brown (1969) described the lag between the perception of differences in speech signals and the production of those speech sounds. In the newborn period the infant does not produce phonated sounds, only cries and physiologic sounds.

Lieberman (1975) identified the range of format frequencies that are necessary to human speech. The well-developed pharynx, with the posterior one-third or so of the tongue forming its anterior wall, is the structural arrangement required for a wide range of formant frequencies. In the newborn and in the nonhuman primate, the hyoid bone is high in the throat, so the tongue lies completely within the oral cavity. There is little or no pharynx. As the larynx and tongue descend, a pharynx is formed and speech sound production becomes possible.

Mother's feedback of the child's sounds lays the groundwork for the first production of a word. The mother imitates the sounds the child makes, and she may add additional speech improvisations. Soon the child imitates the mother's imitations, and speech control is under way. Sometimes, the comprehension of the sound sequence precedes the imitation; sometimes, imitation precedes understanding of the meaning of the sound sequence. Films of babies as young as 2 months reveal a kind of "pre-speech" activity by movements of lips and tongue, with or without sounds (Trevarthen, 1975). Even in the second month the baby may imitate a mouth movement of the mother or a protrusion of her tongue, but this kind of behavior is most often seen after 6 months of age and only after the act is pointedly repeated in a teacher-like way. For Trevarthen, such embryonic speaking confirmed the psycholinguistic theory that language is embedded in an innate context of nonverbal communication.

This tendency of human perceptual systems to combine multimodal information (auditory and visual) to give a unified percept is a robust phenomenon as reported by Kuhl and Meltzoff (1982). In their studies, infants 18- to 20-weeks-old looked longer at a face pronouncing a vowel that matched the vowel sound they heard than at a mismatched face. Young infants apparently have knowledge about both the auditory and the visual information contained in speech. This supports the notion that the stored speech representations of infants contain information of both kinds. Thus, early perceptual learning—primarily auditory but perhaps also visual—may underpin and guide speech production development and account for infants' development of language-specific patterns by the end of the first year. Linguistic exposure is presumably the common cause of changes in both systems: Memory representations that form initially in response to perception of the ambient language input then act as guides for motor output (Kuhl & Meltzoff, 1997).

What do these studies mean in terms of differential development in children? An early study by Irwin (1947) described the early effects of different kinds of auditory input given to infants. He applied both quantitative and qualitative measures to two groups of infants from the time of birth to the age of 1 year. One group was composed of infants of highly verbal, "white-collar" and professional people; the other group was composed of infants of low-verbal, "blue-collar" workers and laborers. The variable was that the first talked a great deal directly to the infant and in its presence; the second group of parents was less communicative both to each other and to the child. The quantity and quality of their vocalizations showed that at about 3 months, something changed the vocalizations of the two groups. The infants of the highly verbal parents began to increase the number of their vocalizations and the quality of the phonemes used more rapidly than the infants of the low-verbal group. It can be inferred that by 3 months, the amount and the quality of the auditory input to these infants were already being transformed into commensurate output. The more highly stimulated infants had greater opportunity to select acoustic information and to apply it to their own auditory feedback loop. Active participation and expression resulted, but differentially in the two groups. What more pragmatic proof can there be that infants are active, not passive, in their utilization of incoming acoustic stimuli?

Carney (1996) noted that the presence of adequate hearing is critical to the development of long-term oral communication competency. The importance of hearing one's own vocalizations to develop speech cannot be overstated. Congenitally deaf infants do not naturally acquire spoken language. Deaf infants show abnormalities very early in babbling, which is an important milestone of early language acquisition. At about 7 months of age, typically developing infants across all cultures will produce this form of speech. The babbling of deaf infants, however, is maturationally delayed and lacks the temporal structure and the full range of consonant sounds of normal-hearing infants (Oller & Eilers, 1988; Stoel-Gammon & Otomo, 1986). The speech of children who become deaf prior to puberty may still deteriorate markedly without appropriate therapy. Thus, even though language production is well developed by late preadolescence, it cannot be well maintained without the ability to hear, which confirms that feedback from the sound of the speaker's own voice is crucial to the development and stabilization of speech production.

Developmental Speech Milestones

Any introductory textbook in normal childhood development or human communication will have extensive information on the development of speech in newborns, infants, and young children. In fact, every new mother's prenatal baby book usually includes ample information regarding baby's speech milestones. Pediatric audiologists must have a firm understanding of the development of speech production and perception in children with normal hearing. The following is a basic framework to aid pediatric audiologists in understanding the general milestones of speech development in the normal child so that they can contrast the typical delays in speech production demonstrated by young children with hearing disabilities. Table 3–1 provides a quick checklist to mark the expected age-specific characteristics of speech, language, and hearing development in children.

Table 3–1. Quick Checklist for Speech-Language-Hearing Milestones

Birth to 3 Months • Startles to loud noises • Calms to familiar voices • Makes vowel sounds "ooh" and "ahh"	*9 to 12 Months* • Responds differently to happy or angry talking • Turns head quickly toward loud or soft sounds • Jabbers in response to human voice • Uses two or three simple words correctly • Gives up toys when asked • Stops in response to "no" • Follows simple directions
3 to 6 Months • Makes a variety of sounds "ba-ba" and "ga-ba" • Enjoys babbling • Likes sound-making toys • Changes voice pitch at will • Turns eyes and head toward sound	*12 to 18 Months* • Identifies people, body parts, and toys on request • Turns head briskly to source of sound in all directions • Can tell you what he or she wants • Talks in what sounds like sentences • Gestures with speech appropriately • Bounces in rhythm with music • Repeats some words that you say
6 to 9 Months • Responds to own name • Imitates speech with nonspeech sounds • Plays with voice repetition, "la-la-la-la" • Understands "no" and "bye-bye" • Says "da-da" or "ma-ma" • Listens attentively to music and singing	*18 to 24 Months* • Follows simple commands • Speaks in understandable two-word phrases • Recognizes sounds in the environment • Has a vocabulary of 20 words or more

Source: Reproduced with permission from Presbyterian/St. Luke's Community Foundation, Denver, CO.

The Newborn

The most common sounds made by the newborn are cries and vowels. By the end of the first month, the cries take on meaning and mothers can differentiate anger and pain from tiredness. The noncrying sounds include normal phonation but lack resonance. Near the end of the first month the infant begins to initiate sounds characterized as "coos" and "gurgles." The newborn can discriminate between different phonemes and different intonational and stress patterns, but this auditory discrimination does not involve sound-meaning relationships.

Two to Three Months of Age

By 2 months of age the infant has developed muscle control to stop and start oral movements and vocalizations. The infant seems to focus on the production of vowel-like sounds such as "ooh" and "aah." By 3 months, babbling and laughter are likely to begin.

Four to Six Months of Age

At this stage, the infant is into strings of sound known as *true babbling* and begins to respond to noisemaking toys. There is definitely more control of the tongue. The infant may spend long periods experimenting and listening to his or her own vocalizations. At about 5 months of age, the infant vocal emissions include consonant-vowel combinations. Glottal and labial sounds are heard from the infant by the age of 6 months.

Six to Ten Months

Babbling slowly decreases at approximately 6 months of age, and during the next few months there is undistinguished progress in vocalizing speech sounds. The speech unit becomes the consonant-vowel. During this period, the mother's feedback of the child's sounds provides the groundwork for the first production of words—yet some 6 months in the future. As the infant gains increasing control of oral movements and vocalizations, speech production progresses to repetitive syllables such as "bababa" and "dadada." Menyuk (1972) showed that the frequency of consonant appearance in babbling is reflected in the order of speech-sound acquisition. With increasing age and vocal experience, the baby's babbling increasingly reflects adult speech in syllable structure and intonation. As mother (or father) imitates the sounds of the infant, and in turn begins to add additional speech improvising, the baby soon begins to imitate the parent's improvisations; the shaping of the infant's speech patterns is underway.

Comprehension of the sound sequence may precede the imitation; sometimes imitation precedes understanding of the meaning of the sound sequence which the parents learn to associate with specific facial expressions or emotions. By now the infant responds to its own name, plays with voice repetition, understands "no" and "bye-bye," may be able to repeat "ma-ma" or "da-da," and listens attentively to music or singing.

Eleven to Eighteen Months

The child's first meaningful word is usually uttered around the first birthday and is dependent on a full year of attentive listening activities. Soon after utterance of the initial word, the child begins to rapidly build a vocabulary. By 12 to 14 months the child can follow simple directions; use two to three words in a meaningful phrase; may correctly identify people, body parts, and toys by name; bounce in rhythm to music; and attempt to imitate words. By 18 months the child should have at least a 6- to 10-word vocabulary.

QUESTIONNAIRES FOR PARENTS

It is useful to get some idea from the parents as to how the child is functioning in terms of communication. The parent can be questioned either by written questionnaire or by oral query, depending on what suits the needs of the population served. A detailed developmental questionnaire for parents is presented in Table 3–2. Use of these questions may bring out facts that do not present themselves during the routine hearing test. The questions presented in Table 3–2 cover auditory behavior, communication skills, and developmental milestones of the child.

Table 3–2. Child Development Questionnaire for Parents. ([a]The pronouns "he" and "his" are used throughout in the generic sense and are intended solely to avoid the redundancy and awkwardness created by using "he or she" and "his or her.")

---

2 Months of Age

Hearing

Have you had any worry about your child's hearing?	☐ Yes	☐ No
When your child is sleeping, does he[a] move and begin to wake up to a loud sound?	☐ Yes	☐ No

Development and communication

Does he lift up his head when he is lying on his stomach?	☐ Yes	☐ No
Does your child smile at you when you are looking face to face?	☐ Yes	☐ No
Does he move both hands together in the same way?	☐ Yes	☐ No
Does he look at your face without you making gestures to him?	☐ Yes	☐ No

4 Months of Age

Hearing

Have you had any worry about your child's hearing?	☐ Yes	☐ No
When your child is sleeping, does he move and begin to wake up to a loud sound?	☐ Yes	☐ No
Does he try to turn his head toward an interesting sound or when his name is called?	☐ Yes	☐ No

Development and communication

Does he lift his head up to 90° and look straight ahead?	☐ Yes	☐ No
Does your child touch his hands together and play with them?	☐ Yes	☐ No
Does he laugh and giggle without being tickled or touched?	☐ Yes	☐ No
Does he coo to himself and make noises when he is alone?	☐ Yes	☐ No

6 Months of Age

Hearing

Have you had any worry about your child's hearing?	☐ Yes	☐ No
When your child is sleeping, does he move and begin to wake up to a loud sound?	☐ Yes	☐ No
Does he try to turn his head toward an interesting sound or when his name is called?	☐ Yes	☐ No

Development and communication

Does he lift his head and chest with his arms?	☐ Yes	☐ No
Does he keep his head steady when sitting? Does he roll over in his crib?	☐ Yes	☐ No
Does he reach for objects within his reach and hold them?	☐ Yes	☐ No
Does he see small objects like peas or raisins?	☐ Yes	☐ No

8 Months of Age

Hearing

Have you had any worry about your child's hearing?	☐ Yes	☐ No

continues

Table 3–2. *continued*

When your child is sleeping, does he move and begin to wake up to a loud sound?	☐ Yes	☐ No
Does he try to turn his head toward an interesting sound or when his name is called?	☐ Yes	☐ No
Does he enjoy ringing a bell, playing with a noisy toy, or shaking a rattle?	☐ Yes	☐ No

Development and communication

Does he support most of his weight on his legs?	☐ Yes	☐ No
Can he sit alone without help for 5 minutes?	☐ Yes	☐ No
Can he sit and look for objects that have fallen out of sight?	☐ Yes	☐ No
Can he pick up two objects, one in each hand?	☐ Yes	☐ No
Can he transfer an object from one hand to the other?	☐ Yes	☐ No
Can he feed himself a cracker?	☐ Yes	☐ No
Does he make a number of different sounds and change their pitch?	☐ Yes	☐ No
Does he clap his hands in imitation and make noises at the same time?	☐ Yes	☐ No

10 Months of Age

Hearing

Have you had any worry about your child's hearing?	☐ Yes	☐ No
When your child is sleeping, does he move and begin to wake up to a loud sound?	☐ Yes	☐ No
Does he turn his head toward an interesting sound or when his name is called?	☐ Yes	☐ No
Does he try to imitate you if you make his own sounds?	☐ Yes	☐ No

Development and communication

Does he play peek-a-boo with you?	☐ Yes	☐ No
Can he stand for at least 5 seconds, holding on to a crib or chair?	☐ Yes	☐ No
Does he try to hold a toy when it is pulled away?	☐ Yes	☐ No
Is he shy or afraid of strangers?	☐ Yes	☐ No

12 Months of Age

Hearing

Have you had any worry about your child's hearing?	☐ Yes	☐ No
When your child is sleeping, does he move and begin to wake up to a loud sound?	☐ Yes	☐ No
Does he turn his head toward an interesting sound or when his name is called?	☐ Yes	☐ No
Is he beginning to repeat some of the sounds you make?	☐ Yes	☐ No

Development and communication

Can he pick up tiny objects with his fingers such as a raisin or candy?	☐ Yes	☐ No
Can he get to a sitting position without help?	☐ Yes	☐ No
Does he wave bye-bye or play pat-a-cake when you encourage him?	☐ Yes	☐ No
Can he say "mamma" or "dada" appropriately?	☐ Yes	☐ No

If any category indicates developmental delay, the child may benefit from referral for additional evaluation. The questionnaire includes information on developmental status and communication abilities in addition to the questions concerning hearing status. It is recommended that this kind of questionnaire be used as a screening device to identify other problems that might benefit from treatment at an early age. The hearing questions are separated from the developmental questions because most of the commonly used developmental milestones are present in otherwise-normal deaf babies and, therefore, would not identify a hearing loss.

Some knowledge of the attributes of the deaf is necessary for the questioner to understand why the questions in Table 3–2 are worded as they are. For example, a deaf child will look around or will wake up when a door slams, when someone stamps a foot on the floor, when a large truck rolls by on the street, or when a loud airplane flies low overhead. Therefore, if the parent states that the child awakens to a loud sound, the parent must be asked to specify the type of sound, because clearly the perception of vibration may actually be the stimulus involved. Another characteristic of the deaf infant is that he or she may be unusually visually alert and may be especially attentive to movements in peripheral vision. Therefore, if the parent reports that the child turns around to an interesting sound or name, the parent must be asked if the sound is out of the child's peripheral visual field.

Profoundly deaf babies do babble, but their productions rapidly become unlike those of hearing infants. Until the age of 6 months the deaf infant sounds to the uninitiated person much like the normal-hearing infant. The deaf infant vocalizes when the parent appears and coos just as the normal-hearing child does. Only an expert phonetician can identify the subtle qualitative differences in the babbling sounds that the deaf child makes.

A common misleading indication is a parent's report that the baby says "mamma" at around the age of 1 year and that, therefore, the baby must be hearing at that point in time. Oddly enough, the parents of most deaf children make just such a report, and it is universally true that a profoundly deaf infant appears to be saying "mamma" at around 1 year of age. Actually, what the baby is saying is "amah," which is the most primitive sound that can be made, involving as it does the almost animal-like "ah" vocalization plus the coming together of the lips. It has been postulated that one of the reasons for the "amah" development is that in infancy the baby is carried close to the mother, feels the vibrations or hears low frequencies of the mother's voice, and thus is stimulated to perpetuate the sounds. At any rate, the sounds soon drop off, and nothing remains except the "ah" vocalization in a strident voice.

To be sure, it is recognized that speech develops at different rates in children depending on a wide variety of factors. The growth in word output is nothing less than astonishing as the child matures. At 1 year of age the toddler is likely to have about 20 words; by 2 years of age, 200 to 300 words; by 3 years of age, 900 to 1,000 words. By age 4, the language acquisition of children has exploded: the 4-year-old will have 1,500 words, and by 5 years of age the child might have as many as 2,500 words with more than 20,000 words in their receptive memory. Often it is the pediatric audiologist, listening to a child's speech patterns for the first time, who is in a position to recognize speech delay or inappropriate speech for the child's age. Generally, when speech problems are identified, the audiologist should be prepared to recommend that a full evaluation be performed by a qualified speech-language pathologist. Matkin (1984) organized some general guidelines as presented in Table 3–3 to assist in knowing when the child's speech patterns require referral for further evaluation.

STUDIES OF SPEECH DEVELOPMENT

The development of speech has been intensively studied at the phonological level and is a topic of focus for speech-language pathologists. Phonetic units are the small-

Table 3–3. Referral Guidelines for Children With Speech Delay

By 12 months
No differentiated babbling or vocal imitation
By 18 months
No use of single words
By 24 months
Less than 10 single words
By 30 months
Fewer than 100 words
No two-word combinations
Unintelligible speech
By 36 months
Fewer than 200 words
No telegraphic sentences
Clarity of speech less than 50%
By 48 months
Fewer than 600 words
No use of simple sentences
Clarity of speech less than 80%

Source: From "Early Recognition and Referral of Hearing-Impaired Children," by N. Matkin, 1984, *Pediatrics in Review, 6*, p. 153.

est elements that can alter the meaning of a word in any language, for example the difference between /r/ and /l/ in the words "rid" and "lid" in American English. Phonemes refer to the phonetic units critical for meaning in a particular language. The phonetic difference between /r/ and /l/ is phonemic in English, for example, but not in Japanese. Each phonetic unit can be described as a bundle of phonetic features that indicate the manner in which the sound was produced and the place in the mouth where the articulators (tongue, lips, teeth) were placed to create the sound. The acoustic cues that signal phonetic units have been well documented and include both spectral and temporal features of sound. For instance, the distinction between /d/ and /g/ depends primarily on the frequency content of the initial burst in spectral energy at the beginning of the sound, and the direction of formant transition change. The temporal acoustic dimension of speech is voice-onset time (VOT), which describes the timing of periodic laryngeal vibration (voicing) in relation to the beginning of the syllable. This timing difference provides the critical cue used to identify whether a speech sound is voiced or voiceless (e.g., /b/ versus /p/, /d/ versus /t/) and is a classic distinction used in many speech studies (Doupe & Kuhl, 1999).

Menyuk (1972) suggests that experimental results comparing primate vocalizations with those of human infants and adults "indicate that speaking is not simply a learned overlaid function on the muscles and structures of breathing and eating, but that man is preprogrammed to develop a vocal mechanism that is specifically adapted to produce speech." Studies of the development of infant vocalization show a logical, orderly sequence of utterances between the initial sounds made by the baby until the first words are achieved. As the infant's one-word vocabulary grows beginning at about 12 months, the frequency of babbling declines until it is entirely omitted between 18 and 20 months of age. Measurements of the fundamental frequency of the baby's voice (*Fo*) were made by Kent (1976). He showed that during the first 3 weeks of life, /b/ is around 400 Hz; then it increases to around 480 Hz by the fourth month, where it stabilizes for 5 months. At 1 year it begins to decrease sharply and levels off at 300 Hz at 3 years.

Babies babble, producing initial vocalizations of consonant-vowel syllables that are strung together (e.g., "bababa" or "mamama"). These beginning sounds are gradually molded to resemble adult vocalizations. The result of this vocal development is that adults produce a stereotyped repertoire of acoustic elements: These are relatively fixed for a given individual, but they vary between individuals and groups (as in languages and dialects). This variability is a reflection of the fact that vocal production by individuals is limited to a subset of all sounds that can be produced by that species. Layered on top of the developing capacity to produce particular acoustic elements is the development of sequencing of these elements: For speech and language this means learning and ordering sounds to create words and, at a higher level, sentences and grammar. Most important in infants is that there exist group differences in vocal production that clearly depend on experience. Obviously, people learn the language to which they are exposed. Moreover, even within a specific language, dialects are mimicked and learned by babies (Doupe & Kuhl, 1999).

Regardless of the linguistic community in which they are raised, babies begin by cooing, then producing reduplicated CV syllables, and finally "variegated" babbling with sentence-like intonational patterns (Oller, 1978, 1980). By 1 month, typical cooing and gurgling sounds are made in addition to the crying; by 3 months, true babbling begins. True babbling consists of the pleasurable repetition of sounds. Babbling is not easily defined in terms of phonetic or acoustic characteristics. Babbling is defined by Kent, Osberger, Netsell, and Hustedde (1987) as "an infant's vocal behavior excepting the so-called vegetative sounds associated with respiratory and gastric events and sounds of obvious distress or discomfort (such as cry or fuss sounds)." Stoel-Gammon and Otomo (1986) define babbling as "relative speech-like utterances." The sounds produced by infants include reduplicated syllables, sustained fricatives and trills, prolonged vocalic phonations, prolonged nasal murmurs, grunt-like short vowels, and complex sequences in which variations can be heard in manner, place, voicing, or any combinations of these (Kent et al., 1987).

The last stage of progress in the vocal capabilities required for the production of speech-like syllables is called the *canonical stage*. Canonical babble is the well-defined mature syllables, a clear vocalic sound with consonant margins that appears between 5 and 8 months of age. The canonical stage is followed typically by strings of syllables that are so speech-like that parents often assert that the infant is talking. These canonical syllables are not used in association with word meaning, but they are certainly the precursors to spoken language (Oller & Eilers, 1988). The differences between the vocalizations of hearing infants and deaf infants are important to note, and considerable new evidence supports the need for early auditory experiences critical to the development of canonical babbling and ultimately speech.

In a convincing study of infant vocalizations from 94 babies with normal hearing and 37 infants with severe to profound hearing impairment, Eilers and Oller (1994) showed that the vocal differences between the two groups were not subtle, but rather were salient and striking. The onset of the canonical stage virtually always occurs by 11 months of age (range, 3 to 10 months) in normally developing, hearing infants. In deaf infants, however, careful studies of the onset of canonical babbling showed significantly delayed development in this speech stage until 11 months or older, often well into the third year of life (range, 11 to 49 months, with a mode onset at 24 months). In their study, no deaf infant ever reached the canonical stage before 11 months of age. The fact that there was no overlap in the distribution of the onset of canonical babbling between infants with normal hearing and infants with hearing impairment led to the suggestion that the failure of otherwise healthy infants to produce canonical syllables before the age of 11 months should be considered a serious risk factor for the presence of hearing impairment. Eilers and Oller noted that as the infants with hearing impairment were fitted with amplification, there was significant correlation between the onset of canonical babbling and the age at which hearing aids were fit.

Up to 5 or 6 months of age, the sounds made by the infant do not seem to be related to the speech sounds heard. The infant's productive capacity for speech lags significantly behind his or her demonstrated ability to perceive differences. From our observations of otherwise normal deaf infants, their vocalizations are identical to those of normal infants until 5 or 6 months. Furthermore, deaf infants increase their vocalizations when parents speak to them, just as normal infants do. It is obvious that the reason for this increase in vocalizations is not the baby's hearing the parent's voice. We postulate that it is a preadaptive, reflexive response stimulated by the presence of the parent's face, much as is the smile response that appears at the same age. The phenomenon of increased vocalization may be a milestone that is predictive of eventual communication skills. Certainly, the established fact that the auditory feedback loop is present at birth indicates that the elementary babbling sounds have a significant prelinguistic function. The lack of auditory feedback in the deaf child deprives him or her of early prelinguistic experiences.

An important research project was conducted by Stoel-Gammon and Otomo (1986) during which they produced phonetic transcriptions of babbling samples from 11 normal-hearing babies aged 4 to 18 months and compared their findings with phonetic transcriptions that they obtained from 11 infants with hearing loss aged 4 to 28 months. The normal-hearing babies showed an increase in size of their consonantal repertoires with age in contrast to the hearing-impaired babies, who had smaller repertoires that decreased over time. A comparison of multisyllabic utterances showed a general tendency for the hearing-impaired infants to produce fewer multisyllabic utterances containing true consonants and for some of the hearing-impaired babies to produce a high proportion of vocalizations with glides or glottal stops. This study confirmed both qualitative and quantitative differences in the babbling development of infants with normal hearing and infants with hearing loss.

Because their study included infants with varying degrees of hearing loss, Stoel-Gammon and Otomo noted that although all the hearing-impaired babies' babbling development was different from that of the normal-hearing infants, the magnitude of difference appeared to be smaller for those with moderate hearing loss compared with those with severe to profound hearing loss. The parental histories obtained in this study suggested not only that normal prelinguistic and early linguistic development (i.e., onset of babbling and meaningful vocal play) was arrested as a result of sudden onset of deafness, but also that the developing speech patterns reverted to behaviors resembling those predominating at earlier stages of development.

This study and others showed the important link between random articulatory movements and the resulting acoustic outcomes to the presence of self-monitoring through the auditory sense. The inability of hearing-impaired babies to hear their own vocalizations prevents them from the acoustic self-stimulation that encourages additional babbling and the consequential expansion of new speech sounds. The results obtained by Stoel-Gammon and Otomo suggest that significant hearing loss affects prelinguistic vocalizations by 8 months of age and possibly earlier. In their analysis of consonantal utterances, the point of divergence between their two groups of subjects was around 6 to 8 months, implying that at that age hearing loss began to influence the development of the consonantal repertoire.

By 5 months of age, Chinese children produce the intonation of the Chinese language. Also, by 5 months of age Polish infants' babbling can be distinguished from the babbling of English infants (Weir, 1966). The later skills of linguistic organization are undoubtedly dependent on these early activities. Field, Woodson, Greenberg, and Cohen (1982) found that infants between 12 and 21 days of age could imitate both facial and manual gestures. Even sequential finger movement (opening and closing the hand by serially moving the fingers) was imitated. The infant enters the world equipped with skills that appear innate to humans. Even facial expressions can be discriminated, according to Field, Woodson, Greenberg, and Cohen (1982). They exposed 74 neo-

nates (average, 36 hours) to three facial expressions (happy, sad, and surprised) and observed diminished visual fixation on each face over trials. The fixations were renewed on presentation of a different expression. What was surprising was that the babies made imitative facial movements that clued observers to the expressions of the model, at greater than chance accuracy.

Speech can be described at many different levels. It can be written, spoken, or signed (using manual language such as American Sign Language or Cued Speech). In all these forms, language consists of a string of words ordered by the rules of grammar to convey meaning. Structurally, language can be analyzed from the standpoint of semantics (conceptual representation), syntax (word order), prosody (the pitch, rhythm, and tempo of an utterance), the lexicon (words), or phonology (the elementary building blocks, phonemes, that are combined to make up words) (Doupe & Kuhl, 1999).

A most intriguing opportunity for research in speech development presented itself to Kent et al. (1987) when they identified two identical twin boys, one of whom had a severe-to-profound, bilateral hearing loss and one of whom had normal hearing. The etiology of the hearing loss was undetermined, although the infant was first suspected to have hearing loss when he failed a routine hospital-screening test. Auditory brainstem evoked response and behavioral testing confirmed his hearing loss, and he was fitted with binaural ear-level hearing aids and enrolled in habilitative services at the age of 3 months. These twin boys offered a rare opportunity to study the effects of hearing loss on vocal development with reasonable control over environmental and genetic factors. The primary objectives of the study conducted by Kent et al. (1987) were to obtain longitudinal information on:

(a) fundamental frequency levels and contours, (b) formant frequencies of vocalic utterances, and (c) spectral characteristics of fricatives and trills. The acoustic data were collected via video and audio while the twins interacted with each other and with an adult (parent or investigator). The twins were evaluated at approximately 3 month intervals, beginning at the age of 8 months, again at 12 months, and again at 15 months.

The results of this unique investigation are presented for syllable shapes, formant patterns, and phonetic inventories obtained from transcriptions of the audiotapes of the twins between 8 and 15 months of age. Histograms of peak fundamental frequencies of syllable productions of the child with normal hearing (called Ned) and the child with hearing loss (called Hal) recorded at the twins' age of 8 months are shown in Figure 3–2. According to the research team, Hal often showed a phonatory pattern in his utterances that was highly vari-

able, and his hearing-impaired twin had a larger range of peak fundamental frequency values and a higher model value as shown in the histograms. The composite data for vocalic formant frequencies Fl and F2 were determined from spectrograms and plotted as shown in Figures 3–3 and 3–4. The composite Fl-F2 results for Ned, the normal-hearing twin (Figure 3–3), show a configuration of the vowel region over the developmental period. A very different pattern is shown for Hal in Figure 3–4, where the developmental pattern is one of marked constriction such that by the age of 15 months the Fl–F2 region is contained within the low-frequency portion of the pattern exhibited at 8 months.

As would be expected from the syllable structure data, Hal and Ned differed significantly in their consonant productions. Of special interest is the fact that unlike the normal-hearing twin—who produced fricatives at several places of articulation, including

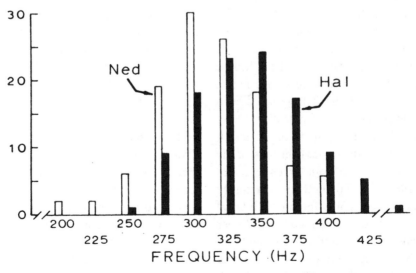

Figure 3–2. Histograms of peak fundamental frequencies of syllable productions of Ned and Hal at 8 months. Reproduced with permission from "Phonetic Development in Identical Twins Differing in Auditory Function," by K. D. Kent et al., 1987, *Journal of Speech and Hearing Research, 52,* p. 66.

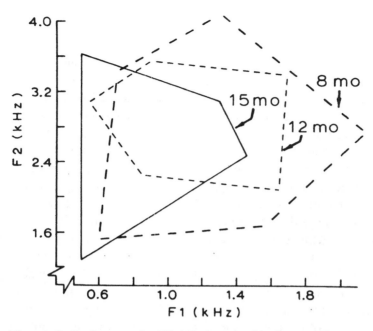

Figure 3–3. Composite F1–F2 data for Ned's vocalic segments at 8, 12, and 15 months. Reproduced with permission from "Phonetic Development in Identical Twins Differing in Auditory Function," by K. D. Kent et al., 1987, *Journal of Speech and Hearing Research, 52,* p. 67.

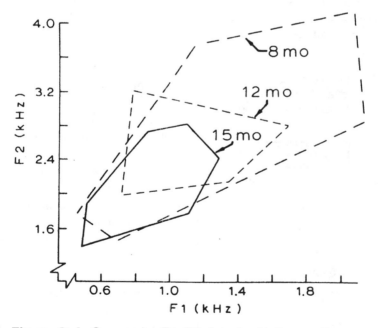

Figure 3–4. Composite F1–F2 data for Hal's vocalic segments at 8, 12, and 15 months. Reproduced with permission from "Phonetic Development in Identical Twins Differing in Auditory Function," by K. D. Kent et al., 1987, *Journal of Speech and Hearing Research, 52,* p. 68.

labiodental, alveolar, palatal, and pharyngeal—Hal was not heard to make even a single fricative sound. Table 3–4 shows the frequency of occurrence data for place of consonant production in the spontaneous vocalizations of Hal and Ned at 24 months. Although Hal's syllable production was greatly diversified at 24 months compared with 8 months, his vocalizations continued to be narrower in range than those of Ned. In their summary, Kent et al. indicate that the spontaneous vocalizations of the twin boys were clearly different as early as 8 months of age. The twin with hearing loss had vocal productions that were much less variable than those of the normal-hearing twin, with a fundamental frequency variability that had a wide range extending from a glottal roll to a shriek. The twin with hearing loss had a restricted range of vowel production and few consonants as late as 15 months of age. This incredible research study has provided the basis of quantitative speech science differences in a unique

Table 3–4. Frequency of Occurrence Data for Place of Consonant Production in the Spontaneous Vocalizations of Hal and Ned at 24 Months of Age

Place	Hal	Ned
Bilabial	12 (15%)	29 (43%)
Dental	1 (1%)	9 (13%)
Alveolar	60 (77%)	15 (22%)
Palatal	4 (5%)	5 (7%)
Velar	0 (0%)	5 (7%)
Glottal	1 (1%)	6 (9%)
Total	78	67

Source: With permission from "Phonetic Development in Identical Twins Differing in Auditory Function," by K. D. Kent, M. J. Osberger, R. Netsell, & C. G. Hustedde, 1987, *Journal of Speech and Hearing Research, 52,* p. 69.

study sample (identical twins) in which genetic and environmental differences can be assumed to be minimal.

Characteristic changes in speech production occur as a child learns to talk, regardless of culture. All infants progress through a set of universal stages of speech production during their first year: Early in life, infants produce nonspeech gurgles and cries; at 3 months, infants coo, producing simple vowel-like sounds; by 7 months infants begin to babble; and by 1 year, first words appear. The capability for vocal motor learning is thus available very early in life. Although speech production skills improve throughout childhood, showing that auditory-articulatory brain maps continue to evolve over a long period, the early vocal imitation capacities of infants indicate that these maps must also be sufficiently formed by 20 weeks of age to allow infants to approximate sounds produced by others (Kuhl & Meltzoff, 1996).

Cross-cultural studies reveal that by 10 to 12 months of age, the spontaneous vocalizations of infants from different language environments begin to differ, reflecting the influence of ambient language (Kuhl, Williams, Lacerda, Stebens, & Lindblom, 1992). Thus, by the end of the first year of life, infants diverge from the culturally universal speech pattern they initially exhibit to one that is specific to their culture, indicating that vocal learning has taken place. The remarkable ability of infants to imitate the speech patterns is evident before the end of their first year.

Research has shown that babies learn the basics of their native language by the age of 6 months, long before they utter their first words. Newborns are "language universalists" in that they can learn any sound in any language and distinguish among all the sounds that adults utter. A language-specific pattern emerges in speech perception prior to its emergence in speech production. For instance, although infant vocalizations produced spontaneously in natural settings do not become language specific until 10 to 12 months of age, the perceptual system shows specificity much earlier (Kuhl et al., 1992). Continued exposure to their native language, however, reduces babies' ability to perceive sounds that are not in that language set. The Kuhl group used computerized speech to generate identical English and Swedish sounds that were presented to 64 6-month-old babies in a double-blind experiment conducted in both the United States and Sweden. The infants showed a significantly stronger preference for and accuracy in identifying the sounds from their own language. This important study demonstrates again that linguistic experience during the first 6 months of life affects an infant's perception of speech sounds.

Studies of auditory localization (identifying the source of a sound in space) of very young infants are also amazing (Bower, 1975). Young babies observed their mothers through a soundproof glass screen, with the voices of the mothers coming at various positions of a loudspeaker. So long as the sound came from where the mother was, the baby was quite happy. But when the voice came from a speaker in another position, the infants manifested surprise and upset, indicating not only auditory localization but also an expectation that voices will come from mouths. Clifton (1998) demonstrated experimentally in newborns that normal-hearing infants show dramatic improvement in precision of localization ability within the first year of life, when the minimum audible angle detectable decreases from more than 20 degrees to approximately 8 degrees. Infants must make constant adjustments between timing and localization based on visual feedback to be able to improve performance over time.

Sininger et al. (1999) state that localization ability is a clear example of the way in which human newborns integrate auditory experience (in this case with visual experience) to rapidly develop near-normal function in the first year of life. Adults seem to be unaware or to have lost such localization, being unaware for example that voices in movies come from a place other than the screen.

The long period of reception of auditory language symbols is the prerequisite to later language formulation. By the time speech and language emerge, there have been 12 to 18 months of receiving complex adult spoken language and distilling it into the matrix of the child language structure. This act of refining out of a complex language structure the basic one- and two-word sentences that are the baby's first speech language utterances must rank as creation's noblest day. Listening to language for a long period is essential to the ultimate usage of language. From the studies described above, it is evident that this listening is not a passive process but one in which the infant participates by acting on the incoming signals. By the time the child's first meaningful word is uttered, miraculously full blown at around 12 months of age, a whole world of listening activity has taken place. Nothing the infant will ever achieve is as intellectually complex as what preceded that first speech utterance.

OPTIMAL PERIODS

Plasticity of the brain is maximal during optimal periods of time during development (also referred to as critical or sensitive time periods). During the critical period, some crucial experience will have its peak effect on development or learning which results in normal behavior attuned to the particular environment to which the organism is exposed. If the organism is not exposed to this experience until after this time period, the same experience will have only a reduced effect or perhaps no effect at all. Optimal theory suggests that after the critical period has passed in time, the brain may never again show the same ability to make big changes in neuronal connectivity (Mundkur, 2005). A critical period for any behavior is defined as a specific phase of the life cycle of an organism in which there is enhanced sensitivity to experience, or to the absence of a particular experience. One of the most universally known and cited critical periods is that for human language acquisition.

Babies learn their complex vocalizations early in life during critical periods. Their vocalizations depend heavily on hearing the adults they will imitate, as well as hearing themselves as they practice. Babies undergo an early phase of learning that is primarily perceptual, which then serves to guide later vocal production. Infants demonstrate innate predispositions for perceiving, learning, and expressing correct sounds. Humans have evolved a complex hierarchy of specialized forebrain areas in which motor and auditory centers interact closely in the production of speech and language (Doupe & Kuhl, 1999).

The urgency of providing appropriate early intervention services is supported by evidence of reduced and limited success of intervention strategies that are initiated after the sensitive period for language and auditory development (Moeller, 2000; Yoshinaga-Itano et al., 1998).

If we apply the optimal or critical period theory to the child with hearing impairment, we might ask how early is it necessary for the hearing-deprived child to receive language input to avoid serious language problems? The critical period of natural language acquisition is the first 6 years of life, and thereafter the ability to acquire language declines gradually. Normal hearing children whose caregivers speak with them regularly tend to develop and display good language skills. However, children who are rarely spoken to tend to have reduced language skills. Researchers have established that there are certain periods in human development when we are programmed to receive and utilize particular types of stimuli, and that subsequently those stimuli will have diminishing potency in affecting development in the function represented. In the case of audition, it means that at a certain developmental stage auditory signals will be optimally received and utilized for important prelinguistic activities, but that once this stage has passed, the effective utilization of these signals gradually declines. An analogous theory for language development holds that language input must be experienced at a certain stage or it becomes decreasingly effective for utilization in emergent language skills. This is probably the basis of the proverb, "You can't teach old dog new tricks." However, knowledge of the plasticity of the brain has opened new doors for various therapies, including sports training, wherein repetition exploits the neuroplasticity of the brain to retrain the cortex and form new pathways.

The basis of vocal learning is the perception of sounds, the production of sounds, and the crucial ability to relate the two. At birth, evidence suggests that infants have an innate perceptual predisposition for the vocal behavior of humans. Vocal perception and production are tightly interwoven in the vocal learning process (Doupe & Kuhl, 1999). It is clear that beyond the critical periods, we do not learn communicative skills equally well at all phases of life. For example, we have all struggled with the learning, perceiving, and expressing of a second language later in life (i.e., high school, college, and senior classes in foreign language), while admiring the abilities of very young children to learn that second language with ease if exposed and experienced during younger and more neuroplastic times of life.

Lenneberg (1967) is of the opinion that puberty marks the last milestone for acquisition of language. With regard to the effects of early deprivation, he cites the difference between the congenitally deaf child and the child who acquires deafness through meningitis after a brief exposure to language. He states that those who lose hearing after having been exposed to the experience of speech, even for as short a period as 1 year, can be trained much more easily in all language arts, even if formal training begins some years after they had become deaf. According to Lenneberg, "It seems as if even a short exposure to language, a brief moment during which the curtain has been lifted and oral communication established, is sufficient to give a child some foundation on which much later language may be based." He formulated the strongest claims for a critical or sensitive period for speech learning, noting that after puberty it is much more difficult to acquire a second language. Lenneberg argued that language learning after puberty was qualitatively different, more conscious and labored, as opposed to the automatic and unconscious acquisition that occurs in young children as a result of mere exposure to language. Late experience, beyond the critical period, misses the window of opportunity for language learning, making it more difficult, if not impossible, to acquire native language patterns of listening and speaking.

In a well-designed study, Templin (1966) compared the language skills of deaf children with the skills of matched groups of normal-hearing children. In some of the language areas the deaf showed no systematic improvement in their performance beyond 11 years. At that point such skills as understanding of word meanings, sentence construction, and analogies reached a plateau and remained there without further insights or improvements. The normal-hearing children went on to achieve to the 14-year language level that was the upper limits of the study. It should be emphasized that there was no substantial difference in intellectual abilities between the deaf and the normal-hearing group and that the deaf had intensive language training in their schools. Their rate of learning up to 11 years was comparable with that of the normal-hearing group. But an irreversible language deficit appeared at this age level and precluded further development. The complexity of language forms and of abstract language symbols takes a great leap around this age and leaves the deaf helplessly behind. The blame was ascribed to early language deprivation covering many periods optimal for language learning.

Yoshinaga-Itano and Apuzzo (1995) compared the language abilities of 46 hearing-impaired children identified before 6 months of age with 63 similar children identified after 6 months of age. All the children had bilateral hearing losses ranging from mild to profound. In longitudinal evaluations of both groups, a consistent advantage existed for the group identified before 6 months of age. The language skills advantage for the early identified children became more pronounced as the children aged. For children assessed between 13 and 18 months, there was only a slight advantage for the early group compared with the late group. For children in the 19- to 24-month-old category, the early group showed a 3-month developmental advantage; for children in the 25- to 30-month category, the early children showed a 4-month advantage. By the age of 31 to 36 months, the children identified early had a 10-month language advantage over the late identified group. Although these studies speak volumes for support of early intervention, they also reflect results that may be interpreted in favor of optimal period theory.

The reports of animal research supporting optimal period theory of development are numerous. Reisen (1947) reported that a chimpanzee raised in total darkness for the first 3 months of life never developed adequate vision. However, if chimpanzees are raised in light for the first 3 months and subjected to total darkness for the next 6 months, they quickly regain perfect vision when exposed to light. The analogous situation in humans is found in the child born with strabismus of one eye (thrown to a side focus). Ophthalmologists report that unless that eye is forced to be used, through patching the other eye, by the age of 4 no useful perceptions can ever be developed in it despite the fact that organically it is a perfect organ of vision. It is the central perception of vision that, untrained during critical periods, can never regain function. There seems to be no demonstrated reason why auditory perceptions do not fall into the same category as the visual modality.

According to Sininger et al. (1999), mice raised in a regular sound environment have, as expected, normal development in the neurons of the auditory nervous system, whereas mice exposed to noxious stimuli throughout development showed non-normal neurons in the auditory pathway. Other animal studies have shown that the type of acoustic stimulation to which the auditory nervous system is exposed determines its mature response pattern. Reisen (1960) reported that chimpanzees showed a reduction in the efficiency of auditory learning following early sensory deprivation of hearing. In addition, he found that in cats deprived of visual sensation, three concomitant manifestations were present: hyperexcitability, increased susceptibility to convulsive disorder, and localized motor dysfunction.

These animal experiments have profound implications for the student of human development with profound deafness. What is the effect of language deprivation on the deaf infant? If biologic theories of language acquisition are correct, then the human infant is just as preprogrammed to develop language skills as to develop motor skills. The effect of early sensory deprivation could then be expected to have far-reaching consequences on CNS functioning in integrative areas of the brain. The concept of language as a biologically predetermined function thus extends the speculation of early sensory deprivation in humans to another plane where animal research cannot apply. What are the effects of early learning deprivation on the CNS? Many clinicians have described symbolic language disorder, minimal cerebral dysfunction, or other kinds of central involvement in the deaf. Can these disorders be a direct result of auditory deprivation?

Edwards (1968) described the educator's attitude toward optimal periods in words that still ring true today: The supremely difficult feat of building language recognition and response which takes place during the first years of life can occur because there is a built-in neurological mechanism for language learning present in every normal human organism. But like the image on the sensitized negative, this potential will not appear as reality unless the proper circumstances develop it. Experience—the right experience—is essential.

Heredity and environment interact. Hereditary possibilities are shaped by the influence that only human culture can provide; they are potentialities that must be developed while the young neurological organism is still rapidly growing, malleable, and open to stimulus. If the "critical periods in learning" hypothesis applies to human beings, then the right experience must come at the right time, or the potential must remain forever unrealized.

Considered from the physiologic point of view, the infant's auditory system is plastic (i.e., it can be modified not only by anatomic alteration but also by variations of acoustic stimuli). Absent or faulty sound stimuli will result in deviant auditory function. According to Ruben and Rapin (1980), the central and peripheral auditory systems exert reciprocal control over each other. As the inner ear matures, its input is necessary to the development of at least part of the auditory nervous system. By the time the peripheral auditory system is fully developed, its input seems to be necessary for the maturation and innervations of portions of the central auditory system (Clopton & Silverman, 1977; Webster & Webster, 1977, 1979, 1980). Therefore, environmental sounds have the greatest effect in shaping auditory ability from the time the inner ear and eighth cranial nerve first become functional to the time when maturation of the CNS is achieved, roughly from the fifth month of gestation to between 18 and 28 months. The consequences of these findings for intervention programs for the hearing impaired are strikingly apparent. The time for action is early in the first year of life, as demonstrated by numerous studies described in this chapter.

Consider the results of a classic study conducted at the Lexington School for the Deaf (Greenstein, Greenstein, McConville, et al., 1976). Thirty children with severe hearing loss who had been admitted to the school before their second birthdays were studied. Two groups were identified: those who had been admitted before 16 months of age and those admitted between 16 and 24 months of age. The children were given standardized tests that revealed that the children admitted before 16 months of age were consistently superior to the later-admitted children in all aspects and at all age levels. Regardless of what caused the differences, its occurrence before 16 months was the variable responsible for the improved speech and language. Here is evidence relating learning ability in the hearing impaired to time of identification of the hearing loss.

Learning is critical to the development of speech. Infants do not learn to speak if they are not exposed to the communication from others. We have looked to studies of children who have been socially and sensorally deprived since infancy to shed light on the periods necessary for acquisition of language. The 1797 "wild boy of Aveyron" remained mute and incapable of even subtle communication even after Dr. Itard attempted to teach and socialize him in his preteen years (Lane, 1977). The description of Genie (Fromkin, Krashen, Curtiss, Rigler, & Rigler, 1974), who was isolated in a closet for 11 years of her life, states that this is "a case of language acquisition beyond the 'critical period.'" However, Genie's history shows that she was exposed to family life for her first 20 months before being placed in isolation until age 13 years, 9 months. The reported language abilities that she acquired after being rescued from a pitiful situation are actually what one could predict for anyone having had 20 months of normal language input. Thus, the critical periods for language during which Genie had exposure laid the matrix from which her ultimate language skills could develop. The need for social auditory experience with others is evident in these rare studies of children raised in abnormal social settings. These instances in which infants with normal hearing were not exposed to human speech provide dramatic evidence that in the absence of hearing speech from other individuals, speech does not develop normally.

LISTENING

In talking with preschool teachers of the deaf, it is commonly agreed that the most important teaching task when hard-of-hearing or deaf toddlers initially arrive in the school classroom, has to do with listening. These young children with significant hearing loss often have little or no awareness of sounds and they have not had the opportunity to learn the association of specific sounds that occur in the environment around them. The prerequisite skill required to learn both receptive and expressive speech and language is listening. Success in listening requires attentive behavior that also must be taught. Once the children begin to learn the concept that attention to sound requires active listening, learning will follow. It may be slow and laborious, one vocabulary word or one environmental sound at a time, but it is a rewarding experience to observe young deaf toddlers develop listening skills (Figure 3–5). Estabrooks and Marlowe (2000) developed a very useful checklist of listening skills formatted in a hierarchy and continuum that begins with noting the ability of the child to respond to the presence or absence of a single sound through a number of listening attributes resulting in the understanding of continu-

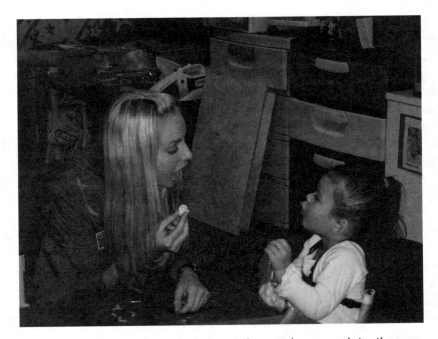

Figure 3–5. Through early intervention and appropriate therapy, the child with hearing loss develops speech sounds into phonemes, then into words, and finally into sentences complete with appropriate expression and speech patterns. Photo courtesy of H.O.P.E. Preschool, Spokane, WA.

ous speech. As the hard-of-hearing or deaf child learns to identify similarities and differences between two or more speech stimuli, and gains the ability to attend to differences among various sounds, and then finally displays appropriately different responses to various sounds, true listening will have been achieved, leading the way to more learning achievements.

Listening and hearing are not the same. Hearing is simply the act of perceiving sound by the ear; listening, however, is an event that includes cortical activity. Listening requires concentration so that the brain processes meaning from words and sentences. The sounds we hear have no meaning until we give them their meaning in context. Active listening, on the other hand, is a process that constructs meaning from both verbal and nonverbal messages. In contrast to active listening, much of our listening is done on an "incidental" basis while we "overhear" ongoing sounds and conversations happening around us.

Hearing can be explained on a scientific and biological basis, but listening is a psychological process requiring internal contextual contemplation of the perceived sound waves. For children with hearing loss, listening must be learned. Listening is so important because it can be considered the doorway to learning. The listening activity can require active, conscious, and alerting effort or exist as a passive process that occurs without our recognizing it. Children require more complete and detailed auditory information than adults in their listening processing, as well as a quieter environment and a louder primary signal (i.e., a helpful signal-to-noise ratio of 10 to 15 dB) (Smaldino & Crandell, 2000).

Barthes (1985) breaks listening into three key elements: (a) comprehension, (b) retaining, and (c) responding. Comprehension is the first step in the listening process. The listener must accurately identify speech sounds, understand them, and synthesize these sounds into words. Because we are constantly flooded with auditory stimuli, the listener has to select which of those sounds are important and which sounds to ignore. The individual with hearing loss faces the challenging task of discerning speech segmentation or the breaks between words as the speech sounds and breaks tend to blur and blend together into a continuous jumble. Determining the context and meanings of each word is essential to comprehending the message (Figure 3–6).

The second element is the retaining in memory that is essential to the listening process. The information we retain when listening is how we create meaning from words. We depend on memory and previous experiences to fill in the blanks as we listen to new or unexpected context during communication. Perhaps, when we receive the information we may not attach importance to it, so it loses its meaning. Using information immediately after receiving it enhances information retention and lessens the forgetting. Retention is lessened when we engage in mindless listening, where little effort is made to listen to a speaker's message.

The third key element of listening is responding, which describes an interaction between speaker and listener. It adds action to a normally passive process. The speaker looks for verbal and nonverbal responses from the listener to determine if the message is being listened to and understood or not. Based on the listener's response, the speaker may choose to either adjust or continue with his or her communication style.

So you might ask, "What is the big deal about listening and what does it have to do with children with hearing loss?" As described by Beck and Flexer (2011), hearing is a sense; listening is a skill that must be taught especially to children with hearing

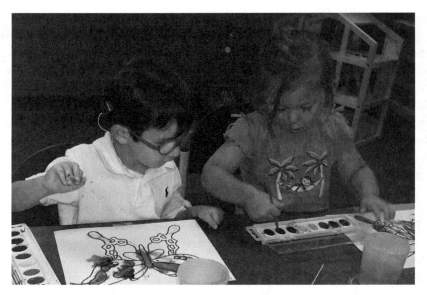

Figure 3–6. Learning from new experiences is critical to the development of speech and language in children with hearing loss. Photo courtesy of H.O.P.E. Preschool, Spokane, WA.

loss. Listening is when we apply meaning to sound; listening requires the brain to organize, establish vocabulary, develop receptive and expressive language, internalize concepts, and the result is that learning occurs. Audiologists have the technology tools to make the sense of hearing easier and better for children with hearing loss, but listening requires attention and focus, elements that must be taught to hard-of-hearing or deaf children. Paying attention through listening is the key for these children to learn.

Listening is a cognitive skill built on learned behaviors and rewards. The cognitive process of elaborating on the meaning of new information is the very best learning strategy, and processing new stimuli improves memory only when processing connects the new information to relevant knowledge. Therefore, development of listening skills in hard-of-hearing or deaf preschoolers will likely set the stage for successful learning. Listening experiences in infancy are the foundation for language

and literacy, as well as cognitive and psychological development (Beck & Flexer, 2011). Early word learning identifies children's use of symbolic communication; the words become the building blocks for the child to express feelings, desires, communications, and allow socializing with others (Moeller, 2010).

Incidental learning occurs when children "overhear" speech that is not directly addressed to them, yet they learn from it. It is the process of learning something without the intention of doing so. Amazingly, it has been estimated that young normal-hearing children learn approximately 90% of the information they acquire through incidental listening. Unfortunately, children with hearing loss are not as likely to benefit from incidental listening as they tend to have difficulties with speech understanding or perhaps loss of loudness and clarity due to their distance from the speaker. Obviously, utilization of appropriately fit amplification can do much to support incidental listening and learning in children with hearing loss. Although we learn "formally" only in some specific situations and periods of our life (i.e., school, training, etc.), incidental and informal learning are much more important for most of the skills and knowledge we learn during the vast majority of life.

In a unique research project designed to study incidental learning of words by children with hearing loss, Moller (2010) established three groups of 3-year-olds, including a group of normal-hearing children ($N = 41$), a group of children with hearing loss wearing hearing aids ($N = 13$), and a group of children using cochlear implants ($N = 19$) and exposed them to two novel words (*toma, neepa*) in a direct teaching condition and a "overhearing" condition. The novel words were associated with unfamiliar kitchen gadgets, and the children were taught a game to find the novel word item several times. During the "overhearing" condition, the test child was seated 3 feet away playing a quiet game with a second experimenter. The finding game was played with the child's mother or teacher, who was exposed auditorily to the target word nine times. The experimenters measured whether or not the subject child learned the novel word by "overhearing" the mother's and teacher's game trials. The results showed that the majority of children learned the novel word from the traditional direct teaching method. However, children with normal hearing were more successful than the children with hearing loss in expressing the name of the novel object ("What is this called?"). In the "overhearing" condition, more than half the normal-hearing and hearing aid wearing 3-year-olds learned the novel word receptively. Of the cochlear implant children, 33% learned the target word in the overhearing task. These results confirmed, within the limitations of the study, that at least some young children with hearing loss and wearing sensory devices do listen and learn words through incidental listening.

In a second study designed to learn how children with hearing loss might listen in on adult conversations, interviews were conducted of 60 mothers of 2- and 3-year-olds with normal hearing and 36 mothers of preschoolers with hearing loss. Survey results suggested that many of the children with hearing loss and amplification demonstrated evidence of overhearing the adult conversations but did so much less often than their normal-hearing siblings. Parents identified the three most difficult conditions for their children with hearing loss to overhear them: (a) car travel; (b) listening from another room; and (c) picking up words or songs from media such as DVDs, radio, or TV. The survey results indicated that the children with normal hearing were indeed successful in overhearing in these same difficult listening conditions. It is worthy of note that the use of FM systems on the children with hearing loss might prove beneficial for overhearing both incidental and direct communications in each of the difficult listening conditions described by the mothers.

AUDITORY PROCESSING IN CHILDREN

Auditory processing disorder (APD), also known as central auditory processing disorder (CAPD) is an umbrella term for central auditory deficits that affect the way the brain processes auditory information. Individuals with CAPD usually have normal structure and function of the peripheral hearing systems. However, due to dysfunction in the central auditory nervous system, they cannot process the information they hear in the same way as others do, which leads to difficulties in recognizing and interpreting sounds, especially the sounds composing speech. Although epidemiological studies of the prevalence of CAPD are difficult to conduct, it has been estimated that as many as 5% of school-aged children have some version of the disorder. It has also been suggested that males are twice as likely to be affected by the disorder as females.

Bellis (2002a, 2002b) aptly describes CAPD as a hearing problem in which "the brain can't hear." CAPD is more formally defined as a deficiency in the perceptual processing of auditory information in the central auditory nervous system (CANS) as demonstrated by poor performance in one or more of the following skills: sound localization and lateralization; auditory discrimination; auditory pattern recognition; temporal aspects of audition including temporal integration, temporal discrimination (e.g., temporal gap detection), temporal ordering, and temporal masking; auditory performance in competing acoustic signals including dichotic listening; and auditory performance with degraded acoustic signals (ASHA, 2005). A similar definition of CAPD was described by the British Society of Audiology (2011) who added that CAPD should be assessed through standardized tests of auditory perception. CAPD may coexist with, but is not the result of, dysfunction in other modalities.

CAPD can be genetic in origin or can be caused by disease processes, neurological conditions, traumatic brain injury, developmental abnormalities including delayed maturation of the central auditory nervous system, and metabolic disorders (Bamiou, Musiek, & Luxon, 2001). There is also growing evidence that in some children auditory deprivation due to early and long-standing otitis media results in impaired development of central auditory pathways and structures with consequential auditory processing deficits (Moore, 2007; Whitton & Polley, 2012).

CAPD is more likely to occur with other conditions than in isolation. Common co-morbidities include dyslexia, attention deficit hyperactivity disorder (ADHD), autism spectrum disorder (ASD), and specific language impairment and reading disorder (Sharma et al., 2009). Sometimes comorbidities may be consequences of the APD. For example, APD may affect language development and reading through its effects on phonological skills. Auditory processing deficits are also a key underlying factor in dyslexia (Burns, 2013). Inattention due to poor ability to hear may sometimes at first be misinterpreted as an attention disorder, but APD can be distinguished by results of auditory tests. Nonetheless, there is considerable comorbidity between APD and ADHD.

The subjective symptoms that lead to an evaluation for CAPD include an intermittent inability to process verbal information, leading the person to guess to fill in the processing gaps. There may also be disproportionate problems with decoding speech in noisy environments. CAPD can manifest in children as problems for them to determine the direction of sounds, difficulty perceiving differences between speech sounds, and the sequencing of these sounds into meaningful words, confusing similar sounds such as "hat" with "bat," "there" with "where," etc. Fewer words may be perceived than were actually spoken, as there can be problems detecting the gaps between words, creating the perception that someone is speaking unfamiliar or nonsense words. Those suffering from CAPD may have problems relating what has been said with its meaning, despite obvious recognition that a word has been said. People with auditory processing disorder sometimes subconsciously develop visual coping strategies, such as lip reading, reading body language, and reliance on other visual cues, to compensate for their auditory deficit. Descriptions of speech perception by adults with APD are informative. They report that speech seems fast, fragmented, and confusing, and that any other sound can seem to drown it out. They often hear the start of a sentence or paragraph but understand less and less as it progresses. They mishear some phonemes or speech sounds, they sometimes jumble the order of sounds, and they may miss pitch or intonation cues that affect the meaning of spoken language. They also report difficulty in localizing sounds.

Children with CAPD are known to exhibit one or more of a wide range of behaviors as they experience language and learning problems (Keith, 2000a):

- inconsistent responses to auditory stimuli;
- inability to follow auditory instructions;
- difficulty with auditory localization;
- inability to differentiate soft and loud sounds;
- unexplainable fear of loud noises, or being overwhelmed by the auditory environment;
- difficulties in learning, discriminating, and remembering phonemes and manipulating them in tasks such as reading, spelling, and phonics;
- poor perception of pitch, intonation, and other suprasegmental features of speech that affect meaning;
- difficulty understanding speech in noisy backgrounds or against any competing sounds;
- impaired ability to recall and repeat simple musical patterns of high- and low-pitch notes or temporal (rhythm) patterns;

- difficulty with auditory memory, either span or sequence;
- poor listening skills with decreased attention, increased distractibility, and restlessness;
- frequent requests to repeat information;
- low academic performance, significant reading problems, poor spelling;
- behavioral problems; and
- withdrawal tendencies, shyness with poor self-concept resulting from multiple failures.

The presence of one or more of the following key symptoms in the presence of normal peripheral hearing is a useful indicator in identifying children who should be assessed for CAPD:

- difficulty following spoken directions unless they are brief and simple;
- slowness in processing spoken information;
- difficulty attending to and remembering spoken information;
- poor listening skills;
- difficulty understanding in the presence of other sound;
- difficulty with language, reading, spelling, writing, vocabulary, or comprehension.

CAPD particularly affects temporal processing of auditory information which in turn affects the recognition and discrimination of phonemes. Impaired phonological awareness in turn may affect auditory memory (if stored templates of sounds are deficient), language, spelling, and reading. The perception of rapid format transitions is impaired in CAPD and dyslexia (Hornick et al., 2012), and research also shows impaired perception of slow temporal aspects of speech (Corriveau, Goswami, & Thomson, 2010).

Approximately half of children with CAPD have amblyaudia, a unilateral weakness or inhibition of one ear affecting binaural integration. Amblyaudia presents as an abnormally large interaural asymmetry on dichotic testing. Amblyaudia may adversely affect any aspect of hearing requiring binaural function for optimal audition (Moncrieff, 2011).

Keith (1988) hypothesized that some basic auditory-perceptual skills (e.g., appreciation of frequency, intensity, and duration of sounds) exist in every child and serve as building blocks of audition, leading to language development through imitation. As language skills are acquired, children also learn to apply auditory-perceptual skills, such as memory, discrimination, closure, and blending to language. In addition, as the child's neuroanatomical pathways mature, the ability to cope with higher level auditory tasks such as dichotic listening and binaural release from masking begins to improve.

A number of screening tests to identify children who might have CAPD have been developed. Although these screening tests are in no way intended to be diagnostic, they can be useful in obtaining information on children too young for formal CAPD assessment. Because CAPD is not a singular entity but rather an umbrella term for a range of central auditory deficits, effective screening is not possible unless the screening tool incorporates a sensitive test for every possible deficit. However, the list of key symptoms presented earlier can be very effective in detecting children who should be evaluated. Groups that warrant almost automatic referral for central auditory evaluation include children with dyslexia and children with reading disorders.

Although a number of questionnaires have been used to screen for CAPD, they gener-

ally have poor specificity, tend to under- or overrefer, and have not been completely validated. A number of CAPD screening tests are currently in use including the Children's Auditory Performance Scale (CHAPS), a 25-item scale that utilizes a scaling continuum related to the child's auditory behaviors (Smoski, Brunt, & Tannahill, 1992); The Children's Home Inventory for Listening Difficulties (CHILD), for use with children between the ages of 3 and 12 which is completed by a parent (Anderson & Smaldino, 2000); the Listening Inventory (TLI) developed by Geffner and Ross-Swain (2006); the Screening Instrument for Targeting Educational Risk (SIFTER) from Anderson and Matkin (1989); and the Listening Inventory for Education (LIFE) (Anderson & Smaldino, 1998). Despite their limitations, these instruments can provide useful background information for the evaluation.

Most tests of CAPD are based on some form of challenging auditory signal for the auditory nervous system to identify as in speech-in-noise or distorted speech tests. These tests, known as *sensitized speech tests*, use various means of distorting speech to reduce the intelligibility of the message. Distortion can be accomplished in many ways including high- or low-pass filtering that reduces the range of frequencies (filtered speech testing). Another approach is to reduce the intensity level of speech above a simultaneously presented background noise (auditory figure ground testing). Speech can be distorted in the time domain by interrupting the speech at different rates, and by increasing the rate of presentation (time-compressed speech). Persons with normal hearing and normal auditory pathways can understand distorted speech messages; however, when a central auditory processing disorder is present, speech intelligibility under difficult circumstances is poor. The construct of sensitized speech testing is extremely powerful and forms the basis of all behavioral speech tests of central auditory function (Keith, 1999a).

It is helpful to note the definitions of the most common central auditory abilities that test developers attempt to measure in order to identify central auditory processing problems in children:

- Auditory Localization. The ability to locate the source of a sound through hearing only. This ability requires simultaneous binaural stimulation.
- Binaural Synthesis. The ability to integrate centrally incomplete stimulus patterns presented simultaneously or alternately to opposite ears.
- Figure Ground. The ability to identify a primary signal or message in the presence of competing sounds. Auditory figure ground can be a monaural or a binaural task.
- Binaural Separation. The ability to listen with one ear while ignoring stimulation of the opposite ear. Dichotic listening, as a binaural separation task, requires the listener to attend to and report back different signals presented simultaneously to two ears.
- Memory. The ability to store and to recall auditory stimuli, including length or number of auditory stimuli, and sequential memory or the ability to recall the exact order of auditory stimuli presented.
- Blending. The ability to form words out of separately articulated phonemes.
- Discrimination. The ability to determine whether two acoustic stimuli are the same or different. In speech, auditory discrimination is the ability to recognize fine differences that exist among phonemes.

- Closure. The ability to perceive the whole (word or message) when parts are omitted.
- Attention. The ability to persist in listening over a reasonable period.
- Association. The ability to establish a correspondence between a nonlinguistic sound and its source.
- Cognition. The ability to establish a correspondence between a linguistic sound and its meaning. Cognition is the highest level of auditory perception and results from a summation of all auditory (and all sensory) tasks.

Before any attempt is made to administer tests for CAPD, the audiologist must be certain that no conductive or sensorineural hearing loss is present in either ear of the child. Generally, patients with CAPD show normal hearing loss for routine audiometric tests, although that is not to say that CAPD does not coexist in children who do have substantiated hearing disorders. It is critical that a complete assessment of the peripheral auditory system, including consideration of auditory neuropathy spectrum disorder (ANSD), occur prior to administering a central auditory test battery. At minimum, this would include evaluation of hearing thresholds, immittance measures (tympanometry and acoustic reflexes), and otoacoustic emissions (OAEs). When contradictory findings exist (e.g., present OAEs combined with absent acoustic reflexes or abnormal hearing sensitivity; abnormal acoustic reflexes with normal tympanometry and OAEs), additional followup should occur to rule out ANSD prior to proceeding with central auditory testing (AAA, 2010; ASHA, 2005). It is possible to carry out some CAPD testing in the presence of mild, particularly conductive, peripheral hearing loss, at increased presentation levels, as long as it is understood that the results may be compromised and conclusions limited by the confounding variables. Tests that involve comparison between ears or conditions may be more meaningful, and the LiSN-S Test (Cameron & Dillon, 2007) has a compensation feature for peripheral hearing loss. Pass results can be taken as suggestive of normal auditory processing, but fail results must be considered ambiguous unless the test incorporates a control condition for comparison.

A child may do poorly on an auditory test for reasons other than poor auditory perception: for instance, failure could be due to inattention, difficulty in coping with task demands, or limited language ability. Factors such as chronological and developmental age; language age and experience; cognitive abilities, including attention and memory; education; linguistic, cultural, and social background; medications; motivation; decision processes; visual acuity; motor skills; and other variables can influence how a given person performs on behavioral tests. Many of these variables also may influence outcomes of some electrophysiologic procedures.

Pediatric audiologists should consider the language, cognitive, and other nonauditory demands of the auditory tasks in selecting and administering a central auditory diagnostic test battery. Screening of cognitive ability, language, memory, and attention should be included in the evaluation. Audiologists must be vigilant to ensure that tasks are understood and attention is maintained by children. If results on cognitive, language, or attention tests are below normal, the validity of any abnormal CAPD test findings must be questioned.

A limitation of some behavioral tests for CAPD is that a minimum developmental age of 7 years is required to perform the tasks involved, or at least a level of cognitive functioning that is consistent with the age level. However, a growing number of tests have norms for younger ages. The AAA Guidelines (2010) recommend using the term *at risk* for CAPD for diagnoses below age 7, but stress that intervention should not be delayed.

Results on the individual tests comprising the diagnostic test battery must be evaluated against appropriate normative standards. Available tests vary considerably in the scientific rigor under which they were developed. Some have limited comparative norm data and some are out of date, being supplanted by more current testing procedures. Testing for CAPD is conducted to determine if an auditory processing disorder is present, and if so, to describe the parameters of the disorder, the child's functional auditory abilities and limitations, neurologic maturation of the auditory system, and hemispheric function. The central auditory evaluation should include: (a) a carefully documented patient history; (b) observation of auditory behaviors; (c) assessment of peripheral hearing; (d) tests of central auditory function including temporal processing skills, localization and lateralization, low redundancy monaural speech, dichotic stimuli, binaural interaction procedures, and electrophysiological tests as appropriate; and (e) cognitive and language evaluation. Comprehensive assessment for CAPD is ideally carried out by a multidisciplinary team including the audiologist, speech-language pathologist, psychologist, educators, physicians, and parents.

A range of behavioral central auditory tests is listed below (ASHA, 2005). A typical test battery will include one test from each category, plus (not listed) a test of hearing in noise (preferably spatially separated noise):

- *Auditory discrimination tests* assess the ability to differentiate similar acoustic stimuli that differ in frequency, intensity, and temporal parameters (e.g., difference limens for frequency, intensity, and duration; psychophysical tuning curves; phoneme discrimination).

- *Auditory temporal processing and patterning tests* assess the ability to analyze acoustic events over time (e.g., sequencing and patterns, gap detection, fusion discrimination, integration, forward and backward masking).

- *Dichotic speech tests* assess the ability to separate (i.e., binaural separation) or integrate (i.e., binaural integration) disparate auditory stimuli presented to each ear simultaneously (e.g., dichotic CVs, digits, words, sentences).

- *Monaural low-redundancy speech tests* assess recognition of degraded speech stimuli presented to one ear at a time (e.g., filtered, time-altered, speech-in-noise, or speech-in-competition).

- *Binaural interaction tests* assess binaural (i.e., dichotic) processes dependent on intensity or time differences of acoustic stimuli (e.g., masking level difference, localization, lateralization, fused-image tracking).

The concept of a test battery to assess a variety of auditory processes and the "cross-check" principle of Jerger and Hayes (1976) should also be applied in CAPD evaluations, thereby eliminating the making of decisions based on results from one testing procedure. According to ASHA (2005), diagnosis of CAPD generally requires performance deficits on the order of at least two standard deviations below the mean on two or more tests in the battery. If poor performance is observed on only one test, the audiologist should withhold a diagnosis of CAPD unless the client's performance

falls at least three standard deviations below the mean or when the finding is accompanied by significant functional difficulty in auditory behaviors reliant on the process assessed. Moreover, the audiologist should readminister the sole test failed as well as another similar test that assesses the same process to confirm the initial findings.

The AAA Guidelines (2010) suggest a diagnostic criterion of a score two standard deviations or more below the mean for at least one ear on at least two different behavioral central auditory tests. This requires the minimum two failed tests to be in the same ear and does not specifically mention an option of diagnosing CAPD on the basis of only one failed test. However, in clinical practice it is not uncommon to see patients who demonstrate only one central deficit (e.g., spatial stream segregation, difficulty hearing against spatially separated noise), or amblyaudia for instance.

One well-standardized test battery is the SCAN-3:C Tests for Auditory Processing Disorders for Children developed by Keith (2009). SCAN-3:C is intended for use with children who are 5 through 12 years of age. The original SCAN was published as a screening test for auditory processing disorders in children (Keith, 1986). It was subsequently revised and published with new norms as a diagnostic test under the name SCAN-C: Test for Auditory Processing Disorders in Children-Revised (Keith, 2000b). The most recent revision was standardized on 525 ethnically, geographically, and gender representative school-aged children ranging in age from 5 to 12 years, 11 months, and titled as SCAN-3 for Children: Test for Auditory Processing Disorders (SCAN-3:C).

SCAN-3 for Children consists of three groups of tests. The screening tests include the gap detection test, auditory figure ground (AFG) testing at 8 dB signal-to-noise (S/N) ratio, and competing words free recall. The screening tests can be used to determine whether the full diagnostic battery is required. The full diagnostic battery should also be administered when the child's referral source or history indicate. The four tests used in diagnosis include filtered words, auditory figure ground at 8 dB S/N ratio, competing words with directed ear instructions, and competing sentences. Those test results are used to compute a composite score that represents the child's overall performance. Four optional supplemental tests not used in calculating the composite score are available to further investigate the child's auditory processing abilities. They include the dichotic word test under free recall conditions used in the screening measure, AFG testing at 0 dB and 12 dB S/N ratio, and time-compressed sentences. Tables are provided to determine from the raw scores the Scaled Score, Confidence Interval, and Percentile Rank of the child's test results. Ear Advantage scoring is included to assist in detecting abnormalities of hemispheric or interhemispheric function. Note, however, that normative values for ear advantage obtained by comparing right and left ear scores can be contaminated by the presence of results from children with stronger performance in their left ears. Ear advantage based on a comparison between the dominant and nondominant ear without regard to right or left is a more accurate determination of lateralization (Moncrieff, 2011).

Auditory evoked responses (AERs) can be used to measure most aspects of auditory processing (Picton, 2013). Electrical potentials can be elicited that reflect synchronous activity generated by the CANS in response to a wide variety of acoustic events (e.g., ABR, auditory middle latency response, 40 Hz response, steady-state evoked potentials, frequency following response, cortical event-related potentials [P1, N1, P2, P300], mismatch negativity, topographical mapping). Hall and Johnson (2007) reported that the ABR elicited with click stimuli is usually normal for children with CAPD associated with developmental disorders but may be more sensitive to children with CAPD secondary to neurological disorders of the brainstem pathways. The speech-evoked ABR shows promise for identifying temporal distortion in the auditory system caused by impaired auditory processing (Hornickel, Zecker, Bradlow, & Kraus, 2012). Research has also shown positive results in identifying CAPD with the P300 and the P1 potentials (Sharma et al., 2006). Electrophysiologic measures may be particularly useful in cases in which behavioral procedures are not feasible (e.g., infants and very young children), when there is suspicion of frank neurologic disorder, when a confirmation of behavioral findings is needed, or when behavioral findings are inconclusive. The AAA (2010) recommended that the use of AERs be limited to the following indicators:

- Behavioral assessment fails to reveal a clear pattern of deficits.
- Behavioral test findings are incomplete or inconclusive or compromised by selected listener variables (i.e., attention, motivation, cooperation, cognitive status, etc.).
- The age of the young child precludes the use of behavioral CAPD measures.
- A neurologic disorder is suspected.
- Information on the site of the dysfunction within the central nervous system is needed for individuals showing a clear pattern of CAPD with the behavioral assessment.

- Behavioral measures of CAPD are not available in the individual's native language.

Auditory processing disorders in children respond well to treatment. Research studies document improvement in auditory skills from a variety of approaches. Treatment approaches are sometimes described as bottom-up or top-down. Bottom-up treatments include strategies to enhance signal quality such as hearing assistance technology and discrimination training, and include training of psychoacoustic and phonological processing skills (Sharma, Purdy, & Kelly, 2012). Top-down approaches use higher level processes such as cognition, language, and metacognitive functions to help interpret the auditory message or to compensate when hearing is deficient. They include therapy to improve vocabulary, word understanding, prosody perception, phonemic perception, inference and reasoning, working memory, verbal rehearsal, summarizing, language, reading, and other high-level skills. Audiologists tend to concentrate on bottom-up treatments and speech-language pathologists on top-down approaches. The two approaches are complementary.

Treatment approaches for APD are also commonly categorized under the headings of environmental modification, compensatory strategies, and direct treatment. Environmental modification includes the use of hearing assistance technology, ensuring the environment is as quiet and distraction-free as possible, and ensuring that the child is seated close to the teacher in school (unless wearing remote microphone hearing aids, in which case position in class should not be critical for hearing). Compensatory strategies include self-advocacy; assistance from a peer assigned as a "hearing buddy"; special assistance with classes, for example a note-taker or technology aids; extra explanation or time for tests; multisensory teaching with utilization of visual cues and supplementary materials to enhance access to the curriculum in school; and metacognitive strategies to use contextual or visual information to help decipher a message with insufficient auditory cues. Direct treatment includes training and therapy, either by therapist, software program, or both, encompassing auditory, phonologic, and language skills, and higher level skills such as memory and reading. Hearing assistance technology should also be included in this category (as well as the environmental modification category) because research has shown the use of amplification by remote microphone hearing aids to be therapeutic as well as assistive (see below). Phonological awareness is a critical area of remediation in most cases of APD, as it is the foundation for reading, spelling, and language and is commonly compromised by difficulties with auditory processing.

Classrooms are difficult listening environments for all children and more so for children with auditory difficulties. Distance from the teacher, noise, and excessive reverberation degrade the auditory signal. Acoustic treatment can reduce reverberation and entry of external noise. Seating within 2 meters of the teacher optimizes signal level. Classroom sound distribution (loudspeaker) systems can provide up to about 5 dB of improvement in signal-to-noise ratio (Schafer & Kleineck, 2009; Wilson, Marinac, Pitty, & Burrows, 2011). But such measures are unlikely to be sufficient to optimize hearing for children with auditory processing disorder (see Chapter 10). There appears to be no peer-reviewed evidence that acoustic improvements or classroom sound distribution systems are beneficial to children with APD. Even the claimed benefits of classroom sound distribution systems to learning in children with normal hearing are not universally supported (Dockrell & Shield, 2012).

Conventional hearing aids are reported by some clinicians to be effective in improving the hearing of children with APD though published evidence is scant (Kuk, 2011; Kuk, Jackson, Keenan, & Lau, 2008). Personal remote microphone hearing aids (RMHAs) are currently the only evidence-based amplification treatment shown to effectively improve hearing in classrooms for children with APD.

Remote microphone hearing aids, often referred to as *personal FM systems*, are hybrid FM receivers/hearing aids designed for children with normal peripheral hearing. The child wears the receivers, usually ear level, and the parent, teacher, or other talker wears the transmitter. Studies of the effects of amplification with RMHAs for children with APD consistently show therapeutic as well as assistive benefits from the amplification. The immediate assistive benefits include improved learning; improved attention, behavior, and participation in class, and improved self-esteem and psychosocial development. The long-term therapeutic benefits, measured without the hearing aids on, after up to 12 months of RMHA use include improvements in cortical auditory evoked potential amplitudes to tone stimuli, auditory brainstem responses to speech stimuli, frequency discrimination, binaural temporal resolution, frequency pattern recognition, auditory working memory, core language, phonological awareness, and speech perception in noise (spatial stream segregation) (Friederichs & Friederichs, 2005; Hornickel et al., 2012; Johnson et al., 2009; Sharma et al., 2012; Smart et al., 2008; Umat, Mukari, Ezan, & Din, 2011). Amplification appears to treat a wide range of auditory skills simultaneously, facilitating neuroplastic change while also providing access to the auditory world. The benefits of RMHAs are generally attributed to the improvement in signal-to-noise ratio (15 to 20 dB) which they achieve. However, given that children with APD do not wear occluding earmolds, the environmental noise level reaching their ears is not reduced. The improvement in signal-to-noise ratio is achieved only by amplification of the signal. The amplification itself may be an important factor in stimulating neuroplastic change in the auditory system. Although there is no specific evidence, it may be beneficial to wear amplification during therapy as is common with other types of deafness. Most children with APD appear to benefit from amplification with RMHAs, and as there is no way to predict which children will benefit, a trial is necessary. Clinical experience suggests that many children only require the amplification for a period of about 2 years.

There is one central auditory deficit that is not improved by RMHA use. Half of children with APD have amblyaudia, which is an abnormal interaural asymmetry on dichotic testing. Amblyaudia is analogous to the visual disorder, amblyopia. It can be effectively treated with auditory training in as little as 4 weeks (Moncrieff & Wertz, 2008; Musiek & Schochat, 1998). It is recommended that the amblyaudia treatment be completed before the fitting of remote microphone hearing aids.

Many training packages, workbooks, and software programs are offered as treatments for APD. Not all are supported by peer-reviewed evidence, and none are likely to provide a total solution for an individual child. Many treatments are promoted for APD that are not evidence based. ASHA and AAA specifically warn that Auditory Integration Therapy and related variations (Berard Auditory Integration, Tomatis Approach, Listening Program, etc.) in which the child listens to processed music are not supported by a peer-reviewed evidence base. They are best used as part of a comprehensive treatment program directed by a qualified therapist who can select suitable difficulty levels and tasks to work on within a program. Some of the popularly recommended programs for CAPD are primarily reading programs with auditory processing and phonics subcomponents. The LiSN & Learn auditory training software developed at the National Acoustic Laboratories in Australia is different in that it is a game-format evidence-based software training program specifically designed to remediate a particular central auditory deficit, spatial processing disorder (hearing in noise). LiSN & Learn produces a virtual three-dimensional environment under headphones. Through a variety of games children learn to attend to target stimuli and improve their ability to hear in background noise. Sound Auditory Training from Plural Publishing, Inc. (San Diego) is a software tool to enable clinicians to customize Web-based auditory skills training for individual clients. Tasks train intensity, frequency, temporal detection, discrimination, and identification using a variety of nonverbal and minimally loaded verbal stimuli.

Additional discussion of CAPD is beyond the scope of this textbook, and the reader is referred to a number of reference texts including Geffner and Ross-Swain (2013), Musiek and Chermak (2007), and Chermak and Musiek (2007). The American Speech-Language-Hearing Association (2005) and the American Academy of Audiology (2010) have published summaries of current knowledge and suggested guidelines for the identification and management of central auditory processing disorder in children.

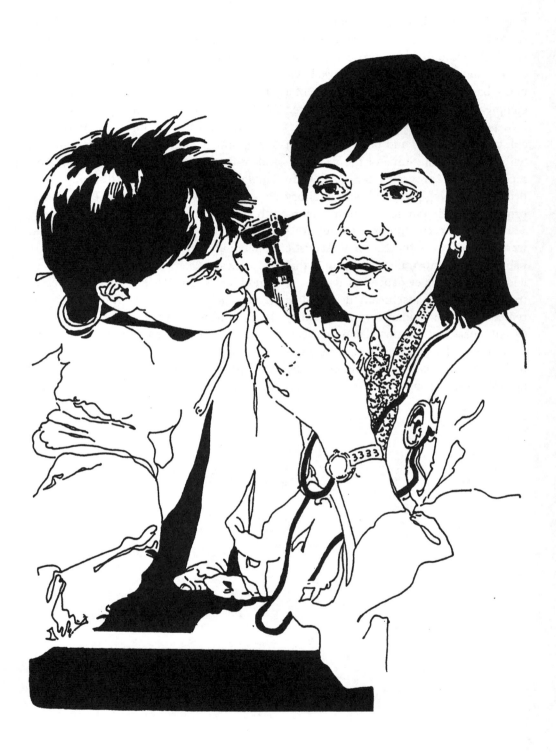

CHAPTER 4

Medical Aspects

The audiologist who evaluates children with hearing loss must be fully aware of the many medical conditions that are associated with hearing disorders. A host of complex medical disorders affect newborns and young infants which can cause or be associated with various types of hearing loss. These medical disorders may be relatively benign, and prompt treatment during the newborn period restores the infant to health with the potential for normal development. Conversely, many ominous conditions result in lifelong disease and disability. Fortunately, techniques for early identification and treatment of infants at risk for these disorders are continually evolving. Diseases that previously affected scores of infants and caused hearing loss (e.g., congenital rubella syndrome, type B meningitis, Rh incompatibility, kernicterus) have been virtually eliminated by effective vaccination and treatment programs. Significant advances in audiologic assessment of infants have resulted in better understanding of the etiology of hearing impairment in newborn infants and very young babies. Improved understanding of the etiology of hearing impairment in these infants and young children hopefully will yield better methods to prevent and to treat these hearing disorders.

Approximately 10% of newborns are at risk for medical problems and developmental disability. Although the risk status of some infants may be known prenatally, most infants at risk are detected either at birth or during the complete physical examination conducted within the first few hours after birthing. Many of these babies with problems will receive their initial care in the newborn intensive care unit (NICU). Hearing loss is much more prevalent in infants who receive care in the NICU than in newborns who thrive in the normal newborn nursery. On average, it has been shown that babies who receive care in the NICU exhibit hearing impairment about 20 times more frequently than infants who receive their care in a well-baby nursery (Simmons, 1982). Although the cause of hearing impairment among the normal newborn population is generally unknown, hearing loss identified in infants from the NICU is often secondary to an identifiable disorder or treatment of that disorder.

Audiologists must possess expertise in the understanding of medical disorders that may, or may not, be associated with childhood hearing loss. With extensive training in behavioral and electrophysiological measurements of hearing, audiologists can determine the extent of a child's hearing loss in terms of degree, audiometric configuration, probable site of auditory dysfunction, ear symmetry, and stability of hearing loss. This audiometric information is enhanced by the audiologist's understanding of the underlying medical problem or disorder. Often the pediatric audiologist will be asked by the family or caregiver for an explanation or clarification of the underlying medical problem. The audiologist's expertise is important in providing family guidance and counseling about the prognosis and recommended management for the child, and to assist in making choices about the most appropriate intervention strategies. Based on ongoing observation and evaluation of the child's hearing problem and development, the audiologist should be involved in identification of other developmental problems that might require referrals for additional evaluations.

For the child with hearing loss, the audiologist must be prepared to advocate prompt medical attention when necessary, and note changes in hearing levels, changes in the quality of sound hearing by the child, as well as the onset of tinnitus or dizziness. Children with hearing loss should be monitored audiometrically on a routine basis whenever they undergo medical examination. Pediatric hearing loss may suddenly become progressive or worsen with ototoxic drug treatment or exposure to noise. Therefore, it is imperative that the child's auditory thresholds be monitored routinely. The importance of every decibel of residual hearing that the child possesses may be in exponential ratio to each decibel of hearing loss. More extensive otologic and audiologic examination will be required if the child shows deterioration in speech production or educational difficulties.

MEDICAL ASSESSMENT OF NEWBORN INFANTS

All newborn infants receive multiple examinations shortly after birth. Typically, the first assessment is completed in the delivery room within moments of birth. During the initial hours of life, the infant receives a complete physical examination. In some instances, formal assessment of estimated gestational age is also made based on specific physical and neuromuscular characteristics.

Apgar Evaluation

At birth, babies are rapidly assessed to detect obvious abnormalities and to determine the need for immediate resuscitation. In 1953, Dr. Virginia Apgar, an anesthesiologist, developed a tool for evaluating an infant's condition in the delivery room. Evaluation is completed at 1 minute and again at 5 minutes following birth. Both evaluations are based on five standardized observations (heart rate, respiratory effort, reflex irritability, muscle tone, and color). A rating of 0 to 2 is assigned to each observation based on the scale summarized in Table 4–1. The maximum Apgar score attainable is 10 (AAP, 1986).

The 1-minute Apgar evaluation provides a rapid method of determining the baby's initial adaptation to extrauterine life. As soon as delivery is complete (baby is completely delivered and umbilical cord is clamped), a timer is started so that the baby can be evaluated at precisely 1 minute. Infants with Apgar scores of 7 or higher require only routine care and observation. Apgar scores between 3 and 6 indicate moderate cardiorespiratory depression. These babies will require some form of resuscitation and close observation for at least 24 hours. Infants with Apgar scores below 3 are severely depressed and will require ventilator assistance and intensive care. The 5-minute Apgar score permits reevaluation of the infant's condition and assessment of the baby's responses to resuscitative efforts (Apgar & James, 1962). Infants who score 7 or less at the 5 minute examination are typically re-evaluated at 10 minutes with hope that they have acclimated better to the extrauterine environment (Hegyi et al., 1998).

Estimating Gestational Age

Both birth weight and gestational age are important determinants of the baby's general condition. Although gestational age can be estimated from the mother's last menstrual period, this calculation is often

Table 4–1. Scoring System for Initial Assessment of Newborn Infants Developed by Dr. Virginia Apgar (1953)

	Score		
Observation	**0**	**1**	**2**
Heart rate	Absent	Slow (below 100)	Over 100
Respiratory effort	Absent; apnea	Slow, irregular, shallow, gasping	Sustained cry, regular respirations
Reflex irritability	No response	Grimace, frown	Sneeze, cry, active avoidance
Muscle tone	Limp, flaccid good tone	Some flexion of extremities	Active motion,
Color	Cyanotic, extremities pale	Body pink and pale	Completely pink

Note: To obtain the Apgar score, the baby is assessed at 1 minute following birth to determine need for resuscitative efforts and again at 5 minutes following birth to evaluate response to resuscitative efforts. Adapted from *Nelson Textbook of Pediatrics*, 11th ed., by V. Vaughan, R. J. McRay, & R. Behrman, 1979, p. 393, Philadelphia, PA: W. B. Saunders.

inaccurate and unreliable. Because certain physical and neuromuscular characteristics emerge in a predictable sequence during fetal development, these characteristics form the basis for an objective estimate of gestational age. These physical characteristics include skin appearance, presence of lanugo (fine hair present on the fetus which largely disappears by 40 weeks' gestation), cartilage development in the ear, and appearance of the genitalia. Neuromuscular characteristics include resting posture and flexion and extension of the extremities. These features yield an estimate of gestational age which can be compared to birth weight to determine if the infant is small for gestational age (SGA), appropriate for gestational age (AGA), or large for gestational age (LGA).

Rh Incompatibility

Rh incompatibility is a condition that develops when a pregnant woman has Rh-negative blood and the baby in her womb has Rh-positive blood. During pregnancy, red blood cells from the unborn baby can cross into the mother's bloodstream through the placenta. If the mother is Rh-negative, her immune system treats Rh-positive fetal cells as if they were a foreign substance and makes antibodies against the fetal blood cells. These anti-Rh antibodies may cross back through the placenta into the developing baby and destroy the baby's circulating red blood cells. When red blood cells are broken down, they make bilirubin. This causes an infant to become yellow (jaundiced). The level of bilirubin in the infant's bloodstream may range from mild to dangerously high. Because it takes time for the mother to develop antibodies, firstborn infants are often not affected unless the mother had past miscarriages or abortions that sensitized her immune system. However, all children she has afterwards who are also Rh-positive may be affected. Rh incompatibility develops only when the mother is

Rh-negative and the infant is Rh-positive. Thanks to the use of special immune globulins, this problem has become uncommon in the United States when access to good prenatal care is available. Owing to improved technology in perinatal care, newborns with access to modern medical treatment of Rh incompatibility are unlikely to have hearing loss, even with complete blood transfusions at birth. Clinical symptoms, when they occur, develop during the immediate neonatal period and include elevated bilirubin, jaundice, and possible brain damage. Rh incompatibility is almost completely preventable.

Jaundice

About 60% of newborn infants in the United States are jaundiced—that is, they look yellow. Excessive jaundice in newborn infants may cause brain damage. Jaundice is caused by a high level of bilirubin in the blood (hyperbilirubinemia) and tissues. When bilirubin gets too high, it can be treated. Norms exist for bilirubin in term and nearly term babies based on the age in hours after birth. Other factors, such as prematurity, blood group incompatibilities between infant and mother including Rh and ABO blood types, and bruising can increase bilirubin production and lead to excessive jaundice. Babies with high bilirubin levels can be effectively treated. Phototherapy (treatment with light) is usually very effective. It is the blue color in visible light that alters the bilirubin from a toxic form to a water-soluble, nontoxic form that can be eliminated. At higher, more dangerous levels of bilirubin, or in certain situations where the bilirubin is expected to rise rapidly, such as Rh or other hemolytic diseases of the newborn, a more extreme treatment may be used, exchange transfusion, to rapidly remove toxic bilirubin from the blood.

Kernicterus

Kernicterus is a serious form of brain damage caused by excessive jaundice. The substance that causes jaundice, bilirubin, is so high that it can move out of the blood into brain tissue. When babies begin to be affected by excessive jaundice, when they begin to have brain damage, they become excessively lethargic. Kernicterus involves a specific part of the basal ganglia, the globus pallidus. It also includes lesions of brainstem nuclei in auditory (hearing), oculomotor (eye movement), vestibular (balance) systems, and the cerebellum (coordination). They are too sleepy, and they are difficult to arouse; either they do not wake up from sleep easily like a normal baby, or they do not wake up fully, or they cannot be kept awake. They have a high-pitched cry, and decreased muscle tone (becoming hypotonic or floppy) with episodes of increased muscle tone (hypertonic) and arching of the head and back backwards. As the damage continues, they may develop fever or arch their heads back into a very contorted position known as retrocollis.

MEDICAL CONDITIONS OF THE EXTERNAL EAR

To recognize the presence of a diseased state, one must appreciate the normal anatomy of the external ear. The pinna or auricle is an appendage attached to the side of the head that is normally level with the middle third of the face. It is composed of a piece of elastic cartilage with numerous convolutions, covered with thin skin, and fixed in position at the lateral aspect of the external auditory canal by its direct continuity with the cartilaginous canal, auricular muscles, and auricular ligaments. Its major convolutions include the helix, anithelix, tragus, antitragus, and concha. The lobule is unique in that it contains no cartilage and, therefore, has been designated by various cultures as the appropriate place through which and on which to hang ornaments for decoration.

An opening, the external auditory meatus, is cartilaginous in the lateral one-third and bony in the medial two-thirds. The cartilage of the external auditory canal is generally continuous with that of the pinna with several fissures to permit flexibility. Hence, the curved path of the ear canal can be partially straightened to facilitate inspection by gently pulling back and up on the pinna. Squamous epithelium lines the external canal and covers the tympanic membrane. This skin is thicker laterally with hair follicles, sebaceous glands, and earwax-producing glands, but it is quite thin over the more medial bony portion of the canal with fewer skin structures present. This skin is unusual because it does not flake, as does other squamous epithelium, but migrates laterally toward the external meatus, providing a self-cleaning mechanism unique to the ear canal.

At the onset of every clinical evaluation or testing procedure, the audiologist should take note of the location, size, and shape of the pinnae and their relationship to the remainder of the structures of the head and face. The making of earmolds and swim-molds, as well as the insertion of acoustic immittance and otoadmittance probe tips during diagnostic and hearing screening testing, make it imperative for the clinician to recognize disorders of the external ear.

Normally, the superior border of the helix is located at the outer canthus of the eye, and the tragus is roughly level with the infraorbital rim (Figure 4–1). Low-set pinnae are frequently associated with other anomalies of the first and second branchial cleft. Although the pinna may have no

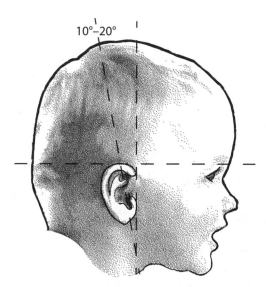

Figure 4–1. Normal position of the pinna in relationship to the eyes and face.

abnormality in its location or basic shape, the alert clinician should be aware of any lump, ulcer, or lesion on the pinna. The child with ears that stick out from his or her head in a prominent fashion faces possible social problems from the ridicule of classmates. Successful surgical treatment of a patient with this deformity before the patient enters school may save a great deal of emotional anguish. Correction of these deformities is easily accomplished through an operation known as otoplasty, which consists of an incision of the back of the pinna, cinched with stitches, to hold the ear in its new position closer to the head.

Malformations of the External Ear and Canal

Early in embryonic life, the auricle develops around the first branchial groove as six knob-like protrusions. These six hillocks soon lose their identity as they coalesce to form the pinna. With six separate growth centers developing at differing rates, it is not surprising that a wide variation exists in final ear configurations that are within normal limits. The shape of the auricle is so different among individuals that European police forces utilize the configuration of the ear much like American police use fingerprints. Supernumerary hillocks, known as *tags* or *preauricular appendages*, may remain with an otherwise normal-appearing pinna (Figure 4–2). However, the presence of tags may suggest anomalies of the external and middle ear systems. A Swedish study established an incidence for preauricular tags of 5.4 in 1,000 live births. Kankkunen and Thuringer (1987) studied 188 Swedish babies with preauricular tags and noted that when the tag was the only facial defect, mild to moderate sensorineural hearing loss was found in 23% of patients. However, in 10 pa-

tients with preauricular tags and associated facial anomalies (facial paralysis, mandibular anomalies), eight patients had conductive hearing loss, one with mixed-type hearing loss, and one with sensorineural hearing loss.

Atresia and Stenosis of the External Ear Canal

Atresia is the complete closing off of the ear canal; stenosis is a narrowing of the canal. Atresia or stenosis of the external ear canal may accompany microtia (congenital malformation of the auricle, see below) or occur in conjunction with a normal auricle (Figure 4–3). Stenosis of the external canal may be congenital or acquired following trauma. In congenital stenosis, the embryonic atresia plate may be solid bone or membranous; radiographic examination distinguishes

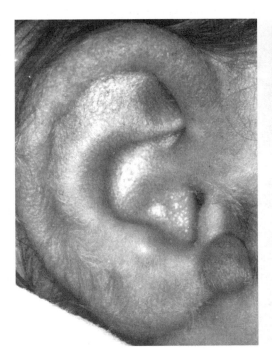

Figure 4–2. Supernumerary hillocks, known as tags or preauricular appendages, may remain with an otherwise normal-appearing pinna.

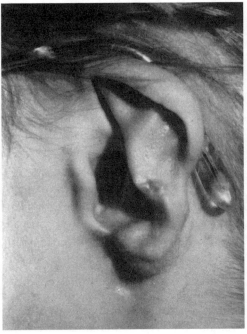

Figure 4–3. Atresia or stenosis of the external ear canal may accompany microtia or occur in conjunction with an otherwise normal pinna.

between these two possibilities. The incidence of aural atresia (with or without abnormalities of the pinnae) is estimated to be between 1 and 5 per 20,000 live births (Cooper & Jabs, 1987). Atresia is frequently observed with cranial, facial, mandibular, or facial dysostoses such as Crouzon disease or Treacher Collins syndrome. Aural atresia may also be associated with facial, labial, and palatal clefts. Abnormalities of the skeletal system and visceral organs or chromosomal aberrations may also accompany atresia. Children with these defects usually suffer conductive-type hearing losses and may do well with bone conduction hearing aids if medical or surgical treatment is not in order. Jahrsdoerfer and Hall (1986) reviewed surgical results and complications from operating on 202 patients with congenital malformations of the external ear. They noted that defects of the external ear and canal may be apparent without damage to the middle or inner ear structures, or in some cases severe middle ear anomalies or aplasia of the middle ear may be associated with the external defects. External ear and canal anomalies may be visible at birth, but they are often overlooked, and the defect is not noted until hearing loss is suspected or discovered. Sometimes the auricle and the opening to the external auditory meatus appear normal, but the meatus may narrow and funnel down (atresia) to complete closure (stenosis). Surgery to open the external ear canal occasionally reveals thick soft tissue where the tympanic membrane should be; more often, a bony atresia plate of varying degrees of thickness causing closure of the external canal is present.

Microtia

Microtia is an abnormally formed, or absent, pinna. Fortunately, this occurs only once in about 20,000 births (Holmes, 1949).

The congenitally microtic ear varies from the mildly deformed ear, to total absence of pinna with no external auditory meatus, to complete atresia of the canal. Unilateral microtia is about six times more frequent than bilateral microtia (Dupertius & Musgrave, 1959), is more common in males than females, and is found predominantly on the right side (Brown, Fryer, & Morgan, 1969).

When a patient has one normal-hearing ear, obviously the problem of unilateral microtia is not so bad. When hairstyles are long, the deformity of the auricle is easily covered. Patients who wish to do something about the microtia have a choice between attempted surgical improvement or the use of a prosthetic-type pinna that is attached to the side of the head by special adhesive material. Regardless of the surgical techniques used, parents should be aware that the reconstructed ear seldom has the appearance of a normally developed pinna, and the result is not totally inconspicuous. For improved hearing benefit, however, as in the patient who has bilaterally stenosed ear canals, surgical intervention may be successful. If the atresia is bilateral, the child should be fitted with a bone-conduction hearing aid as soon as possible. If the atresia is unilateral and normal hearing can be validated in the opposite ear, treatment or habilitation is generally deferred. Aural atresias may accompany other defects of the cranium, face, skeleton, or mandible. The etiology of aural atresia may be due to a chromosomal aberration. Bone-conduction hearing aids work very well for patients with bilateral atresia.

Congenital Middle Ear Malformations

Malformation of the middle ear may be due to hereditary factors or to disturbances during embryonic development. Because the middle ear is largely formed during the first trimester of fetal life, gross developmental anomalies of the middle ear are often related to factors that influence the fetus during that time. Failure in the proper development of the first and second branchial arches may result in the absence of the ossicles or a fusion of the ossicles. A malformation of the stapes footplate, however, is related to the development of the otic capsule. A disturbance in the fetal growth of the first branchial pouch may affect the eustachian tube, middle ear cavity, and the ultimate pneumatization of the mastoid air spaces.

Isolated anomalies of the middle ear ossicles are not particularly rare. Malleus anomalies include fixation or deformation of the malleus head and bony fusion of the incudomalleolar joint or absence of the malleus. Incus deficiencies may exist in isolation or in conjunction with other middle ear ossicular problems and range from total absence to a deficiency of the lenticular process. The incus may have only a fibrous connection to the malleus or be fused to the lateral semicircular canal wall. Stapes anomalies may involve fusion of the stapes head to the promontory, absence of the head or crura, absence of the entire stapes itself, or presence of a columellar ossicle. Congenital absence of the oval window or the round window may also exist as a unilateral or bilateral defect.

Middle ear anomalies should be suspected whenever other branchial arch anomalies are observed and are often noted as part of congenital syndromes. Branchial arch disorders include atresia of the external auditory canal, cleft palate, micrognathia, Pierre Robin syndrome, Treacher Collins syndrome, and low-set auricles. Disorders that feature other skeletal defects may also include middle ear anomalies such as Apert syndrome, Klippel-Feil syndrome, and Crouzon, Paget, and van der Hoeve diseases. Middle ear anomalies have been reported in disorders of connective tissue such as gargoylism or Hunter-Hurler syndromes, Mòbius syndrome, and dwarfism. See Appendix A, "Pediatric Hearing Disorders," for additional information.

Discharge From the Ear Canal

The presence of fluid running from the external auditory meatus should give the clinician concern. Fluid from the external auditory canal may be divided in three categories: (a) clear; (b) cloudy, whitish, or yellow; and (c) bloody. Presence of these fluids in the ear canal requires immediate medical referral.

Clear fluid may represent cerebral spinal fluid leaking from a temporal bone fracture. This is a serious condition as it provides a ready route for access of the infection into the cranial cavity. This condition requires prompt otologic consultation for physical examination, radiographic studies, and perhaps surgical exploration to confirm and repair the spinal fluid leakage.

Cloudy fluid usually represents inflammation of the external auditory canal, a condition known as external otitis (see below). Less often, cloudy discharge may result from an inflamed middle ear space with existing perforation of the tympanic membrane.

Spots of blood in the external ear canal frequently result from self-instrumentation of the ear canal to relieve itching or attempts to self-remove cerumen. More significant amounts of blood found in the ear canal require immediate medical consultation.

Cerumen

Cerumen, commonly known as earwax, is a yellowish, waxy substance secreted in the outer third of the cartilaginous portion of the ear canal of humans. It protects the skin of the human ear canal, assists in cleaning and lubrication, and also provides some protection from bacteria, fungi, insects, and water. Excess or impacted cerumen can press against the eardrum and occlude the external auditory canal and cause conductive-type hearing loss. Cerumen is a combined product of the apocrine and sebaceous glands located in the skin of the ear canal.

Cerumen comes in two varieties: wet and dry. Wet earwax varies from yellowish to dark brown and, at times, even resembles blood. Dry earwax tends to be whitish scales or powdery feathery-like material. Most people's ear canals are self-cleaning of cerumen because the migratory pattern of the epithelium hairs sweep the cerumen outward through the external auditory meatus. Cerumen may usually be easily wiped away with a washcloth. People with excessive production of cerumen or inadequate self-cleaning mechanisms may accumulate wax in the external auditory canal, which can cause hearing loss. These individuals need to have their wax removed by an audiologist or trained specialist. The self-use of a water pressure system or the use of the infamous Q-tip applicator is to be condemned. Use of cotton-tip applicators, in the hands of an aggressive parent, is a major source of lacerated ear canals and perforated eardrums, and occasionally leads to conductive and sensorineural hearing loss.

Foreign Bodies

Children are the leading candidates to appear with foreign objects in their ear canals. Young children commonly place foreign bodies in the ear canal and nose. Objects may include broken crayons, food, cereal, beans, peas, beads, small toys, pieces of jewelry, or sometimes insects. If an organic foreign body is present, do not use eardrops because they will cause the foreign body to swell. If the foreign body is a hearing aid battery, eardrops may cause an electrical reaction that can cause severe burns to the ear. This produces hydroxides that will cause a severe alkaline burn. Hearing loss is usually not a major concern with foreign bodies in the ear canal unless the foreign object has ruptured the tympanic membrane or totally occludes the external canal. Most foreign objects can be carefully removed with forceps in the hand of a trained audiologist, although referral to a medical specialist for removal of the object may also be appropriate.

Bony Growths of the External Ear Canal

Occasionally, bony outgrowths in the external auditory canal may create problems. These come in two forms: (a) multiple growths termed *exostoses* and (b) single growths termed *osteomas*. Bony exostoses manifest as a gradual narrowing of the bony canal by broad-based mounds of bone that arise from the anterior and posterior canal walls. They are most often observed in individuals with a history of cold-water exposure (such as swimmers or surfers). The bone mounds usually occur bilaterally and are generally asymptomatic. Symptoms such as conductive hearing loss and otitis externa can arise if the canal becomes occluded. These appear as smooth, hard, round nodules in the external ear canal covered with normal skin. Exostoses do not require removal unless they cause cerumen accumulation, impair hearing, or create canal obstruction. Osteomas usually continue to grow and ultimately may require surgical removal.

External Ear Inflammatory Conditions

Occasionally, just touching the pinna will cause the child to wince or react with noticeable discomfort. Conditions most frequently responsible for this phenomenon are: (a) external otitis, (b) perichondritis, or (c) furunculosis of the external auditory canal. Each of these conditions is usually quite painful, and the patient needs prompt medical attention.

Perichondritis is an inflammation of the cartilage of the ear or ear canal. It is usually secondary to trauma to the cartilage, as in a blow to the pinna. The pinna may be red and tender with generalized swelling. Repeated episodes of perichondritis may lead to cartilage deformities of the pinna known commonly as *boxer's ears* or *cauliflower ears*.

A furuncle of the external ear canal is a boil or pimple. It is exquisitely tender because the skin of the ear canal is tightly applied to the cartilage. It usually clears without treatment, but painkillers and antibiotics are sometimes needed. Other symptoms may include itch, irritation, and possible temporary hearing loss while the infection is present. If the boil bursts, there may be a sudden discharge from the ear. If this happens, the pain eases dramatically and the symptoms soon abate.

Otitis Externa

Otitis externa is an inflammation of the skin of the external ear canal, most frequently due to bacterial or fungal infection. Often known as "swimmer's ear," the continual presence of water in the ear canal provides ideal circumstances for bacterial growth. The skin of the canal with acute external otitis is usually red and quite tender. External otitis is not uncommon in children who wear hearing aids. The use of an occlusive earmold may trap moisture in the ear canal and contribute to external otitis. The condition may be quite painful and the child will not let you insert an insert earphone or immittance probe tip into the inflamed ear canal.

Acute otitis externa is a sudden onset bacterial infection usually caused by *Pseudomonas aeruginosa*. The outer ear canal may be partially or fully swollen shut, and the auricle is very painful to touch. Treatment is to open the ear canal, place a temporary wick, and treat with eardrops. The wick is made of cloth or foam rubber which allows the eardrops to penetrate the swollen canal. This condition requires prompt otologic consultation by physical examination, radiographic studies, and perhaps surgical exploration of the ear to confirm and repair the leakage. It may be necessary for the patient to use a unilateral hearing aid in the opposite ear or go without the hearing aid until the condition clears. The increase in the use of open-type earmolds and receiver-in-the-canal hearing aids may help prevent this condition.

Perforation of the Tympanic Membrane

A perforated or "punctured" eardrum or tympanic membrane is a rupture or perforation (hole) that can occur as a result of otitis media infection or some type of trauma (Figure 4–4). Trauma episodes leading to perforation of the tympanic membrane might include a blow to the side of the ear, a water-skiing fall, underwater diving, sudden changes in surrounding air pressure, an accidental mishap while trying to clean the ear with a sharp instrument, a nearby explosion, a loud noise, or even secondary to otoscopic surgery. Flying with a severe cold can

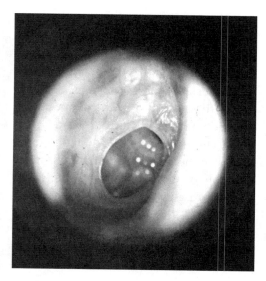

Figure 4–4. A perforated tympanic membrane can result from acute or recurrent otitis media infections or trauma to the ear.

also cause perforation due to changes in air pressure. Perforation of the eardrum leads to conductive hearing loss, which is usually temporary. Other symptoms may include tinnitus, earache, or a discharge of mucus.

The tympanic membrane is about 8 mm in diameter, and perforations are usually much smaller. Because the outer layer of the tympanic membrane is squamous epithelium, small traumatic perforations of the pars tensa area of the tympanic membrane will often heal spontaneously within a matter of days. The perforation may heal spontaneously within a few weeks, or may require a few months. Some perforations require otologic intervention. This may take the form of a paper patch placed over the perforation to promote healing, or in cases reticent to self-healing, tympanoplasty surgery may be necessary. However, in some cases, the perforation can last several years and will be unable to heal naturally. Such cases are usually a result of a perforation being surgically induced during an operation involving the ear. Hearing is usually

recovered fully, but chronic infection involving perforation over a long period may lead to permanent hearing loss.

Conductive hearing loss occurs as a consequence of poor vibration of the tympanic membrane. The degree of loss, however, is variable and dependent on the size of the perforation and its location on the tympanic membrane. Small perforations may be obvious with hearing levels within normal limits. Complications from perforations may be serious, and all such children should be immediately referred to a medical specialist. Parents should be advised to practice aural hygiene by keeping water out of the ear when the child is swimming or bathing until proper medical care of the ear has been given.

OTITIS MEDIA

Otitis media refers to inflammation of the middle ear, commonly termed *middle ear infection*. Otitis media is the most common of childhood diseases and one of the most frequent reasons for concerned parents to take their child for medical care. Typically, this inflammation of the middle ear follows, or is accompanied by, a cold or upper respiratory infection (URI). After a few days of a stuffy nose, the child notes that his or her ear hurts and complains of pain. The pain may quickly become severe or may settle down within a day or two, but pain can be prolonged as long as a week. Sometimes the pain can be reduced by home applications of heat compress applied to the ear. In the event that the infection continues without proper treatment, it may lead to rupture of the tympanic membrane, followed by discharge of pus from the ear. In some occurrences the ruptured drum will self-heal within a few days, but in other cases surgical repair of the tympanic membrane is necessary.

Ear infections can be very distressing in a child, and prompt, effective evaluation and treatment are necessary. Children younger than 2 years of age with otitis media have the highest rate of visits to physicians' offices. Statistics reported by the U.S. National Ambulatory Medical Care Survey of 2010 show that the number of medical office visits with otitis media as the primary diagnosis shows a general decline from a baseline of 34.4 per 100 children per year in 1997 down to 24.3 per 100 children in 2005. The steepest decline has occurred for young children under 3 years of age where the prevalence of ear infections is highest. Introduction of the pneumococcal conjugate vaccine in 2000 is credited in part for this decline.

Parental concern is foremost because otitis media is usually a disease of infants, toddlers, and young children. The disorder is particularly difficult for parents to deal with because the symptoms can have a sudden, unexpected onset or a quiet and long-term course without complaint from the child. Preverbal children are especially problematic because they are unable to localize and describe the source of their pain. It has been estimated that 25% to 40% of all upper respiratory infections (URIs) in children younger than 3 years of age are associated with acute otitis media (Karver, 1998). Many parents have come to believe that ear pulling is a reliable sign of an ear infection; however, ear pulling, in the absence of other symptoms, is not necessarily related to ear infections (Baker, 1992).

Otitis media has many degrees of severity, and various names are used to describe each. The terminology is often confusing because of multiple terms being used to describe the same condition. The disorder is characterized by the presence of negative middle ear pressure and the possible presence of fluid (effusion). The disorder may be present in a child without obvious clinical signs or symptoms of infection. Otitis media creates a mild-to-moderate degree of conductive hearing loss by compromising the traditional air-conduction sound pathway. A current hypothesis about the natural history of the pathology is that the clinical variations of otitis media form a continuum of the disease process and are dynamically interrelated—that is, the simple beginning forms of otitis media, if untreated, may lead to more complex and severe disease processes.

The economic considerations of otitis media as a public health issue have tremendous influence on national health expenditures. It is estimated that the total cost related to the identification and treatment of otitis media in the United States is more than $5 billion annually. This figure includes physician fees and surgery, prescribed medications, audiology, and speech-language evaluations. More than 30 million office visits per year to physicians for treatment of otitis media are estimated to take place in the United States. It is possible that on any winter day in the United States, up to 30% of children may be suffering ear infections and missing school. Before the age of 6 years, approximately 85% to 90% of all U.S. children have had at least one ear infection. Half of the children who have one ear infection before the age of 6 months will go on to have at least six or more episodes of otitis media before the age of 2 years. And, nearly 20% of children who suffer repeated ear infections will require surgery to correct the problem. Thus, it should not be surprising that otitis media is one of the most common indicators for outpatient use of antimicrobial agents in the United States resulting in an astronomical cost. Pediatric patients and their parents are often caught in the middle between policies of cost-oriented health care management and the recommendations for treatment provided by patient-oriented physicians.

Nearly every aspect of childhood otitis media, from diagnosis to treatment to sequelae, raises controversy and debate among professionals (Paradise, 1976a). Whereas recurrent otitis media is a well-recognized medical problem in children, the treatment and the management of this common disorder have been the focus of numerous research efforts. Questions regarding the short-term and long-term effects on child development of the otitis media continuum and the effect of the accompanying mild-to-moderate conductive hearing loss continue to raise unresolved questions.

Etiology of Otitis Media

Eustachian tube dysfunction has long been recognized to be a significant factor in the development of otitis media. The underlying cause of otitis media is nearly always the result of poor eustachian tube function, which leads to the production of sterile fluid by the mucosal lining of the middle ear. The eustachian tube has three general purposes: (a) protection of the middle ear from invading microbes; (b) clearance of middle ear secretions through the nasopharynx; and (c) equalization of pressure between the middle ear space and the nasopharynx. However, the most important function of the eustachian tube is ventilation of the middle ear space. When the eustachian tube malfunctions, from either a mechanical blockage or some functional cause, the air trapped in the middle ear cavity is absorbed by the mucosal lining of the middle ear, creating negative middle ear pressure and, ultimately, transudation of fluid into the cavity.

The child's eustachian tube is short, horizontal, and composed of relatively flaccid cartilage, whereas the adult eustachian tube lies in a more vertical position (Figure 4–5). The adult vertical position provides more effective protection for the middle ear. The nearly horizontal position of the child's eustachian tube more easily permits retrograde reflux of bacteria from the nasopharynx into the middle ear. Otitis media is most common during the first 2 years of a child's life and then decreases in incidence as the child grows older. As the young child ages, the inclination of the eustachian tube increases to about a 45-degree angle between the middle ear and nasopharynx, thereby decreasing the incidence of ear infections.

A thorough audiometric study was conducted by Fria, Cantekin, and Eichler (1985)

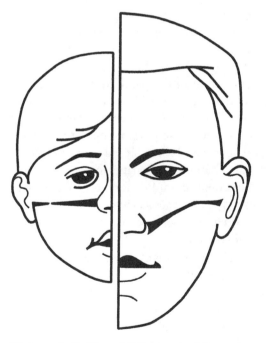

Figure 4–5. The child's eustachian tube is short, horizontal, and composed of relatively flaccid cartilage, whereas the adult eustachian tube lies in a more vertical position.

which carefully measured air conduction thresholds, based on 762 children with documented middle ear effusion (MEE). The average audiogram results were reported to be 27 dB HL at 500, 1000, and 4000 Hz, with a better hearing threshold of 20 dB HL at 2000 Hz. Hearing sensitivity in this study was approximately 10 dB worse in children with bilateral effusion than in children with unilateral effusion.

Diagnosis of Otitis Media

The diagnosis of otitis media is based on clinical manifestations, physical examination of the tympanic membrane, as well as acoustic immittance, otoacoustic emissions, and routine audiometry. But the mainstay of the diagnosis of otitis media by pediatricians is pneumatic otoscopy, a procedure in which a hermetically sealed otoscope is used to visualize the tympanic membrane with magnification while the air pressure in the external ear canal is varied. This permits evaluation of tympanic membrane mobility that is not possible by simple inspection through a simple otoscope. Many medical offices now use portable operating microscopes with binocular viewing to examine ears. Although hearing loss is the most prevalent complication associated with otitis media, the hearing usually returns to normal following resolution of the middle ear effusion.

The symptoms of otitis media can be classified as either specific or systemic. Specific symptoms include earache, rubbing or tugging at the ears, otorrhea (drainage), hearing impairment, and balance disturbance. Of these, only earache and otorrhea are generally associated with active infection. The systemic symptoms include fever, temperament disorders, restless sleep, irritability, or

low-grade discomfort. The goal of effective treatment is to provide rapid symptomatic relief and to reduce the likelihood of long-term sequelae such as hearing loss, permanent middle ear damage, and development and learning dysfunction. Difficult cases of otitis media require aspiration of the fluid, which is then cultured to identify the specific organism responsible for the infection (Figure 4–6).

Risk Factors for Otitis Media

The incidence of otitis media has been found to be a function of age, gender (more otitis media in boys), race (Native Americans, Eskimos, and Caucasians have higher incidences than Blacks), genetic factors, socioeconomic status, season, allergies, and climate influences. A number of research studies have identified risk factors that may make certain children more likely to have recurrent otitis media. Children living in households with many members have more episodes of otitis media than children living in households with fewer members. Children with siblings or parents who have a history of otitis media show a higher incidence of otitis media than children with family members without a history of the disease. Other risk factors include certain socioeconomic factors such as overcrowding with poor sanitation, inadequate diet, and the absence of routine health care; secondary cigarette smoke exposure; use of pacifiers; and possibly sleep position. Breast-feeding and group day-care play roles in URIs in general, leading to possible bouts of otitis media (Aniansson, Aim, & Andersson, 1994; Duncan et al., 1993; Paradise, Elster, & Tan, 1994). Infants who are bottle-fed in the supine position are more at risk for otitis media than infants who are fed

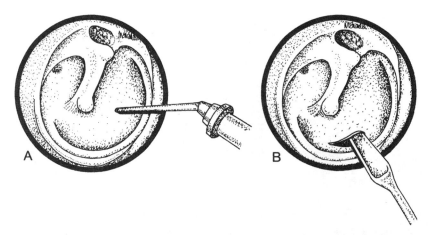

Figure 4–6. A. Tympanotomy, or surgical puncture of the tympanic membrane, is used to aspirate fluid by suction for culture. **B.** Myringotomy, or surgical incision of the tympanic membrane, is performed in the lower quadrant to avoid damage to middle ear ossicles. Myringotomy is conducted to provide instant relief from pain, to drain fluid from the middle ear space, and thus to help initiate rapid recovery from middle ear disease.

while being held upright. Children placed in day care have more otitis media than do children who are cared for at home because of endemic URIs passed among children (Teele, 1994). Allergies in young children have also been described as a major risk factor for otitis media because upper respiratory mucosal swelling during an allergic episode may cause eustachian tube dysfunction, similar to that observed during an upper respiratory infection.

Classification of Otitis Media

The general definitive and descriptive categories of otitis media are: (a) otitis media without effusion, (b) acute otitis media, (c) otitis media with effusion, and (d) otitis media with tympanic membrane perforation. Each of these categories may be classified by duration into acute (0 to 21 days), subacute (22 days to 8 weeks), and chronic (more than 8 weeks). In otitis media with effusion, with or without tympanic membrane perforation, the fluid or discharge may be characterized as serous (thin, watery liquid), purulent (pus-like liquid), or mucoid (thick, viscid, mucus-like liquid). An otoscopic view of a normal tympanic membrane is shown in Figure 4–7 with normal landmarks clearly visible.

Acute Otitis Media

Acute otitis media presents with sudden onset accompanied by severe ear pain, redness of the tympanic membrane, and fever. Other symptoms may include pain that causes general irritability and disruptive sleep patterns. Acute otitis media is an inflammatory disorder caused by microorganisms in the middle ear, usually as a sequel to an upper respiratory infection (URI). Acute otitis media (AOM) is often self-limited, following mild congestion

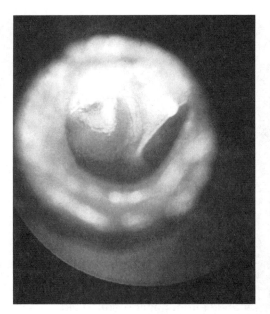

Figure 4–7. View of a normal tympanic membrane through an operating microscope with normal landmarks clearly visible. Viewed posteriorly through the translucent eardrum, the malleus, incus, and, stapedius tendon can be seen.

of the ears and perhaps mild discomfort and complains of popping sounds, but the symptoms resolve with the underlying URI. The seasonal incidence of acute otitis media is associated with seasonal upper respiratory illness during the cooler fall and winter months.

Otitis media without effusion is usually present in the early stages of acute otitis media. The diagnosis of acute otitis media is usually made with otoscopy based on the color, decreased mobility, and outward bulging contour of the tympanic membrane. Painful acute otitis media may be associated with a spontaneous perforation of the tympanic membrane, resulting in otorrhea that parents describe as "discharge found on the child's pillow in the morning." Approximately 50% of all children have had three or more episodes of acute otitis media by the age of 3 years, and 16% have experienced six or more episodes (Bluestone, 1998).

Should there be a spontaneous rupture of the tympanic membrane, the acute pain typically ceases immediately. Although generally an obvious diagnosis, sometimes acute otitis media presents without a red tympanic membrane, without fever, and without pain. Treatment is usually dependent on eliminating the infecting organism through adequately prescribed antibiotic treatment. When the diagnosis of acute otitis media is in doubt, or when determination of the causative agent is in question, aspiration of the middle ear fluid is performed with tympanocentesis or myringotomy. In patients with unusually severe earache and pain, myringotomy may be performed to provide immediate pain relief.

Bullous Myringitis

This disorder is extremely painful and may be accompanied by a feeling of pressure in the ear. Patients with bullous myringitis will typically not tolerate the pressure of earphones or any testing procedures that involve touching the pinna or ear canal as this creates unbearable pain. This disorder is created when blisters form on the tympanic membrane in association with a coincident upper respiratory infection and acute otitis media. The blisters, or bullae, represent an accumulation of fluid between the layers of the tympanic membrane and may appear to the untrained observer to represent acute otitis media. Hearing levels may be within normal limits. Bullous myringitis is an inflammatory response that causes symptoms of swelling, itching, and burning sensations in the ear. The most common causes of bullous myringitis are the bacteria *Mycoplasma pneumoniae*. This painful condition generally develops quickly over 1 or 2 days secondary to bacterial otitis media, and treatment includes administration of antibiotics and analgesics and possible surgical draining of the tiny blisters.

Serous Otitis Media

This is the most common form of otitis media and refers to the presence of middle ear effusion that is clear, thick, or sticky but not infectious. This condition generally is without pain and the effusion may be asymptomatic in most children. However, if pain is present in this disorder, it is usually intermittent and mild. Older children may complain of muffled hearing or a sense of fullness in the ear. Younger children may turn up the television volume because of hearing loss. Serous otitis media goes by many names including secretory otitis media, silent otitis media, and may become "glue ear" that is recalcitrant to medical treatment. The tympanic membrane is usually opaque, and there may be relatively normal mobility to applied heavy positive and negative pressure from the pneumatic otoscope. Following an episode of acute otitis media, an effusion may persist despite antibiotic treatment of the condition. Otitis media with effusion usually goes away on its own over a few weeks or months. Medical treatment may speed up this process. Some cases require surgical treatment of myringotomy with tympanostomy tube insertion. About 50% of pediatric cases of serous otitis media show no significant hearing loss (Cohen & Sade, 1972). However, children with middle ear effusion and hearing loss should be given periodic hearing tests and routine tympanometry until the fluid clears and the hearing returns to normal. Additional monitoring with age-specific language developmental tests may also be an appropriate monitoring tool. The otoscopic photomicrograph shown in Figure 4–8 was taken from an ear with serous otitis media

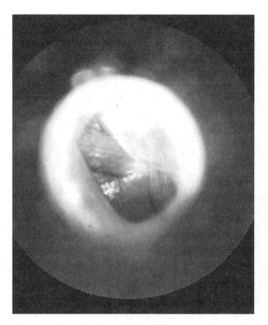

Figure 4–8. An otoscopic view of a tympanic membrane with serous otitis media characterized by the absence of all normal landmarks. The eardrum is retracted, with the short process of the malleolus prominent and the long process foreshortened in appearance. Inferiorly, the eardrum is sucked inward from effusion into the middle ear space.

characterized by the absence of all normal landmarks.

Adhesive Otitis Media

This form of otitis media is the result of chronic inflammation of the middle ear and prolonged presence of middle ear effusion. This condition may lead to the growth of fibroblasts and the formation of scar tissue in the middle ear space. The thickening of the fibrous tissue in the middle ear space may create negative middle ear pressure leading to severe retraction of the tympanic membrane (Figure 4–9). The proliferation of the fibrous material frequently impairs movement of the tympanic membrane

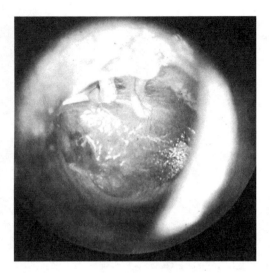

Figure 4–9. Adhesive otitis media with severe retraction of the tympanic membrane. The eardrum is draped around the incus posteriorly, and the stapedius tendon is clearly seen. The thickening of the fibrous tissue in the middle ear space may create severe negative middle ear pressure leading to adhesive retraction of the tympanic membrane.

and middle ear ossicles. The long-standing negative middle ear pressure causes atelectasis of the tympanic membrane binding the eardrum tightly to the ossicles. When a retraction pocket forms in the posterior-superior portion of the pars tensa of the tympanic membrane, the development of a retraction pocket leading to cholesteatoma (see below for definition) is probable. Successful treatment of adhesive otitis media is sometimes difficult as it represents a long-standing disorder that is nonresponsive to antibiotics and general pharmacological agents. Surgical intervention with myringotomy and placement of ventilation tubes can be successful unless the tubes are naturally extruded before adequate ventilation and healing of the middle ear can take place. Some physicians recommend various techniques of auto-insufflation (i.e., simple procedures for forcing air into the middle ear

space through the eustachian tubes). Adhesive otitis media generally creates a significant conductive hearing loss (Allen, 2004).

Chronic Suppurative Otitis Media

Chronic suppurative otitis media (CSOM) is the specific diagnosis of long-term and recurrent middle ear disease with drainage (otorrhea) through a perforation of the tympanic membrane. This is a late stage of ear disease in which there is active infection of the middle ear (and possibly the mastoid) as well as a central perforation of the tympanic membrane accompanied by variable discharge usually described as foul smelling, purulent, and "cheese-like." This condition most often has its onset in childhood, between the ages of 5 and 10 years. CSOM is the result of middle ear cyclic activity of inflammation, ulceration, and infection with granulation tissue, which can ultimately destroy the middle ear ossicles and the bone surrounding the middle ear space. This disease may occur with or without accompanying cholesteatoma, although it inevitably leads to serious complications of otitis media. Mastoiditis is invariably a part of the pathologic process. Long-term recurrent otitis media may negatively impact the normal process of mastoid pneumatization or cause mastoid sclerosis. Severe forms of chronic otitis media may damage the middle ear ossicles, depending on the severity and duration of the disease. Treatment of CSOM is often challenging usually beginning with various medical procedures and applications followed by surgical removal of the tympanic membrane and repair of the perforation when necessary.

Treatment of Otitis Media

During the 1930s and 1940s, otitis media and its suppurative complications, such as cholesteatoma and mastoiditis, constituted common severe medical problems for infants and young children. With the advent of effective antimicrobial agents during the 1950s and 1960s, control of otitis media became commonplace in medical practice. However, the overapplication of antimicrobial treatments during more recent decades has produced antibiotic-resistant strains of the most common bacterial pathogens creating growing alarm and concern among physicians and parents alike. The concern regarding the growth of antibiotic-resistant bacterial strains created reluctance for immediate prescription of antibiotics, and new approach to treatment of otitis media during the 1980s was developed, known commonly as "watchful waiting." By 2004, major medical associations were recommending that initial routine observation rather than immediate antimicrobial therapy for the management of acute otitis media should be followed in selected children. Audiology professionals, on the other hand, voiced outspoken concern about the potential problems created by unresolved fluid in the middle ear causing long-term conductive hearing loss and adverse effects on a child's speech-language and educational development. Middle ear effusion may persist following completion of recommended medical treatment (Waldman & Brewer, 2007). According to Teele, Klein, and Rosner (1989), middle ear effusion may persist following completion of traditional antibiotic treatment for 2 weeks in 60% to 70% of cases, 4 weeks in 40% patients, and as long as 8 weeks in 10% to 25% of individuals.

Tonsillectomy and Adenoidectomy

The tonsils and adenoids have traditionally been implicated in the pathophysiology of otitis media, although current medical research questions this assumption. Tonsils and adenoids are part of a ring of glandular tissue encircling the back of the throat. The tonsils are the two masses of tissue on either side of the back of the throat. The adenoids are located high in the throat behind the soft palate and are not visible through the mouth without special instruments. It is thought that they help form antibodies as part of the body's immune system to resist and fight future infections, although they often become infected themselves. Chronic infections in the tonsils and adenoids can affect nearby structures, and their swelling may create blockage around the base, or opening, of the eustachian tubes. This situation may lead to mechanical blockage or interference in the function of the eustachian tube. Eustachian tube blockage or dysfunction leads to ineffective aeration of the middle ear spaces, and thereby ear infections and subsequent hearing loss.

Recurrent tonsillitis and enlarged adenoids were once thought to be the major cause of otitis media. A tonsillectomy is a surgical procedure in which the tonsils are removed from either side of the throat. The procedure is performed in response to cases of repeated occurrence of acute tonsillitis or adenoiditis in children; the adenoids are typically removed at the same time, a procedure called adenoidectomy. Experts agree that tonsillectomy alone is not recommended as routine treatment for otitis media, although the role of adenoidectomy in treating otitis media is somewhat more controversial. The surgical removal of the tonsils and adenoids of children has generated considerable controversy among health professionals for many years. In the United States, the number of tonsillectomies has declined annually since the 1970s. In 2006, an estimated 530,000 tonsillectomies (with or without adenoidectomy) and 132,000 adenoidectomies (without tonsillectomy) were performed in children younger than 15 years of age with most of these operations performed as ambulatory, same-day procedures (Cullen, Hall, & Golosinskiy, 2009). The American Academy of Otolaryngology-Head and Neck Surgery (2011) recommends that children who have three or more tonsillar infections a year undergo tonsillectomy.

Pneumococcal Conjugate Vaccine (PCV13)

Although on the decrease since 2000, infections with *Streptococcus pneumoniae* bacteria can make children very sick. It causes blood infections, pneumonia, and meningitis, mostly in young children. Children younger than 2 years of age are at higher risk for serious disease than older children. *Pneumococcal* bacteria are spread from person to person through close contact. *Pneumococcal* infections may be hard to treat because some strains of the bacteria have become resistant to the drugs that are used to treat them. This makes prevention of *pneumococcal* infections through vaccination even more important.

Considerable research has resulted in the development of the *pneumococcal conjugate vaccine* to prevent otitis media; clearly, this protective strategy for children at risk for otitis media will be beneficial in reducing this enormous health problem from the points of view of human suffering and economic consequences. Klein (2011) pointed out four factors that have recently led to a reverse in recommended medical treatment of otitis media in children: (a) access to medical care has increased considerably over the years reducing the probabilities of adverse complications from otitis media; (b) diagnostic techniques have improved to permit more certain and accurate diagnosis of otitis media; (c) there has been a change in the virulence of the bacterial pathogens from the preantibiotic era (i.e., streptococcus is now a rare cause of acute otitis media

due to an aggressive vaccine program); *Haemophilus influenzae* and *Moraella catarrhalis* cause almost half of the cases that, fortunately, produce a relatively mild form of the disease; and (d) the growing number of new antibiotics that have been introduced to treat otitis media. No single antimicrobial agent appears to be suitable for all patients with otitis media. At least 19 antimicrobial agents for treatment of middle ear effusions have been approved by the FDA as of 2010.

Klein summarized the results of two meticulously designed large sample studies of treatment protocols for acute otitis media in children less than 2 years of age (Hoberman et al., 2011; Tahtinen et al., 2011). In these two important, randomized, double-blind studies of antibiotic and nonantibiotic treatment regimens, only children with a clear, certain diagnosis of acute otitis media served as subjects. The results of each study showed a significant benefit among children who received antibiotic treatment with respect to the duration of acute signs of illness. The disease rates of clinical failure were higher in the placebo groups than in the antibiotic treatment groups. Children treated with antibiotics had fewer associated side effects of the disease process. Accordingly, Klein concludes that children with a certain diagnosis of acute otitis media recover more quickly when they are treated with an appropriate antimicrobial agent.

Tympanic Membrane Ventilation Tubes

When middle ear fluid becomes persistent, and antibiotics have not been effective, surgical insertion of ear ventilation tubes is usually recommended. Otitis media due to eustachian tube dysfunction is commonly treated indirectly by a simple surgical procedure to insert tiny, hollow, plastic tympanostomy tubes into the tympanic membranes. The hollow plastic tubes are also known as pressure equalization tubes or PE tubes (Figure 4–10). The tubes, inserted into the tympanic membrane, serve to aerate the middle ear space until the eustachian tube recovers and functions normally. The tubes are left in place for several months until they naturally extrude, in hopes that the eustachian tube dysfunction, which initially caused the otitis media, has resolved naturally. There is a wide variety of tubes available that differ by lumen size, tube length, and retention styles and time.

Treatment of otitis media with tympanostomy tubes is the most common surgical operation performed in children in the United States with more than 700,000 children undergoing the procedure each year. The insertion of tympanostomy tubes for recurrent ear infections has increased 35% in the past decade, while the number of office visits for otitis media has decreased by about 25% during the past 10 years. During

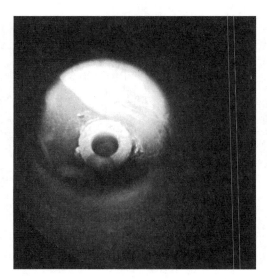

Figure 4–10. Hollow ventilating tubes known as pressure equalization tubes or PE tubes are placed in the tympanic membrane to provide aeration to the middle ear.

this period of time tympanostomy surgeries increased from 2.1 procedures per 100 outpatient medical visits for otitis media in 1996 to 3.8 procedures per 100 visits in 2006. Considerable controversy exists as to the reasons for these changes in the treatment of otitis media between pediatricians, who typically oppose surgical treatment of otitis media, and otolaryngologists, the surgical specialists. In 2006, children from birth through 2 years of age received 64% of the ear tube operations, while children from 3 through 5 years underwent another 24% of the surgical procedures.

Gates (1988) points out that surgical treatment for otitis media should be recommended only when recognized standard of care medical treatment fails. Thus, medical and surgical therapies for otitis media should be sequential, not alternative, treatments. If otitis media is likely due to inadequate ventilation of the middle ear, then insertion of tympanostomy tubes is the recommended surgical treatment. If infection of the middle ear from reflux of nasopharyngeal organisms is the problem, adenoidectomy may be the appropriate surgical treatment. In most cases of chronic otitis media, both pathophysiologic conditions exist concurrently; thus, the combined operation of tympanostomy tubes with adenoidectomy may be recommended. Rosenfeld (1997) dispelled several common myths about tympanostomy tubes:

- Tympanostomy tubes do not cause significant scarring of the eardrum, and the tiny scar that may form when the tube falls out does not affect hearing.
- A properly placed tympanostomy tube does not usually fall into the middle ear. Instead, the tube is naturally pushed into the external ear canal between 6 and 18 months.

- Water precautions are typically unnecessary for most children with tympanostomy tubes. Water precautions may be necessary for those children who swim in lake water or spend a substantial amount of time immersed underwater.

- The tympanostomy tube placement does not cure the ear infection; it simply controls the infection by temporarily ventilating the middle ear. Hopefully, by the time the tube falls out naturally, the majority of children will have outgrown their tendency for middle ear problems.

Opposing points of view regarding the use of tympanostomy tubes for treatment of otitis media with effusion cite the lack of convincing evidence linking otitis media early in life to either otologic or developmental difficulties later in life. That is, if the majority of patients with otitis media spontaneously recover, why is surgical intervention necessary? Other considerations to be weighed before surgical intervention include the cost and risk of surgery as well as the potential complications resulting from tympanostomy tube insertion. Comparison of preoperative threshold audiometry with postoperative auditory thresholds measured after tympanostomy tube placement is important to document improved hearing.

Complications Associated With Otitis Media

Although complications from otitis media were commonplace in the years preceding the advent of antibiotic treatment of otitis media, in more recent years occurrences of complications have diminished due to improved access to medical care, better training of physicians, and the growth of the audiology profession. Of course, the recent presence of specific-target antimicrobial agents to treat acute episodes of otitis media has also helped reduce complications. Nonetheless, however, complications do occur and cause serious ear and hearing considerations. Complications of untreated or nonresponsive otitis media (Figure 4–11) may include hearing loss, perforation of the tympanic membrane (with or without effusion), tympanic membrane retraction, cholesteatoma, mastoiditis, adhesive otitis media, tympanosclerosis, ossicular discontinuity, facial paralysis, and labyrinthitis. Serious intracranial complications may include meningitis, encephalitis, brain abscess, and sinus thrombophlebitis.

The most prevalent adverse sequel to surgical insertion of tympanostomy tubes is purulent otorrhea or infected drainage from the tube itself. Treatment of otorrhea consists of a topical steroid and oral antibiotic that are usually sufficient to clean up the discharge. In some 15% of patients, the tympanic membrane fails to heal following extrusion of the tympanostomy tube, leaving a small perforation in the eardrum. The persistent perforation rate has been shown to be significantly higher when the tympanostomy tubes are retained longer than 36 months (Nichols, Ramadan, Wax, & Santrock, 1998). The treatment of the persistent perforation generally requires a minor surgical procedure, known as a myringoplasty, to seal the perforation.

Tympanosclerosis

Although not a "complication" of otitis media, per se, tympanosclerosis is a common finding in individuals who have had a long history of middle ear infections. Following recurrent episodes of otitis media, the tympanic membrane, and possibly also the middle ear space, may develop *tympanosclerosis,* defined as easily observed shiny

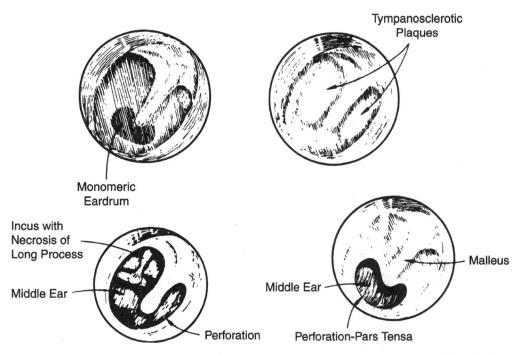

Figure 4–11. Otoscopic illustrations of the tympanic membrane showing sequelae of chronic otitis media. Chronic and recurrent otitis media may damage the tympanic membrane and middle ear ossicles depending on the severity and duration of the disease.

white deposits of hyalinized and calcified scar tissue. Tympanosclerosis deposits may cause stiffening of the tympanic membrane or fusion and fixation of the middle ear ossicles. Middle ear granulation tissue, polyps, and monomeric membrane formation are also associated with various types of chronic otitis media, as shown in Figure 4–11.

Paparella and Brady (1970) and English, Northern, and Fria (1973) reviewed patients with chronic suppurative otitis media and mastoiditis. In each study there was found a definite increase in the incidence of sensorineural hearing loss that they suggested was due to a cochlear biochemical change created by toxic materials passed into the inner ear through the round window. These studies noted that bone conduction thresholds worsened with the severity and duration of chronic otitis media, confirming that

sensorineural hearing loss can be sequelae of chronic otitis media.

Cholesteatoma

Cholesteatoma is a growth of skin from the external ear canal which invades the middle ear space by pressing into a retraction pocket in the tympanic membrane. The technical definition of cholesteatoma is an inclusion of keratinizing squamous epithelium that proliferates within the temporal bone; cholesteatoma is a misnomer because the growth is not made of cholesterol and it is not a tumor (Waldman & Brewer, 2007). Repeated infection and persistent negative middle ear pressure may create a retraction pocket (also termed a *pouch* or *sac*) in the posterior-superior portion of the tympanic membrane. The continuing growth of the squamous epithelium (skin) into this retraction pocket takes the form of a cyst formed by new layers of skin growing over older layers of skin. Over time, cholesteatoma can increase in size and destroy the surrounding tissues and structures of the middle ear. In otitis media with perforation, the tissues of the middle ear intermittently undergo destruction, healing, and scarring during the recurrent infection process.

Congenital cholesteatomas can, on rare occasion, grow behind the intact tympanic membrane, from an aberrant embryonic inclusion of squamous epithelium of the middle ear. Congenital cholesteatoma is a difficult diagnosis as its early growth does not necessarily impede motion of the tympanic membrane or middle ear ossicles. Accordingly, there may not be noticeable hearing loss, and the diagnosis is based on otoscopic identification of a white mass observed behind the eardrum. Acquired cholesteatoma is the more common disease occurring secondary to chronic suppurative otitis media (CSOM). Initially, the symptoms of cholesteatoma include drainage (sometimes accompanied by a foul odor), conductive hearing loss, fullness or pressure in or behind the ear, dizziness, and facial weakness. Cholesteatoma is usually, but not always, a unilateral problem. This is a very serious ear condition that must be examined and evaluated by an otolaryngologist. Cholesteatomas that are undiscovered or untreated can be dangerous, with resultant bone erosion leading to significant hearing loss or deafness, brain abscess, and meningitis; and, in fact, death can sometimes occur as a complication of the untreated disease. Because of the seriousness of this disorder, audiologists must be extremely careful in the evaluation and referral of children with unilateral conductive hearing losses that do not respond to traditional medical treatment.

The cross-sectional diagram shown in Figure 4–12 illustrates an attic and a middle ear cholesteatoma. Moisture and bacteria may gain access to the cholesteatoma, creating infection and drainage. Initial treatment may consist of careful cleaning of the debris, topical eardrops, and antibiotics to clear up the infection process. Large or complicated cholesteatomas usually require surgical removal to protect the patient from more serious complications. The purpose of the surgery is twofold: to remove the cholesteatoma and infection, as well as to preserve or improve hearing. In some cases, these goals are accomplished through two separate operations. Following surgical removal of the cholesteatoma, routine visits are scheduled to examine the ear for possible recurrence of the tumor. In some patients, an open mastoid cavity is surgically created, and office visits every few months (perhaps for life) are necessary to clean out the cavity and prevent new infections.

Mastoiditis

Mastoiditis is categorized into either acute or chronic stages. The terms represent the degree of involvement of the infected mastoid air cell system. The anatomic continuity between the middle ear and the mucosal lining of the mastoid antrum allows for the coexisting inflammatory process associated with these structures. With the onset of edema or insufficient drainage of the mastoid mucosa, pressure is created within the air cells, causing localized discomfort. Some of the clinical manifestations of mastoiditis are fullness, pain, otitis media, tenderness, edema, and conductive hearing loss. Other clinical findings may consist of tympanic membrane and middle ear ossicular destruction.

Acute mastoiditis is an inflammation of the ciliated mucosa of the antrum. Until the

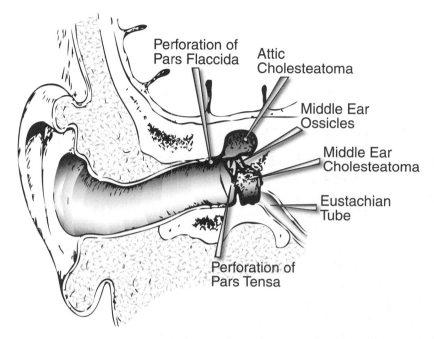

Figure 4–12. A cross-section of the external ear showing two forms of cholesteatoma growing through perforations and retraction pockets of the tympanic membrane. Reprinted with permission from "Chronic Otitis Media as a Cause of Sensorineural Hearing Loss," by G. M. English, J. L. Northern, and T. J. Fria, 1973, *Archives of Otolaryngology, 98*, pp. 17–22.

1940s, acute mastoiditis was a complication of acute otitis media in 25% to 50% of cases. With the advent of antibiotics such as penicillin, the incidence of acute mastoiditis has been lowered considerably. However, antibiotic therapy has been said to "mask" the presence of mastoiditis, whereby the disease is suppressed enough to reduce the symptoms but not enough to resolve the ongoing destructive process.

Chronic mastoiditis occurs with chronic inflammation of the membrane lining the mastoid antrum and ciliated cells. The bone structure is often involved in the infection. Generally, chronic mastoiditis is associated with a history of otitis media and the possible presence of cholesteatoma, which may be active or inactive, depending on whether purulent discharge is present or absent. The symptoms of chronic mastoiditis are similar to those of acute mastoiditis, with the exception of the type of hearing loss noted. Acute mastoiditis may be accompanied by normal hearing or mild conductive hearing loss; chronic mastoiditis likely is associated with a mixed hearing loss composed of a significant conductive hearing component as well as sensorineural loss.

During the pre-antibiotic era, some of the most life-threatening complications of mastoiditis were meningitis, brain abscess, and cerebellar abscess. Current complications still include facial nerve paralysis, labyrinthitis, meningitis, and cholesteatoma. In cases in which antibiotics have been ineffective in treating acute mastoiditis, a simple mastoidectomy is performed with surgical drainage of the mastoid air cells. Patients with chronic mastoiditis are initially treated nonsurgically to dry the ear and prevent factors that would complicate surgical treatment. When medical management fails, a surgical mastoidectomy is performed.

Otitis-Prone Neonates and Infants

The diagnosis of middle ear effusion (MEE) in neonates and infants presents special problems because of the small and narrow external ear canal, the presence of vernix caseosa, and the difficulty in visualizing the infant tympanic membrane. It is well acknowledged that middle ear effusion occurs commonly in neonates, both in the outpatient population and in the intensive care nursery. In the infant, the external ear canal is flexible and often collapsed, and the tympanic membrane lies in a nearly horizontal plane (Figure 4–13). Balkany et al. (1978) reported results from 125 consecutive infants from the neonatal intensive care unit (NICU) and found MEE to be present

in 30%. They concluded that this finding was especially important because unrecognized middle ear fluid may act as a focus for the dissemination of bacteria into the circulation or central nervous system. They also found that nasotracheal intubation of longer than 7 days was highly associated with effusion.

Howie, Ploussard, and Sloyer (1975) studied the whole of his private practice caseload and noted that one group of children could be identified as "otitis-prone." These children had had six or more recurrent bouts of otitis media before the age of 6 with their first episode during the first 18 months of life. This finding has been replicated in numerous other subsequent studies that verify that if a child has an initial bout of otitis media very early in life, the chances of recurrent episodes of MEE are high. On the other hand, the research shows that if a child's first bout of otitis media occurs after 18 months of age, the child is likely to have only a singular or perhaps a few isolated occasions of MEE during childhood.

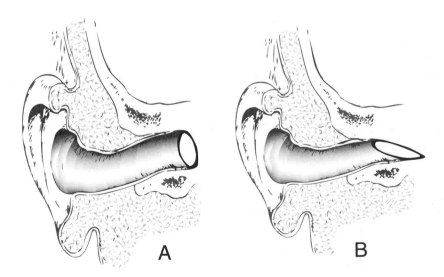

Figure 4–13. Orientation of the tympanic membrane in the adult (**A**) and in the infant (**B**). Note the horizontal plane of the infant eardrum which makes visualization of the tympanic membrane difficult in infants. Used with permission from T. J. Balkany, S. A. Berman, M. A. Simmons, et al., 1978, *Laryngoscope, 88*, p. 399.

Native Americans

Otitis media continues to be a serious health problem among the native populations of North America. Health problems exist among Native American populations because of poor living conditions, harsh physical and psychological environments, inadequate water facilities, crowded living conditions, unsanitary waste disposal, inadequate refrigeration, nonexistent insect control, and poor nutrition. With federal financial support, significant strides in the health care for American Indians and Eskimos have been accomplished. However, cultural barriers, genetics, poverty, poor transportation, and lack of education about health issues make solutions to health problems difficult. The widespread health problems associated with otitis media are not uncommon in many of the developing countries around the world. Research methodological difficulties preclude precise statistical data regarding otitis media in native populations, because studies often report data for "otitis media" without specifying the type of disease being evaluated, without noting that different diagnostic methods are represented, and without having complete audiological information. Accordingly, incidence and prevalence data among native populations are limited and ambiguous, especially among subcultures such as indigenous tribes, but there is little doubt that otitis media remains a major health issue.

It has been suggested that the small and closed genetic pool among the Navajos is a major cause of increased abnormal otologic findings such as bifid uvula, microtia, and aural atresias. For example, one hundred years ago there were only 5,000 Navajos; the Navajo population has grown to more than 300,000. Reports have been published on various American Indian tribes confirming the high presence of conductive hearing loss in children associated with various forms of otitis media (Fischler, Todd, & Feldman, 1985; Hunter, Davey, Kohtz, & Daly, 2007; Johnson, 1967; Johnson & Watrous, 1978).

Ear disease has been so endemic among native Eskimo children that parents did not consider otorrhea (drainage from the ear) to be a serious problem. Brody (1964) and Brody, Overfield, and McAlister (1965) reported that 31% of an Eskimo village population had at least one episode of draining ears within the evaluation year, with two-thirds of the ear disease group indicating more than one episode of otorrhea. It has been shown that ear pathology in Eskimo children is established by the age of 2 years, and those children who by age 2 did not have draining ears were unlikely to develop ear pathology. Several additional studies on Eskimo populations have been published confirming the extraordinarily high incidence of middle ear disease (Bowd, 2005; Reed, Struve, & Maynard, 1967; Reed & Dunn, 1970; Moore, 1999). The identification and treatment of otitis media in these native groups are especially important due to the impact that early hearing loss may have on the children's abilities to learn their native language and English and subsequent educational achievement.

MEDICAL DISORDERS AND SENSORINEURAL HEARING LOSS

Connexin 26 (Cx26) Hearing Loss

Advances in genetics have enabled researchers to identify a significantly large number of genes that cause sensorineural hearing loss. A considerable portion of people with nonsyndromic sensorineural hearing loss have Connexin 26 (Cx26) disorder. Connexin 26 is a protein found on the GJB2 gene and is the most common cause of congenital sensorineural hearing loss. Although the technical name of this gene is GJB2 (gap junction beta 2), the protein name, Connexin 26, is a more recognizable name. It is also referred to as DFNB1 deafness (Morton & Nance, 2006). This is a complex genetic disorder caused by defective copies of the gap junction beta 2 (GJB2). Connexin 26 mutations are responsible for at least 20% of all genetic hearing loss and 10% of all childhood hearing loss; some scientists believe that Cx26 is the underlying cause of nearly 50% of all cases of hereditary deafness (Nance & Kearsey, 2004). In certain ethnic populations and population cohorts, more than 80% of cases of nonsyndromic recessive deafness may be caused by mutated Connexin 26 genes.

Connexin 26 is a protein made in the cochlea, coded in our DNA by a gene identified as GJB2. The GJB2 gene contains the instructions for manufacturing a number of proteins, including Connexin 26. Connexin proteins, in general, are known as gap-junction proteins that are necessary for cells to communicate with each other. Without sufficient levels of Connexin 26, the potassium flow from hair cells in the cochlea is disrupted, resulting in extremely high levels of potassium in the organ of Corti leading to profound sensorineural hearing loss. The exact purpose of the protein is not known, but it is thought to help regulate the balance of potassium in the supporting cells. If the potassium balance is wrong, the supporting cells die, followed by the death of the sensory hair cells.

Connexin 26 mutations are genetically transmitted from parent to child in an autosomal recessive pattern, which means that the child with hearing loss must inherit one copy of the nonfunctioning gene from each parent. Carriers who have only one copy of the gene (i.e., one normal gene and one mutated gene) do not have any of the

signs of the hearing loss, but they have a one in two chance of passing on the defective gene to their children (who would then also be nonsymptomatic carriers), and a one in four chance of having an affected child if the other parent is also a carrier. Thus, everyone has two copies of the Cx26 gene; if each birth parent has a single flawed copy of the GJB2/Connexin 26 gene, their baby has a 25% chance of being born with a hearing loss. In the typical case, each parent, usually unknowingly, has one healthy and one mutated copy of the gene. If their child inherits a mutation-carrying copy from both parents, the child will have sensorineural hearing loss (Cohn & Kelley, 1999).

There have been at least 80 different mutations identified in the gene for Cx26 that cause hearing loss since it was first discovered in 1997. Research has suggested that these different mutations can have different hearing loss effects. Those that stop the protein from being made are the most damaging and usually cause more severe hearing loss. Those Cx26 mutations that cause the protein to be made in an altered form may cause less severe hearing loss. Cx26 mutations are nonsyndromic, meaning that the mutation produces only isolated hearing loss, and there is no increased risk for other medical problems commonly associated with hearing loss. However, there is in a minority of cases a higher incidence of skin disorders in patients with a Connexin 26 mutation. In a comprehensive study of 126 children with GJB2 mutations seen at Boston Children's Hospital, 56% demonstrated some hearing loss progression, generally gradually but occasionally precipitously (Kenna et al., 2010).

Children born with bilateral significant sensorineural hearing loss without identifiable etiology are candidates to be referred for genetic testing for Connexin 26 mutations. To perform the Cx26 test, a DNA sample is obtained from the child and sent to a special laboratory where the gene sequence is compared to that of the regularly occurring sequence to look for flaws or mutations. If two Cx26 identical mutations or two different mutations are found, it can be assumed that the patient's hearing loss is caused by the Cx26 mutations.

When a mutation analysis is positive with Cx26 testing, there will usually be no need for further investigations such as imaging and ophthalmological tests, because other causes of congenital deafness no longer have to be excluded (Kemperman, Hoefsloot, & Cremers, 2002). Cx26 testing can help identify the cause of the hearing loss as well as help predict the prognosis of the hearing loss. Confirming Cx26 hearing loss can also help with management decisions as most of these children do well with hearing aids and cochlear implants.

Unilateral Sensorineural Hearing Loss in Children

As infant screening programs have become the standard of care across the United States, there has been an increase in the early identification of children with unilateral hearing loss, and many audiologists are faced with making management recommendations. Parents, physicians, the educational community, and policymakers have questions about how these hearing losses can be expected to impact child development and how this relates to needed early intervention services, educational management, and school readiness. There certainly is a need to have a habilitation protocol for this group and a need to monitor them for any progressive hearing loss that might occur. Unfortunately, at this time, once these children have been identified, the best course of management is still undetermined.

Single-sided deafness, also described as unilateral hearing loss (involvement of one ear only) is a fairly common problem among children, with a prevalence of 3 to 14 in 1,000 according to Porter and Bess (2011). Fitzpatrick et al. (2010) identified 46 children with unilateral hearing loss in a review of 670 (14.5%) of their pediatric clinical patients. The definition of unilateral hearing loss is described as a one-sided, pure-tone, three-frequency average (500, 1000, 2000 Hz) of 20 dB HL or greater or hearing thresholds greater than 25 dB at two or more frequencies at 2000 Hz or higher in one ear only (Eichwald & Gabbard, 2008).

Known causes of severe-to-profound single-sided hearing loss include physical trauma, measles, microtia, meningitis, or mumps. In many instances, the child and family are unaware of the problem, and the parents do not discover the loss until some sequence of events suggests the presence of a hearing loss in one ear such as the realization that the child only hears and follows conversations when presented on the good ear side. Parents will finally realize that their child can only hear on the telephone with one particular ear, or the child cannot be awakened when the normal-hearing ear is pressed into a pillow.

Problems experienced by children with unilateral hearing loss were brought to light by Bess and Tharpe (1984) and Bess, Klee, and Culbertson (1986) of Vanderbilt University. They identified 60 children with unilateral hearing loss enrolled in the Nashville Metropolitan School System and closely examined their educational records. Bess and Tharpe found that approximately one third of this group had failed at least one grade during their school years and that nearly 50% of the group needed special resource assistance in the schools. In studies in which unilaterally hearing-impaired children were matched with normal-hearing children, Bess's group showed that the children with unilateral hearing loss performed much poorer on localization tasks and syllable recognition tasks. Oyler, Oyler, and Matkin (1987, 1988) challenged the Vanderbilt data on unilateral hearing loss by conducting a similar study in a large school district in Tucson, Arizona. They found a remarkably similar academic failure rate, proving again that children with unilateral hearing loss are at a risk factor approximately 10 times greater than that for the general school population for academic difficulties resulting in grade failure. In both the Nashville and Tucson studies, the recurring profile among the unilateral hearing loss students who experienced academic difficulties included: (a) early age of onset, (b) severe to profound hearing impairment, and (c) right-ear impairment.

From these research efforts, it is clear that children with unilateral hearing loss experience considerably more difficulty in communication and in education than was previously supposed (Tharpe, 2009). When the unilateral hearing loss is confirmed by testing, the audiologist should take time to explain the ramifications of the problem. These patients, with only one hearing ear, have significant difficulties in localizing the source of a sound. They have pronounced difficulties in listening in backgrounds of noise creating overall and ongoing communication difficulties. Fitzpatrick et al. (2010) found that there is considerable uncertainty among audiologists (and parents) about the appropriate management of these children.

Ototoxicity

Unfortunately, almost every available drug effective for treatment of disease has the potential to compromise the human system through possible side effects. Hearing loss and tinnitus due to the administration of certain drugs are not uncommon side effects. Drugs that damage the cochlea and vestibular portion of the inner ear are known as ototoxic. Ototoxic drugs (including loop diuretics) may cause permanent sensorineural hearing loss that may be accompanied by vertigo, nausea, and, occasionally, gait instability. Considerable individual susceptibility to ototoxic drugs exists and is generally unpredictable. The resultant hearing loss is usually sensorineural, bilaterally symmetrical impairments of varying degree, audiometric configuration, and severity. The physician's management of illness with drugs and chemotherapy becomes a fine-line judgment, weighing the potential benefit to the patient against the potential risk of adverse side effects.

The drug family of antibiotic aminoglycosides, such as kanamycin, neomycin, and gentamicin are the most commonly used ototoxic drugs. Other ototoxic aminoglycosides, including vancomycin, amikacin, and tobramycin, have also been documented to cause hearing loss. Streptomycin, long the front runner for the treatment of tuberculosis, is well known to be destructive to the cochlea and vestibular system. Because aminoglycosides are cleared more slowly from the fluids of the inner ear than from the bloodstream, the high concentration of the drug in the perilymph of the inner ear may result in ototoxic effects long after the drug has been discontinued (Fausti, Henry, & Frey, 1996). Physicians monitor drug dosages by determining serum drug peak and trough concentrations routinely to achieve and maintain serum levels within a therapeutic range.

Various aminoglycosides are commonly used in the treatment of infection in newborns. The evaluation of aminoglycoside ototoxicity in infants presents a problem, because these babies are usually receiving medical therapy for severe life-threatening problems. Infants with low birth weight who contract systemic infection may also experience jaundice or other health disorders associated with deafness. Salamy,

Eldredge, and Tooley (1989) examined very-low-birth-weight infants and found a significant association between the long-term administration of the diuretic, furosemide, and aminoglycosides with sensorineural hearing loss. Genetically predisposed susceptibility to aminoglycoside ototoxicity has been identified as a risk factor by Prezant, Shohat, Jaber, Pressman, and Fischel-Ghodsian (1992). Other drugs are known to be ototoxic and may lead to hearing loss. Several cancer platinum-based chemotherapeutics are also damaging to hearing. They include cisplatin, carboplatin, caroplatin, nitrogen mustard, and difluoromethylornithine (DFMO). Cisplatin is used commonly in cancer treatment for both children and adults, and irreversible ototoxicity is well documented.

Aspirin (salicylates), quinine, and some loop diuretics produce temporary hearing loss, which may be fully or partially reversed when the medication is stopped. Impaired kidney function may result in increased serum levels for drugs that are poorly metabolized; thus, the potential for ototoxicity is increased. Renal failure, concomitant use of loop diuretics such as ethacrynic acid and furosemide, and a prolonged course of drug therapy are the most important factors in the development of ototoxicity. Other important factors include mode of drug administration, dose per treatment, length of administration, and cumulative dosage. Ingestion of ototoxic drugs by pregnant women can result in a multitude of congenital abnormalities, including hearing loss, because of passage of the drugs across the placenta (Siegel & McCracken, 1981).

The ototoxic pathology in the cochlea begins with cell damage in the innermost row of the outer hair cells at the basal turn. As the damage progresses toward the apex of the cochlea, it also involves the outer rows of hair cells. This cell damage is consistent with the onset of high-frequency sensorineural hearing loss. Campbell (2011) identifies the three primary methods of monitoring for ototoxic hearing losses: (a) basic or conventional audiometry threshold measures, (b) high-frequency audiometry, and (c) otoacoustic emissions (OAEs). Campbell points out that no consensus exists on determining significant changes in otoacoustic emissions secondary to ototoxic drugs. There is some suggestion in the literature that distortion-product OAEs tend to provide an earlier warning than transient OAEs. However, in comparative studies in children receiving platinum-based chemotherapeutics, high-frequency audiometry generally detected ototoxic change in hearing earlier than OAEs (Knight, Kraemer, & Neuwelt, 2005; Knight, Kraemer, Winter, & Neuwelt, 2007). Infants receiving such drugs should be evaluated as early as possible before drug application to establish a baseline of hearing levels, and then be scheduled for extensive audiologic follow-up, otoacoustic emission tests. Very young infants may need evaluation with ABR to establish and follow hearing threshold levels. Information on ototoxic drugs and hearing loss is available for audiologists by Fausti et al. (1996), American Speech-Language-Hearing Association (1994), and the American Academy of Audiology (2009).

It is worth mentioning that although 45% of infants treated in the NICU receive treatment with potentially damaging ototoxic medications, only a small percentage actually incur hearing loss (Vohr et al., 2000).

Enlarged Vestibular Aqueduct (EVA)

The vestibular aqueduct is a tiny, bony canal that connects the inner ear with the cranial cavity. The canal contains a miniscule tube called the endolymphatic duct, which normally carries endolymph from the inner ear to the endolymphatic sac in the cranial cavity. A vestibular aqueduct is abnormally enlarged if it is larger than 1 mm, roughly the size of the head of a pin. When the endolymphatic duct and sac are larger than normal, termed enlarged vestibular aqueduct (EVA) syndrome, endolymph can flow back from the endolymphatic sac into the inner ear. EVA is hypothesized to result from abnormal or delayed development of the inner ear during early childhood. Although large vestibular aqueduct syndrome is a congenital condition, hearing loss may not be present from birth. Age of diagnosis ranges from infancy to adulthood, and symptoms include fluctuating and sometimes progressive sensorineural hearing loss and disequilibrium. Enlarged vestibular aqueduct syndrome is often associated with other inner ear development problems, such as cochlear deformities. Studies show that genetic defects such EVA can result from abnormal or delayed development of the inner ear (nonsyndromal) or may be associated with syndromes such as Pendred syndrome, brancio-oto-renal syndrome, CHARGE syndrome, or Waardenburg syndrome (Pryor et al., 2005). Hearing loss caused by large vestibular aqueduct syndrome is not inevitable, although individuals with it are at a much higher risk of developing hearing loss than the general population (Madden, Halsted, Benton, Greinwald, & Choo, 2003).

It is generally accepted that most children with enlarged vestibular aqueducts (EVA) will develop some amount of hearing loss. EVA is not an uncommon finding in young children with sensorineural hearing loss, and as many as 5% to 15% of children with sensorineural hearing loss have EVA (Callison & Horn, 1998). The associated hearing loss is usually progressive and may lead to profound deafness. EVA also may be linked to balance problems in a small per-centage of individuals. Magnetic resonance imaging (MRI) and computed tomography (CT) of the inner ear are used to identify and confirm EVA. EVA should be considered in children with progressive hearing loss, unilateral or bilateral sudden hearing loss, or in light of a significant difference in hearing between ears. No treatment has proven effective in reducing the hearing loss associated with EVA or in slowing its progression.

Perilymph Fistula

A perilymph fistula (PLF) is a leak of inner ear fluid through a tear or opening or hole in either the round window membrane or the oval window annular ligament. This defect permits an open communication between the middle ear and the fluids of the inner ear. Rarely, these fistulas can be congenital, leading to progressive hearing loss and vertigo in childhood. The perilymph leak is associated with certain cases of stapes footplate defect or may occur through the otic capsule bone from trauma or cholesteatoma erosion. It is estimated that 6% to 11% of unexplained pediatric sensorineural hearing loss is the result of PLF (Reilly, 1989). In data for children with progressive sensorineural hearing loss, estimates of PLF increase to nearly 25% (Pappas et al., 1998). It is believed by some that the perilymph leak can occur spontaneously, but it more typically occurs as the result of trauma to the head or from heavy lifting. The diagnosis of PLF is often tenuous and difficult in children and may be a diagnosis of last resort when other possible etiologies are systematically eliminated (Balkany & Pashley, 1986).

Because sensorineural hearing loss results from PLF, many otologic surgeons perform exploratory operations to seek evidence of fluid leakage that can be repaired by patching the defect. Petroff, Simmons, and Winzelberg (1986) summarized several facts about PLF, including the following: (a) the relationship between fistulas and hearing loss is not completely understood, (b) PLF may occur in normal-hearing ears, and (c) surgical repair of PLF may not restore or improve hearing, although a successful repair may stabilize progressive sensorineural hearing loss. Some physicians believe that PLF may self-heal without surgery and with sufficient bed rest.

Diagnosis of PLF is difficult at best, because it is a condition with a wide variety of signs and symptoms. There is no consistent pattern of diagnostic findings, but "typical" symptoms may be as subtle as fluctuation in speech recognition scores, aural fullness, dysequilibrium, positive fistula test, or fluctuating severe hearing loss, which may be unilateral or bilateral. Factors that suggest PLF include precedent history of head trauma, hearing loss in the presence of craniofacial anomalies, radiographic evidence of inner ear dysplasia, signs of enlarged vestibular aqueduct, unexplained vestibular or balance abnormalities, progressive or fluctuating hearing loss, and history of previous meningitis or labyrinthitis (Marple & Meyerhoff, 1998). Caution must be exercised to separate fluctuating hearing loss from test-retest normal variations noted during testing in children (Myer, Farrer, Drake, & Cotton, 1989). PLF should be considered in any child with a progressive sensorineural hearing loss and intermittent dizziness, because total hearing loss can result if the condition is left untreated (McCabe, 1989; Parnes & McCabe, 1987).

Temporal Bone Fracture

The temporal bone is one of the most complex bones in the human body. It houses many vital structures, including the cochlear and vestibular end organs, the facial nerve, the carotid artery, and the jugular vein. A temporal bone fracture can involve none or all of these structures. Associated trauma to cranial nerves other than the facial nerve might include the abducens, glossopharyngeal, vagus, and spinal accessory that can also cause paralysis. The spectrum of temporal bone trauma is extremely varied, ranging from minor concussion without functional deficits to severe blunt or penetrating trauma with multifunctional deficits that involve the auditory and vestibular nerves, the facial nerve, and the intracranial contents. The clinical presentations specifically related to temporal bone trauma include facial nerve paralysis (partial or complete), hearing loss (conductive, sensorineural, mixed), vertigo, dizziness, cerebrospinal fluid (CSF) otorrhea, tympanic membrane perforation, and hemotympanum and canal laceration.

Amnesia and loss of consciousness usually accompany a blow to the head that is severe enough to cause a temporal bone fracture. Skull fractures of the occipital or squamous portion of the temporal bone may extend into the petrous portion of the temporal bone and involve the otic capsule. Temporal bone fractures are classified as longitudinal and transverse. The longitudinal fracture often results in mild to moderate sensorineural hearing loss that exhibits the audiometric pattern of acoustic trauma. Should the fracture line cross the external auditory canal, laceration of the skin and bleeding of the external canal may occur with no loss of hearing. More medial fractures may produce bleeding in the middle ear or disruption of the ossicular chain. When the middle ear ossicles have been dislocated, severe conductive hearing loss will be present, requiring correction by reconstructive middle ear surgery.

The transverse temporal bone fracture typically passes through the vestibule of the inner ear, causing extensive destruction of the membranous labyrinth accompanied by complete loss of cochlear and vestibular function. Severe vertigo and facial nerve palsy may exist for a few weeks following the traumatic event (Schuknecht, 1993). Meningitis may occur as a late complication of temporal bone fracture months or years later, usually associated with upper respiratory infection.

Even relatively moderate trauma to the occiput of the skull can cause a permanent sensorineural hearing loss. Trauma to the head may produce temporary or permanent sensorineural high-frequency hearing loss. A sharp blow to the head creates a pressure wave in the skull that is transmitted through bone to the cochlea, often causing hearing loss on the contralateral side (known as the contrecoup effect). When the head strikes a fixed object, the coup injury occurs at the site of impact, and the contrecoup injury occurs at the opposite side. Coup and contrecoup injuries can occur individually or together. In a contrecoup injury, the head stops abruptly and the brain collides with the inside of the skull. The contrecoup hearing loss often mimics a noise-induced 4000 Hz notch in the opposite ear from the traumatic insult.

Noise and Hearing Loss

The topic of noise-induced hearing loss in children is a growing problem. It is well established that a sound of sufficient intensity and duration can cause injury to the cochlea producing a temporary or permanent hearing loss. Such auditory injuries may occur accidentally from a single exposure to very high sound pressure levels (noise trauma hearing loss) or as a result of gradual, long-term exposure to loud sounds (noise-induced hearing loss). Different ears

vary in their resistance to noise-related hearing loss. The extent of noise-induced or traumatic noise-inflicted hearing loss in children is difficult to ascertain, but its presence is relatively common.

A dangerous sound for the human hearing system is anything 85 dB SPL or higher. The World Health Organization (WHO) has set a standard that children should be exposed to sounds that are 70 dBA or less for only a 24-hour period to be safe with no exposures over 120 dB peak SPL (1999). According to the National Institute for Occupational Safety and Health (NIOSH), exposure to sounds of 85 decibels (dBA) or less is safe for up to 8 hours over a 24-hour period. For every additional 3 dBA, the safe listening time is cut in half (i.e., at 91 dBA "safe" listening is reduced to 2 hours per 24 hours). However, since the advent of amplified sound in the music and entertainment industries, and the growing popularity of portable music and gaming devices among the younger population, noise-induced hearing loss in children is a serious and growing concern. Hearing loss due to noise exposure typically consists of sensorineural impairment at 4000 Hz in the affected ear, regardless of the type or frequency spectrum of the noise exposure.

With an estimated 10 million Americans suffering from irreversible noise-induced hearing loss, and 30 million more exposed to dangerous noise levels each day, very little evidence-based data have been reported on the risk of noise-induced hearing loss in children. Of course, the real concern is that noise-induced damage in early years may not immediately manifest itself as a hearing concern, but may become a serious hearing problem later in life. Noise-related hearing loss can be both cumulative and progressive over time. Thus, over the short term, the effects of noise overstimulation may not be obvious, but the accumulated effects of damaging episodes may eventually lead to significant hearing deficits (Mills, 1975). Early noise research in school-aged children suggested that noise-induced losses are first identified in junior-senior high school boys who have a history of experience with firearms and farm machinery. Litke (1971) evaluated higher frequency hearing among 1,516 South Dakota school children. He found high-frequency hearing loss in 6% of the population, with five times more boys involved than girls.

Noise exposure is increasingly common in the age of ear-level or head-worn personal music players, and it has been commonly noted that some 50% of adolescents listen to music through earphones at dangerously high volume settings The maximum sound from personal music devices has been measured at 115 dBA, a level that can cause hearing loss to listeners of all ages. A survey sponsored by the Australian government found that about 25% of people using portable stereos had daily noise exposures high enough to cause hearing damage. Researchers at Boston Children's Hospital in the United States determined that listening to a portable music player with headphones at 60% of their maximum volume for 1 hour a day is relatively safe (Fligor & Cox, 2004). The maximum volume limit is adjustable on many current personal music players, and many devices now carry warnings about the use of high-intensity music as potentially damaging to hearing. Our rule of thumb is that if the speaker has to shout to be heard and understood at an arm's length away, then the music player is too loud.

Literally thousands of children have permanent hearing losses caused by the acoustic impulses of excessively loud toys. Numerous toys are developed and marketed each year that produce sound levels capable of producing acoustic injury. Toys and devices with sufficiently high sound levels include fireworks, model airplane engines, and toy firearms. Examples of noisy toys include certain rattles and squeaky toys (110 dBA), some musical toys (120 dBA), toy telephones (125 dBA), and toy firearms (150 dBA). For noise-emitting toys to conform to the safety requirements of the American Society of Testing Materials, they should not produce impulsive noises with sound pressure levels exceeding 138 dBA which is as loud as a jackhammer. If a toy produces a sound that "seems too loud," it probably is too loud. Parents should pay attention to noise exposure in children's recreational activities, encourage children to lower the volume on stereos and noisy computer games, remind them to take hearing defenders to loud movies and rock concerts, and monitor the volume of personal stereo systems.

Concerned parents often ask if listening to or playing loud music can damage the hearing of their children. Various studies have found sound levels at rock concerts generally to be significantly higher than 85 dBA, with sound intensity peaks that reach 90 dBA to 122 dBA. Although evidence-based research in the issue of hearing loss and music is somewhat conflicting, there is little doubt that exposure to loud music can produce temporary threshold shift and tinnitus. Jerger and Jerger (1970) reported that eight of nine rock-and-roll musicians, aged 14 to 23 years, showed temporary threshold shift in excess of 15 dB on at least one frequency between 2000 and 8000 Hz. Significant hearing threshold shift was measured in students attending a typical school dance with loud, live music (Danenberg, Loos-Cosgrove, & Lo Verde, 1987).

A thorough patient history, or an audiogram with a 4000 Hz noise-induced hearing loss, may identify unrecognized youngsters exposed to excessive noise. Those youngsters routinely exposed to high noise situations must be counseled carefully regarding the potential hazards of additional noise exposure and fitted with ear/noise defenders as soon as possible. Hearing protection (i.e., ear plug inserts or over-the-ear muffs) worn correctly can reduce the noise reaching the cochlea to safe levels. There are a number of public awareness campaigns that have been developed to warn of the dangers of noise exposure, with educational programs for schools that teach children that hearing loss can result from listening to loud sounds. Useful Web-based information, coupled with innovative age-appropriate programs to educate and protect young people from loud music, have been developed by non-profit groups such as Dangerous Decibels (http://www.dangerousdecibels.org), Hearing Education and Awareness for Rockers (HEAR at http://www.hearnet.com), and Sound Sense (http://www.soundsense.com).

Congenital Inner Ear Malformations

Failure of the inner ear to reach full development is known as aplasia. Accordingly, inner ear aplasia is always a congenital malformation. Of course, the embryonic time of developmental failure determines the ultimate structure and appearance of the deformity. An individual may possess different degrees of aplasia in the two ears. Aplasia of the inner ear is a relatively uncommon aberration. Although wide variety exists in anatomic abnormalities of the inner ear, three classic types exist. These include Michel (complete failure of development of the inner ear), Mondini (incomplete development and malformation of the inner ear), and Scheibe (membranous cochleosaccular degeneration of the inner ear).

Knowledge of these inner ear anomalies is important for accurate diagnosis, proper treatment, and genetic counseling for the parents of the handicapped child, as well as for the child when he or she is old enough to become a parent. Therefore, differentiation and specific diagnosis of the inner ear problem are crucial in the determination of whether the hearing loss in question is of a genetic or an acquired origin. The degree of abnormal development that is actually involved in any specific patient may vary considerably from other patients with similar inner ear malformations. Diagnostic considerations must include petrous pyramid polytomography of the inner ear and a complete evaluation of the hearing impairment.

Michel Aplasia of the Inner Ear

Michel first described the macroscopic description of this temporal bone anomaly in 1863. This type of anomaly is represented by a complete absence of the inner ear and auditory nerve. The outer ear may be completely normal with a narrow middle ear cavity. The malleus and incus may be present, but the stapes and stapedius muscle may be absent or abnormal. Audiometric patterns in the Michel ear should show no hearing, because no true inner ear exists. True hearing is impossible, and a hearing aid for such a patient is of limited, if any, value.

Mondini Aplasia of the Inner Ear

Mondini described a temporal bone in 1791 that showed incomplete development of a flattened cochlea that consisted of only a single basal coil. In 1904, Alexander added more detail to this type of anomaly, indicating involvement of the auditory nerve and the vestibular canals. Characteristic of this anomaly is that it involves both the bony capsule and the membranous labyrinth. Middle ear anomalies may be present in these cases, and atresia of the external canal has also been reported. Many temporal bone studies have described this deformity, which varies considerably from one case to another and may be unilateral or bilateral. It is possible for the Mondini malformed inner ear to have some hearing, because the basal coil of the cochlea may be present; thus, a cochlear implant may be a consideration. The Mondini ear is often a candidate for cochlear implantation.

Scheibe Aplasia of the Inner Ear

The Scheibe abnormality of the inner ear, originally described in 1892, is characterized by involvement of only the membranous portion of the cochlea and saccule. This type of dysplasia is the most common of the inner ear aplasias. Histopathology of these inner ears shows atrophy of the stria vascularis, degeneration of the organ of Corti, and rolling up of the tectorial membrane, especially in the basal turn of the cochlea. This anomaly has been identified in cases of Waardenburg syndrome, the cardioauditory syndrome of Jervell and Lange-Nielsen, Usher syndrome, Refsum syndrome, and maternal rubella. The Scheibe ear may show residual hearing in the low frequencies because the major damage is in the basal coil of the cochlea.

CHILDHOOD INFECTIONS ASSOCIATED WITH HEARING LOSS

At birth, the infant's immune system must respond to the challenges of extrauterine life. Although many defense mechanisms are present, the newborn infant's immune system is not as effective as that of older infants, children, and adults. Newborn infants and premature infants, in particular, are at risk for acquiring infection during the prenatal and neonatal period (birth through 28 days of age). Mothers with active birth canal infections may transmit disease to their infants during the birth process. Whenever possible, infants of infected mothers are delivered by caesarean section to prevent exposure of the infant to these diseases. In addition, premature infants are at increased risk for acquiring generalized infections due to immature immune system development. Hearing impairment in infants with peri- or postnatally acquired bacterial infections is most often secondary to meningitis. However, an important consideration in the treatment of sepsis and bacterial meningitis is the potential cause of sensorineural hearing loss from treatment by ototoxic drugs including the commonly used aminoglycosides.

Meningitis

Meningitis is inflammation of the protective membranes covering the brain and spinal cord, and known collectively as the meninges. Their inflammation may be caused by infection with viruses, bacteria, or other microorganisms. Meningitis can be life threatening because of the inflammation's proximity to the brain and spinal cord; therefore, the condition is considered a medical emergency. The most common symptoms of meningitis are headache and neck stiffness associated with fever, seizures, vomiting, and an inability to tolerate light (photophobia) or loud noises (phonophobia). Sometimes, especially in small children, only nonspecific symptoms may be present such as irritability and drowsiness. Meningitis caused by meningococcal bacteria may be accompanied by a characteristic rash.

A lumbar puncture is needed to confirm the diagnosis of meningitis. This involves inserting a needle into the spinal canal to extract a sample of cerebrospinal fluid (CSF) which is then examined for causal agents. The usual treatment for meningitis is prompt application of antibiotics or antiviral drugs. Meningitis can lead to serious long-term consequences such as sensorineural deafness, epilepsy, hydrocephalus, and cognitive deficits, especially if not treated quickly. The infection is so serious that if not treated as an emergency, death can occur within 48 hours. Fortunately, there is a vaccine for two of the three known types of meningitis. Vaccination against meningitis for individuals receiving cochlear implants is generally required.

Viral meningitis is milder and occurs more often than bacterial meningitis. Most infections occur in children under the age of 5 years. The bacterial infections that cause meningitis include *Haemophilus influenzae, Neisseria, meningococcal, pneumococcal,* and *staphylococcal.* The infecting organisms travel from the meninges to the inner ear through the cochlear aqueduct and along vessels and nerves of the internal auditory meatus. Serous or purulent labyrinthitis may follow with partial or complete destruction of sensory receptors in the cochlear and eighth nerve elements. Subsequent replacement of the membranous labyrinth in the cochlea and vestibular divisions of the inner ear with fibrous tissue and bone ossification is common. In recent years, West Nile virus, spread by mosquito bites, has been identified as a cause of viral meningitis.

Gallaudet University's Research Institute 2006 survey notes that 3.2% of U.S. deaf and hard-of-hearing pupils lost their hearing due to meningitis. Earlier studies from Kaplan, Catlin, Weaver, and Feigin (1984), Dodge et al. (1984), and Arditi et al. (1998) showed significantly higher percentages of meningitic deafness in deaf and hard-of-hearing populations, demonstrating the beneficial effect of vaccine protection to diminish the hearing problems caused by this disease. The percentage of meningitis as a cause of deafness is likely much higher in developing countries where meningitis vaccines are less accessible.

Sensorineural hearing loss is the most common complication from viral and bacterial meningitis in infants and young children. The severity of the sensorineural hearing loss ranges between mild and profound degree, and the audiometric pattern is typically, but not always, bilateral, symmetrical, and irreversible. Conductive hearing loss may be present due to associated acute otitis media and upper respiratory infection. Although ABR is likely the choice of audiometric evaluation of sensorineural hearing loss in infants and toddlers, clinicians need to be reminded that the ABR tests hearing only in the higher frequencies and may be insufficient as a singular hearing test. Behavioral testing is the best means by which to determine hearing levels with certainty at all frequencies in each ear in all children. Because hearing loss is so common in patients with bacterial meningitis, a hearing evaluation is recommended as routine practice prior to hospital discharge. Follow-up audiometrics are required for those patients who show presence of hearing loss.

Herpes Simplex Virus (HSV)

Herpes simplex virus is one of the most common sexually transmitted diseases. Herpes simplex virus 1 and 2 (HSV-1 and HSV-2) are two members of the herpes virus family, *Herpesviridae,* that infect humans. Two types of HSV infect humans. HSV-I is acquired during childhood and isolated from the mouth, nose, and oropharynx (cold sores). HSV-II is usually acquired in adolescence or adulthood as a sexually transmitted disease and is isolated from the genitalia mucosa (genital herpes). Symptoms of herpes simplex virus infection include watery blisters in the skin or mucous membranes of the mouth, lips, or genitals. Lesions heal with scab characteristic of herpetic disease. Sometimes, the viruses cause very mild or atypical symptoms during outbreaks. HSV-1 and HSV-2 persist in the body by becoming latent and hiding from the immune system in the cell bodies of neurons. In an outbreak, the virus in a nerve cell becomes active and is transported via the neuron's axon to the skin, where virus replication and shedding occur and cause new sores.

The transmission of HSV to the fetus is possible during birth if the mother is actively infected. HSV may cause severe generalized disease in the neonate, with high mortality rates and devastating sequelae (Rudnick & Hoekzema, 2002). HSV infections in the newborn are rarely subclinical or asymptomatic. The majority of cases are acquired during passage through the birth canal. A cesarean section delivery is indicated for mothers with a known genital infection at the time of delivery. When HSV infection does occur in the neonate, more than 50% are fatal; only 4% of neonatal infected HSV infants survive without sequelae (Nahmias & Norrild, 1979). Infants with herpes infection may demonstrate symptoms ranging from localized skin lesions to severe generalized infection involving major organ systems. Neurologic and sensory system complications are common, including sensorineural hearing loss.

Bacterial Sepsis

Bacterial infections are not uncommon in the newborn period and result from exposure to common microorganisms. Older children typically are not so easily affected because they have developed immunities to these ubiquitous bacteria. Postnatally acquired bacterial infections are often life threatening in newborn and premature infants. In infants, bacterial infections are often observed following significant obstetrical histories (premature rupture of membranes, premature onset of labor, or maternal fever). In general, the infant acquires the infection from the birth canal during delivery. Early-onset (e.g., within the first few days of life) bacterial infections can result in fulminant, multisystem illness with high mortality, especially in premature infants. Organisms commonly responsible for early onset bacterial infections are *Group B streptococcus, Escherichia coli,* and *H. influenzae.* Early onset disease may mimic respiratory distress syndrome. Without prompt treatment, the infant may develop increased oxygen requirement and PPHN. The most common presentation of late-onset disease is bacterial meningitis with septicemia (manifestation of system illness with infectious organisms present in the bloodstream). Treatment consists of immediate broad-spectrum antibiotics (may be an ototoxic aminoglycoside) until the specific organism is identified. Overall mortality from bacterial infections has been reported as high as 20% with the greatest problems occurring in small, preterm infants. Complications in survivors include mental retardation, spastic quadriplegia, cortical blindness, hydrocephalus, uncontrollable seizures, and sensorineural deafness.

Mumps

In years past, mumps was the most common cause of unilateral sensorineural hearing loss. Before the development of vaccination and the introduction of a vaccine, mumps, caused by the mumps virus, was a common childhood viral disease worldwide. It is still a significant threat to health in the third world, and outbreaks still occur sporadically in developed countries. Painful swelling of the salivary glands (classically the parotid gland) is the most typical presentation. The symptoms are generally not severe in children. The disease is generally self-limiting, running its course before receding, with no specific treatment apart from controlling the symptoms with pain medication. Mumps is a contagious disease that leads to painful swelling of the salivary glands, usually on one side of the cheek at a time, although bilateral mumps is also possible. The salivary glands produce saliva, a liquid that moistens food and helps you chew and swallow. The mumps virus is spread from person-to-person by respiratory droplets or by direct contact with items that have been contaminated with infected saliva. Mumps most commonly occurs in children ages 2 to 12 who have not been vaccinated against the disease. The mumps vaccine was introduced into the United States in December 1967; since its introduction there has been a steady decrease in the incidence of mumps and mumps virus infection. Currently the MMR immunization (vaccine) protects against measles, mumps, and rubella. However, the infection can occur at any age, including adulthood. The time between being exposed to the virus and getting sick (incubation period) is usually 12 to 24 days. After the illness, lifelong immunity to mumps generally occurs; reinfection is possible but tends to be mild and atypical.

Viral Diseases and Hearing Loss

It has long been recognized that numerous viral diseases are known to cause deafness including measles, chickenpox, influenza, and even the viruses of the common cold. Deafness occurs when the inner ear is damaged as a result of direct infiltration of the virus from the bloodstream or meninges via the internal auditory meatus. Viral infections may cause any degree of hearing loss from mild hearing impairment to profound deafness. Residuals of postnatal viral infections can also include optic nerve atrophy, cerebral palsy, developmental mental problems, disturbances of respiration, muscular atrophy or paralysis, convulsions, disturbances of autonomic system, and disturbances of metabolism.

Diabetes Mellitus

Diabetes mellitus is a chronic hormonal disorder of carbohydrate metabolism that is believed to result from insulin deficiency. There are two types of diabetes mellitus: juvenile onset and maturity onset. Juvenile onset is the more severe of the two and usually appears suddenly in childhood or in the teenage years. Daily insulin injections are required to compensate for a lack of native insulin. The young, untreated diabetic is often quite thin and experiences excessive hunger, thirst, need to urinate, weakness, and weight loss. Diabetics are more susceptible to infection. Long-term complications of this disorder include blindness; kidney, urinary tract, and bladder dysfunction; hearing loss; and gangrene of the extremities. Deafness is not an invariable accompaniment to juvenile diabetes, but when it occurs it is usually mild-to-moderate, progressive, bilaterally symmetrical sensorineural hearing loss. The incidence of hearing loss has been shown to be higher in diabetics than in nondiabetics of the same age (Cremers, Wijdeveld, & Pinckers, 1977; Friedman, Schulman, & Weiss, 1975).

CLEFT PALATE

Deformities of the lip and palate are among the most common major congenital malformations. Cleft lip, cleft palate, or both appears in approximately 1 per 700 births. Clefting is associated with many problems including cosmetic and dental abnormalities, as well as speech, hearing, and facial growth difficulties. Oral clefts happen very early during pregnancy as the fetus' lips are formed by about 6 weeks and the palate is formed by about 10 weeks of pregnancy (see Chapter 2). Oral clefts happen when the lips or palate or both do not come together completely. Some babies with cleft lip have just a small notch in the upper lip. Others have a complete opening or hole in the lip that goes through the upper gum to the bottom of the nose. A cleft lip can happen on one or both sides of a baby's mouth. A cleft palate can affect the soft palate (the soft tissue at the back of the roof of the mouth) or the hard palate (the bony front part of the roof of the mouth). A cleft palate can happen on one or both sides of a baby's palate. Some babies have just a cleft lip. But most babies with a cleft lip also have a cleft palate. Some babies have only a cleft palate, which is called an isolated cleft palate. There are about 400 syndromes that are related to oral clefts. The incidence of hearing problems in children with cleft lip or palate is very high and requires special attention in the audiology clinic. A substantial number of articles have been published concerning the otologic and audiologic problems of children with overt cleft palate. The incidence of recurrent otitis media in such children is quite high and has been reported to be from 50% to 90% by various investigators.

Paradise and Bluestone (1974) identified the "universality" of otitis media findings in 50 infants with cleft palate. Hearing loss as a secondary problem to the middle ear disorder related to cleft palate is so common that it may exist in nearly all such patients. Sterile inflammatory effusions that vary in viscosity are commonly found in the ears of these infants. Paradise (1980) recommended that infants with cleft palate receive myringotomy and tympanostomy tube insertion within the first 6 months of life, if possible, especially if hearing loss seems to be present or discomfort or infection is present. Repeat myringotomy and tubes may be necessary to keep the infant's ears clear and hearing normally. Complications such as cholesteatoma and adhesive otitis may accompany repeated middle ear effusion in children with a cleft palate. The incidence and severity of middle ear problems related to cleft palate decrease as the patient grows older.

Otologic and hearing problems may also be associated with submucous cleft palate. Although overt cleft palate is diagnosed at birth, submucous cleft palate may not be diagnosed until years later. The submucous cleft palate is an imperfect union of muscle across the soft palate that tends to "tent" when the patient phonates. The area may appear bluish because it is covered by only nasal and oral mucosa. The dehiscence of muscle and bone may be obvious with palpation and is often accompanied by a bifid uvula. Most clinicians agree that the deficiency of palate musculature is the probable cause of poor eustachian tube function. This results in inadequate middle ear ventilation, effusion of fluid, tympanic membrane retraction, and hearing loss.

Medical and surgical treatment is often necessary for these children who may qualify for repeated myringotomy and ventilation tubes. Mild power output hearing instruments may be in order for children who do not respond well to medical treatment, especially during the school years.

Hearing loss related to cleft palate is most common between 3 and 8 years of age, which also corresponds to the increased exposure and susceptibility to upper respiratory infections found in this age group. Audiologists must be aware of this increased incidence of hearing difficulty and recurrent middle ear disease in children with cleft palate. The hearing and speech-language development of the child with cleft palate must be monitored on a regular basis by a team of specialists. It is important that the audiologist be included on the cleft palate team, because routine hearing evaluations contribute substantially to the total management of these children.

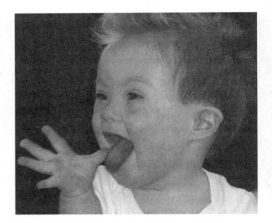

Figure 4–14. Savanna, with Down syndrome and hearing loss, loves signing. Courtesy of Colorado Children's Hospital.

DOWN SYNDROME

Down syndrome, also known as trisomy 21, is due to a mutation with the zygote formed by three copies of the 21st chromosome (see Chapter 2). Down syndrome is one of the most common causes of intellectual disability, occurring in 1 in 600 live births with approximately 5,000 new cases born each year in the United States. These individuals exhibit a warm and happy characteristic personality and are noted for their affectionate friendliness (Figure 4–14). There are more than 50 characteristic features of Down syndrome. Each child's symptoms vary in number and severity, but there is a common appearance to all of them. The risk of occurrence increases with the age of the mother from 1:1,200 at mother's age 25 to 1:100 at mother's age 40. But because younger women have most of the babies, 80% of children with Down syndrome are born to women under 35. More women, age 35 and older, are having babies later in life due to their higher education, birth control opportunities, fertility treatments, and changing attitudes toward marriage.

The audiologist must be aware that the child with Down syndrome is likely to have a high incidence of hearing loss that may contribute to developmental delay. The child with Down syndrome often has a narrow external auditory canal making otoscopic examination, tympanometry, and otoacoustic emissions measurements difficult. Developmental delay and subnormal intellect make it difficult to obtain valid hearing test results without careful testing protocols, and an affable personality makes the child with Down syndrome an overresponder during the traditional hearing test. External ear abnormalities such as small or deformed pinnae are also frequently noted in the child with Down syndrome. There is a high incidence of otitis media with complications causing conductive hearing loss. The degree of hearing loss is usually mild to moderate and may also be associated with a sensorineural component creating a mixed-type hearing impairment. A child with Down syndrome may be more susceptible to upper respiratory infection than is the normal child because of abnormal nasopharynx and eustachian tube development that adversely affects proper drainage of the sinuses and middle ear spaces. Approximately

50% of individuals with Down syndrome also have a cardiac defect. Modern medical developments have increased the average life expectancy for a child with Down syndrome from 25 years in 1983 to 60 years in 2010.

Without question, any audiologist who has evaluated children with Down syndrome realizes many of them have persistent conductive hearing loss. Downs (1980) published one of the first comprehensive studies of the high incidence of hearing problems in children with Down syndrome. She noted that the child with Down syndrome is usually treated medically for persistent middle ear effusion; however, her clinical experience showed that conductive hearing loss often persisted after medical treatment. She conducted a comprehensive study of 107 noninstitutionalized children with Down syndrome and found 78% to have hearing loss in one or both ears. Fifty-four percent of children had conductive loss, 16% had sensorineural loss, and 8% had mixed-type hearing loss. Otologic examinations were conducted on each of the 107 children. According to Balkany et al. (1978), middle ear effusion or chronic otitis media could not explain approximately 40% of the children with conductive hearing loss. On microscopic pneumatic otoscopy, the patients had normal-appearing tympanic membranes suggesting the presence of middle ear anomalies as the etiology for the conductive hearing loss. Seventeen operative procedures on carefully selected patients with Down syndrome revealed congenital ossicular malformations and ossicular destruction caused by inflammation due to chronic infection. These findings lead us to recommend that children with Down syndrome and persistent conductive hearing loss be treated aggressively to normalize their hearing, break the cycle, and prevent recurrent and chronic ear disease.

Roizen, Walters, Nicol, and Blondis (1993) recommend that auditory brainstem response (ABR) audiometry be performed routinely during the initial 6 months of life, as their evaluation of 47 unselected young children with Down syndrome resulted in finding 66% with significant hearing loss. The high incidence of conductive hearing loss in the Down syndrome population makes immittance and otoacoustic emissions measures imperative parts of the hearing evaluation (Northern, 1980a). Audiologists conducting hearing tests on a child with Down syndrome should utilize insert earphones or sound field testing to avoid erroneous "conductive loss" due to collapsed ear canals common in these children caused by traditional earphones. Some children with Down syndrome who have persistent hearing loss may do well with mild hearing aid amplification. In addition, a total team approach including an ear, nose, and throat specialist, pediatrician, audiologist, and speech-language pathologist is recommended for the child with Down syndrome to provide optimal opportunities for advancement.

AUTISM SPECTRUM DISORDER (ASD)

Autism spectrum disorder is classified as one of the pervasive developmental disorders (PPD). Autism is diagnosed by observation of a cluster of behaviors, usually with early onset (often before 18 months of age), disturbances of social relationships, disturbances of speech and language, and extremely deviant behaviors characterized by preoccupation with particular objects or self-destructive activities, insistence on sameness, fixation on repetitive movements, abnormal preoccupations, ritualistic behaviors, and resistance to change. A decrease or loss of language or social skills can be present in 25% to 35% of children with autism and can occur between 12 and 24 months of age. Of interest is the fact that this regression in language and social skills in toddlers with autism has led to the hypothesis that toxins or vaccines lie at the cause of autism spectrum disorder despite overwhelming scientific evidence that this is not the case (Lindsay, 2005).

Audiologists may be among the earliest health care professionals to encounter the child with ASD and must be prepared to identify symptoms and make appropriate referrals (Egelhoff, Whitelaw, & Rabidouxs, 2005). There has been a general increase in awareness of ASD related to an actual increase in the incidence of this disorder. The current occurrence rate is 35 to 40 per 10,000, and autism affects boys three times more often than girls, and generally follows a steady course without remission (Rutter, 1978). Overt symptoms gradually begin after the age of 6 months, become established by age 2 or 3 years, and tend to continue through adulthood, although often in more muted form.

Autistic patients show a pervasive lack of responsiveness to other people and gross deficits in language development and inabilities for symbolic or imaginative play. When speech is present, it is characterized by peculiarities such as echolalia, metaphorical language, and pronoun reversal (Wing, 1993). Autistic individuals may exhibit bizarre responses to various aspects of the environment and failure to use or comprehend verbal and nonverbal messages, with illogical and inconsistent responses to sensory, especially auditory, stimuli. Autistic children may be easily distracted, enraged, or frightened by normal background noises. About a third to a half of children with autism do not develop enough natural speech to meet their daily communication needs. Differences in communication may be present from the first year of life, and may include delayed onset of babbling, unusual gestures, diminished responsiveness, and vocal patterns that are not synchronized with the caregiver. In the second and third years, autistic children have less frequent and less diverse babbling, consonants, words, and word combinations; their gestures are less often integrated with words. Children with ASD are less likely to make requests or share experiences and are more likely to simply repeat others' words (echolalia) or reverse pronouns.

Many believe the basis of autism to be a neurodevelopment disorder with abnormalities of the limbic system, thalamus, basal ganglia, and cerebellum. Although minor differences in ABR patterns have been reported between normal and autistic patients, the differences are not consistent across studies, and the reports are difficult to compare because control conditions and experimental variables are often not well described. Some authors have attempted to use central auditory tests to speculate about the specific loci of dysfunction in autistic children (Wetherby, Koegal, & Mendel, 1981). Although it is probable that the organic dysfunction is clearly implicated in autism, no precise etiologic mechanisms have been identified. Audiologists should be aware that autistic children consistently fail to point at objects in order to comment on or share an experience which limits testing procedures.

AUDITORY NEUROPATHY SPECTRUM DISORDER (ANSD)

Auditory neuropathy spectrum disorder (ANSD), formerly termed *auditory neuropathy*, describes a type of hearing loss that is caused by an abnormality in the transmission of nerve impulses traveling from the inner ear to the brain. Both ears are usually affected, and the disorder is usually (but not always) associated with mild-to-severe sensorineural hearing loss. Children with normal or near-normal hearing have also been diagnosed with ANSD. Children with auditory ANSD may have days of good hearing followed by periods of seemingly "poor" hearing. Regardless of the level of the hearing threshold levels, auditory neuropathy is always associated with impaired ability to understand speech. The affected individual may be able to hear everyday sounds fairly normally, but inevitably has difficulty in understanding spoken words, particularly in noisy environments.

The symptoms of auditory neuropathy vary greatly from one affected individual to the next, and may even fluctuate in the same individual from time to time, often resulting in puzzling reports from parents about the child's hearing difficulties. The course and the prognosis of the condition are totally unpredictable. Although the precise cause of ANSD has yet to be determined, researchers suspect that a number of interrelated factors may be responsible including damaged hair cells within the inner ear, damage to the synapse connections between the hair cells and the cochlear nerve, damage to the cochlear nerve, damage to the eighth cranial nerve, or damage or malfunction along the auditory pathways in the brainstem. ANSD has an effect, directly or indirectly, on the neural processing of auditory stimuli which requires physiological measures to accurately identify and assess hearing problems (Hood, 2011).

ANSD first came to audiologists' attention when Worthington and Peters (1980) published a paper with the intriguing title of "Quantifiable Hearing and No ABR: Paradox or Error?" The authors described a patient who presented the paradoxical findings of a child who clearly could hear normally, but demonstrated no auditory evoked responses (AERs). Kraus, Ozdamar, Stein, and Reed (1984) also reported a patient with absent auditory brainstem response and questioned whether the findings were

due to peripheral hearing loss or brainstem dysfunction. Although the study of this unusual phenomenon in clinical patients remained somewhat dormant for a decade, by the mid-1990s the advent of otoacoustic emissions measurements as a means to differentiate among sensorineural hearing loss identified a number of clinical patients with a "typical" grouping of auditory test results. The term *auditory neuropathy* was suggested by Starr, Picton, Sininger, Hood, and Berlin (1996) to describe a group of 10 patients who exhibited common symptoms including hearing loss, normal otoacoustic emissions, absent or severely abnormal ABR waveforms, and poor speech perception. Sininger and Star (2001) described in great detail a patient with an auditory disorder that did not fit into our well-established patterns of audiometric diagnosis. They described a young patient they identified as "Eve" who could hear the click ABR test stimulus but surprisingly showed no auditory brainstem response waveforms. Although initially it was thought that these auditory findings applied to only a few unique patients, it has turned out that the disorder, now known as auditory neuropathy spectrum disorder (ANSD) is not such an uncommon diagnosis, and now presents new challenges to the field of audiology. It has become clear that individuals diagnosed with ANSD are a heterogeneous group even though they may exhibit some common audiological findings (Roush, 2008). The ANSD diagnosis refers to patients with a profile that includes normal otoacoustic emissions (OAEs) and absent or grossly abnormal ABR waveforms. The normal otoacoustic emissions suggest normal outer hair cell function, and the abnormal ABRs are consistent with a higher level neural disorder.

Hood (1998) reported that infants and children with ANSD may appear to have repeatable ABR responses, but their ABR latency does not increase with decreasing intensity as expected with normal ABR testing. Hood pointed out that when the polarity of the stimulus is reversed (i.e., changed from condensation to rarefaction clicks), the recorded responses also reverse, which is characteristic of the cochlear microphonic rather than the ABR. Sininger, Hood, Starr, Berlin, and Picton (1995) suggested a set of salient clinical features that distinguish the patient with auditory neuropathy spectrum syndrome that includes mild to moderate sensorineural hearing loss, absent to severely abnormal ABR to high-level stimuli, normal otoacoustic emissions that do not suppress with contralateral noise, absent acoustic reflexes to both ipsilateral and contralateral tones at 110 dB HL, and inconsistency of middle and late evoked auditory potentials. These patients may also show a loss of speech comprehension in quiet that is out of proportion to their pure tone auditory threshold configuration. Although neither organic evidence of auditory neuropathy nor the exact anatomic loci of the disorder have been identified, the symptoms are not unlike disruption of neural synchrony (Starr, 2008). The presence of normal otoacoustic emissions and cochlear microphonics leads to the conclusions that the outer hair cells and general cochlear mechanics are normal, whereas the absence of the auditory nerve action potential (no wave I of the ABR) suggests a more central lesion (Stein et al., 1996).

Rance et al. (1999) published the clinical findings for a large group of infants and young children with auditory neuropathy in Australia in an attempt to determine the prevalence of this newly described disorder. There is large variability in estimated prevalence data regarding ANSD in the population of children with sensorineural hearing loss from 1.8% (Vohr et al., 2000) to an estimate of 14.6% (Kraus et al., 1984). Prevalence in the high-risk population is just as varied ranging from 0.2% (Rance et al., 1999; Uus, Bamford, Young, & McCracken, 2005) to 4.0% reported by Stein et al. (1996). This variation in predicting prevalence of ANSD is likely due to the specific study definition of the disorder, as well as the characteristics of the underlying population studied (Uus, 2008).

ANSD likely has multiple etiologies in different children, that the disorder affects all age groups, and that the severity of the symptoms may vary considerably between mild and profound. The course of the disorder varies from being stationary, progressing, improving, or even disappearing (Madden, Rutter, Hilbert, Greinwald, & Choo, 2002; Attias, Muller, Rubel, & Raveh, 2006; Starr, 2008). Risk factors for ANSD in newborns are typically metabolic abnormalities as many are critically ill with low birth weight, hypoxia, hyperbilirubinemia, and infections (Starr, 2008). Healthy newborns with ANSD are likely due to genetic factors. As children enter school and receive hearing screening, more cases will be no doubt identified with various etiologies including genetic, immunological, infectious, neoplastic, congenital, and metabolic causes (Sininger & Starr, 2001).

Poor understanding of speech in normal or near-normal hearing is a consistently reported consequence of ANSD. Studies of speech understanding in children show wide variability with some individuals performing at levels similar to their peers with sensorineural hearing loss, while others show little or no capacity to understand speech despite having complete access to the normal speech spectrum in their hearing sensitivity (Rance, 2008). Additional difficulties have been noted for patients with ANSD when the speech is presented in a background of noise, a common clinical symptom of the disorder (Kraus et al., 2000; Rance et al., 2008; Starr et al., 1996).

Proper identification of this disorder in children calls for routine use of cross-check audiology including otoacoustic emissions, acoustic immittance measurements, and ABR evaluation.

Treatment and management of pediatric patients with ANSD has been a controversial topic since the disorder was identified. This disorder is often confused with sensorineural hearing loss and treated in the traditional manner with hearing aids. Some children with ANSD have gained success with the use of hearing aids, whereas others have gone on to cochlear implantation with mixed results. Johnston, John, Kreisman, Hall, and Crandell (2009) evaluated 10 children (average age 11 years) with normal hearing and confirmed auditory processing disorder (APD) and recruited them and fitted them with FM systems. Thirteen normal-hearing children served as controls (mean age 10 years). Subjects were fitted with nonoccluding, ear-level style FM systems. Parameters evaluated included speech perception, academic performance, and psychosocial status. Upon conclusion of their study, Johnston et al. (2009) noted that speech perception benefits (such as speech in noise tasks) from FM systems were greater for children with APD than for the control group—and the benefit improved significantly over time for the APD group. With regard to academic performance and psychosocial performance, children in the APD group showed improved performance in both categories after 5 months. The authors reported potential long-term benefits from FM systems for the children in the APD group with regard to academics, emotional issues, psychosocial status, and improved speech perception ability.

The literature includes considerable debate over the benefits of hearing aids or cochlear implants with ANSD patients. Success in learning language using a purely auditory mode certainly seems questionable in light of the neural auditory dysfunction of these children. Because ANSD individuals vary significantly in both their audiometric findings and general response to sound, it is recommended that the management of children with auditory neuropathy should be flexible and take into account individual differences. Evidence-based research for treatment of ANSD patients is limited with few peer-reviewed studies available. Sininger (2008) comments that methodologies that emphasize "auditory/oral" communications such as auditory-verbal therapy tend to minimize visual information in the speech signal. Roush (2008) concludes that considering the realm of varied etiologies, possible sites of lesion, age of identification, and risks of cognitive developmental delays, it is unlikely that a single management strategy will apply for all infants and young children with ANSD. Hood (2011) discusses future challenges in understanding the bases of ANSD and suggests that progress in this area will depend on developing diagnostic methods that can accurately distinguish normal from abnormal function at the inner hair cell, synaptic juncture, and neural levels of the auditory system.

Hayes and Sininger (2008) organized an international conference of leading scientists and clinicians to share information and develop practical guidelines to help clinicians identify, diagnose, and manage infants and young children with auditory neuropathy. In fact, the outcome of the conference resulted in an important and valuable monograph entitled, "Guidelines for Identification and Management of Infants and Young Children with Auditory Neuropathy Spectrum Disorder" which is presented in its entirety as Appendix B.

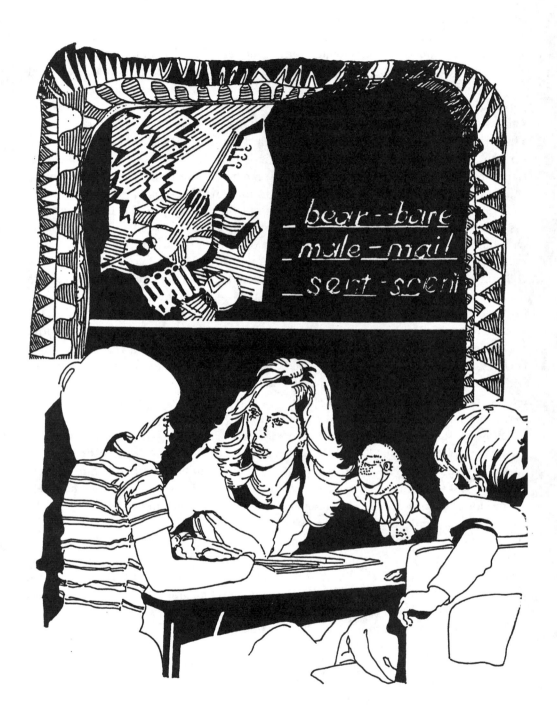

CHAPTER 5

Early Intervention

Early intervention is a broad term that describes the need to begin habilitation services as soon as a disability is confirmed. Early intervention is the course of action taken to achieve the proper steps to obtain services needed by a child. Intervention refers to services for infants and toddlers who have conditions that may cause delays in the development of five general areas including physical development, cognitive development, social or emotional development, adaptive development, and communication. For deaf and hard-of-hearing babies, early intervention services usually focus on communication skills although other interventions may be necessary. Communication skills can be learned through sign language, spoken language, or both. Family members are the most important people in babies' lives, so early intervention services must include support for family members, too.

Babies that are diagnosed with hearing loss should begin to get intervention services as soon as possible, but no later than 6 months of age (JCIH, 1994). Hearing screening and confirmation that a child is deaf or hard-of-hearing are largely meaningless without appropriate, individualized, targeted, and high-quality intervention. For the infant or young child who is deaf or hard-of-hearing to reach his or her full potential, carefully designed individualized intervention must be implemented promptly, utilizing service providers with optimal knowledge and skill levels, providing services based on research, best practices, and proven models.

EARLY INTERVENTION SERVICES

No single model of intervention is the answer for every child or family. Good intervention plans include program planning, close monitoring, follow-up visits, and flexibility in changes needed along the way. There are many different options for children with hearing loss and their families, such as working with a professional or a team of specialists, joining support groups with similar interests and issues, and taking advantage of resources available to children with a hearing loss and their families. In children with hearing loss, early intervention inevitably begins through the provision of counseling and supportive services to parents and primary caregivers to help them accept and understand the child's diagnosis and management plans. Early intervention can take many forms, such as fitting the child with hearing aids, evaluating for cochlear implants, arranging home visits to evaluate the child's progress and provide support, providing advice and training for parents, and teaching and encouraging parents how to stimulate speech and language in their child. Early intervention services are provided in different ways and in different locations, always with consideration to maintaining cultural values. The goal is to provide services in the baby's natural environment so that many of the necessary services may be provided in the home. Additional services may be provided in schools, clinics, or medical centers.

The pediatric audiologist may be the first informant to the parents that their child has a hearing loss. Following confirmation of the hearing loss and a medical specialist's evaluations, the audiologist may again be the first professional to discuss intervention steps with the parents. Parents report that their physicians are generally not well informed about hearing loss in children (Meadow-Orlans, Mertens, & Sass-Lehrer, 2003). As pointed out by Luterman (1996), this may present a challenge because the ability to impart knowledge and expertise to parents, without imposing personal opinions, is a delicate art. It takes time and confidence to build a trusting relationship with parents so that all parties are comfortable sharing and disagreeing about strongly held beliefs. Intervention planning requires ongoing sharing of information in interactive sessions that allow the audiologist and parents to respect, react, and respond to each other.

With early identification and the use of advanced hearing technologies, deaf and hard-of-hearing children can access audition and follow an intervention approach focused on achieving typical developmental milestones in listening, speech, language, cognition, and conversational competence. Parents' communication choices should be based on their long-term desired outcomes for their child. Once those decisions are made, professionals providing early intervention and habilitative services must support the parents' choices and provide the necessary support and intervention to ensure, to the greatest extent possible, that the child achieves those outcomes.

The basic components related to early hearing intervention that should be initiated by the pediatric audiologist as soon as possible include the following: (a) immediate counseling to support the parent's adaptation to the diagnosis and provide a forum in which they can express and work through their feelings; (b) the infant's impaired auditory system should be attended to and supplemented as quickly as possible through the appropriate fitting of hearing aids; and (c) encouragement should be given to the early development of a rich symbolic communication system between family members and the infant (Greenberg, Calderon, & Kusche, 1984). Early identification and intervention allow the family members to feel that they are doing all they can to assist the child and to bolster the child's sense of being. Such a program provides direct intervention with the child and a psychotherapeutic counseling experience for the parents to help them achieve satisfactory emotional adjustment to the birth of an infant with hearing impairment (First & Palfrey, 1994).

IMPLEMENTATION OF EARLY INTERVENTION

A number of studies and thoughtful publications have influenced the acceptance of early intervention by administrative authorities regarding children with hearing loss. The pertinent points include the following (Gallaudet Research Institute, 2008; Yoshinaga-Itano, 1995; Yoshinaga-Itano et al., 1998):

- The age of identification has steadily decreased since the 1960s as assessment and assistive technologies have improved.
- Pediatric hearing aid strategies and fittings have improved dramatically.
- Advances in computer technology have influenced nearly every aspect of pediatric audiology.

- Changes have occurred in the modes of communication used in the education of children with hearing loss.
- The widespread provision of parent-infant intervention and preschool education changed from the private sector to the public sector.
- Assessment tools for hearing, speech, and language development have improved.
- The types of school placement and service delivery systems have improved.
- The educational philosophies of parent-infant and preschool intervention have shifted to the family.
- The basic etiologies of pediatric hearing loss have changed during the past three decades.

Of significant concern, however, is the fact that the incidence of multiple handi-capping conditions has increased over the years. In fact, it has been estimated that 35% to 40% of all children who are deaf or hearing-impaired have disabilities in addition to deafness (Yoshinaga-Itano, 1995). These additional disabilities often affect the child's ability to access and use language. Estimates are available for hearing loss associated with other disabilities as reported by Roush, Holcomb, Roush, and Escolar (2004) as shown in Table 5–1.

An extremely important issue that affects the outcomes of early identification and intervention is the time interval between age of detection of the hearing loss and the age at which the initiation of intervention services begins. Fortunately, this time interval has decreased dramatically during the past three decades. In 1984, Bergstrom reported data showing that although the average age of parental suspicion of deafness in a group of children was 10 months of age, it took until the children reached an average age of 21 months before a medical diagnosis of the

Table 5–1. Distribution of Conditions That Occur in Addition to Deafness

Condition	Percent (%) of Children
No condition in addition to deafness	60.1
Learning disability	10.7
Intellectual disability	9.8
Attention deficit disorder	6.6
Blindness and low vision	3.9
Cerebral palsy	3.4
Emotional disturbance	1.7
Other conditions	12.1

Note: *n* = 42,361; 11.9% not reported. Gallaudet Research Institute, 2003; Roush et al., 2002.

hearing loss was determined. Further delay was noted because amplification and other intervention services were not initiated in these families until the children reached an average age of 27 months. The pattern of delays in these earlier years seemed to be due to three factors: (a) initial parental disbelief or denial of the fact that their child was hearing-impaired, (b) delays due to physician scheduling and referrals to other specialists, and (c) some babies had multiple handicaps in which hearing was only part of the total concern of the parents.

By the mid-1970s, statistics from the infant hearing screening program at the University of Colorado Medical Center (Downs, 1986) proved that the average time between confirmation of the hearing loss and initiation of habilitation procedures could be reduced to as little as 6.5 months. However, the situation in the United States in the early 1990s was a typical average interval of 12 months between the time of diagnosis to the initiation of intervention. At that time, the average age of identification was 2.5 years, and the average age of intervention was 3.5 years (Strong, Clark, & Walden, 1994). The need to reduce the time of identification and intervention was of sufficient concern that the 1994 and the 2000 Joint Committees on Infant Hearing issued strong declarative statements that called for infant hearing screening programs to identify infants with hearing loss and initiate early intervention services prior to 6 months of age.

A major government-sponsored consensus meeting was held in Washington, DC, in 1993 to address the problems faced in the early identification of children with hearing loss and problems related to their subsequent enrollment in early intervention. The committee of experts' deliberations resulted in a strong statement calling for all infants born in the United States to be screened for hearing status prior to discharge from the hospital. In addition, the committee identified the need for research to evaluate and improve methodologies for early intervention for those infants identified with hearing loss (NIDCD Consensus Statement on Early Identification of Hearing Impairment in Infants and Young Children, 1993).

This epic consensus statement changed forever the outlook for infants and young children with hearing loss, as the federal government recognized the need for improvements in infant hearing screening and intervention and provided authorization and funds to establish Early Hearing Detection and Intervention (EHDI) programs in all states. Between 1999 and 2002, EHDI programs were established in all 50 states and the District of Columbia, providing a new emphasis on providing hearing services for deaf and hard-of-hearing babies and young children. The new law required the Secretary of Health and Human Services to assist in the recruitment, retention, education, and training of qualified personnel and health care providers and to support efforts to ensure that babies who are suspected of being deaf or hard-of-hearing receive an appropriate hearing evaluation and are not lost to follow-up; it also required EHDI programs to establish and foster family-to-family support mechanisms.

Clearly, infants who are identified at birth with hearing loss have an important advantage over their later-identified peers (Fitzpatrick et al., 2007; Nicholas & Geers, 2008; Sharma, Dorman, & Spahr, 2002; Sharma et al., 2004; Sininger et al., 1999, 2009; Wake et al., 2005; Yoshinaga-Itano et al., 1998). Optimal intervention should begin as soon as the hearing loss in an infant is confirmed. Those infants identified early must receive intervention services so that they will have the opportunity to be exposed to a more abundant language environment that will enable them to achieve maximal language skills. The current universal infant hearing screening programs are helping to identify infants with hearing loss at birth so that their hearing losses may be confirmed and diagnosed by the age of 1 month, fitted with amplification no later than 3 months of age, and intervention begun immediately but no later than 6 months of age. Early identification of hearing loss can only be efficacious if quality early intervention is provided at the earliest possible time, certainly within the first year of life.

FEDERAL MANDATES

Of vital importance to the family, the pediatric audiologist must be prepared to discuss the opportunities provided through Part C of the Individuals with Disabilities Education Act (IDEA, 2004). Through this law the federal government ensures that there is a system for deaf and hard-of-hearing babies and their families to receive early intervention services. Under Part C of the Individuals with Disabilities Education Act, each state receives funds to make early intervention services available to infants and toddlers under the age of 3 years and their families. To be eligible for services provided by the state EHDI program, proper application must be made through appropriate referral sources to the state EHDI coordinators' offices. All early intervention services are identified in a baby's formalized Individualized Family Service Plan (IFSP). Each baby's IFSP is different, depending on the baby's and the family's needs. Deaf and hard-of-hearing babies with other needs or additional disabilities may qualify for services such as occupational therapy or physical therapy as needed. Many, but not all, services are free but program support

may vary between states. State-supported programs for early interventions services may include any or all of the following:

- an evaluation of the baby's needs,
- home visits from early intervention professionals,
- sign language instruction for family members,
- audiology services,
- speech-language services,
- special instruction,
- assistive technology devices and services, and
- social work services.

Each state IDEA-supported early intervention program has a number of specific pre-referral and post-referral requirement procedures that have been developed to establish a high standard of care for infants and toddlers under 36 months age. IDEA requires referral of the child with hearing loss to the Part C program "as soon as possible but in no case more than seven days after the child is identified." Furthermore, within 45 days after the lead agency has received referral of a child, the screening (if applicable), initial evaluation, initial assessments (of the child and family), and the initial IFSP meeting for that child must be completed. The EHDI program has a comprehensive website with information on early intervention services available in each state (http://www.cdc.gov/ncbddd/hearing-loss/ehdi-goals.html).

Although all states are now required by federal law to provide appropriate early intervention programs for children with disabilities, the earliest state-funded early intervention programs were developed before hospital-based newborn hearing screening programs became widespread (White, 2004). Accordingly, most programs at that time were serving mostly children with severe-to-profound bilateral hearing loss. Many of the children being identified in the hospital-based hearing screening programs were children with mild, moderate, and unilateral hearing losses. State Early Hearing Detection and Intervention (EHDI) coordinators estimated that only 53% of infants and toddlers identified with hearing loss in 2004 were referred to an appropriate early intervention program by 6 months of age. White noted the need for early intervention services for infants and toddlers with hearing loss to be redesigned and refocused to help children with mild-to-moderate hearing loss.

Currently, federal law provides funds for states to participate in early intervention services for infants with hearing loss through Public Law 105-17. When hearing loss is identified, evaluation and early intervention services should be provided in accordance with the Individuals with Disabilities Educational Act (IDEA), Part H, Public Law 102-119 (formerly PL 99-457). Components of an early intervention program for children with hearing loss and their families should include the following:

- Family support and information regarding hearing loss and the range of available communication and educational intervention options. Such information must be provided in an objective, nonbiased way to support family choice. It is recommended to use consumer organizations and persons who are deaf or hard-of-hearing to provide such information.
- Professional, consumer, state, and community-based organizations should be accessed to provide ongoing information regarding legal rights, educational materials, support groups and networks, and other relevant resources for children and families.
- Implementation of learning environments and services designed with attention to the family's preferences. Such services should be family centered and should be consistent with the needs of the child, the family, and their culture.
- Early intervention activities that promote the child's development in all areas, with particular attention to language acquisition and communication skills.
- Early intervention services that provide ongoing monitoring of the child's medical and hearing status, amplification needs, and development of communication skills.

CORNERSTONES OF EARLY INTERVENTION

Many attempts have been made over the years to prove the efficacy of early intervention for hearing loss. The early research was limited by the fact that few children with hearing loss were identified before the age of 2 to 3 years. These early studies were weakened because nearly all of them were retrospective rather than prospective. Fortunately, the past few years have been especially profitable in terms of prospective research in the area of early intervention, and a great many valuable insights have been established.

Evidence-based early intervention research studies are challenging, and few comparative effectiveness studies have been conducted. Randomized controlled trials are particularly difficult for ethical reasons, making it challenging to fully establish causal links between interventions and outcomes. Certainly, preliminary studies have strongly related the importance of the early developmental years for the well-being and normal development of each individual. The goal for deaf and hearing-impaired children is the development of language skills commensurate with their normal-hearing peers, regardless of the degree of hearing loss, the mode of communication, socioeconomic status, cultural ethnicity, or gender. Yoshinaga-Itano (1999) stated that the focus should be on prevention of developmental delay through early identification and appropriate early intervention services. Educators strive to achieve language development that is commensurate with the child's cognitive potential, rather than focusing energy on closing the developmental delay. The manner in which individuals are able to function in preschool, adolescence, and even adulthood often depends on their experiences before the young age of 30 months.

A classic study by Levitt, McGarr, and Geffner (1987) reported measures on the development of speech and language in 120 children with hearing loss in the 10- to 14-year age bracket over a 4-year period. The children's hearing losses ranged from moderate 40 dB HL levels to profound hearing losses in excess of 80 dB HL. All the children in the study cohort were identified after 30 months of age. Following numerous longitudinal testing procedures, it was clear that the highest language skills were found in the children with the earliest intervention. A surprising finding in this research, however, was that the degree of hearing loss did not constitute a significant factor in later language skills and educational performance. The children with milder hearing losses showed the same reduced language skills as those children with profound hearing loss. The answer to this paradoxical finding is, of course, that

none of these children had been identified at an age young enough to take advantage of the optimal periods for language learning. The equivalence of the language scores represented only the intense educational training that the children received and did not reflect any benefit from a truly early intervention course of action. However, speech intelligibility, as would be expected, was directly proportional to the children's degree of hearing loss. Those children with the mildest hearing losses had the best speech; the children with the most severe hearing losses had the poorest speech. This finding is related to the fact that speech is an overlaid function, derived from a number of organs and structures that were developed for other uses, and dependent on accurate auditory reception for its production. The pathway to normalized speech and language patterns for the child with significant hearing loss is a long journey.

In another study of "earlier versus later," Watkins (1987) studied three groups of children with hearing loss who received intervention services at different times in their developing years. Group 1 children received 9 months of home intervention before 30 months of age; group 2 children attended preschool beginning at 36 months of age; group 3 children did not receive any intervention services until they began school at 60 months of age. When all three groups of children were 10 years old, the results of a number of evaluations showed that for all variables assessed, the children who received the earliest, and therefore the most intervention, performed the best. The average child in this study who received early intervention performed better than 75% to 92% of the children in the groups that received later or no intervention.

In England, Robinshaw (1995) described a group of five young children whose deafness had been confirmed between 3 and

5 months of age, and who received intervention with hearing aids before the age of 7 months. He compared these deaf children with five normally hearing children and 12 similarly deaf children whose average age of identification was later than 24 months. His results showed that by 5 years of age, the earlier-identified group of children developed speech and language skills similar to the normal-hearing control group of children. These results buttress the argument for early intervention.

There is a growing body of research demonstrating that intensive early intervention can alter positively the cognitive and developmental outcomes of young infants with disabilities and reduce the levels of family stress reactions, as cited in a valuable tutorial review prepared by Carney and Moeller (1998). They concluded that enriched intervention programs provide some children with hearing loss with the ability to overcome developmental lags in language and academic skills. There has been considerable evidence that the natural give-and-take of communication that typically occurs with parents and infants can be disrupted when childhood hearing loss is present. In contrast, deaf parents of deaf infants appear to be effective interventionists for their children because of their understanding of deafness, their ability to communicate at the earliest ages with sign, and their lack of conflict with deafness as a disability (Meadows-Orlans, 1987).

Moeller (2000) contributed a significant study showing that better language outcomes are clearly tied to early intervention. Moeller reported results from 112 children with mild to profound hearing loss who communicated through various methods. She evaluated the children with a variety of language tests including the PPVT for vocabulary, Preschool Language Assessment Instrument for verbal reasoning, and a rating scale of family involvement in the intervention program. Moeller's results showed that early enrolled children had significantly better vocabulary and better reasoning skills at 5 years of age than later-enrolled children regardless of degree of hearing loss or mode of communication. She also reported that the most successful children with better vocabulary and nonverbal intelligence scores were those with high levels of family involvement.

Research in Early Intervention

Under the direction of Christine Yoshinaga-Itano, a professor at the University of Colorado, a number of important research studies were conducted during the last half of the 1990s that have had a profound effect on the acceptance of early identification of children with hearing loss and the concomitant value of early intervention. These research projects were largely made possible by the fact that several newborn hearing screening programs had been in effect in Colorado for nearly 20 years, making a large sample of children with hearing losses of varying degrees available for studies. These now classic studies provide an impressive framework in which to develop additional studies as more is learned about the importance of early intervention in the lives of children with special needs.

Apuzzo and Yoshinaga-Itano (1995) reported one of the earliest evidence-based verifications to prove the efficacy of early intervention. They compared the language abilities at 40 months of age across four sets of children grouped by their age of hearing loss identification: (a) 0 to 2 months; (b) 3 to 12 months; (c) 13 to 18 months; and (d) 19 to 25 months. The degree of hearing loss of the children in all groups ranged from mild to profound, and all of the children received the same intervention services shortly after their hearing loss was identified. The analysis of data showed that those children identified before 3 months of age had significantly higher language scores than those children identified later than the age of 2 months despite all the children receiving similar intervention therapy.

Yoshinaga-Itano et al. (1998) extended their earlier study with a report on a group of children with hearing losses gleaned from a database of nearly 500 Colorado children with hearing impairment who had been carefully monitored for 10 years. From this series of subjects, 150 children with varying degrees of hearing losses and varying ages of identification and intervention were enlisted for her study. Approximately 50% of the group were identified and entered intervention activities before the age of 6 months; the remaining 50% were identified, and of course intervened with, at later ages. The children in both groups all had bilateral, congenital hearing losses ranging from a 27 dB HL average to hearing losses greater than 110 dB HL. Particular attention was given to matching the two groups of subjects, early identified and later identified, as closely as possible to be sure that all of the children had received intervention immediately as soon as they were identified to have significant hearing loss.

All study children were given the Minnesota Child Development Inventory (MCDI) when they were between 13 and 36 months of age (Ireton & Thwing, 1974). The MCDI is a 320-item questionnaire that is filled out by the child's primary caregiver. It is composed of eight subtests that evaluate different areas of development including general development, gross motor skills, fine motor skills, expressive language, comprehensive-conceptual (language understanding), personal-social, comprehensive-situational (nonverbal understanding), and self-help scales. Children are considered to be functioning within normal developmental limits if their developmental age is greater than 75% of their chronologic age. The MCDI identifies children as "borderline delayed" (delay between 25% and 30% of chronologic age) and "delayed" (developmental age lower than 70% of chronologic age). Yoshinaga-Itano used the MCDI to compare the developmental scores of the children who were earlier-identified versus later-identified by a number of variables that included cognitive ability, age at time of testing, communication mode, minority status, gender, degree of hearing loss, socioeconomic status, and presence or absence of other disabilities in addition to hearing impairment.

The positive effects of early identification and early intervention showed consistently across all the variables analyzed by Yoshinaga-Itano's research group. The group of children with hearing losses identified between birth and 6 months of age had significantly higher developmental functioning at 40 months of age than the group of later-identified children. Both the receptive language and expressive language scores reflected a significant difference between the two groups in favor of the early identified-early intervened children. In addition, those children with normal cognitive abilities who were identified and received intervention before the age of 6 months achieved language skills well within the normal range of functioning for their age. Even children with lower cognitive quotients showed positive benefit from early identification and intervention. Somewhat surprisingly, when the early identified children with mild hearing losses (26 to 40 dB HL) were compared with children in their cohort with profound hearing losses (greater than 90 dB HL), there was no appreciable difference in language skills. Personal-social quotients were significantly lower in the mild hearing loss group than for the profound hearing loss group, suggesting a greater need for attention to those children with milder hearing losses than previously thought necessary.

Finally, analysis of speech perception concurred almost exactly with the earlier Levitt et al. (1987) findings. Speech perception in the children of the Colorado study was found to be directly proportional to the degree of hearing loss, regardless of the age of identification or the age at which intervention services were initiated. However, the early identified children with all degrees of hearing loss (except the profoundly deaf) ultimately achieved normal range of speech perception, albeit on different time lines. The children with milder hearing losses acquired good speech perception by 31 to 36 months of age, whereas the children with moderate and severe hearing loss took 37 to 61 months to achieve optimal speech perception. The effects of other demographic variables such as ethnicity, maternal education level, and communication mode were generally nonsignificant.

The findings of the important studies from Colorado demonstrate that early identification of infants with hearing problems, when followed by immediate and appropriate intervention, does improve the outcomes for these children by resulting in significantly better performances in language, speech, and educational progress. Although mean language scores for early identified children were within the low normal range, their developmental quotients were lower than those reported for normal-hearing children. The collective analysis of these studies proves that regardless of the degree of hearing loss present, the trend for significant improvement in the children of the study cohort is related to early identification and early intervention (Yoshinaga-Itano & Apuzzo, 1995; Yoshinaga-Itano, 1999).

LENA

The LENA system (an acronym for "Language ENvironment Analysis"), developed in 2008, is a powerful tool that can provide objective data for early interventionists to screen the language environment of children with language delay and disorders and use the information to make significant changes to accelerate the child's language development. Data collected in an intensive longitudinal study and described in *Meaningful Differences in the Everyday Experiences of Young American Children* (Hart & Risley, 1995) revealed that the number of adult words spoken to children from birth to age 3 predicted almost all of the variance in the children's language ability and IQ at age 3. The LENA Research Foundation, founded in 1998 by Terrance and Judith Paul, was established on the premise that the more talk and conversational engagements a child experiences in the first 4 years of life, the better off the child will be in academics and society. The LENA Foundation realized that with the application of advanced speech recognition technology, a digital accessory could be developed to streamline the data acquisition process and provide therapists and parents a simple tool that can thoroughly chart a child's natural language environment on a 5-minute, hour, daily, or weekly basis (http://www.lenafoundation.org/).

Initially designed for research and treatment of language delays and disorders in children 0 to 5 years of age, LENA has proven useful in numerous applications of data collection and especially useful in early intervention programs for children with hearing loss (Aragon & Yoshinaga-Itano, 2012). Use of LENA provides language environmental analysis data that have been nearly impossible to acquire without costly and lengthy methods. The LENA System provides more than 25 different metrics on the natural language environment of children, including estimates and percentile scores for adult words spoken to the child, conversational turns, and child vocalizations. The system also generates an automatic expressive language developmental age and percentile score based on a child's voiceprint.

The LENA system uses a small recording device, the LENA Digital Language Processor, worn by the child to monitor, collect, analyze, and sort a child's language environment into multiple categories and analyzes variables such as child vocalizations, adult words, and conversational turn taking. The device also can monitor and measure the audio sounds in the child's natural language environment such as time spent with television (LENA Foundation, 2011). Data are analyzed through specially developed computer software. The LENA system is truly a breakthrough technology which has the potential to help parents communicate with their children and to assist clinicians and therapists in planning clinical sessions and data to coaching parents and to monitor their progress in talking with their children. Researchers are using the system to find means to close the gap in language development between advantaged and disadvantaged children (Evans, Gonnella, Marcynyszyn, Gentile, & Salpekar, 2005; Hoff, 2012; Rowe, 2008; Rowe & Goldin-Meadow, 2009). This new technology allows us to document how much language a child is exposed to with their daily environment, and provides opportunity to estimate how much language a child with hearing loss is exposed to within his or her daily language environment so that we can provide parents with concise information that they need to improve their communication efforts to benefit their child.

OPTIMAL EARLY INTERVENTION STRATEGIES

Technological advances have helped in many ways to improve the communication impediments between families and their deaf and hard-of-hearing child. But the skills of the intervention providers really make the difference in the success and progress of the child with hearing loss (Stredler-Brown, 2008). Optimal early intervention strategies provide appropriate services for the child with hearing loss and assure that families receive a full complement of consumer-oriented information. Families should be informed of organizations that enhance informed decision making such as peer models, persons or mentors who are hard-of-hearing or deaf, as well as consumer and professional associations. The 2000 Joint Committee on Infant Hearing Position Statement summarized some important principles of effective early intervention:

- *Developmental timing* refers to the age at which intervention services are initiated with the knowledge that programs that enroll infants at younger ages and continue longer are found to produce the greatest intervention benefits.
- *Program intensity* refers to the amount of intervention provided. This is measured by multiple factors such as the number of home visits or individual contacts per week.
- *Direct learning* implies that learning experiences are more effective when

center-based educational activities are provided by trained professionals in addition to indirect home-based training.

- *Program breadth and flexibility* refer to the fact that successful intervention programs offer a broad spectrum of services and are flexible and multifaceted to meet the unique needs of the infant and family.
- *Recognition of individual differences* refers to the basic principle of education that states that individual progress and benefits from programs are functions of infant and family differences (i.e., not everyone progresses or benefits at the same rate).
- *Environmental support and family involvement* refers to the fact that the benefits of early intervention continue over time depending on the effectiveness of existing family and other environmental support (i.e., home, school, health, and peer).

The 2013 JCIH and Early Intervention

The Early Intervention Supplement to the Year 2007 Position Statement was developed by the Joint Committee on Infant Hearing (JCIH) and published by the American Academy of Pediatrics (2013). This lengthy and detailed Intervention Supplement codifies best practice statements to advocate for the implementation of coordinated, statewide systems with the expertise to provide individualized, high-fidelity early intervention programs for children who are deaf and hard-of-hearing and their families. Consistent monitoring of child and family outcomes is an essential step toward ensuring optimal outcomes for the majority of children. The establishment of practice stan-

dards, implementation of developmentally appropriate protocols for the monitoring of outcomes, and commitment to research collaborations are critical steps toward this goal. The JCIH Intervention Supplement presents 12 specific goals for clinicians and state-empowered EHDI programs to strive to achieve the optimal outcomes for children who are deaf or hard-of-hearing:

Goal 1: All children who are children with hearing loss and their families have access to timely and coordinated entry into early intervention programs supported by a data management system capable of tracking families and children from confirmation of hearing loss to enrollment into early intervention services.

Goal 2: All children who are children with hearing loss and their families experience timely access to service coordinators who have specialized knowledge and skills related to working with individuals who are children with hearing loss.

Goal 3: All children who are children with hearing loss from birth to 3 years of age and their families have early intervention providers who have the professional qualifications and core knowledge and skills to optimize the child's development and child/family well-being.

Goal 4: All children who are children with hearing loss with additional disabilities and their families have access to specialists who have the professional qualifications and specialized knowledge and skills to support and promote optimal developmental outcomes.

Goal 5: All children who are children with hearing loss and their families from culturally diverse backgrounds and/or from non-English-speaking homes have access to culturally competent services with provision of the same quality and quantity of information given to families from the majority culture.

Goal 6: All children who are children with hearing loss should have their progress monitored every 6 months from birth to 36 months of age, through a protocol that includes the use of standardized, norm-referenced developmental evaluations, for language (spoken and signed); the modality of communication (auditory, visual, and augmentative); social-emotional and cognitive issues; and fine and gross motor skills.

Goal 7: All children who are identified with hearing loss of any degree, including those with unilateral or slight hearing loss, those with auditory neural hearing loss (auditory neuropathy), and those with progressive or fluctuating hearing loss, receive appropriate monitoring and immediate follow-up intervention services where appropriate.

Goal 8: Families will be active participants in the development and implementation of EHDI systems at the state/territory and local levels.

Goal 9: All families will have access to other families who have children with hearing loss and who are appropriately trained to provide culturally and linguistically sensitive support, mentorship, and guidance.

Goal 10: Individuals who are children with hearing loss will be active participants in the development and implementation of EHDI systems at the national, state/territory, and local levels. Their participation will be an expected and integral component of the EHDI systems.

Goal 11: All children with hearing loss and their families have access to support, mentorship, and guidance from individuals who are children with hearing loss.

Goal 12: As best practices are increasingly identified and implemented, all children with hearing loss and their families will be assured of fidelity in the implementation of the intervention they receive.

FAMILY-CENTERED SERVICES

Family-centered care provides an expanded view of how to work with children and families. Family-centered service is made up of a set of values, attitudes, and approaches to services for children with special needs and their families. Family-centered service recognizes that each family is unique; that the family is the constant in the child's life; and that they are the experts on the child's abilities and needs. The family works with service providers to make informed decisions about the services and supports the child and family receive. In family-centered service, the strengths and needs of all family members are considered. Family-centered practice recognizes the strengths of family relationships and builds on these strengths to achieve optimal outcomes for themselves and their children. Family-centered practice is characterized by mutual trust, respect, honesty, and open communication between parents and service providers. Families are active participants in the development of policy, program design, and evaluation; and they are active decision makers in selecting services for themselves and their children. Family and child assessment is strength-based and solution-focused. Services are community based and build upon informal supports and resources.

During the 1960s and 1970s, the process for managing children with hearing loss was generally disease centered. That is to say, the focus was on diagnostic specifics with careful delineation of syndromic or nonsyndromic symptoms, moving directly into intervention and educational recommendations based on the professional's background, training, and experience and with limited consideration of the family parent's role in the child's development. This period was followed in the 1980s by a gradual change in philosophy, to be known as the patient-centered focus, whereby the management provided by health care professionals was directed to whatever seemed best for the child. Decisions were still made by the professionals who advised parents based on whatever the child's needs would be, and the family followed directions as best as possible. By the 1990s, family-centered management in health care was widely adopted by professionals, whereby the family was provided ample information to make the necessary decisions regarding their child. The professional's role was to provide nonbiased information about all the choices available and encouraging contact with other parents of children with hearing impairment, or attendance at support groups, to help the family reach meaningful decisions. Of course, the pediatric audiologist must demonstrate full support for the decisions reached by the family by doing everything possible to make the family's choices best serve the child.

Family-centered service reflects a shift from the traditional focus on the biomedical aspects of a child's condition to a concern with seeing the child in context of their family and recognizing the primacy of family in the child's life. "Family" means any person(s) who plays a significant role in an individual's life. This may include individuals not legally related to the individual. Members of "family" include spouses, domestic partners, and both different-sex and same-sex significant others. The principles argue in favor of an approach that respects families as integral and coequal parts of the health care team. The overall goal of this approach is to improve the quality and safety of a child's care by helping to foster communication between families and health care professionals. Furthermore, by taking family/patient input and concerns

into account, the family feels comfortable working with professionals on a plan of care, and professionals are "on board" in terms of what families expect with medical interventions and health outcomes. Family-centered approaches to health care intervention also generally lead to wiser allocation of health care resources, as well as greater patient and family satisfaction.

The changing roles of the parents and the professionals reflect the important fact that the child is always an extension of the family. Family-centered services emerged as an important concept in health care, but the implementation of family was met with a variety of snags. Prior to the early 1990s, the relationship between care providers and patients was distant. The traditional model of care centered on directions issued by physicians, and an expectation existed that patients and their families would assume passive roles as observers, rather than participants. The audiologist or speech pathologist acted as an outside expert who imparted selected, and oft-times biased, information to the parents and then directed decisions to the family on behalf of the child. However, it is now recognized that family, close friends, and educators are more likely to identify slight variations in the patient's behaviors and mental or physical health that health care professionals, largely unfamiliar with the daily activities of the child, may miss. Furthermore, health care professionals view the child during brief snapshots of time, whereas a patient's family lives full-time with the child. Enlisting a patient's family as a part of their health care team helps enable their ability to assist, manage, and assess the child's auditory, speech, and language performance. Children with hearing loss and their families often need special help to learn methods to facilitate communication. These methods might be used together, or possibly at different times depending on the environment, preferences, and immediate needs. This leads to the fact that many families move between two or more methods of communication with their child.

The cornerstone of family-centered services requires that the audiologist acknowledge that the child cannot be viewed apart from the family. Accordingly, the family-centered approach to intervention and habilitation is individualized on the basis of each family's beliefs, resources, priorities, and concerns (Bailey, 1994). Key components of family-centered practice include: (a) working with the family unit to ensure the safety and well-being of all family members; (b) strengthening the capacity of families to function effectively; (c) engaging, empowering, and partnering with families throughout the decision- and goal-making processes; (d) providing individualized, culturally responsive, flexible, and relevant services for each family; and (e) linking families with collaborative, comprehensive, culturally relevant, community-based networks of supports and services. Furthermore, it must be recognized that families have the right to retain as much control as they desire over the intervention process (Roush & McWilliams, 1994).

Parents and families of children with special needs play a pivotal role in the successful development of the child. It has become increasingly clear that parents are the best advocates and facilitators for their child and must be actively involved in decision making. Involving the family from the initial contact with the audiologist is critical, creating an open and equally flowing communication system. In view of the newborn with strongly suspected or confirmed hearing loss, immediate involvement with the family is crucial. The basic components related to this family intervention should include:

(a) immediate counseling to support the parents' adaption to the diagnosis and provide a forum in which they feel free to ask questions and express and work through their feelings; (b) an orientation to the facts that the infant's impaired auditory reception might benefit from or require fitting with hearing aids; and (c) encouragement given to the early development of a rich symbolic communication system between infants and family members (Greenberg et al., 1984). Early identification and intervention allow the family members to feel that they are doing all they can to assist the child and to bolster the child's sense of well-being. Such a program provides direct intervention with the child and a psychotherapeutic counseling experience for the parents to help them achieve satisfactory emotional adjustment to the birth of an infant with hearing impairment (First & Palfrey, 1994).

Parents are their children's first and most important teachers; parents have a profound impact on development and ultimate success in education. Parents have the ability and opportunity to enrich their child's early language environment. Accordingly, the role of parental and family involvement with the child with hearing loss is absolutely crucial and is tied to success in all areas of the child's life. Although early intervention based on this premise has been suggested since the early 1950s, PL 94-142 mandated the shift to family-centered practices. In the family-centered paradigm, the basic concept is that parents, or the primary caregivers, will be able to make appropriate decisions if they have sufficient information and understand the factors involved in reaching these decisions. The audiologist performs the role of guide as an educator and facilitator in the provision of resources and in answering questions. Because of the enormous learning potential of infants, early parent intervention training programs have received considerable attention in recent years (Laughton, 1994).

For most parents, their child's hearing loss is unexpected. Parents likely need time and support to adapt to the child's impaired hearing and need to be made aware that their child may have other developmental delays, especially in the area of language development. When parents learn that their child has a disability or chronic illness, they begin a journey often filled with emotion, difficult choices, and interactions with many different professionals with an ongoing need for information and services. Parents react in ways that are entirely predictable and often documented. Parents are likely to go through periods of denial, grief, fear, and guilt followed by confusion, helplessness, disappointment, and even rejection (Luterman, 1996). Not all parents go through each of these emotions, but it is important for parents to know that they are neither alone nor unique in all of these feelings.

Table 5–2 provides suggestions for constructive actions that may help parents or primary caregivers through their rampant emotional reactions to learning that their child has a hearing loss. Family support groups can play an important role in helping parents and caregivers understand the special problems presented by the child with hearing impairment. Support is anything that helps a family and may range from just providing advice and information, and helping locate a deaf mentor, to finding

Table 5–2. Constructive Suggestions and Actions for Parents

Seek assistance from other parents of children with hearing loss.

Talk with your spouse, significant other, and family members.

Rely on positive sources in your life.

Take one day at a time.

Learn the terminology.

Seek information from all sources.

Do not be intimidated.

Show and express emotions; learn to deal with natural feelings.

Maintain a positive outlook; keep in touch with reality.

Remember that time is on your side.

Find programs for your child.

Take care of yourself.

Avoid pity; recognize that you are not alone.

Decide how to deal with others.

Keep daily routines as normal as possible.

Remember to love your child.

Source: Adapted from "National Parent Network on Disabilities," by P. M. Smith, 1997, *News Digest*, 2nd ed., February, Washington, DC.

appropriate child care or transportation, and giving parents time for personal relaxation. The family's main initial need may just be finding a supportive listener. Families who have children and young people with special needs very often deal with similar lifestyles, face the same problems and challenges, and share the same concerns with communication preferences, education access, availability of local services, family recreation possibilities, and limitations and numerous other issues directly related to their children's needs. Support groups for parents of children with special needs bring families together for friendship, to share information, and to support one another. Soloman et al. (2004) surveyed six different support groups to confirm that membership and involvement were reported by the majority of parents to be very helpful and supportive in many ways such as providing opportunities for expression and group discussion of pertinent issues. The goal of family support groups is to provide useful and practical information aimed at parents and families through a variety of means including education and training, advocacy support, parent-to-parent networking, print media such as bulletins and newsletters, website with blogging and chat room availability, special event and activities for children and their families, as well as references to other useful and practical resources.

Parents can easily become overloaded by the onslaught of information that is communicated when they learn that their child has a disability. The process is part of the effort to initiate early intervention services and must be handled with confidence and skill. The parents or primary caregivers are suddenly immersed in information regarding management of their hearing-impaired child, application of personal amplification devices, recommended changes in their daily living, concerns for social interac-

tions, and communications within the family structure, as well as decisions that must be made regarding educational approaches and placements. The role of the audiologist is an important one in this context, and a thorough understanding of the many complexities, potential diversions, and personal conflicts that may arise among family members must be taken into account in each counseling session.

The pediatric audiologist must develop a keen sense of appropriate timing and respect for the family's role in determining future directions for their child newly identified as having a hearing loss. Families are a collection of unique individuals, usually related but not always, who represent certain cultural and social histories. Most importantly, successful families alter their lifestyles to accommodate a child with special needs. Unfortunately, not all families can be considered successful in this ability to adjust to the needs of the hearing-impaired child. The audiologist needs to understand the complexities of a specific family unit, such as its size, health, interaction patterns, and socioeconomic factors, to assist effectively in developing a habilitation program that best fits its members. Added to these complexities presented by the traditional family are the special problems faced by lower socioeconomic families, working parents, broken families, the single parent, and various other nontraditional home environments (Rushmer, 1994).

The changing roles of the parents and the professional reflect the important fact that the child must always be considered an extension of the family. Typically, hearing-impaired children are born to parents who have little knowledge of the child's disability. In the past, the professional acted as an outside expert who imparted selected information to the uninformed parents and then made critical decisions on behalf of the child. However, in the 1980s a new awareness developed for the importance of the family in the successful habilitation of the child with special needs. The professional's role changed to being involved in a collaborative process with the parents to determine what is best for both the child and the family. The professional must understand that a family-centered approach to intervention and habilitation is individualized on the basis of each family's resources, priorities, and concerns (Baily, 1994). According to Roush and McWilliam (1994), the family-centered approach assumes that the child's needs are best met by meeting family needs, and that families have the right to retain as much control as they desire over the intervention process. The basic tenet underlying family-centered counseling is the understanding that what affects one member of the family affects all family members, and that the child's needs are best met by meeting family needs (Roush & Matkin, 1994).

An important part of the family-centered service is the focus on being advocates for children. Audiologists need to be cognizant of the basic principles of children's rights: (a) above all children must be protected and safe, and their well-being must be protected; (b) children have the right to a fair chance in life and the essentials of healthy development, including a sense of belonging, continuity of care, safety, nurturing, socialization to constructive societal norms, and access to opportunities; and (c) children who are at risk have the right to community protection (McCroskey & Meezan, 1998). The following basic principles provide a good summary of the family-centered approach to intervention (Dunst, Trivette, Starnes, Hamby, & Gordon, 1993):

- Recognize that the family, not the individual, is the unit of intervention.

- Foster the family's sense of competency and independence.
- Respect the parents' right and responsibility to decide what is best for their child.
- Help mobilize resources for coordinated, normalized service delivery.
- Develop a collaborative relationship with the family.

BREAKING THE NEWS TO PARENTS

Historically, the diagnosis through hearing evaluations of childhood deafness was attained when the child was 2 to 3 years of age. In those days, parents ended up at the audiology clinic because of their concern that their child's speech and language were not developing normally. The audiologist's task was to determine the presence of normal hearing and refer the child on to a speech-language pathologist for developmental testing, or to confirm the parent's suspicions that something was wrong with their child's hearing. Accordingly, acknowledging the parents' expectations of hearing loss in their toddler-aged child did not come as a total surprise, and in fact, was often received with some relief by the parents to know that their child did not have some more significant or threatening disability. However, with today's audiometric technologies that can identify hearing loss in newborns, "breaking the news" to parents that their new baby has a hearing loss usually comes as a complete surprise followed by shock and disbelief.

Luterman, Kurtzer-White, and Seewald (1999) described the feelings that parents go through after learning the diagnosis of their child's deafness. Parents' feelings are often below the level of awareness, and except for denial and shock, may not be able to express themselves until the emotions come in a flood. Feelings of inadequacy, anger, guilt, vulnerability, and confusion are certain to surface with time. Luterman's view is that these feelings are neither good nor bad, but need to be acknowledged and accepted. The audiologist must be nonjudgmental toward the parent's emotional behaviors and expressions and be prepared to participate in these normal processes, providing support through empathetic listening.

It is important to remember that nearly 95% of all deaf children are born to hearing families and that it is likely that 90% of these families have absolutely no knowledge of deafness (Mitchell & Karchmer, 2004). Thus, it is often the audiologist who informs the parents that their child has significant hearing impairment. This presents an important responsibility for the pediatric audiologist which requires the utmost in professionalism and genuine concern for the child and the involved family. Accordingly, the audiologist must be open and sensitive to the feelings and needs of families as the hearing loss in their youngster is revealed through the audiometric testing experience. Each clinician has to develop his or her own techniques for addressing this important issue. If possible, it is beneficial to have the parents observe the child's responses in a free-field situation; they will see for themselves that their child does not hear or respond appropriately to normally audible sounds. This firsthand, controlled experience will help the parents realize what their child can and cannot hear. In some instances with older children, the parents may have a strong suspicion that their child has a hearing problem, and confirmation of the handicap will help them in whatever

intervention procedures are appropriate. Whether the parents show concern, grief, or contain their feelings initially within themselves, the audiologist can be sure that they will, no doubt, be deeply disturbed over this new knowledge. As they discover their child is hearing-impaired or deaf, they will no doubt have a thousand questions that will immediately raise their stress levels. It is the role of the audiologist, under these circumstances, to put the parents at ease while reassuring them that future steps with their child will follow well-established protocols implemented by you, but requiring their decision-making involvement and cooperation.

Breaking the news to parents that their child has significant hearing loss is a huge responsibility and must not be taken lightly. Even under the best of circumstances, this information will be an important intervening factor in the family's daily life and in all future family actions. The audiologist should utilize proven counseling techniques to inform the parents about what test results found about their child's hearing, what it means for the child and for the family, followed briefly by what needs to be done in the immediate future. Clearly, this conversation must be delivered with tact and sensitivity.

This counseling information will likely have long-term influence and be long remembered by the parents, and therefore should be unemotional and supported with evidence-based facts. The pediatric audiologist must consider carefully every statement and interaction with parents and families of their young patients. The initial parent discussion should be clear and concise while conveying true interest in the child and in the parents. Ample and sufficient time should be scheduled for this session, as it is not uncommon for parents to complain in later years that this first discussion from the audiologist was way too short in time, too technical for them to comprehend the key important facts, and presented in a cold, nonsensitive manner without much feeling for the importance of the problem. Therefore, it is crucial that the audiologist create an atmosphere of mutual respect, immediately make the parents part of the process, and be prepared to support the parents by listening to their statements, questions, and expressions of concern. In fact, listening to the parents is even more important than presenting the facts of the case to them.

It is the usual tendency of parents to want to find out immediately everything that concerns the future of the child and his or her functioning. The audiologist must resist the temptation to go into great detail about the prognosis for the child's development. Whatever is said will be only half-absorbed and perhaps misunderstood or distorted on the first visit. One should limit the amount of information to the relative degree of loss that seems to be present—mild, moderate, severe, or profound—and concentrate on the implications of the loss and what is going to be done for the child. If the parents press the question as to whether the child will speak, what kind of school he or she will attend, or how and whether the child will ever communicate, they should be assured that their questions will be answered completely in due time. Do not let the parents focus on the hearing loss itself or the technology that might be applied to the child. Instead center the discussion on suggestions to stimulate and encourage the communication process within the family. Suggest to the parents that the main issue is not about the child's ears or hearing, per se, it is about doing whatever it takes with their child to develop spoken speech and language. During this appointment period, the audi-

ologist should listen as a receiver rather than a critic, demonstrating noncontrolling, empathetic, direct, and honest communication while patiently providing personal confirmation to the parents and family. It may be useful to direct parents to outside support groups for additional information and resources to cope with their own personal inadequacies as well as with the needs of the child.

Most parents will need assistance to progress positively and without debilitating delay through the stages of adjustment in understanding and accepting their child's hearing loss. Their progress toward a level of reasonable acceptance, closure, and reconstruction includes an accurate understanding of reality, as they reach the usual and customary benchmarks in their child's development. The pediatric audiologist must help parents achieve a balance between their hopes and reality in terms of their child's hearing abilities. For example, there is no need to engage in speculation about what a 2-year-old child will be able to do when he or she has reached school age, teenage years, or adulthood. While most parents want and have a need for professionals to be truthful as a prerequisite to being recognized as trustworthy persons with credibility, they do not need information that is bleak and replete with dismal prognosis. The majority of parents will come to understand the realities and implications regarding their child's achievements. This is especially true if parents are involved in all stages of the child's development and they put the child's needs foremost in seeking appropriate audiologic, health care, educational, and related services as needed (Healey, 1996).

There is perhaps no way to cushion the shock to the family learning for the first time that their child is hearing-impaired. Any attempt to minimize the problem would be a disservice and would avoid the reality of the situation. Nevertheless, a sympathetic attitude and an understanding of the parents' feelings will help as much as possible. The audiologist could say things such as, "You probably feel pretty upset about this news," or "It's perfectly natural for you to feel badly about this." The parents should be allowed sufficient time to express their feelings and fears and to ask questions. The audiologist should offer to be available for any future questions and let the parents know that they will be closely involved in the process of discovering their child's capabilities. It should be emphasized that he or she is a child first, has a hearing loss only secondary, and is just as lovable as any other child. Stein and Jabaley (1981) stated that the two factors in the environment of deaf children that can account for their emotional or behavioral differences are: (a) the lag in the child's language development and its strong effect on family communication and socialization, and (b) the psychological response of parents to the diagnosis of a hearing handicap in their child. They described three stages of parental responses that are useful for the audiologist to acknowledge and be aware of: (a) an initial expression of anger toward the professionals who diagnose the deafness in their child, (b) subsequent expressions of anger toward the child as they find it increasingly difficult to deny the existence of the hearing loss, and finally (c), the acceptance of the hearing-impaired child by the parents, which marks the transition from sadness and anger to the development of adaptation and coping behaviors. The audiologist must develop a mutual working relationship with the involved parents to reduce emotional and behavioral problems, while helping to establish the important parent-infant or parent-child bond.

Counseling Parents

The parents of children with hearing loss have to adjust to a wide variety of emotional and psychological problems when first confronted with the problems presented by their child. Counseling is a formal or informal procedure or transaction in which both the audiologist and the parents work together to find a mutually acceptable plan of adjustment. Jerger (personal communication, 2010) described counseling as the process of telling people what you found, what it means, and what needs to be done, and doing so with tact and sensitivity. Informational counseling provides the parent with relevant facts to understand the child's disorder and how to manage it, and might include, over a reasonable time period and several appointments, an explanation of audiogram, the effects of childhood hearing loss, and the various choices for communication including various limitations and guidelines of each. It must be remembered that each set of parents represents a unique set of circumstances regarding their educational background, their socioeconomic factors, how much they know about normal hearing and speech milestones and child development, and their overall motivation and desire to know more about their child's hearing status, limitations, management, educational choices, and communication skills. It behooves the pediatric audiologist to have a prepared and carefully thought-out simple presentation of information with visual aids and printed materials in an easy-to-read format, summarizing each discussion and counseling session, for the parents to take home and review. In terms of personal counseling, issues such as dealing with the emotional impact of the child's hearing loss on the family, helping parents through and beyond the grieving process, and intervening with the impact of the child's problems on the family lifestyle, are often better left to professionals working in the mental health fields who are professional counselors.

In ongoing conversations with the family, the audiologist has a responsibility to thoroughly interpret and explain what the audiogram means, and what the child can and cannot hear; describe the type and degree of the child's hearing loss, whether conductive or sensorineural, and what it means in terms of whether medical treatment may or may not be possible; provide a thorough explanation of the intervention choices and educational programs that are available for the child; provide suggestions and options to encourage communication within the family to stimulate the child's speech and language development until the child is entered into a formal speech-language therapy program. The parents should be encouraged to visit various intervention and educational programs so that they may knowledgeably participate in the decision as to which program will be best for their child. The family may benefit from joining a support group to help the parents accept the situation of hearing impairment in their child and have opportunities to observe how other families have dealt with similar problems. This may take the form of a one-to-one relationship, or the parents may require group programs or even professional counseling. Pratt (1999) points out that hearing loss in children substantively increases stress levels in normal-hearing families, and that this situation can have deleterious effects on parent-child interactions. The increase in stress levels puts the children at risk for attachment problems and has implications for emotional, cognitive, and linguistic development—all of which may affect the stability of the family. Pratt describes the audiologist as working "beyond the audiology clinic doors" to provide an accepting and supportive environment for parents and families of children with hearing impairment. All students of audiology, as well as practicing clinicians, should read the classic books written by Luterman (1979), Luterman, Kurtzer-White, and Seewald (1999), and Bodner-Johnson and Sass-Lehrer (2003) for additional insight and understanding into working with parents and families.

It is an interesting exercise to examine the retention of information by patients of medical information. Pediatric audiologists should be cognizant of the fact that parents and families who are under the duress of learning that their heretofore "perfect child" has a significant hearing loss, are probably not in the best mental condition to retain much of the facts and discussion elements presented in early appointments. In fact, studies conducted by audiologists of their clinic patients have shown that only about 50% of the information communicated to them during an appointment is actually retained in memory. Furthermore, and clearly disheartening, is the fact that only about one half of the 50% retention is recalled correctly (Kessels, 2003; Margolis, 2004).

Researchers have also determined the importance of "primacy" and "recency" factors which means that the very first facts presented and the last facts (most recent) are the most likely to be retained as particularly memorable, while most of the middle conversational material is forgotten or lost to memory. In planning parent counseling sessions, audiologists would be advised to keep these retention markers in mind. Sometimes shorter, clearer conversations will have better and longer parental impact than longer, more detailed presentations. Of course, there are many tools used by public speakers and teachers for improving the recall of their listeners as follows: (a) keep the information simple, to the point, and specific to the topic; (b) use repetition of main ideas throughout the conversation; (c) limit the use of technical and professional jargon, acronyms, and abbreviations; (d) emphasize important points at the beginning and end; and (e) provide customized handout summaries of pertinent facts and information.

THE AUDIOLOGIST'S SELF-UNDERSTANDING

In the zeal to help the child with hearing loss and the child's parents, the audiologist often overlooks his or her own motivations and how they will affect relations with the parents. These relations may be critical to the parents' acceptance of the problem. Quite without meaning to, and without proper preparation and training, the audiologist may leave the parents with fears and pent-up emotions that can adversely affect the habilitation process. At some point the audiologist must look inward to see what his or her own feelings are in relation to the way information is given to the parents. The audiologist, who enters the profession with an emotional service-oriented zeal, may see himself or herself as the authoritarian figure who directs the lives of people; or the audiologist with an objective interest in the scientific manifestations of hearing may shy away from becoming emotionally involved and committed to the parents' problems. In either case, it behooves the audiologist to take a good look inward and examine his or her own motives and consider thoughtfully how his or her own personality fits into the

manner of dealing with pediatric patients and their parents and families.

It may be that the audiologist, too, may have problems in feeling comfortable in the role as protagonist in the drama of the parent-clinician interplay. To parents who are anxious to hear that their idealized child is perfect, the statement that, "Your child has a hearing loss" may be painful words. In order to avoid this uncomfortable experience, some audiologists may inadvertently choose a personally painless method of reporting the diagnosis. Although it is painless for the pediatric audiologist, the words may have devastating effects on the outcomes of the parents and their child with hearing loss. You may be sure this will be a moment in the parents' lives that will never be forgotten and remembered exactly as it happened, and they will discuss and relive it again and again. The importance of this announcement and this moment cannot be understated.

After listening to many parents relate their experiences and frustrations over the years, we realized that the act of reporting the diagnosis was not only of paramount importance, but also that it was the beginning of a process that would influence the habilitation and education of the child and the crucial involvement of the parents. A seemingly minute detail, but incredibly important, for effective reporting of the hearing loss diagnosis is an ample allotment of time. One of the most consistent complaints of parents in their dealings with audiologists initially is that the situation was regarded lightly by the audiologist as though it was not a significant matter and not enough time was devoted to this important conversation.

There are ways, of course, to help parents accept their child's hearing loss. If the child is about preschool age, there may already be a suspicion by the parents that the child does not hear normally. Nonetheless, the audiologist must relay the hearing loss diagnosis with compassion and with an appropriate degree of hope for the child and parents. The initial explanation from the audiologist in this early encounter may have a profound and prolonged effect on the parents' attitudes toward the child, motivations for helping the child, and long-range dealings with other professionals. The parents should be encouraged to ask questions and express their doubts, concerns, and emotions. Try to determine the most effective and preferred means of communicating with the parent, and make the explanations in language easy for them to follow and understand. Attempt to determine how much the parents are absorbing and understanding, and assess what they have internalized regarding the topics you have discussed with them. Be honest in admitting those things you do not know and be prepared to provide them with local resources and suggested actions they can take prior to the next appointment. Be prepared to help the parents though the stages of adjustment, and show your full empathy, understanding, and support without being condescending.

Schlesinger and Meadow (1972) described four ineffective and inappropriate professional stances that have no place in the reporting of the diagnosis to parents and family:

- *The "Hit-and-Run" Approach.* The diagnosis is reported quickly, coldly, and matter of factly in passing. "Your child didn't respond too much today . . . his or her hearing loss is probably severe-to-profound. I'll see your child in 6 months for another evaluation to firm up the presence of hearing loss." The parents are left with feelings of bewilderment as to what to do next.

The reporting of the diagnosis to them appears to be a dead end with no source of help or how to proceed.

- *Minimizing the Problem.* The audiologist lightly infers to the parents and family that there is really nothing to worry about. "In this day and age, deaf children use hearing aids (or cochlear implants) and go to regular school just like any other child." Actually, these words may give false hope to the parents, but the audiologist says them in order to make the parents feel better and to avoid going deeper into the discussion.

- *The Objectivity Approach.* This approach is used by audiologists who are somewhat entranced with their own knowledge and love to use all the "big words." In 1 hour, they report to the parents the child's diagnosis, explain the audiogram and how the hearing mechanism works, show how their child differs from normal, describe methods of habilitation, demonstrates the use and maintenance of a hearing aid, and schedules the child for the first habilitation session. The audiologist does most of the talking, often using technical and professional jargon and acronyms, leaving the parents confused and feeling lost. There is no time for the audiologist to listen in this approach.

- *The Action-Oriented Approach.* The audiologist states the problem, completes the reporting of the diagnosis, and immediately tells the parents what they need to do to take care of the problem. The action-oriented audiologist tends to take over the situation and pushes the parents for commitments to deal with the various issues presented by their child. Again the audiologist does little listening and most of the talking. It may be that some action is required, but only if there is adequate provision for exploring the feelings of the parents and including them in the decision-making process.

These less than stellar approaches, as described above, have given parents plenty to complain about regarding the profession of audiology and how the audiologist "broke the news" to them about their child's hearing loss. These inappropriate communications from the audiologist will greatly interfere with the process for the parents to openly accept the child's handicap. And, a lack of acceptance of the problem will prohibit the parents from helping their child grow both emotionally and educationally.

The parents may choose to deny the information and "shop around" to seek a professional who will tell them that their child is normal. Meadow (1968) pointed out that parents are more likely to listen to and integrate painful and unpleasant information from concerned, interested, and feeling professionals. Parents may experience a number of feelings at the outset, the most frequent being shock. The feeling of shock may then be followed by anger, guilt, and depression. It is very important not to tell parents what they may feel because people experience different emotions. It is important to provide an open-ended approach, however, such as, "Today I have told you about your child's hearing loss. Over the next few weeks and months, you may experience some uncomfortable feelings as many parents naturally do. We are available to you to discuss whatever feelings you may be having. Let's plan to talk again in a few days, a week, a month or any time should you desire. Please feel free to contact me with your questions."

The audiologist may lack knowledge of, experience with, and an understanding of the grieving and habilitative processes. The audiologist may be uncomfortable with the range of emotions that these parents may feel and need to express. Often audiologists state that they simply do not have the time to devote to reporting and holding proper communication sessions with the parents and family. This reasoning, however, may actually be a way of avoiding the fact that the audiologist has not yet worked out in his or her own mind what it means to deliver painful news. It is natural for individuals to want to avoid painful conversations. However, there is no painless way to inform parents that they have a child with a hearing loss. Pain does not necessarily have to be regarded negatively; it is part of a process that gains the parents' attention and facilitates and encourages the family's involvement. Even though there is no way of softening the blow, there are ways to help parents accept the realities of the situation:

- *Deliver a clear statement of the facts.* Obviously it is important to state the audiometric facts and their implications as clearly and as emphatically as possible. The initial discussion of the child's diagnosis should be given by the audiologist who administered hearing tests to the child. Preparation should be in place to ensure privacy and adequate time with no interruptions. Parents want up-to-date and accurate scientific information about their child's problem presented to them authoritatively, but in language they can understand. If an alliance is going to be created between the pediatric audiologist and the child's parents, it is important to admit to any lack of information or knowledge about the problem confidently and without strain. Throughout the giving of this information, the audiologist must convey a true interest in the child and in the family. The tone of voice and nonverbal behavior of an audiologist can convey callousness, or it can convey concern. It is essential to convey concern, empathy, and understanding rather than the idea that you are just doing your job.

- *Be supportive through attentive listening.* Perhaps the most important path to successful communication with parents and family is to provide support through listening. By listening patiently and nonjudgmentally, you may be able to bring some of the parents' feelings out into the open—possibly they will relate feelings in their statements of which they may not have been aware. Many parents are understandably anxious about their child's diagnosis, progress, and prognosis, but may not have shared that anxiety with anyone, not even their spouse. This may be the first opportunity they have had to express what they have been feeling for months, and thus it is so important that the audiologist take time to listen and provide support when necessary. Although it is not always possible, for many reasons, it is best if both parents are present for these discussions to discuss the diagnosis, progress, and prognosis of their child. Understandably, having both parents present may be physically impossible. During these discussions, the alert audiologist should begin to assess the parents' interactions. This assessment will help decide whether the parents have the kind of relationship that will provide support to one another or whether they will require some help from outside. It is important that the audiologist note and report the initial impression of the parents, as these notes may be valuable to others involved with the family.

- *Be truly empathetic to the parents.* Another important goal of communication is to convey to the parents that they have an important role to play and a great deal to offer, even though they may have little formal knowledge about hearing loss and child development. They may need some time to consider future directions and actions that may be necessary to accommodate the new needs of their child. Focusing on the parents' interaction with their child can give them some confidence. "You seem to sense Joey's needs very well." "That's perfect; you called Joey's attention to that sound." "That's one of the most important ideas you will learn and you already appear comfortable with it." The audiologist can provide initial reinforcement of attributes that the parents are already equipped with that will help their child's development.

Parents will likely want to be involved right away to feel as though they are doing something to help. Help them arrange for a follow-up appointment. It might be helpful at this point to provide parents with concrete activities to complete while waiting for the follow-up appointment. Providing a list of online resources and websites can be useful and effective to get the parents started.

Referral to a strong parental support group such as Hands and Voices (http://www.handsandvoices.org) can be an important and useful starting point for parents. Roush and Kamo (2008) cite Buckman (1982) for suggesting three more valuable tips in counseling parents:

1. *Don't promise anything you can't deliver.* Overassurance is misleading and may be condescending to the family. It is important to be realistic with your statements, but at the same time assure the family that much can and will be done for their child.

2. *Allow the parents to express their concerns and feelings.* Encouraging honest expressions of emotions gives parents permission to speak out and not contain their distraught feelings or concerns of doubt.

3. *Let the parents know that you will be available and your relationship with them will continue.* This will be reassuring to parents and they will remember and appreciate the idea that you will be helping them through the process with their child.

Parents clearly need and want lots of information, but they do not necessarily want to make decisions by themselves (Laugen, 2013). It is necessary to acknowledge that the family has the right to decide what information is important and what is not. It is not appropriate for the pediatric audiologist to "filter" information to the parents as this would clearly violate the non-bias obligation in parent counseling. Laugen points out that it is important for the professional to be fully aware of the responsibility to participate in the decision-making process; at the same time the audiologist has to be mindful as to not get in the way of the parents' thinking, their discussions with each other, and their final decisions. The pediatric audiologist should provide high-quality information but be attentive to incorporating the parents' knowledge, attitudes, and cultural feelings to help them reach common decisions. There is a reciprocal information exchange relationship that allows the parents and the audiologist to reach a solution that both can agree upon. It is to be remembered, and perhaps reminded to the parents, that decisions are not forever; decisions can be changed at any time to take advantage of new knowledge, different circumstances, or advanced technologies.

Some audiologists may be sensitive and concerned about their role in helping families, but this does not necessarily mean that they feel comfortable in dealing with feelings. Sensitivity can potentially be a valuable tool and an asset for the audiologist, but just because the potential is there does not mean that it will automatically be used in a facilitative way. To learn how to use one's sensitivity effectively is a delicate process and cannot be taught. It is the universal observation of those who have constructed programs for special groups of young disabled children that unless the parents' emotional needs are adequately dealt with, the programs themselves have limited benefit for the children. Thus, it is critically important that an atmosphere of mutual respect and honesty be created—an atmosphere that allows the expression of feelings in nonjudgmental and accepting ways. It may happen that the atmosphere of mutual respect is interrupted when the parents' depression explodes into external anger sometimes directed at the audiologist. The audiologist must understand that this expression of anger is only an indication of the parent's internal struggles.

Counseling parents requires tact and sensitivity to their feelings and behaviors. In her study of families in newborn hearing screening situations, Laugen (2013) stresses the importance of comprehensive information given at an early stage, although this also may be overwhelming to many families. From the point of screening and throughout audiological, medical, developmental, and educational follow-up, parents react to the quality of information provided by the pediatric audiologist, which in turn, affects their trust in professionals. Audiologists should treat every parent or caregiver of a child with hearing loss as if he or she is a member of your immediate family—with kindness, concern, and of course, with the highest standard of care. Other counseling keys to keep in mind are that listening is your greatest attribute; often "less is more" and "humility is a virtue" in terms of talking to parents; above all, remain within the bounds of your training. Other important considerations in counseling parents are to be meticulous, methodical, and complete in your advisements; use evidence-based information whenever possible; and track and document every visit. Be fully aware that your words and actions may often be the turning point in people's lives; what you say and how you say it may last forever in parents' memories.

A group of six providers of highly successful family-centered services were identified and studied from a pool of over 40 service providers by McWilliam, Tocci, and Harbin (1998) Common to the success of all of the providers of family-centered services were the following underlying components: (a) positiveness and a philosophy of thinking the best about the parents; (b) sensitivity and an ability to put oneself in the parents' shoes; (c) responsiveness in terms of paying attention to parents and taking action when parents expressed a need or a complaint; (d) friendliness through the development of rapport between family and service provider; and (e) child-level skills and competence in integrating their work with the broader community.

It is important to the parents during this early period of time to understand that they have opportunities to make choices for communication with their child and their child's educational program, and that their choices can be altered or changed at any time. Parents need to be made aware of the resources available to them—not only resources for habilitation and educational programming, but also resources available to help with emotional needs. Ideally, the audiologist will remain in contact with the family periodically, in order not only to give repeated evaluations, but also to act as a coordinator of professionals working with this family. It is vital that there be an interface between the person delivering emotional supportive services and those people primarily responsible for the intervention and habilitation programs. This interaction will provide an opportunity to share and be aware of mutual concerns and will prevent the traditional approach of professionals working in isolation of each other. The prognosis for the hearing-handicapped child to obtain maximum benefit from intervention has a direct relation to the level of support provided by the immediate family.

Family behavior can be observed over time and modified when necessary through careful and appropriate counseling. Evidence of strong family support can actually be noted with empiric observation by the audiologist and should not be made solely on subjective intuition. Keys to strong family support are demonstrated by the following indexes:

- Family accepts and understands the child's hearing loss.
- Family shows responsibility for scheduling and keeping all medical

and educational appointments on behalf of the child.

- Family is knowledgeable about the etiology of and the prognosis for the child's hearing loss.
- Family communicates well with the child by encouraging conversation under all circumstances.
- Family has appropriate expectations about the amplification devices used by the child.
- Family displays high interest and motivational levels in child-related activities.
- Family spends ample, constructive time with the child.
- Family has genuine concern for the child's educational and physical development.

INTERVENTION STRATEGIES FOR THE CHILD WITH OTITIS MEDIA

A substantial number of studies have been published that strongly suggest a correlation between middle ear disease with hearing impairment and concurrent delays in the development of speech, language, and cognitive skills. Wallace et al. (1988) conducted an important prospective study of neonates from birth until 1 year of age that demonstrated language deficits in those infants who had recurrent bouts of otitis media in the first year of life. These researchers concluded that infants who suffer repeated episodes of bilateral otitis media during the first year of life are more likely to have reduced hearing and to be at risk for expressive language difficulties. The astute pediatric audiologist will identify these children and refer them for a thorough speech and language screening or evaluation. During this short period of critical language learning, 3 months of poor hearing is an eternity in the development of language skills.

Medical treatment, of course, is the first line of defense in otitis media, although the treatment philosophy and regimen may vary considerably among physicians. Otitis media symptoms may be subtle and easily overlooked by busy parents, or the increased frequency of occurrence may not be noted. When a child has frequently recurring otitis media with middle ear effusion persisting for longer than 3 months, hearing thresholds and tympanometry should be assessed and the development of communicative skills should be monitored routinely. It is important that both the managing physician and the parents understand that a child with middle ear disease may not hear normally. The parents should be encouraged to continue communicating by touching and seeking eye contact with the child when loudly and clearly speaking. Such measures, along with prompt restoration of hearing whenever possible, may help to diminish the likelihood that a child with middle ear disease will develop a communicative disorder. Depending on the course of the otitis media disease, physicians may take a "careful observation" treatment plan, or choose to treat the child with longer pharmaceutical treatment, or more aggressive treatment might be surgical placement of ventilation tubes in the child's tympanic membranes.

Audiologic Management

According to the American Academy of Audiology (AAA), a thorough analysis of the voluminous research available demonstrates a causal relationship between communication disorders and early, recurrent, episodes of otitis media in infants and young children (1992, 1997, 2008). The disease process itself must be medically managed by physicians, but the identification, assessment, and management of any concomitant hearing loss falls within the scope of audiologic practice. It must be recognized that there are children who do not function to their full communicative and developmental potential because of hearing loss associated with early, recurrent episodes of otitis media with effusion. Accordingly, AAA has recommended specific audiologic guidelines as an effort to decrease substantially the number of children who will be burdened with persistent communicative and learning deficits related to undetected or untreated otitis media.

The hearing assessment should include complete audiologic evaluation to characterize the audiometric profile including the configuration and degree of hearing loss for each ear independently with air and bone-conduction testing, acoustic immittance tests including tympanometry and acoustic reflex measurement, along with speech audiometry tests when possible, including higher-order central auditory processing when indicated. The otitis media hearing deficit is inherently fluctuant; that is, it exists only during the duration of the otitis media episode. Between otitis media episodes, the child's hearing presumably returns to the "normal" range unless sensorineural hearing loss is also present. Therefore, hearing sensitivity may vary within the same episode of otitis media, as well as between episodes within the same child; the actual number of episodes the child experiences within a particular time period is an additional consideration. Finally, asymmetries in hearing sensitivity may exist between the child's two ears, thereby potentially disrupting critical binaural auditory processing skills.

Any child whose parent questions whether his or her child hears normally or not, should receive audiometric evaluation without delay. The audiologist may also wish to administer a formal screening test of the child's receptive and expressive language abilities. Children failing this screen should be referred to a certified/licensed speech-language pathologist for a formal comprehensive evaluation and for the determination of the need for therapeutic intervention. The management of infants and young children with otitis media must ensure parent/caregiver and teacher awareness of the implications of hearing loss on the communication process.

Audiologic management considerations might include: (a) providing information optimizing auditory-based communication strategies during bouts of otitis media when hearing sensitivity might be compromised; (b) monitoring auditory behaviors that might signal subsequent episodes of otitis media; and (c) providing suggestions for optimizing the classroom environment for all children who might experience "minimal fluctuant hearing loss" through the reduction of classroom noise and the provision of a sound field amplification system (Gravel & Wallace, 1998).

Language and Speech Screening

Delayed early language milestones are often the keystone for identifying possible developmental delay in children and may indicate slow cognitive development or the presence of hearing loss. Children who are experiencing otitis media with effusion may score poorer on tests of language than those children who are otitis free. Speech-language pathologists often note that children with a significant history of otitis media have phonologic or articulation deficiencies. A large number of well-normed language screening tests to identify both receptive and expressive delays are available for children of all ages such as the Illinois Test of Psycholinguistic Abilities (ITPA), the Peabody Picture Vocabulary Test, the Templin-Darley Tests of Articulation, the Mecham Verbal Language Development Scale, and the Early Language Milestone Scale (American Speech and Hearing Association, 1993; Coplan, Gleason, Ryan, Burke, & Williams, 1982; Walker, Downs, Gugenheim, & Northern, 1989). Because language delay can be a significant factor in the identification of young children with mild-to-moderate hearing loss or history of otitis media with effusion, the pediatric audiologist must develop competency in the observation of normal speech-language milestones as well as skill in administering language screening tests. Naturally, when a child is noted to be functioning at a level significantly less than normal for his or her age, referral should be made for a comprehensive language evaluation and a thorough hearing evaluation. Children who have significant communication deficiencies identified in screening tests should be referred for diagnostic language evaluation and possible remediation from a speech-language therapist.

Educational Intervention

Traditionally, the approach to delivering services to very young children has focused on identifying strengths and weaknesses, then remediating deficits and "teaching" the child the needed skills. In recent years, however, the focus in many early intervention programs offers a more positive approach for children, their families, and the professionals who work with them. This approach, often referred to as prevention-intervention, recognizes that not all problems or deficits can be "fixed" through many of the medical or educational therapies available, and that parents and professionals cannot change the long-term problems that occur at birth, such as brain damage or severe hearing loss. Parents and professionals can, however, minimize or prevent hearing loss in children by working through a child's strengths in home intervention programs to help the child develop alternative or compensatory learning strategies. In home intervention activities, professionals serve as consultants to families, helping them determine the goals and activities they want for their child. The changes in the approaches taken and attitudes adopted by professionals working with parents reflect the focus on family needs, with an emphasis on enhancing the child's growth, development, and sense of well-being, rather than a singular focus on correcting a problem. Parents need to be fully involved and valued as prime contributors in decisions made about their child's program and progress.

The American Academy of Audiology suggests the following interventions for children with recurrent otitis media: (a) the provision of information on optimizing auditory-based communication strategies during bouts of otitis media when hearing sensitivity might be compromised; (b) the monitoring of auditory behaviors that might signal subsequent episodes of otitis media; and (c) suggestions for optimizing the classroom environment for all children who might experience "minimal fluctuant hearing loss" through the reduction of classroom noise and the provision of soundfield amplification systems (AAA, 1997).

It has been suggested that some children might benefit from the use of a mild gain hearing aid, with appropriate limitations on maximum saturation and gain, during periods of otitis media caused hearing loss. The obvious drawbacks to hearing aid fittings are that it is difficult to convince parents of the necessity for such an extreme antidote, and there are problems in keeping such an instrument on an infant or toddler. Hearing aid placement is a feasible procedure only if: (a) the parents are highly motivated; (b) continual guidance by an audiologist or speech therapist is obtained; (c) a total support system by physician, parent, and therapist is in effect; and (d) a period of diagnostic therapy with a loaner hearing aid is initiated to judge the effectiveness of the aid.

Oyler et al. (1987) suggested several management recommendations for supporting the child with unilateral hearing loss. These recommendations are equally applicable for communicating with all children who have hearing loss:

- Gain the child's attention before beginning to speak.
- Use familiar vocabulary and less complex sentence structure.
- Rephrase statements that are misunderstood, rather than just repeating them verbatim.
- Provide visual supplement to the communication to improve understanding.
- Provide students preferential classroom seating to take advantage of the better hearing ear.
- Minimize noise interference generated from within or outside the classroom.
- Routinely monitor the child's speech and language development and academic progress.
- Consider use of a personal FM or a classroom amplification system to enhance the signal-to-noise ratio.
- Pay particular attention to the hearing of the good ear.
- Provide hearing conversation rules to protect the good ear.

- Stay away from loud noises.
- Get prompt medical care for any ear infection.
- Avoid putting anything into the ear.
- Avoid ototoxic drugs unless absolutely necessary.
- Take special care of general health, especially during flu seasons.
- Have an otologic and audiologic check once a year, or more often if needed.
- Do not get advice on treatments for hearing impairment from anyone except qualified otolaryngologists and audiologists.

TELEPRACTICE AND TELEAUDIOLOGY

Telepractice services can deliver hearing health care to children with hearing loss and their families with effectiveness and efficiency. With today's advances in communications systems, there has been growing interest and experimentation with providing hearing services through remote and distance telepractice. The definition of telepractice is the use of electronic information and telecommunication technologies to support remote and distance clinical health services and professional and public education among many other uses (Northern, 2012). For the purposes of pediatric audiology, telepractice is already in use for infant hearing screening, hearing evaluations, hearing aid fittings and management, early intervention, counseling, and just about any other clinical activities that might be of benefit to the hard-of-hearing or deaf child and the child's parents and families.

At the basic level, telepractice, or perhaps in this case the term *teleaudiology* might be a better descriptor, involves Internet chats, videoconferencing, or telephone conferencing that might be person-to-person or involve several other interested persons or the health team members, online education purposes, and even the use of social media or face-to-face electronic conversations. Telepractice is any electronic communications means by which we can bring professional services to those who are in need and are located in remote or distant areas. Advanced communications technologies allow constant connectivity from a range of devices and the ability to see and hear others in real time, whether they are just down the street or thousands of miles away (Houston, Stredler-Brown, & Alverson, 2012). The proliferation of computer technologies and "smart chips," along with broadband Internet connections, laptop and tabletop computers, smartphones, teleconferencing websites, teleconference and face-to-face telephone conversations, and the widespread use of videoconferencing, opens up entire new worlds of applications useful to children with hearing loss and their families, professionals who provide hearing, speech, and language services, and universally accessible educational and resource materials. Although we are now on the creative and innovative edge of applying telepractice services to deliver hearing health care, clearly the future is bright for these new technologies to change the lives of our patients and their families.

It is widely acknowledged that there are not enough trained professionals to provide needed hearing services to meet the needs of the hard-of-hearing and deaf communities. The result of this problem is that many children with hearing loss and their families are either underserved or not served at all (Behl, Houston, & Stredler-Brown, 2012). So telepractice is a growing entity and is recognized as a viable service delivery model for families of children with hearing

loss who might be located far from a clinical service center. Telepractice is a welcome alternative as it allows for direct interaction with an audiologist while saving the family travel costs and time, down time from work, and the need for babysitters for the other children in the family while the child with hearing loss is traveling to a far-away clinic.

Nearly every aspect of audiology can be delivered through telepractice. Swanepoel (2012) of South Africa was one of the first to utilize teleaudiology to conduct hearing evaluations and hearing aid fitting over vast distances between remote villages in his country. Reports of telepractice with audiologic services have also been reported from other countries, such as Brazil (Ferrari, 2012) and Australia (McCarthy, Duncan, & Leigh, 2012), where long distances between cities and limited numbers of professionals have made remote hearing services invaluable. Successful outcomes for children identified early with hearing loss have been treated through "virtual home visits" which are telepractice services delivered by professionals trained in parent-infant intervention (Olsen et al., 2012); Galster & Abrams (2012) describe hearing aids designed to be remotely programmed, adjusted, or fined-tuned by their dispenser through personal mobile phones; the use of remote technology to provide cochlear implant services is describe in detail by Goehring, Hughes, and Baudhuin (2012). They point out that cochlear implants can now be routinely tele-tested for speech-processer programming levels as well as electrode impedance measures and electrically evoked compound action potentials with equivalent results as obtained in traditional face-to-face conditions. Hayes (2012) and Hayes, Eclavea, Dreith, and Habte (2012) describe an innovative telepractice program where infants born in Guam who fail the infant hearing screening tests receive follow-up diagnostic audiologic evaluation through ABR by audiologists in Colorado. The follow-up audiologic testing is completed in real-time using commercially available software and personal computers to control the diagnostic equipment remotely, while simultaneously videoconferencing with support personnel in Guam and the baby's family. And, finally, Gans (2012) has developed tele-educational online teaching programs to help prepare students and assistants to work in the fields of audiology and vestibular clinical services.

As videoconferencing technology has become more widely available, the associated equipment costs have declined, and these services have become more cost efficient. According to Houston & Stredler-Brown (2012), advances in telecommunication and distance technologies offer to eliminate many of the barriers to services that continue to affect young children with hearing loss and their families. By leveraging the use of technology with innovative communication-service models, young children with hearing loss and their families will have greater access to well-trained practitioners. Telepractice is, no doubt, here to stay; and future audiologists must be aware and trained accordingly as it seems extremely likely that in the future, remote and distant hearing services programs will be developed, expanded, and implemented more fully.

HEARING DOGS

Parents might wish to give consideration to procuring a trained "hearing dog" as a pet for their child with hearing loss. It is well agreed among child specialists that there are many good reasons for a child to be responsible for a personal pet dog. The relationship between a child and his or her dog can be beneficial to the child's emotional and mental well-being. It makes quite good sense that a child with hearing loss would benefit from having a specially trained dog for friendship, and the dog will provide an increased awareness of the child's environment. Typically, the hearing dog is trained to alert to household sounds that are necessary for everyday safety and independence. They are trained to make physical contact with the child and lead the child to the source of the sound. By providing sound awareness and companionship, the hearing dog provides greatly increased freedom and independence for children.

Hearing dogs come in all breeds and sizes and they are skillfully and carefully selected from animal shelters for their intelligence, friendliness, alertness, trainability, and willingness to work and be with people. Training generally takes 4 to 6 months to undergo temperament evaluation, and then on to obedience training, socialization, and sound training. The dogs are taught to work for toys and affection. The hearing dog is typically taught to respond to home sounds such as fire and smoke alarms, telephone, oven timer, alarm clock, doorbell, door knock, name call, and baby cry. Hearing dogs are trained not to bark; rather they are trained to use their nose or paw to nudge, and then lead to the source of the sound. Once placed with their deaf partner, the dogs easily learn to respond to additional sounds such as commands and family names.

By law, the Americans with Disabilities Act ensures that hearing dogs must be allowed to accompany their owners into businesses and other places that serve the public, and must be permitted to stay with their owners in public transportation (i.e., trains and airplanes). Hearing dogs are identified by a bright orange or yellow leash or harness. There is usually a co-pay cost for the dogs, and sometimes, because of the high demand for hearing dogs, a lengthy wait may be required before a dog can be trained and delivered to the deaf or hard-of-hearing child (Olsen, 2008).

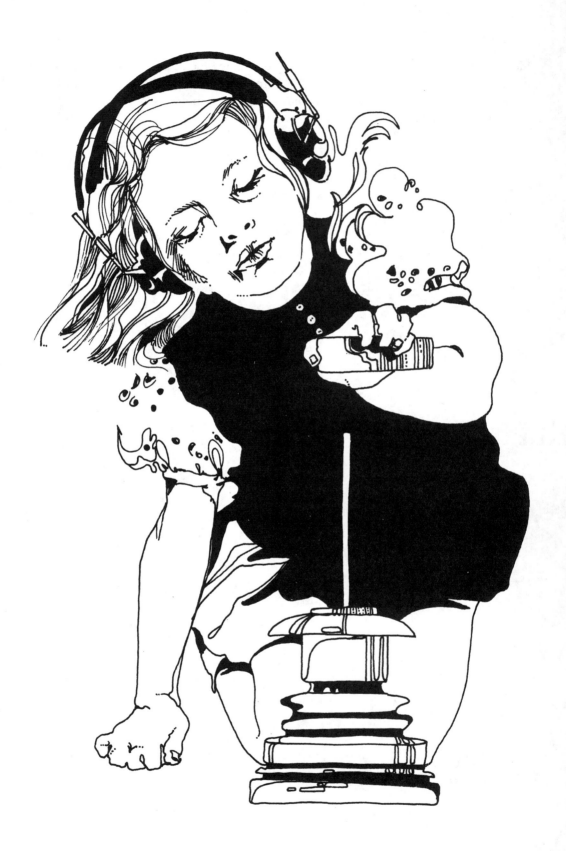

CHAPTER 6

Behavioral Hearing Tests With Children

The essence of pediatric audiology is behavioral hearing testing. The most fun you can have in a sound booth is working with a happy, cooperative young child who is both intrigued and challenged with the "hearing test." Fortunately children are all different and the pediatric audiologist never quite knows for sure what to expect from any particular child on the first visit or a follow-up visit. The delight in the eyes of the child as he or she enthusiastically responds to hearing that "little soft sound in their ear" is quite rewarding (Figure 6–1). Some routine pediatric visitors to the ear clinic become familiar enough with the test situation and the listening tasks to know in advance what is expected of them, and to jump happily into the chair and help set up the test paraphernalia. Of course, there will be times when you will find a timid or apprehensive child who needs joyful enticements just to enter the sound booth.

Regardless of the application of advanced technologic procedures to evaluate hearing in children, most audiologists who work with pediatric patients realize that the "gold standard" of hearing test results is achieved through behavioral measurements. However, it must be made clear that the behavioral test approach with children

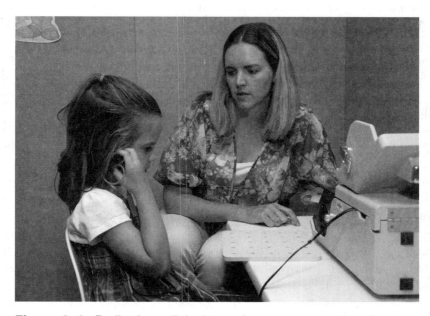

Figure 6–1. Pediatric audiologist performs pure tone hearing test. Photo courtesy of Colorado Children's Hospital, Aurora, CO.

is not always easy. It is often a very challenging task to determine the hearing levels of infants and children who can be difficult to test for a wide variety of reasons. Nonetheless, professional satisfaction is its own reward when testing a young child who smiles and cooperates throughout the testing procedure as well as when obtaining accurate test results from a child who might be less than fully cooperative. Every child presents a new, interesting, and different personality to work with, and the audiologist has opportunities to use skills and knowledge while being flexible with each child to meet the challenge.

Testing the hearing in infants and young children was not given much credence prior to a report from Sir Alexander and Lady Ewing of England in 1944. Although their goal in those early years was to teach speech to children with deafness, it was imperative that they evaluate the hearing of their young students so they could apply appropriate therapies. The Ewings used various percussion sounds and pitch pipes to elicit "aural reflex responses" in young children. They reported that auditory responses could be easily observed in infants during the first 6 months of life, but these reflexive responses to sounds were actually more difficult to observe as the infants grew older, as though the children were actually inhibiting their reactions to the noisemakers. The Ewings also reported that children with profound deafness did not show any responses to sound regardless of intensity.

Modern technology has greatly increased the number of options available to test the hearing of infants and young children. However, regardless of how sophisticated testing techniques become, there will always be a need for the behavioral hearing evaluation. Many of the newer testing procedures require expensive equipment or lengthy time commitments. Audiologists must use

caution regarding the sense of confidence provided by hearing test results obtained with physiologic "objective" techniques (discussed in Chapter 7). Every clinician must be well versed in the understanding and application of basic behavioral pediatric audiometry. With experience in pediatric audiology, a battery of special testing procedures becomes available for use in the clinical setting, and on-the-spot decisions need to be made for cost- and time-effective protocols to be used with each infant and child. Although electrophysiologic tests can be used to estimate auditory sensitivity, they are not "true" tests of hearing; thus, they should be considered as part of the pediatric test battery but not as a substitute for behavioral audiometry in children.

Auditory evaluation of hearing in children should not be considered complete until specific thresholds are obtained for octave interval frequencies from 250 to 4000 Hz in each ear. Determining the hearing sensitivity in each ear at each frequency is valuable for establishing reference for medical and surgical interventions and treatments, selecting and fitting of amplification, and identifying progressive hearing loss. A variety of testing procedures might be needed to obtain this final result, and more than one test session may be necessary to achieve the complete hearing examination. Parents need to be advised that the pediatric hearing examination, especially when hearing loss is suspected, is an ongoing, age-specific activity, so that as the child grows older, more accurate hearing results can be obtained during subsequent evaluations.

Jerger and Hayes (1976) defined the now well-accepted protocol of using a cross-check methodology in pediatric audiometry. They caution that simple behavioral observation of auditory behavior in children based on one test can be misleading and result in misdiagnosis of auditory problems and, ultimately, delay or cause mismanagement of the child with hearing loss. The cross-check principle uses the entire test battery of physiologic tests, such as auditory brainstem response (ABR) audiometry, acoustic immittance, and otoacoustic emissions procedures as cross-checks of behavioral test results. They reason that behavioral test results need to be confirmed by independent test measures to reduce the potential errors of using behavioral results alone. In most cases, acoustic immittance audiometry and otoacoustic emissions will serve as cross-checks for behavioral audiometry (Baldwin, Gajewski, & Widen, 2011). Diefendorf (2003) advised against the use of any single test alone in evaluating the hearing of pediatric patients. In addition to test results, consideration of the case history and parents' reports and observations of the child's behaviors should be considered integral to the cross-check methodology.

The standard of pediatric testing recommends the use of insert earphones that are placed into the ear canal of the child to perform air conduction testing. The use of traditional earphones with some children creates collapse, or a folding closed, of the ear canal from which then can be produced a pseudo-conductive-type hearing loss. In such instances, the audiometric testing will show an erroneous air-bone gap and false conductive hearing loss. The potential for the pseudoconductive hearing loss is eliminated with the use of insert earphones as shown in Figure 6–2.

The experience of the audiologist is the main key to successful evaluation of the pediatric patient. A broad test battery approach with children is the recommended clinic protocol and both the ASHA and AAA have developed guidelines for assessing hearing in children describing multitest approaches. Audiologists who work with

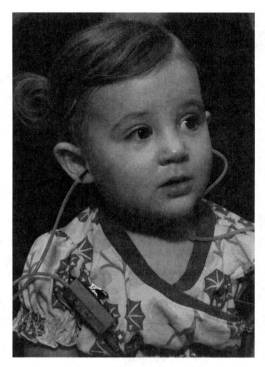

Figure 6–2. Use of insert earphones is recommended whenever possible. Photo courtesy of Colorado Children's Hospital, Aurora, CO.

pediatric patients must have the skills and flexibility to incorporate any and all of the testing procedures at a moment's notice as well as the knowledge and experience to know when to change approaches during the testing period. Behavioral testing of children and infants is the cornerstone and foundation of pediatric audiology.

THE AUDIOLOGIST AND THE CHILD

Too often audiologists say, "I don't like to work with young children—I can't depend on their responses, and they are too inconsistent to be relied upon." Nothing could be less true. Babies and young children usually do just what they are supposed to do; the clinician often does not. The audiologist has to give the right stimulus in the right structured situation to get the right response. There are no poorly responding babies—only inadequately prepared clinicians.

What are the general rules about working with children of all ages? The audiologist should begin by quickly establishing an easy relationship with the parents by speaking pleasantly and in a relaxed manner with them, particularly in front of the child. During this "hallway conversation" (as named by Renshaw & Diefendorf, 1998), the child will look back and forth between the audiologist and the parent(s). As the child watches the interaction develop, he or she will finally recognize that all is well and will likely relax. In other words, the child absorbs the cathexis between the audiologist and the parents and becomes at ease. Many clinicians work with a child alone without the parents present in the testing sound suite. This is fine if there is enough time to establish a relationship with the child. It may be quicker and easier to include the parents in the testing situation so that the child is less apprehensive and stays relaxed during the session. Parents are usually (although not always) quite cooperative, genuinely concerned, and entirely rational. The most important piece of advice for every pediatric audiologist is to tell the child what to do in each listening task—not to ask. In this respect, the very young and the very old are alike, and one handles them both not by asking whether they would like to do something (they never do) but by telling them firmly and pleasantly that this is what they are going to do. Children do just what is expected of them, and if the audiologist firmly expects them to do what he or she wants them to, they usually oblige. Occasionally, of course, a child balks and yells like a banshee anyway—you can't win them all, but give it a try! The sound room is not a place for negotiations with a child to obtain cooperation. Do not give up too quickly or easily. There is nothing a child enjoys more than controlling any uncomfortable situation by whining and crying. We have seen many unruly and uncooperative children unexpectedly quiet down, show interest in the test environment, and suddenly become happy, cooperative patients enabling a quick and easy completion of the hearing test. Children are a great deal easier to handle than most people think.

The pediatric audiologist should develop a staunch and fervid confidence that when children hear a sound, they will react in a stereotyped way that is consistent with their level of mental functioning. This holds true for the child with hearing loss and for the normal-hearing child. The child with a threshold of 80 dB HL for a given sound will respond at 85 dB HL like the normal-hearing child who hears the same sound at 5 dB above their normal-hearing threshold. A 2-year-old child with cognitive difficulties, operating at a mental age of 1 year, will respond near his or her threshold in the way a normal-hearing child of 1 year responds near his or her threshold. There is no mystique about observing the child's responses; the answer, if there is any, is to become confidently familiar with the auditory behavior of normal-hearing children so that the lack or absence of normal responses will be immediately evident and suggest the need for additional testing.

At the risk of becoming maudlin, another principle should be added—love every child as a human being. The clinician is often hard-put to develop any charitable feelings toward the wall-climber, the temper tantrum expert, and the withdrawn child, or in some cases the syndrome-ridden child with misshapen, contorted face and limbs. The same humanity underlies all these children, the kicker, the screamer, the silent one—all of them humanly acting out their protests at a world that has given them less than it has to others. They too can be loved.

Knowing What to Expect From Children

The auditory responses of infants less than 6 months of age can also be described in terms of reflexive or attentive behaviors. Reflexive behaviors include the startle (body) response, arm or leg jerks, slow limb movements, the auropalpebral reflex, intensity or latency change in sucking behavior, eye blinks, and facial twitches. Attentive behaviors are described as quieting responses (decrease in ongoing activity), increase in ongoing activity, breath-holding or a change in breathing rate, onset of vocalization, sudden stopping of vocalization, starting or stopping crying, eye widening, searching or localization, head turning as in searching or localizing the sound source, smiling or other change in facial expression, brow furrowing, or shriek of surprise. A commonly seen attentive behavior in response to the presentation of a speech sound is when the child looks directly at the parent's face as though in expectation of finding the source of the sound.

As normal-hearing infants grow older, they respond to auditory stimuli at lower (softer) levels. Audiologists must gain experience testing infants and young children with normal hearing to recognize the expected responses with various noise-makers and sound field auditory stimuli. This experience will be different for each clinician depending on individual style of eliciting auditory responses with acoustic stimuli and performing the test on literally hundreds of infants and young children

with normal hearing. Only then can the audiologist feel confident with this simple but effective means of separating children with normal hearing from those with possible hearing problems.

At about 6 months of age, the infant begins to turn the head and eyes toward the sound source. During this period of growth, muscle strength and eye-motor coordination show substantial improvement. By 6 months of age, the baby might laugh out loud, hold a rattle tightly, reach for objects and grasp them, turn over without help, and sit with only minimal support. By 7 months of age, the baby should be able to transfer an object from hand to hand and sit up without support momentarily.

When the infant reaches the 7- to 9-month period, there will be improvement in strength and motor coordination that allows the infant to sit steadily and to change position without falling. The child can now manipulate two objects simultaneously and transfers objects from hand to hand to mouth. This is the explore-everything-in-the-mouth stage, and the well-advised clinician gives the infant only clean items to hold or play with. This stage is not uncommonly seen in older children with developmental delay who function at this mental age. The child of 7 to 9 months is able to play peek-a-boo and perhaps a pat-a-cake game with you. However, at this age, a child begins to be initially shy with strangers and may take a few moments to warm up to the audiologist. The baby probably can respond to the "bye-bye" game with a wave of the hand and arm but may need some encouragement to perform this act for a new or strange person. "Dada" and "mama" may be heard in vocalizations but without specific referents. Imitation of gross sounds should be in place by the age of 9 months.

The older infant and toddler, 9 to 12 months of age, tends to be somewhat afraid or suspicious of strangers if they come too close or offer to hold the child. "Strangeness" is one of the psychic organizers described by Spitz (1959). In fact, the child who comes easily to the arms of a complete stranger at this age may suffer a lack of psychic development. The parent should handle the child exclusively for the auditory evaluation period. The audiologist may need to do his or her work from outside the sound-treated booth in a darkened room, because as long as the child can see this "stranger," suspicion reigns. Without this visual presence, the child will relax and feel secure in the lap of the parent. Normal babies do not object to the quiet of the sound-treated booth, and only occasionally have we seen a youngster object violently to going into the sound-treated booth.

By 12 months of age, the baby should be standing firmly and perhaps walking by holding on to furniture or the parents. The child may begin making single-word utterances, perhaps with an appropriate referent. The baby knows his or her own name easily by now, and a speech awareness response level can be determined by using the name in an ascending intensity approach until the child localizes briskly to the correct loudspeaker. Typically, the child in this age range is extremely interested in the environment and will localize rather briskly and quickly to auditory signals occurring out of silence from soundfield speakers. The average minimal response level at this age is 10 dB HL.

The child of 6 to 12 months or older can be tested with visual reinforcement audiometry (VRA). Accordingly, it is possible to obtain frequency-specific minimal response levels for each ear in the soundfield situation or the child may accept insert-type earphones. Remember that our goal in the hearing evaluation is to obtain as much audiometric frequency-specific information as possible in each ear, verified by speech awareness minimal response levels in each ear, before the child grows tired and becomes irritable about the testing situation. Ample time should be anticipated at the end of each audiometric test session to cross-check the VRA behavioral hearing test results with immittance audiometry to include tympanometry and acoustic reflex measures, and otoacoustic emission measurements.

By 18 months of age, the toddler should know a few simple objects well enough to identify them by command. This skill and ability can be used in the speech stimulus to establish speech reception threshold (SRT) in each ear by asking the child, at lower and lower intensity levels, to identify by looking at a few simple toys, such as, "Where is the kitty cat?" or "Where is the baby doll?" or at the appropriate parent, such as, "Where is mama (or daddy)?" By 24 months of age, it may be possible to have the child pick up certain simple toy objects and hand them to the parent at the audiologist's instruction through the loudspeakers. Some children at this age are clever enough to identify simple body parts on suggestion, such as, "Where is your nose?" or "Show me your teeth," or "Show mama (or daddy) your shoes." A final behavioral response may be obtained by asking, "Do you want to go bye-bye?" To establish minimal speech response levels it is necessary to present the carrier phrase in the soundfield ("Give mama [or daddy] the . . . ") at 20 dB speech level and then quickly to shift down to the level you want to test for the key word. The minimal response level for speech audiometry in a toddler of this age is 5 dB HL for normal hearing.

The pediatric audiologist need be forewarned and cautious in approaching the 2-year-old child as it is difficult to know what to expect with these youngsters. This is the age when "no" is the answer to every question and direction. Around the age of 24 months, the child may try to avoid direct eye contact and actually hide away in the parent's arms or behind mother's skirt rather than acknowledge the audiologist. The 2-year-old may actually inhibit response behaviors, especially without reinforcement of some type. It is a good time to utilize the "hallway conversation" technique to question the parents at this time about the vocalization skills of the child so they can be related to normal speech development milestones. It may also be important to ask the parents about possible previous history of ear infections with medical or surgical treatment. It is not surprising for a child in this 2-year-old age category to suddenly stop responding because he or she has lost interest in the activity.

A quick and simple developmental questionnaire for use with parents of pediatric patients is presented in Table 6–1. Care should be taken in interpreting some of the landmarks as indicative of normal hearing (see Chapter 3). A baby with severe-to-profound deafness coos and chuckles quite normally at 2 to 3 months of age, laughs aloud at 4 months, babbles in two sounds before 6 months, and may say something like "ma-ma" at 9 months of age and "da-da" by 12 months of age. When reported by parents, this sequence of events can be misleading. We interviewed a set of parents who insisted that their child had normal hearing at 1 year of age because all of his vocalizations were on time at the correct age milestones. Yet, radiographic studies of the child's temporal bones showed congenital gross bony abnormalities of both inner ears that precluded the possibility of any hearing at birth. It is well to view such parental reports of early speaking abilities in their child with healthy skepticism.

One challenge of pediatric audiology is to learn when the child has had enough and the limits of attention have been exceeded.

The audiologist must be prepared to change the game or activity to re-interest the child and prolong the test session so that additional information about the hearing response levels can be obtained. The use of a darkened instrument room is still indicated for children up to 24 months of age. The purity of the child's responsiveness is an unquestioning reaction to the voice signal. At this stage, the child may be initially confused by the presence of a voice originating in loudspeakers without visualizing a person doing the speaking. However, it is likely that the unquestioning obedience of a child of this age will serve the practitioner of pediatric speech audiometry well. The need to apply the cross-check of immittance audiometry with tympanometry and acoustic reflex measurements, otoacoustic emissions, and ABR to confirm behavioral testing cannot be emphasized enough.

Once the child has reached the age of 3 years, the child generally wants to be cooperative and will perform as a happy helper. The child may only briefly and initially be interested in the VRA system until he or she quickly loses interest in the game. However, by this age the child should easily take to game tasks associated with the presentation of auditory signals through insert earphones permitting the audiologist to incorporate play conditioning paradigms. A full audiogram, complete with thresholds four to five test frequencies for each ear, should be easily attainable from the 3-year-old in one clinical session. By the age 4 to 5 years, the child should be able to perform by finger-raising when threshold sounds are heard. The pediatric audiologist should be aware, however, that the child in an effort to please the tester and "get the task done correctly" may not respond to threshold sounds that are barely perceivable, but rather will wait until the stimulus pure tone is presented at a level of 5 to 10 dB above actual thresholds.

Table 6–1. Pediatric Audiology Developmental Screening Questionnaire for Parents

---

I. Chief complaint _____

   When was the problem first noted? _____

   Extent of problem _____

   Previous examinations and evaluations _____

II. Prenatal history _____

   Exposure to viral diseases during pregnancy? _____

   Which viral disorder? _____

   During which pregnancy month? _____

   Drugs during pregnancy? _____

   Trauma during pregnancy? _____

III. Birth history _____

   Gestation age at birth _____

   Birth weight _____ Bilirubin level high? _____

   Asphyxia? _____ Meningitis? _____

IV. Family history _____

   Childhood deafness in family? _____

     Relationship to patient _____

   Birth defect or abnormalities _____

     In any other relatives? _____

V. Developmental history _____

   Age of first smile response? _____

   Age when sat up alone? _____

   Age when first crawled? _____

   Age of "stranger anxiety?" _____

   Age of walking? _____

VI. Physical history

   Cleft lip or palate_____ Submucous cleft _____

   Low-set ears_____ Poorly formed ears _____

   High fevers with illness_____ Seizures _____

   Ear infections_____ How many? _____

   Previous treatment for ear conditions? _____

VII. What do you (parents) really think caused this hearing problem? _____

   Name of child's pediatrician _____

   Names of other physicians who have seen this child _____

Speech audiometry may confirm the accuracy of the child's auditory threshold levels. Tympanometry and acoustic reflex measures, along with otoacoustic emissions evaluation, should be an integral part of every pediatric hearing evaluation.

THE CASE HISTORY

In addition to the actual hearing test, audiologists can contribute insight into the auditory and oral behavior of children. No one understands better than the experienced clinician the effect of a certain degree of loss on the child's behavior and how the history of auditory development relates to the onset and degree of hearing loss. The audiologist's time will most valuably be spent in observing and analyzing these aspects of the child's history and the child's behaviors. Very often, simple questions presented to the parent or caretaker will help the audiologist anticipate and understand problems presented by the pediatric patient. Of course, the accurate diagnosis of a child's hearing loss needs to include thorough consideration of the early developmental and medical history of the child.

The case history can be particularly important as it may guide the selection of a particular testing protocol or sequence of audiological procedures to be conducted during the behavioral test period. The case history should be recorded in the patient record and follow a standard format to ensure that the information collected is orderly and complete. The audiologist asks the questions and leads the discussion but may need to guide the parents or caregivers with their responses to avoid them going off course and supplying extraneous and insignificant information. That is not to say there may be information revealed in the responses that has to do with the child's hearing issues, but in terms of time it is generally better to stay within the standard case history questions.

The dialogue involved in obtaining the case history can be helpful in setting the stage for working with the parents and caregivers. Introduce yourself in a friendly manner if this is the first time you have seen this patient. For example, say, "Hi! I'm Kathy Smith (or " . . . I am Dr. Kathy Smith") and it is nice to see you today. I am the audiologist who will be evaluating the hearing of your child. I would like to ask you a few background questions that will help me understand what brings you here today and what problems your child might be having." The presentation of case history questions by the audiologist should be gentle, calm, and asked with confidence in a nonchallenging manner. It may be that the child is present and observing this initial interaction between the pediatric audiologist and the responsible parties.

The opening questions should be brief and easy to answer, and the responses will likely let the pediatric audiologist know what to anticipate in the testing session. Therefore, the sequence of the audiologic case history interview might be as follows: Question the parents or caregivers as to the chief concern that precipitated the visit: "What brings you and your child into the audiology clinic today?" "Do you believe your child has hearing problems?" "Who referred you to the audiology clinic and why?" From this beginning, additional questions should pursue family history for hearing loss, the child's developmental history with focus on speech and language milestones, any general health issues of the child, and previous medical treatments or surgeries. Table 6–2 contains a sample case history form of questions that comprise a basic history that includes the primary items that place a child at risk for hearing loss.

Table 6–2. Sensorineural Hearing-Impaired Child Assessment

Name _____

Age _____

Date of birth _____

Hospital # _____

Age child identified by M.D. (months) _____

Age suspected of loss by mother (months) _____

Family History

Were parents relatives before marriage	Yes	No
Family history of kidney disease	Yes	No
Family history of thyroid problems	Yes	No
Family history of progressive blindness	Yes	No
Family history of previous stillbirths or miscarriages	Yes	No
Family history of hearing loss	Yes	No
Another affected child in family	Yes	No
Mother worked outside home	Yes	No
Specify _____		
Father worked during pregnancy	Yes	No
Specify _____		

Maternal Factors

Drugs (incl. antibiotics)	Yes	No
Specify _____		
Exposure to chemicals	Yes	No
Specify _____		
Exposure to radiation	Yes	No
Specify _____		
Amniocentesis	Yes	No
Rh immunoglobulin given Rh or ABO incompatible	Yes	No
Maternal illness during pregnancy	Yes	No
Specify _____		
Bleeding	Yes	No
Anemia	Yes	No
Diabetes	Yes	No
Toxemia	Yes	No
Paternal illness during pregnancy	Yes	No
Specify _____		

During pregnancy, mother exposed to:

Measles	Yes	No
Mumps	Yes	No
Chickenpox	Yes	No
German measles	Yes	No

During pregnancy, mother diagnosed with:

Syphilis	Yes	No
Herpes virus	Yes	No
Influenza	Yes	No
Cytomegalovirus (CMV)	Yes	No
Toxoplasmosis	Yes	No
Other	Yes	No
Specify _____		

Delivery/Labor

Full-term pregnancy	Yes	No
Labor induced	Yes	No
Labor less than 3 hr	Yes	No
Labor longer than 24 hr	Yes	No
Premature membrane rupture	Yes	No
Bleeding	Yes	No
Forceps/assisted delivery	Yes	No
Cesarean section	Yes	No
Other	Yes	No
Specify _____		

Infant/Newborn Factors

Small birth weight (<2 kg/5 lb)	Yes	No
Birth weight (lb/oz _____)		
Apgar low at birth	Yes	No
In an intensive care unit	Yes	No
How long (wk) _____		
Breathing problems	Yes	No
O_2 given	Yes	No
How long (wk)_____		
Bilirubin >15 mg/100 mL	Yes	No

Table 6–2. *continued*

Congenital rubella	Yes	No	Dizziness problems	Yes	No
Defect of ear, nose, throat	Yes	No	Cerebral palsy	Yes	No
Specify _____			Seizures	Yes	No
Congenital heart disease	Yes	No	Head trauma/skull	Yes	No
Drugs (incl. antibiotics)	Yes	No	Ever hospitalized for:		
Specify _____			Meningitis	Yes	No
Exposure to chemicals	Yes	No	Encephalitis	Yes	No
Specify _____			Influenza	Yes	No
Exposure to radiation	Yes	No	Rubella	Yes	No
Specify _____			CMV	Yes	No
Paralysis	Yes	No	Chickenpox	Yes	No
Seizures	Yes	No	Septicemia	Yes	No
Septicemia	Yes	No	Diabetes	Yes	No
			Sickle cell disease	Yes	No
Infant/Childhood History			Other (including conductive loss)	Yes	No
Eye problems	Yes	No			
Specify _____			Specify _____		
Balance/gait/incoordination	Yes	No			

A very informative first question that can be asked of the parents of any child presented for hearing evaluation is, "Do you have any concerns about your child's hearing, speech, or language?"

Obviously, an infant with a family history of permanent childhood sensorineural hearing loss in blood relatives is at risk for inheriting that same trait. Not so simple, however, is the task of eliciting family history from the baby's parents. Unfortunately, family history information is typically sparse for generations earlier than the infant's grandparents. Often, only one parent is available for interview, so little information is available from the other side of the family. Information about relatives with disabilities is often glossed over by relatives, so that considerable uncertainty exists about the true nature, degree, onset, or diagnosis of the condition. A parent once told us that no deafness existed in his family, although a cousin did attend the state deaf school. The parent was quick to add that the cousin was not "deaf," he "wore a hearing aid and could hear normally." In another case history interview, the parent implicated his uncle, who "was not hearing-impaired—but totally deaf since birth."

Therefore, questions must be phrased carefully to avoid misunderstandings or erroneous responses. The authors ask, "Do you know any of the baby's relatives who now have a hearing loss, which started before the age of 4 or 5 years? Please think hard about all of your family and the baby's father's (or mother's) family." If the answer is "Yes," the parent is asked who the relative was (is) in relationship to the baby. The parent is then asked, "Do you know what caused the hearing loss? Did he or she still wear a hearing aid before age of 4 or 5? Does the relative still wear a hearing aid? Did he or she attend a special school for the deaf or public school?" It is important to remember the potential progressive nature or possible late onset of hereditary hearing loss. Careful follow-up and parental counseling may be advised for those youngsters who have risk indicators but who pass the initial hearing screening test.

If the infant or child has previously confirmed hearing loss, and currently is wearing hearing aids or using a cochlear implant, it would be important to query the parent as to where and when the amplification assistive hearing devices were obtained, how long they have been in use, and what benefits the child derives from their use. Does the child wear them full time or just on occasion? At this point, you might wish to inquire if any speech or language test records or audiograms obtained previously could be made available for you to review. We prefer not to actually see previous audiograms until our own testing of the child is complete to avoid being influenced in any way. Of course, comparison of our own testing results with previous hearing tests is an important consideration as the case proceeds. Table 6–3 presents a detailed developmental milestones checklist and questionnaire. Perhaps you will be able to elicit a brief speech sample from the child with a simple question like, "How are you today?" "How old are you now?" "Do you go to school?" with the intent that you can listen to the child's voice quality and speech or at least determine the child's preferred communication method. The pediatric audiologist might be able to derive clues as to the onset time of the hearing loss and its degree as well as an initial judgment about benefits from the amplification systems. If the voice quality is strident and only vowel sounds are made, an early onset severe hearing loss might be suspected. If the voice quality is good, in the presence of an evidently severe hearing loss, a later onset would be more

likely. Important clues can be obtained from a short dialogue with the child. For example, if the child has some words or sentences expressed in normal intonation in the presence of hearing loss, or if the child has difficulties expressing speech that is understandable, these will lead to additional questions. The responses may lead the pediatric audiologist to ultimately administer a pediatric standardized speech and language screening test. Such clues are helpful in determining the etiology and onset of the hearing loss as well as indications as to how the parents and caregivers are dealing with the child's hearing problem.

The Ear Examination and Otoscopy

Every pediatric hearing evaluation must be preceded by careful examination of the external ear prior to performing otoscopy. Examination of the outer ear should be accomplished in a friendly and casual approach as to not upset the child. Consideration should be given to determining if the external auditory canals fold shut or collapse when external pressure is applied. Collapsing canals can create a pseudoconductive component easily misinterpreted as hearing loss. Use of insert receivers for the subsequent hearing tests should alleviate this potential problem.

Observable anomalies associated range from the very obvious to slight, subtle defects of the head, ears, mouth, and neck. Typical indications of a neonate with syndromal stigmata include malformed, low-set, or aberrant pinna configurations (microtia or atresia); preauricular or postauricular tags and pits; cleft lip or palate (including submucous cleft palate); first-arch or second-arch anomalies including mandibular and maxillary variants; and

Table 6–3. Rapid Developmental Screening Checklist

NAME: _____ D.O.B: _____ 1st Visit.		
AGE _____ DATE _____		

1 mo:	Can he raise his head from the surface in the prone position?	Yes	No
	Does he regard your face while you are in his direct line of vision?	Yes	No
2 mo:	Does he smile and coo?	Yes	No
3 mo:	Does he follow a moving object?	Yes	No
	Does he hold his head erect?	Yes	No
4 mo:	Will he hold a rattle?	Yes	No
	Does he laugh aloud?	Yes	No
5 mo:	Can he reach for and hold objects?	Yes	No
6 mo:	Can he turn over?	Yes	No
	Does he turn toward sounds?	Yes	No
	Will he sit with a little support (with one hand)?	Yes	No
7 mo:	Can he transfer an object from one hand to another?	Yes	No
	Can he sit momentarily without support?	Yes	No
8 mo:	Can he sit steadily for about 5 minutes?	Yes	No
9 mo:	Can he say "ma-ma" or "da-da"?	Yes	No
10 mo:	Can he pull himself up at the side of his crib or playpen?	Yes	No
11 mo:	Can he cruise around his playpen or crib, or walk holding onto furniture?	Yes	No
12 mo:	Can he wave bye-bye?	Yes	No
	Can he walk with one hand held?	Yes	No
	Does he have a two-word vocabulary?	Yes	No
15 mo:	Can he walk by himself?	Yes	No
	Can he indicate his wants by pointing and grunting?	Yes	No
18 mo:	Can he build a tower of three blocks?	Yes	No
	Does he say six words?	Yes	No
24 mo:	Can he run?	Yes	No
	Can he walk up and down stairs holding rail?	Yes	No
	Can he express himself (occasionally) in a two-word sentence?	Yes	No
2½ yr:	Can he jump lifting both feet off the ground?	Yes	No
	Can he build a tower of six blocks?	Yes	No
	Can he point to parts of his body on command?	Yes	No
3 yr:	Can he follow two commands involving "on," "under," or "behind" (without gestures)?	Yes	No
	Can he build a tower of nine blocks?	Yes	No
	Does he know his first name?	Yes	No
	Can he copy a circle?	Yes	No

continues

Table 6–3. *continued*

4 yr:	Can he stand on one foot?	Yes	No
	Can he copy a cross?	Yes	No
	Does he use the past tense properly?	Yes	No
5 yr:	Can he follow three commands?	Yes	No
	Can he copy a square?	Yes	No
	Can he skip?	Yes	No

Note: Developed by the Committee on Children with Handicaps, American Academy of Pediatrics, New York Chapter 3, District II. This checklist is a compilation of developmental landmarks matched against the age of the child. These are in easily scored question form and may be checked "Yes" or "No." "No" responses at the appropriate age may constitute a signal indicating a possible developmental lag. If there is a substantial deviation from these values, then the child should be evaluated more carefully, taking into consideration the wide variability of developmental landmarks. (Adjust for prematurity, prior to 2 years, by subtracting the time of prematurity from the age of the child, i.e., a 2-month-old infant who was 1 month premature should be evaluated as a 1-month-old infant.)

branchial cysts. Not all infants with such defects will have hearing loss. The presence of such abnormalities, however, certainly increases the risk of hearing problems in that particular child.

An informative study was conducted by Hayes (1994) of 145 infants with cranial or facial anomalies (CFAs) and included ABR evaluation to determine the presence of hearing loss. Although the presence, type, and degree of hearing impairment varied by the type of CFA involvement, approximately 50% of infants demonstrated at least mild bilateral hearing loss; 20% of infants with isolated external ear anomalies (ear tags, pits, isolated microtia) exhibited various degrees of hearing loss. In 92% of infants with hearing loss, the results of ABR evaluation were consistent with conductive dysfunction.

Otoscopy can be conducted with a handheld otoscope with good lighting and visibility or with a video otoscope. The video otoscope has some advantages as the parents or caretakers can simultaneously view the images of their child's ear canals and tympanic membranes. During the otoscopy examination the audiologist should determine the size and direction and general anatomy of the ear canal as well as any obstructions in the ear canal that might interfere with the hearing test such as excessive wax, foreign bodies such as beads, broken crayons, Q-tip debris, or ear canal skin lesions or osteomas (Figure 6–3). In some newborns, vernix might be present in the ear canals which could affect tympanometry, acoustic reflex, or otoacoustic emission measurements. In addition, the purpose of otoscopy is to evaluate the appearance of the tympanic membrane including an appropriate light reflex and any abnormalities such as perforations, ventilation tubes, or membrane retraction with or without the presence of middle ear fluid. Accurate evaluation of the ear canal and tympanic membrane will help the pediatric audiologist anticipate and correctly interpret the child's hearing test results.

Use of an Assistant in Pediatric Audiology

Although many audiology clinical settings require that the audiologist work alone,

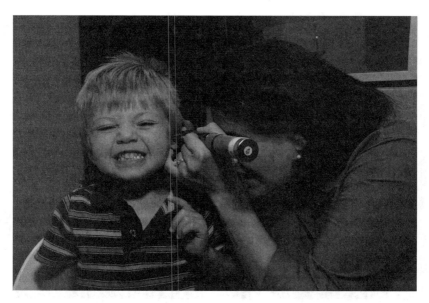

Figure 6–3. The pediatric hearing evaluation begins with an otoscopic examination of the ear. Photo courtesy of Colorado Children's Hospital, Aurora, CO.

the hearing testing of children is often enhanced by the use of an extra observer or a trained audiometric assistant or perhaps a second audiologist. Each of these helpers serves as an assistant to the tester. The assistant remains in the test room with the child to help control the test paradigm, to monitor and direct the behavior of the child under evaluation, and to communicate with the tester as necessary. Communication from the assistant with the parents or caregivers should be limited. Cooperation guidelines are in order, as well as sufficient training, so that the assistant can be of maximum use in the pediatric audiologic evaluation.

To be a successful team, the tester and the assistant must have clearly defined roles and areas of responsibility understood before testing begins. One person is identified as the "tester" and typically is the person in charge and responsible for the task at hand. The other person is the "assistant" and follows the directives of the tester. Both should be in continuous contact by earphones and the talkback circuit of the audiometer, through the soundfield system, or even by closed circuit video when available. The designated person has the task of all major communication with the parents. It is very disruptive to have both the tester and the assistant talking to the parents at different times during the test session.

The assistant is in charge of the test room as much as possible and maintains the behavior of the child and the parents (see Figure 6–4). It may be appropriate for the assistant to talk briefly to the parents during the session to warn them of what is about to happen in the test sequence, to guide their communication with the child, or to caution them about influencing the responses of the child unless specifically asked to do so. The team must often make an educated estimate about whether to include the parents in the sound room during the test session, based on a variety of observations including the behavior of the parents, the relationship

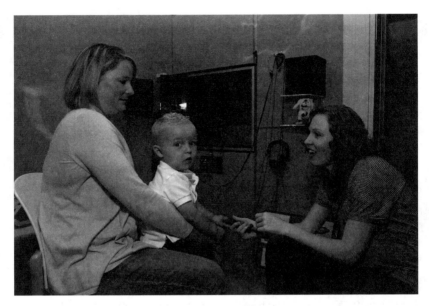

Figure 6–4. The use of an experienced assistant is helpful during pediatric hearing evaluations. Photo courtesy of Colorado Children's Hospital, Aurora, CO.

between the parents and the child, and the number of accompanying relatives, friends, neighbors, and siblings as well as the mood and preferences of the child.

Before the start of the test session, the sound room environment needs to be well organized. Toys must be kept out of sight until they are ready to be introduced to the child, one at a time, under control of the assistant. The test room should be as visually bland as possible to keep distractions to a minimum. Careful consideration must be given to the arrangement of chairs, tables, soundfield speakers, and visual reinforcers as well as the positions of the parent(s), assistant, and child, all so that the tester will have an unobstructed view of the child.

The test session should be started when the infant or child is showing a moderate amount of interest in a quiet toy used as a distractor. The timing of the test signal presentations and the time interval between signal presentations are very important to the success of the test session. Generally, the initial test presentations are slow and methodical, and as the child's performance improves, trials can be generated with shorter intertrial intervals. "Time out" may be used following false responses from the child, allowing the youngster to "settle down" again. One of the most common errors made by inexperienced testers is to run through the test session too quickly, too soon. Well-conditioned infants and children can perform quite well with rapid trial presentations, but the tester must be sure that the desired response relative to the stimulus presentations has been adequately shaped.

The assistant's task is to keep the child in a moderate state of alertness—not so absorbed in the toys that he or she will not be responsive to the auditory stimulus, yet not so uninterested that he or she will continuously visually search the room or fixate on the reinforcer. It is to be expected that there is tremendous variability among children's behavior in the test room environment. There is also wide variation in the child's attention level during the test session. The real challenge is for the assistant to judge precisely when the signal is presented and understand the state of the child at that time and to have the ability to manipulate and maintain the child's state at the desired level.

The choice of toys is important. Toys vary in how much attention they demand from children. Sometimes a child will have no preconceived idea of what a specific toy is supposed to do, so the imagination of the assistant has much to do with how successful a toy can be during the test session. Toys that generate noise and action toys that become too intriguing should be avoided. Toys should be introduced only one at a time, with all other toys being kept out of sight. When a child is done with a toy, it should also be put out of sight and out of reach. Toys in use should be kept directly in front of the child to eliminate false head turns. The manipulation of the toys by the assistant is very important to the timing and the eventual success of the hearing evaluation.

Response bias by testers and observers is one of the most difficult errors to avoid in the clinical hearing evaluation of children. Several studies have confirmed that there is a tendency for judges to score responses when no auditory signals are presented (Langford, Bench, & Wilson, 1975; Ling, Ling, & Doehring, 1970; Moncur, 1968). To help eliminate the tester bias problem, Weber (1969) suggested using two persons to test the child, with one observer in the room with the child while the tester operates a tape recorder in the control room. The operator selects a randomized stimulus schedule with 20 stimulus presentations—10 of which are heard only by the child. The observer wears earphones and hears all 20 stimulus presentations but cannot tell which sounds are presented to the

child under evaluation. The operator and observer each make judgments about the responses of the child, which are compared with the stimulus presentation schedule following the test session.

The bias condition can exist when only one audiologist is working with the child and has inherent anticipation of what the child's hearing should or might be. It is easy to see behavioral responses when they are just random responses from the child. Thus, it is crucial to accept only well-defined responses time-locked to the stimulus presentation. Sometimes, during the hearing evaluation process, the single-examiner audiologist might incorporate the parents' help when necessary to shape the child's conditioning behavior. Although we prefer having the managing audiologist outside the test room, many pediatric audiologists prefer working in the test room with the child (and parent). The pediatric audiologist who understands and is cautious about the potential bias that can exist with a single tester presenting stimuli and judging the child's responses should not significantly alter the accuracy of the hearing test. An experienced single-examiner audiologist is able to engage the infant's (or child's) forward attention with a simple toy, select and present a test signal, vary its presentation intensity as appropriate, judge the child's behavioral response, and activate the reinforcement. A careful and thoughtful clinician guarding against the potential hazards of single-examiner assessment may obtain reliable and accurate audiograms (Gravel, 1989).

Gans and Flexer (1982) investigated observer bias in behavioral observation audiometry (BOA) with profoundly involved multiple-handicapped children. Their findings implicated clear observer bias in 85% of children. At low test intensities, observers aware of the stimulus events tended to score fewer responses than those judges unaware of stimulus intensity. In cases of high sound intensities, judges tend to "see" more behavioral changes to sound than actually occur. Gans and Flexer were disappointed that even when observers were told that they exhibited biased scoring responses, this information did not influence the observer's subsequent scoring tactics.

Behavioral observation is a subjective procedure generally limited to use for the hearing screening of newborns and infants between birth and 6 months of age. Behavioral observations of these infant responses to sound are in no way an attempt to actually measure or determine hearing threshold levels. Experienced pediatric audiologists may choose to extend this hearing screening technique, when appropriate, to screen toddlers and young children through 24 months of age. However, it is recognized that unconditioned behavioral observation techniques with infants and young children are often confounded by poor test-retest reliability, high inter- and intra-subject variability, and quick habituation by the child to the acoustic stimulus.

Although there is no standard accepted technique for performing behavioral observations, in general terms the audiologist presents some type of calibrated auditory stimulus and observes the infant's or toddler's response to the onset and presence of the sound. Depending on the response of the infant or toddler, the audiologist then interprets whether or not the child "heard" the stimulus. The audiologist watches for a clear reflexive or active response from an infant or toddler who might be passively sitting on a parent's lap or quietly involved in a simple quiet task. An example of this technique is the presentation of an auditory stimulus to a lightly sleeping baby while observing behavioral changes that are time-locked to the stimulus presentation. The response magnitude is dependent on many variables, including the state of the infant or child during the procedure, the parameters of the acoustic stimulus, especially its intensity, the definition of an acceptable response, and the subjective decision by the audiologist as to whether a "hearing" response occurred following presentation of the stimulus.

Kevin Murphy of Reading, England (1962, 1979), developed the concept of an auditory maturation index that was expanded into clinical age-appropriate protocols by Northern and Downs (1974). This technique was based on predictable behavioral responses of children with normal hearing to noisemakers as a function of their chronological age. The value of such an index lies in its description of the normal maturation process that all normal-hearing infants go through during specific periods in their development. Some variability is to be expected around the age periods described for each auditory behavior, but one must be impressed with the consistency and predictability of the age limits at which certain developmental auditory responses are noted. The audiologist who works with infants, babies, and very young children should be familiar with the normal auditory maturation index as a helpful aid in screening the hearing of infants and babies. However, the auditory maturation is not a threshold procedure, and accordingly it should not be considered a hearing test, per se.

The auditory maturation of infants and babies is quite interesting to observe. During the first 4 months of life, the newborn's behavioral responses to auditory stimuli are limited to reflexive actions such as arousal from sleep, eye widening, and eyelid blinks that may, or may not, be associated with limb or body movements. However, between 4 and 12 months of age, the infant with normal hearing progresses through an orderly auditory maturation process. From 4 to 7 months of age, the normal infant response to a sound is a horizontal head turn toward the side of the sound source. The head turn becomes more robust as the infant's neck muscles strengthen but remains on the horizontal plane regardless of the level of the sound source. At 4 months of age the head turn is slow and labored, but by 6 months of age the horizontal head turn becomes definite and brisk. At approximately 7 months of age, the infant begins to localize to the sound source when it is presented on a lower plane. As this auditory maturation process proceeds, the baby may turn first on the horizontal level and then seek the sound source by looking downward. By 9 months of age the baby should be mature enough to locate the sound source when presented above head height. And, by 12 months of age, the infant with normal hearing should be able to locate the sound source in any plane on either side of the body easily and briskly.

A valuable clinical spin-off of the use of the maturation index has been its value in identifying developmental delay in children. Zigler (1969) described two theories of childhood maturation in children with handicaps that are known as the *difference theory* and the *developmental theory*. The difference theory predicts that the auditory responsiveness displayed by developmentally delayed children compared with normal children will be unexpected, deviant from the normal, and nonpredictable. The developmental theory assumes that the child with developmental delay passes through the same maturation sequence as the normal child, although much more slowly. Flexer and Gans (1986) verified the developmental theory for the auditory behavioral testing of children with multiple handicaps, showing that the expected audi-

tory responses follow the normal sequence of auditory maturation in normal-hearing children but are significantly delayed. Thus, if an 8-month-old baby shows only arousal and basic eye widening to acoustic stimuli but does not show even rudimentary head turning for localization, his or her auditory behavior is less than expected for the age level. If an 18-month-old toddler shows only lateral head-turning localization behavior and does not seek out sound sources presented below or above eye level, the child is performing on a 6- to 9-month auditory maturation stage.

Further logic suggests that if one can correlate auditory behavior with mental age, with a reasonable level of confidence, then the audiologist who is testing a developmentally delayed youngster with a chronologic age of 6 years but a mental age of 2 years or less should expect the child to have auditory responses appropriate to the limited mental age. Thus, a 6-year-old with an IQ of 60 will not respond with hand-raising behavior but will respond with the auditory localization responses expected from a child of approximately 2 years of age. The auditory responses of children with developmental delay are much closer to their mental age than to their chronologic age. Although not a perfect solution, the application of the auditory maturation knowledge to the difficult-to-evaluate child with developmental delay can provide useful and predictive information. Wilson and Thompson (1984) noted that even though behavioral observation lacks precision as an indicator of hearing thresholds, it may be the only available behavioral procedure for some children with profound delay and involvement without a more advanced evaluation with ABR. Gans (1987) reported results from behavioral observations used successfully to test 82 children with profound mental handicaps.

Behavioral Response Observation in the 0 to 6-Month-Old Infant

Most infants in this age group will be brought to the audiology clinic due to failing the hospital newborn hearing screening test seeking follow-up screening testing and possible diagnostic ABR hearing evaluation. Typically, infants are presented either in an infant carrier, bassinet, or in the arms of a parent. Although reactions from an awake baby to outside sounds can be observed, Ling et al. (1970) point out, the chance is too high for the audiologist to observe random responses and judge them to be valid responses to sound. Behavioral observation can be initially used to monitor auditory responses while the infant is in a light sleep. In the observation of responses it is useful for the audiologist to be able to see the baby's face clearly, with both ears visible, and with all blankets, wraps, coats, and so forth, peeled off the infant so that responses of the body, limbs, hands, and facial expressions can be noted. Lack of responses from the infant to loud noise sounds certainly speaks to the necessity for additional testing and likely referral for diagnostic auditory brainstem response (ABR) test to be completed.

The behavioral response screening of young babies, less than 6 months of age, is accomplished without reinforcement and results rely on the audiologist's subjective, and experienced, observation of responses under structured conditions. The use of sudden-onset speech signals and narrow bands of noise from soundfield speakers while observing the infant's behaviors allow calibration of stimulus intensity and frequency spectrum. The disadvantages of behavioral observation include the oft-subtle and questionable infant's responses, and the presence of tester bias or misin-terpretation of responses. In addition, the auditory responses of infants and young children are quick to reach extinction without reinforcement, and a wide variance of extraneous responses may be noted. Behavioral observation is useful for initial hearing screening with infants and very young children, but some form of operant reinforcement audiometry such as visual reinforcement audiometry (VRA) should be used to establish ear-specific hearing threshold data in children older than 6 months of age.

For lightly sleeping infants between birth and 4 months of age, a moderately loud, sudden-onset sound is usually required to elicit behavioral responses. The recommended stimulus is speech or speech-shaped noise or narrow bands of noise complex acoustic stimuli presented between 60 and 90 dB HL. We prefer to start with the softer stimulus presentations and slowly increase intensity as necessary to observe a reactive response. The duration of stimulus presentation should be between 3 and 4 seconds. There should be a brief period of quiet between stimulus presentations. Younger infants may be slower to respond to the stimulus presentation than older infants. Acceptable responses include a definite eye blink immediately following the presentation of the stimulus, a slight shudder of the whole body, an opening or widening of the eyes, or a marked movement of the body, arms, or legs. The infant's response should be seen within 2 seconds of the stimulus presentation. It may be helpful to use an associate to confirm these subtle responses.

Prior to presentation of the stimulus, it is important to maintain complete quiet for at least 30 seconds to "set the stage" for the sudden onset of the stimulus to evoke a response of large magnitude. If the infant is in deep sleep, there is less chance for good behavioral responses than when the baby is in a lighter stage of sleep. The recommended procedure is to wait at least 30 seconds between stimulus presentations to permit the infant to again relax and settle down. Do not rush the stimulus presentations. The stimuli lose their novel effect very quickly as the infants habituate to the sounds and their responses soon extinguish.

Thompson and Thompson (1972) noted that for infants of 7 to 12 months of age, speech and high-pass filtered speech produced the most behavioral observation responses over other types of auditory stimuli. They found that with 22- to 36-month-old infants there is no testing advantage of one auditory stimulus over another. Samples and Franklin (1978) observed the responses of 7- to 9-month-old infants to speech signals, warble tones, and noise bands. They found that the intensity level required for a response was lower, and the number of responses was significantly higher to speech signals than to either the warble tones or broadband noise stimuli.

Auditory localization testing of infants of 6 months of age may be attempted by having the baby sit in the parent's lap, facing the audiologist. A small, passive toy (such as a book or a soft animal) can be given to the baby as an entertaining device. The parent or caretaker should be instructed not to talk to the baby, not to provide any cues to the baby during the test, and not to make any undue noise. In fact, we sometimes put hearing conservation earmuffs on the parent to ensure that the parents do not participate in any way when the sound stimuli are presented in the sound booth.

Babies around 6 months of age and older should localize to novel speech and narrowband noise stimuli presented from soundfield loudspeakers. Typically, sound stimuli (speech or narrow bands of pulsed noise) are presented from one loudspeaker at a 45-degree angle to the child until a slow but deliberate head-turn response is

elicited. Then a similar or different stimulus is quickly presented from a loudspeaker located 45 degrees on the other side of the child until a head turn is noted. It is important that the observed behavior responses, or head turns, are time-locked to the auditory stimulus presentations and should be noted only as "present" or "absent" and not interpreted as a threshold or minimum response level.

There will be times when it is beneficial to use behavioral observation with children older than 6 months of age. In terms of auditory maturation, the 7- to 9-month-old is able to find a sound source located below eye level and off to the side but only by looking first to the lateral side and then down to the sound source. The 9- to 12-month-old child should briskly and directly localize to the softer stimulus presentations at 60 dB. The transitional stage of the auditory maturation sequence is clearly evident in this age range. Be warned, however, as these young children are normally visually very alert, and it is difficult to do any activity without attracting visual attention from the baby. A child of this age will usually sit quietly in the parent's lap and be mildly amused with a passive toy or book, or a few blocks. As in all of the tests with young children, the audiologist needs to develop a calm presence and steady pace and to be fully aware of an opportune moment to present the auditory stimuli. If the child is still exploring the environment, the audiologist should allow a few moments until the child is comfortable and relaxed before starting the testing sequence. If the child becomes too engrossed in the toy to be aware of the auditory environment, it may be necessary to change toys (if possible) or to wait until the enthusiasm for the item diminishes. At this age, an effective speech stimulus is to use the child's name: "Hi, Johnny! Hi, Johnny! Look this way, Johnny." Of course, always find out exactly what name the parents use with the child, as it does little good to say, "Hi, Johnny!" to John Edwin who is called "Eddie" by his family. The use of speech or noise band localization may produce a series of quick head turns from side to side. The infant may also be responsive to a speech stimulus of "bye-bye," and a voluntary, but somewhat reflexive, wave may be elicited from the baby.

The use of calibrated soundfield speech stimuli, and alternating from the loudspeakers on either side of the sound suite, accompanied by visual reinforcement, may actually turn a well-conditioned child's head from side to side like that of a person watching a tennis match. Not for long, however, even with visual reinforcement of some type, this is not an interesting enough activity to sustain the child's interest. The audiologist may wish to engage the child in some vocalization responses to speech stimuli at various levels, and the child may actually imitate the speech sounds, such as "oh-oh," if presented with singsong inflection. At this age, the child is normally happy and outgoing and very curious about everything going on in the environment. Once again, the cross-check techniques of VRA, acoustic immittance, otoacoustic emissions, and ABR should be conducted to confirm behavioral observations.

Some pediatric audiologists may wish to observe the baby's startle response that is usually reserved until all other behavioral observations have been completed. The startle response is elicited by presenting a sudden speech stimulus between 60 and 90 dB HL, although we generally find the 65 dB HL level to be a sufficiently loud stimulus. A simple technique is to have the baby seated quietly on the parent's knees as far forward as possible with minimal support. The startle reflex is easily observed as a brisk, whole-body Moro response as soon as the baby hears the loud speech sound. This procedure is conducted when all else is finished as the baby may be scared into sudden crying. The presence of a strong startle reflex by no means is indicative of normal hearing, as an infant with sensorineural hearing loss and abnormal loudness appreciation might also startle at 65 or 75 dB HL. The absence of a startle reflex, however, should be interpreted cautiously and in conjunction with other observations and test results and suggests the need for additional audiology evaluation.

REINFORCEMENT THEORY

Successful behavioral hearing evaluation in children is heavily dependent upon the audiologist's understanding and application of reinforcement theory. Reinforcement theory, also known as behavioral modification, is the shaping of behavior by controlling the consequences of the behavior. That is, applying a combination of rewards to encourage certain wanted behaviors or withholding reinforcement to extinguish unwanted behaviors. This is in contrast to *classical conditioning* that focuses on responses that are triggered by stimuli in an automatic fashion. The noted psychologist of the 1960s and 1970s, B. F. Skinner, was a key contributor to the development of modern ideas about reinforcement theory. Skinner's view was that individual behaviors were not the result of internal needs and drives, but rather were shaped by what happens to the individual as a result of his or her behavior. Behaviorists, as Skinner's followers were known, produced a huge volume of experiments, publications, and books to prove that individuals placed in a position to choose from several responses to a given stimulus will inevitably select the response that has been associated with positive outcomes. Any behavior that elicits a consequence is called *operant behavior* because the individual operates on his or her own environment based on reinforcement possibilities. These principles can be summarized by what has become known as "the law of effect," whereby all other things being equal, responses to stimuli that are followed by satisfaction will be strengthened, but responses followed by dissatisfaction will be weakened.

Generally speaking, there are two types of reinforcement: positive and negative. Positive reinforcement results when the occurrence of a valued behavioral consequence strengthens the probability of the behavior being repeated (i.e., parents give children with good behaviors candy). Negative reinforcement does not mean punishment; rather negative reinforcement results when an undesirable behavioral consequence is withheld (i.e., good children do not receive "time-out" periods). For purposes of pediatric audiometric evaluations, our focus is primarily on positive reinforcement techniques designed to strengthen the child's responses to auditory stimuli presentations.

Pediatric audiology has been developed around behavioral modification protocols based on reinforcement techniques. Audiologists have specific desired behaviors that we work to elicit from the children in our sound-treated rooms, and when we observe these behaviors, we provide positive reinforcement (i.e., hand-clapping, expressions of excitement and pleasure, or perhaps more tangible events). The timing of these reinforcement events is important to shaping and maintaining desired behaviors and is known as the reinforcement schedule. Basically, there are two types of reinforcement schedules: continuous reinforcement and intermittent reinforcement. When a behavior is reinforced every time it occurs,

we speak of continuous reinforcement. Research has shown that continuous reinforcement is the fastest way to establish new behaviors or eliminate undesired behaviors. However, children may find continuous reinforcement leads to satiation and is thus insufficient to hold their interest over time. An intermittent reinforcement schedule implies each instance of a desired behavior is not reinforced, and thus the behavior is learned more slowly. Both continuous and intermittent reinforcement schedules are used in pediatric audiology: continuous reinforcement is used to quickly establish the desired responses from children, followed by intermittent reinforcement to maintain their responses over time.

Intermittent reinforcement can be applied in four general protocols: (a) fixed intervals of reinforcement are applied after consistent set periods of time; (b) a fixed ration schedule of reinforcement applies the reinforcement after a set number of responses of the desired behavior; (c) variable interval reinforce schedules are employed when desired behaviors are reinforced after varying periods of time; and (d) variable ration reinforcement schedule applies the reinforcement after a number of desired behaviors have occurred. The intermittent reinforcement schedules will elicit the desired behavioral responses that are consistent and resistant to extinction. Gambling is a good example of the power of intermittent reinforcement. Gamblers will sit at a casino table for long hours if they have a winning hand every now and then.

Wilson and Thompson (1984) classified the behavioral audiologic testing of children into two major divisions: procedures without reinforcement and procedures that utilize reinforcement of the child's responses. The conditioning approach to assessing hearing levels in infants and children uses a stimulus-response-reinforcement paradigm to elicit repeatable responses. In these procedures, the response is predefined and cued by the presentation of auditory stimuli through soundfield speakers or insert earphones. The child's response is strengthened through the use of various positive reinforcements. In this approach, the infant or child is an active participant in the testing situation. Studies have confirmed that under proper conditioning procedures, 6-month-old infants can be evaluated with conditioning techniques. Typically these conditioning techniques are used with children older than 6 months of age through 12 months of age.

The study of operant reinforcement focused the attention of psychologists for nearly 30 years. It is well accepted that "operant consequences" are so specific that they can be used to increase desired behaviors and decrease unwanted behaviors. Audiologists realized that operant theory applied precisely to pediatric hearing testing paradigms, and thus, operant conditioning became the cornerstone of pediatric hearing evaluations. Operant reinforcement audiometry for children between 6 months and 3 years of age is a particularly valuable clinical tool for the pediatric audiologist. Stimulus, response, and reinforcement parameters and techniques have been developed to be consistent with each child's developmental level and response capability. The use of reinforcements for the child's behavioral responses made to audiometric stimuli strengthens the test paradigm, maintains the child's responses longer, reduces habituation and extinction to the stimulus, and thus allows for a more precise estimate of hearing thresholds for all test frequencies in each ear of young children.

Wilson and Thompson (1984) were strong proponents of the operant discrimination paradigm in hearing testing. They described two modes of operant conditioning termed *operant discrimination* and the *conjugate procedure*. In operant discrimination, the stimulus precedes the responses and acts as a discriminative signal that reinforcement is available. In the conjugate procedure, the stimulus follows the response as a consequence. The intensity of a continuously available reinforcing stimulus varies as a function of the rate of the response. Because the stimulus is a consequence of the response, in the conjugate procedure the stimulus itself must have reinforcing value to the child.

An example of a conjugate reinforcement technique is the innate sucking response in infants, which was originally developed by Siqueland and DeLucia (1969) and described by Madell and Flexer (2014). This procedure relies on a natural newborn response and capitalizes on the reinforcing properties of the stimulus. The spontaneous behavior (sucking) is brought under stimulus control through the use of response-contingent stimulation. The auditory stimulus is then made contingent on a criterion-level sucking response, and the auditory stimulus takes on reinforcing properties for the infant. Disadvantages to the sucking response are the physical demand placed on the infant, a baseline criterion level of 20 to 40 sucks per minute so that criterion level changes may be noted, and the fact that the general length of time required to complete studies is substantial. Eisele, Berry, and Shriner (1975) generated threshold hearing data from 100 infants by observing the rate of sucking as a function of stimulus intensity.

Primus (1987) investigated response and reinforcement features of two operant discrimination paradigms with normal-hearing 17-month-old children. He found more success in a paradigm that based the response task on complex central processing skills (i.e., localization and coordination of auditory/visual space) over a simple detection task. His use of animated toy reinforcement resulted in more than a twofold increase in responses. In a 1985 research project, Primus and Thompson (1985) tested the response strength of young children in operant audiometry. One- and 2-year-old children reinforced on a variable-ratio schedule of intermittent reinforcement and a 100% schedule demonstrated equivalent response habituation and consistency. Primus and Thompson reported that the use of novel reinforcement had a strong influence in eliciting conditioned responses from normal-hearing 2-year-old children and that an audiologist can delay the habituation and extinction of responses by the use of novel (different) reinforcements.

The use of behavioral and conditioning procedures with infants and young children may lack sufficient precision to establish valid auditory sensitivity thresholds. Accordingly, Matkin (1977) suggested the use of minimum response level (MRL) to describe the lowest intensity of auditory stimulus that produces the desired response. Use of the term *minimal response level* rather than *auditory threshold* for pediatric hearing evaluations serves as a reminder that improvement in response behavior might be anticipated as the child matures and test results become more accurate.

Procedures using computer technology have influenced operant conditioning paradigms (Eilers, Widen, Urbano, Hudson, & Gonzales, 1991). Computerized stimulus presentations can be programmed to include preprogrammed catch trials or control presentations when no auditory signal is actually presented. This technique is especially useful when using an audiometric assistant in the sound room with the child who cannot observe when the stimulus is being presented or withheld. Computerized scoring response criteria also can be estab-

lished to limit the time window of the child's response in other ways and can be used to define the "correctness of response," with the assistants blinded as to the presentation of control (no signal) trials.

VISUAL REINFORCEMENT AUDIOMETRY (VRA): 6 MONTHS TO 2 YEARS OF AGE

Suzuki and Ogiba (1961) were the first to report that a visual reinforcer could be used to shape auditory localization to establish hearing thresholds in young children. Their initial study utilized children from 3 to 5 years of age. Suzuki and Ogiba termed their procedure *conditioned orientation reflex* (COR) as the child was conditioned to correctly orient to a sound presented from one of two speakers in corners of the sound booth. The child's head turn was reinforced with a blinking lighted toy. Liden and Kankkonen (1969) of Sweden coined the term *visual reinforcement audiometry* (VRA) that described a conditioning technique that did not require localization, but merely a notable response to the presence of the sound stimulus. In the early years, VRA referred to a procedure utilizing a single soundfield speaker. When the child made any motion of awareness of the presentation of the stimulus sound, a blinking light reinforcer drew the child to localize to the speaker. Awareness, rather than conditioning, was the appropriate and rewarded response. Subsequent studies with the use of visual reinforcement of auditory localization proved that the technique could be used successfully with children in the 5- to 12-month age range. Moore, Thompson, and Thompson (1975) found that the use of animated toys hidden in smoked Plexiglas boxes and lit with flashing light following the presentation of an audible auditory signal worked well for reinforcing the auditory localization head-turn response in infants 12 to 18 months of age. The terms *conditioned orientation reflex* and *COR audiometry* have been largely abandoned in favor of the use of the term *visual reinforcement audiometry* (VRA). A brief review of the history and procedures involved in VRA is presented below, but for an excellent and more thorough discussion of VRA, the reader is referred to Widen (2011).

Moore et al. (1976) and Moore, Wilson, and Thompson (1977) confirmed the success of VRA in eliciting responses in infants as young as 5 months. Wilson and Thompson (1984) established auditory thresholds in 90 infants between 5 and 18 months of age. Their results showed the VRA responses to be significantly better (i.e., lower intensity) than comparison behavioral observation levels. Gravel and Traquina (1992) utilized VRA to evaluate hearing in a cohort of 211 babies and toddlers ranging in age from 6 to 24 months, obtaining ear and frequency-specific thresholds from more than 80% of these children.

The technique of VRA is to seat the child in the parent or caregiver's lap or in a nearby high chair (Figure 6–5A–C). Observers in the sound room are warned not to help or cue their child in any way during the testing procedure. VRA should be conducted with the child wearing insert earphones whenever possible (Day, Bamford, Parry, Shepherd, & Quigley, 2000). If the child refuses the insert earphones, earphones or soundfield presentation of the stimuli can be used. However, under soundfield conditions it is more difficult to ascertain independent ear hearing levels. The VRA task is established through the use of a few training trials during which the child's attention is usually spontaneously directed toward the side of the stimulus (auditory sound) presentation and held there while the reinforcer (flashing and animated lighted toy) is presented. Thompson and Folsom (1984) found no difference between 30 and 60 dB HL conditioning tone presentations, whereas more recently Widen et al. (2005) reported that the actual type of stimulus used in conditioning children for VRA had little to do with the success of the procedure.

If the child does not initially and voluntarily turn toward the source of the sound, it may be that he or she does not hear it or needs help in making the association between the presence of the sound and the need for a head turn to view the flashing light toy. Obviously if the child does not hear the conditioning trial stimulus, the intensity of the sound needs to be increased before proceeding. The important fact, however, is to ensure that the child is able to clearly hear the conditioning auditory stimuli; children with hearing loss will likely require louder conditioning trials. Parents or other observers in the test room with the child may wish to wear ear defenders during loud training trials of 75 dB HL or greater. Perfunctory classic conditioning may be necessary to help the child associate the onset of the auditory stimulus with the lighting of the toy. The visual reinforcers should be at least 90 degrees from the midline and require the child to make a full head turn to the side to observe a lighted animated toy or brief video that is illuminated or activated remotely located to one side. In most clinical settings, the pediatric audiologists use speakers and reinforcers on both sides of the child, whereas in other clinics only one speaker and reinforcer location is utilized. The success of VRA will depend somewhat on the novelty of the reinforcer to maintain the child's interest and attention; reinforcers should provide positive reward by creating a fun

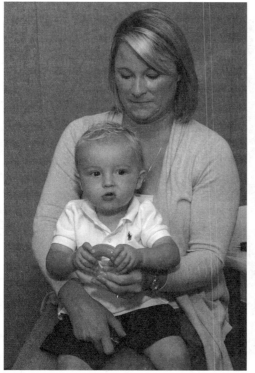

A

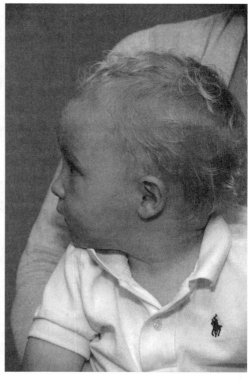

B

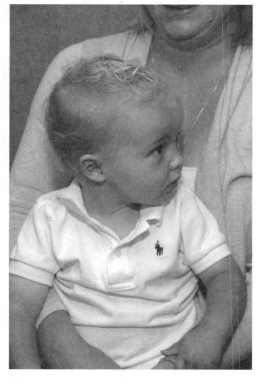

C

Figures 6–5. A–C. Child sits quietly in mother's lap for visual reinforcement audiometry (VRA): Note toddler's head turn toward soundfield auditory for right side and left side stimulus presentations. The toddler sees a brief activated and lighted toy from source of the sound which reinforces the toddler's head turn. Photos courtesy of Colorado Children's Hospital, Aurora, CO.

and pleasant experience (Pehringer, 2011). Some children will respond as minimally as possible to see the reinforcer out of the corner of their visual field and they may need behavior shaping to make a full 90-degree head turn. Limited head turns can be shaped into full head turns by the experienced pediatric audiologist controlling the reinforcement with each trial to require stronger and more overt responses following each stimulus presentation.

When a response to the auditory stimulus alone is not elicited, the transducer should be changed to a bone vibrator and a low-frequency signal (e.g., 250 Hz) or speech should be presented at a level known to provide tactile stimulation (e.g., 50 to 60 dB HL) through the bone oscillator (AAA, 2012). If the child does not respond to the stimulus/reinforcer combination or to the vibrotactile stimulus alone, it is likely that the task is not developmentally appropriate for the child (usually at the younger end of the age range) or that the task is not sufficiently interesting to the child (usually at the older end of the age range). In such circumstances, alternative hearing assessment procedures (i.e., physiological) should be considered. If the child is unable or refuses to localize to tonal or noise signals, the audiologist should modify the testing procedure to determine the lowest level at which the child initially perceives speech, thereby establishing a speech awareness threshold (SAT).

When the audiologist is confident that the child's head-turn responses are well established following a few conditioning trials (perhaps only two or three trials will be necessary), the search for hearing thresholds may begin. A systematic bracketing protocol with predetermined start level and step sizes is recommended (Widen et al., 2000, 2005). Typically, the auditory stimulus may be presented at a supposed below threshold level and be stepped up until

a head-turn response is obtained, or the stimulus can be decreased in steps until no response is elicited. Working from below the child's thresholds, minimum response levels (MRLs) can be established with fewer head-turn responses, thereby holding the child's interest in the visual reinforcements longer.

The order of stimulus presentation recommended by AAA Pediatric 2012 Assessment Guidelines is that MRLs should be obtained initially for easy speech stimuli (e.g., monosyllables, individual speech sounds, the child's name), followed by pure tones or complex signals centered at frequencies of 0.5, 1.0, 2.0, and 4.0 kHz. The order of stimulus presentation can be flexible depending on the purpose of the VRA evaluation. For example, starting with high frequencies has the advantage of making an early determination of the need for amplification in case the child cannot participate for testing of all test frequencies. Consideration should be given to alternating ears between stimuli to ensure that at least partial or complete data can be obtained for both ears. Alternating signals between ears may help focus the child's attention for a longer period of time. One approach might be to obtain MRL for speech in right ear, then in left ear; MRL for 1.0 or 2.0 kHz tone in right ear, then in left ear; and so on until the audiogram is as complete as possible. Thresholds or minimum response levels consistent with normal hearing sensitivity vary depending on the age of the child and are available in the literature. Normative data are available for TDH-39 earphones at a limited number of frequencies (Nozza & Wilson 1984; Sabo, Paradise, Kurs-Lasky, & Smith, 2003), for soundfield stimuli (Gravel & Wallace, 2000), and for insert phones (Parry, Hacking, Bamford, & Day, 2003; Widen et al., 2000; Widen et al., 2005).

Diverting the child's attention between trials to the midline and away from the visual reinforcer is easily accomplished with a visually appealing toy held by an assistant stationed in the full-on front view of the child. The auditory stimulus presentation and head-turn response must always precede delivery of the visual reinforcement. Although the "on" time between trials for stimulus presentation should be varied, the reinforcement (illuminating and activating the toy) must immediately follow the desired head-turn response. The auditory stimulus should not be terminated until the desired head-turn response occurs. Culpepper and Thompson (1994) recommend short stimulus duration of 0.5 seconds rather than longer presentations of 4 seconds to decrease habituation time and increase the overall number of responses from the child. Primus (1992) reported that the most valid responses from a child during VRA occur within 4 seconds after the stimulus onset, although in clinical practice this seems like a "long" wait.

Matkin (1977) found that VRA can be successful with 90% of both normal-hearing and children with hearing loss between the ages of 12 and 30 months. Hodgson (1985) suggested that the child with a severe-to-profound hearing loss might not have learned to localize sound. He suggested that where there is confusion in localization, it is best to use only one loudspeaker in testing. In the huge multicenter survey project reported by Norton et al. (2000), 96% of more than 3,000 infants (mean age 10 months) provided at least one threshold in one ear with VRA; astoundingly, 92% of the total cohort completed a three-frequency threshold test and speech detection level in each ear; 56% of the infants were tested in one session while an additional 30% required two sessions to complete the VRA hearing test. Norton et al. reported that the average test session lasted 15 minutes and required 45 reinforced stimulus trials.

Children with asymmetrical hearing loss or a significant unilateral hearing loss might have difficulties localizing the source of a sound, and this should be a consideration in children who seem to have difficulty with VRA for no other apparent reason. Children who have unilateral hearing loss sometimes can actually localize sound, albeit more slowly than children with normal hearing by moving their head slightly between the presentations of stimuli. Localization skills among children vary considerably and seem to be a function of the child's age and the parameters of the stimulus. For example, warble tone signals are much more difficult to localize than speech or narrowband noise stimuli. Moore et al. (1977) determined rank order of signals according to their effectiveness in producing VRA localization responses in 12- to 18-month-old infants: (a) an animated toy, (b) a flashing light, (c) social reinforcement, and (d) no reinforcement (Figure 6–6).

Eilers, Wilson, and Moore (1977) used VRA techniques in a speech discrimination paradigm designed to show developmental changes of discrimination ability that they termed visually reinforced infant speech discrimination (VRISD). They demonstrated that infants aged 1 to 3 months could discriminate some of the easier phonemic contrasts, but that closer phonemic contrasts are more difficult for very young children than for older infants. Thus, VRA conditioning procedures have been successfully used in the study of the development of auditory prelinguistic skills.

Thompson, Thompson, and Vethivelu (1989) noted a paucity of information about the relative effectiveness of audiometric procedures for testing hearing in younger 2-year-old children. They evaluated 2-year-old subjects and found that a higher percentage of children could be conditioned to VRA than to play audiometry. However,

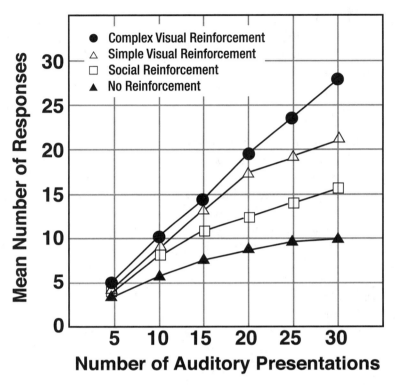

Figure 6–6. Response curves for operant conditioning audiometry. Reprinted with permission from "Visual Reinforcement of Head-Turn Responses in Infants Under Twelve Months of Age," by J. M. Moore, W. R. Wilson, and G. Thompson, 1977, *Journal of Speech and Hearing Disorders, 42*, p. 328.

in terms of response habituation, play conditioning had a longer response activity period. In their conclusions, these researchers noted that under general clinical conditions, the use of VRA can be used to quickly answer the question in 2-year-olds as to whether hearing loss might be a factor in their delayed speech and language development. Under this circumstance, VRA is recommended because the vast majority of 2-year-olds readily condition to this task for purposes of hearing screening to establish the presence of normal hearing or hearing loss.

VRA is a valuable technique for assessing minimal response levels (MRLs) in young children when used correctly following conditioning protocols. VRA is the primary method to assess hearing sensitivity in children between 6 and 24 months of age (Widen, 2011). The cross-check protocol of tympanometry and acoustic reflexes, evoked otoacoustic emissions, and ABR when necessary, may be required to confirm degree and configuration of hearing loss in a baby or toddler in this young age group. Within this age range, the pediatric audiologist will likely find a wide diversity of childhood behaviors. Usually the older children in this age range will condition to VRA more easily and quicker than the younger children.

Commercially available VRA systems generally have a pair of illuminated or animated reinforcement boxes. These systems are especially useful for the audiologist working without an assistant as the equipment often includes a third (orientation) toy, to be placed in front of the child, which can be illuminated remotely between stimulus presentation trials to bring the child's head back to the center position in readiness for the next stimulus presentation. In addition to the infant and toddler, the VRA technique is especially viable for older, developmentally delayed children who may be functioning at a level too low for the hand-raising response task.

Computerized and automated VRA systems are also available that use interactive video images as the reinforcement for correct responses in an application of visual reinforcement operant conditioning audiometry (VROCA), initially developed and introduced by Keith and Smith (1987) to facilitate hearing assessment in 3- to 7-year-old children. Currently there are a variety of VRA systems available with colorful toys and animals that move and light up on activation. Other systems use colored blinking lights to serve as a mid-line attention holder. There are also video VRA systems that utilize short-action video images of colorful cartoon characters displayed on a flat-screen television. The television is kept dark until remotely activated when the child makes the desired and accurate localization response. A changing multitude of images and vignettes can hold the child's attention and enthusiasm until the testing period is complete (Pehringer, 2011).

Other computer-mediated VRA procedures have been reported to obtain complete audiometric data more efficiently than is possible using standard behavioral techniques. With the Keith and Smith system (1987), the child was conditioned during practice trials to quickly depress a bright red button on the response box immediately following presentation of an auditory stimulus. A brief, animated color video presentation occurs after each correct response made within a short time window. False responses produce no visual reinforcement of any kind. This pediatric VRA audiometer adapts the test signal presentation speed to the response speed of the child and in the automatic mode includes several validity checks. Such systems can also include silent control trials interspersed at random intervals. Tharpe and Ashmead (1993) evaluated several parameters in computerized simulations leading to various test outcomes using adaptive testing procedures. Berstein and Gravel (1990) described a three-frequency Interweaving Staircase Procedure, and Eilers et al. (1991) developed a four-frequency Optimized Hearing Test Algorithm. We can likely expect more advancement with these innovative VROCA systems, suggesting great promise for future pediatric hearing assessment.

CONDITIONED PLAY AUDIOMETRY WITH CHILDREN AGES 2 TO 4 YEARS

Conditioned play audiometry is the preferred behavioral technique to determine ear-specific and frequency-specific hearing thresholds in children between 2 and 4 years of age.

During these years, the child grows into the independence of early maturity. The child begins to separate from mother without much fuss and to dress alone, first with supervision and then without. The youngster now becomes a wanderer and can quickly delve into the audiologist's toys and equipment. The child begins to understand some abstract words, such as cold or hungry, and can give a full name when asked.

Actually, the child becomes eager and happy to please the audiologist. As a result of this strong desire to please, the child may give the clinician a difficult time in testing. Once children know that cooperation in responding pleases the audiologist, they may forget what they are supposed to listen for, in their eagerness to be praised.

Conditioned play audiometry is a form of operant conditioning in which the child is taught to wait and listen carefully for a pure tone, narrow band noise, or speech stimulus, and then to perform a task that is actually a sort of child's game in response to the presentation of the stimuli. The motor task itself is fun for the child, and the activity actually serves as the reinforcer. The learning of play-conditioning techniques can begin with youngsters of 2 years of age, although some children may be able to perform the tasks a few months earlier. However, one should not be deceived by the bright, talkative 2-year-old who appears certain to be able to learn the procedure but is not yet sufficiently mature to do so.

The clinician should still obtain all the information possible from the observation of behavior as the child waits in the waiting room, walks into the sound booth, and watches the interaction with the parents during the case history conversation. Until the child is 4 or 5 years old, the audiologist's ingenuity is challenged to complete the definitive and complete hearing test. Remember that the goal is to achieve pure tone thresholds at all test frequencies in each ear. However, the child should not be traumatized so much that he or she will be frightened the next time in the sound-treated booth. If the process does not go well with the child, for whatever reason, there is always another day for a new appointment and a new try at the hearing test.

The darkened instrument room is often helpful when testing the young child. A shy, immature child of 2.5 years may learn play-conditioning techniques easily, but the odd situation of a stranger's face in the window staring at them may create too much distracting stress. The bodiless voice over the speaker can be coped with; it takes the stranger (audiologist) out of the situation. All the necessary instructions to the child can be given through the speech circuit (insert earphones or loudspeakers) without being seen by the child. A friendly assistant or parent can be working with the child in the test room.

Because this technique is such an important part of the pediatric audiologist's skills, a detailed step-by-step description of our recommended protocol, along with numerous clinical tips, is presented in the following paragraphs. The younger child may choose to sit on the parent's lap while the parent holds the necessary objects for the play conditioning task (although possible, this can be cumbersome). The more confident 3- or 4-year-old may prefer to sit alone in a child-size chair in front of a child-size play table with a parent nearby in another chair. The parent's closeness may be important for successful play conditioning, although when the child is experienced with numerous hearing tests, he or she may be willing to come to the sound suite alone without the parent.

The audiologist should establish rapport with the family initially by talking to the parents first, developing an easy relationship. Opening comments can be about the weather, the parking issues at the clinic, or more directly asking about the child's problem as in, "What brings you to the audiology clinic today?" or "What seems to be Parker's problem?" The parents should be given time to tell briefly why the child is being tested, but the child's case history should not be belabored at this particular moment. The child is the chief interest and target. The audiologist should turn casually to the child and ask some simple questions such as, "How are you today?" or "How old are you?" Further conversation might include comments about the child's clothing, hair, or a toy that the child brought along. The child should then be told that there are some special and fun listening games to play today.

During this period of talking with the child, the experienced pediatric audiologist should carefully attend to clues regarding the child's potential speech and language levels as well as potential hearing loss. Attention should be paid to the child's voice quality and articulation of words. Does the child substitute for the high-frequency consonants? If he or she omits or substitutes for the unvoiced consonants, either mild sensorineural or a conductive loss can be suspected. If the child misses the voiced consonants and some of the vowel sounds in addition, a more severe sensorineural loss may be expected.

The conditioning phase includes review of the planned play task which will require a gross motor response from the child following each presentation of an auditory pure tone stimulus. Explanation and demonstration of the motor task (i.e., dropping marbles into a can, putting pegs into a peg board, building a block tower, etc.) should be accomplished with sufficient number of trials to ensure the child understands the instructions. This brief initial training session (i.e., play conditioning) should be conducted to ensure that the child understands the game. The child should reliably provide two or three consecutive, unprompted correct responses to the presence of an auditory stimulus before beginning the threshold testing procedures.

When verbal instructions cannot be used because of language, age, or severity of hearing loss, the task may be demonstrated using the parent as the patient, or the audiometric assistant acting out the required response. The audiologist should maintain control of the session and gently tell the child what is going to happen in simple, clear terms that are easily understandable for the language-age of the child (our golden rule is: "Never ask the child if he or she wants to play the game—unless you want to hear the "no" word). The audiologist should say something like, "Now we're going to play a telephone (or cell phone) game. We'll let you listen through this special telephone (foam-covered insert receivers), and you can talk back to me. Hello!" The clinician should then put the ear inserts gently but firmly into the ear canals, saying at the same time, "Can you hear me now? Wait and listen because I'm going to talk to you from the other room." The audiologist should move quickly before the child balks. However, if he or she balks, the parent can hold the inserts or earphones to the child's ear ("Like a special telephone"). With the very young and the shy child, it may be preferable to start with soundfield auditory signals. A trial run can be done in soundfield initially, allowing the child to become familiar with the situation and the play task, then the placement of inserts or earphones may be reattempted. Another way to demonstrate the test session is for the audiologist to put the earphones on himself or herself or the parents for the child's observation.

There should be available a number of sets of motivational toys geared to different ages: plain blocks for building a tower, a graduated ring tower, beads to throw into a container, and a peg board with colored pegs, perhaps a horse or other animal or a car to be in the center of the peg board while the child builds a perimeter fence or a garage (Figure 6–7). A popular game is to drop pennies into a bank. The ingenious audiologist can devise other motivational

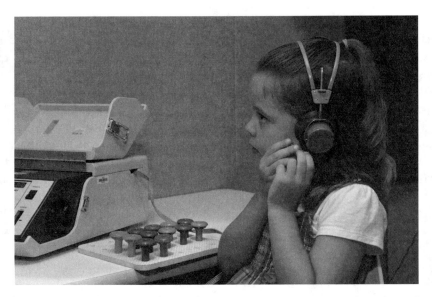

Figure 6–7. Conditioned play audiometry using pegs and pegboard as the child's response mode. Photo courtesy of Colorado Children's Hospital, Aurora, CO.

games. Usually, a single game is sufficient to accomplish the task, but one must be ready to switch to another game at the first sign of boredom. It is largely the enthusiasm of the clinician that keeps the child attending, but occasionally novelty must be used. Although it is perhaps more motivating to use different-colored beads, pegs, or plastic rings, it can slow the process down considerably if the child decides to select and dig around to use only the red (or green or some other specific color, or only the biggest or the smallest) toys in the conditioned motor task. Once again, it is important to remember that infection control procedures should be followed including cleaning and disinfecting any furniture, equipment, or toys that come into contact with the patient prior to reuse with another patient.

The pediatric audiologist needs to show the child what the game is about, using instructions and demonstrations at the child's verbal level. Simple instructions can be communicated without talking much.

Facial expression, body language, and clear demonstrations can transmit even to the nonverbal child what is to be expected. The child can also be told in words, "We're going to hold this peg (or block, etc.) up to our ear and listen for a little bell (beep or sound). Oh! I hear it, so I can put the peg quickly into the board. Now, I'm going to listen for another little soft bell or beep-beep. Oh! I hear it, so I put another peg in. Now you can do it, and build a fence for the horse (or car)." In the case of the 2- and 3-year-old, the parent should be instructed to actually hold the child's hand with the peg at the test ear and to guide the child's hand to the pegboard when the sound is heard. This should be practiced through soundfield even to the extent of establishing a quick threshold for a 2000 Hz tone or narrowband noise centered at 1000 or 2000 Hz stimulus until the clinician is confident that the child understands the task. Three or four trials should be sufficient for the child to learn. Be cautioned not to use so many conditioning trials that the novelty of the task is worn out before the hearing threshold search is begun.

The child should then be instructed to perform the task alone, preferably with earphones testing one ear at a time. The tone should be presented at 40 to 50 dB above the expected threshold. The audiologist should quickly switch to the speech circuit and praise the child for a correct action. The parent should be instructed to have another peg ready to give to the child the moment the child has responded accurately. The challenge in play audiometry is teaching the child to wait, listen, and respond with the play activity only when the auditory signal is audible. Testing should descend in intensity as rapidly but carefully in 10- or 15-dB steps, indicating to the child to listen for a "tiny little bell (or beep)" prior to each presentation. A systematic bracketing protocol with audible starting level, and predetermined step sizes is recommended; for children of this age, this typically means down 10 dB, up 5 dB step size, but the audiologist should be flexible enough to change to a larger step size (down 20 dB, up 10 dB) if speed is required. The testing should be done quickly to obtain thresholds, accepting two responses on the ascending presentation. The clinician must guard against presenting the test stimuli in any sort of predictable pattern, occasionally waiting a few extra seconds after the urge to present the tone. Children are very good at anticipating a pattern or picking up subtle cues as to when they are "supposed" to respond.

It is most important to establish hearing thresholds at 500 and 2000 Hz in each ear as quickly as possible. The initial practice tones should be loud enough for the child to hear easily based on their SRT levels. Sometimes a child will seem to be cooperative at first but soon forget what to do. In this case, the child should be reconditioned, with the parent's help, at levels at which it is certain that he or she can hear. Several reconditioning periods may have to be run during a test. The audiologist should not give up until it is apparent that the child is not about to stay with the task. If the child stays with the task nicely, the clinician should fill in the 1000 and 250 Hz thresholds and then 4000 Hz threshold for each ear. It is important for the clinician to know when to stop, because there is likely additional testing to be done, and there must be some reserve of the child's attention and interest in subsequent audiologic tests.

The play conditioning goal is to obtain independent ear hearing thresholds to tonal stimuli of 500, 1000, 2000, and 4000 Hz. The order of stimulus presentation may be altered depending on the purpose of the evaluation. If the hearing test suggests the need for hearing aids, then determining thresholds at the higher frequencies first may be important for hearing aid selection and fitting. If the testing is going well and time permits, additional frequencies might be helpful in hearing aid programming (e.g., addition of 1500 and 3000 Hz). For very young children of 2 or 3 years developmental age, consideration should be given to alternating ears between stimuli to keep the task interesting to the child in order to obtain partial or complete data on both ears.

When the child persistently refuses to wear the earphone headset or even one insert earphone, the audiologist should move quickly to soundfield audiometry. Warbled pure tones or narrow bands of noise, precalibrated to the location where the child is sitting, should be presented by using the play conditioning techniques. The thresholds will represent the hearing in the better ear only but will give essential information about how the child is hearing, at least in the better ear. Conditioned play audiometry is useful when evaluating hearing in children older than 4 years old who might be delayed in maturity and uneasy in the sound suite situation.

Play conditioning audiometry can also be used to determine bone conduction thresholds. The bone conduction oscillator is placed on the child's mastoid ("We're going to use another kind of telephone—one that goes behind your ear. But you can hear the sounds just like the other telephone. That's like airplane pilots [or astronauts] use!") The clinician should repeat the procedure as described above for air conduction testing, completing the more important frequencies first, and filling in with the other frequencies when possible. Bone-conducted testing can be masked effectively in the opposite ear without affecting the validity of the child's responses, but the child must be warned of the masking noise presence and directed to pay no attention to it but rather listen for the tone (or beep-beep). At the end of each test procedure, the child should be praised with some token such as a sticker or toy. This tangible token is insurance for future cooperation. The audiologist may have to see this child many times, so groundwork should be laid for happy return visits.

The successful evaluation of a child ultimately depends on the observational skills, interpersonal skills, and experience of the audiologist. Regardless of the confidence the audiologist might have following play conditioning testing, it must be remembered that adequate confirmation of an infant's or child's hearing status cannot be obtained with a single test (i.e., sometimes near-normal hearing will be found in a child with otitis media). Rather, a test battery is required to cross-check the results of both behavioral and physiologic measures (Jerger & Hayes, 1976). The cross-check procedures include tympanometry, acoustic reflex measurement, and otoacoustic emissions. When test results are still questionable about the child's actual hearing levels, an ABR evalu-

ation may be in order. However, ABR evaluation is not a necessary component to be incorporated into every pediatric patient's workup. Because of the time and expense associated with ABR evaluation, this procedure should be reserved for those children whose hearing levels cannot be determined precisely through any other method.

Tangible Reinforcement Operant Conditioning Audiometry (TROCA)

During this operant conditioning paradigm, the auditory stimulus cues the child that a behavior-specific response will immediately produce a positive and tangible reinforcement. The positive reinforcement is a tangible (i.e., solid and real) item such as candy, cereal, or a trinket of some sort that is automatically dispensed from specifically designed audiometric equipment. Negative reinforcement such as a brief "time out" without the tangible reinforcements for false-positive responses from the child can be incorporated in difficult situations to shape the desired response behaviors. Typically, the child's response behavior is conditioned to push a response button whenever a sound is perceived in soundfield or under insert earphones. The tangible reinforcement item is usually accompanied by an outburst of exaggerated secondary social approval reinforcement by the audiologist, the audiologist's assistant, and the parents or caretaker. Fulton, Gorzycki, and Hull (1975) reported success using the TROCA technique to assess hearing levels in young children. TROCA is useful with children between 2 and 4 years of age and generally requires more total testing time than traditional conditioning techniques. Lloyd, Spradlin, and Reid (1968) described success with TROCA, using edible positive reinforcement, with a group of developmentally delayed children. Although not a common technique for play conditioning as most clinics do not have TROCA audiometers, the TROCA technique might be best used with difficult-to-test children or those children with developmental delay or mental challenges.

PEDIATRIC SPEECH AUDIOMETRY

Pediatric audiologists use a hierarchy of hearing tests based on speech materials. After all, speech is the signal of interest to most young children, and they often react positively to speech stimuli in a way that helps audiologists gauge their ability to hear and understand. The simplest of the speech tests is the speech awareness threshold, followed by the speech reception threshold, and culminating with a variety of standardized test procedures to determine the understanding abilities of the child with hearing loss.

The most elementary of sound suite procedures is the speech awareness threshold (SAT), sometimes known as the speech detection threshold (SDT). Actually, this informal procedure establishes a minimal response level for awareness of speech. The awareness or detection level is recorded as the lowest decibel level at which the child makes any response or acknowledgement to the onset of speech through loudspeakers or insert earphones. During this procedure the child does nothing but listen; it is a matter of presenting speech stimuli slowly in 10 dB steps from below the child's hearing thresholds and noting exactly the decibel hearing level when the child indicates "awareness" as speech or tonal stimuli are presented. The SAT response can vary greatly from a surprise eye widening, or a head movement, or a slight head turn toward the speaker, or facial change when the stimulus signal is heard. The speech signal used is generally presented by live-voice and informally calls the child's name or gives a soft command to "look here" or the audiologists asks, "Where's mommy? (or daddy?)." The SAT is especially useful for patients too young to understand or repeat words or the mentally challenged or developmentally delayed. It may be the only behavioral measurement that can be made with these special needs populations. The SAT may also be used for patients who speak another language or who have impaired language function because of neurological insult. The SAT does not lend itself to a true bracketing procedure, but rather is more successful if the initial sounds are presented at subthreshold levels and increased in 5 dB steps until an awareness response is noted. The SAT is typically measured in the soundfield and reflects the level of hearing in the better ear.

Pediatric Speech Reception Threshold (SRT)

The speech reception threshold procedure is used with children as a quick estimate of hearing levels in each ear. The SRT can also be used to validate pure-tone thresholds because of a high correlation between the SRT and the average of pure-tone thresholds at 500, 1000, and 2000 Hz. In clinical practice, the SRT and three frequency average should be within 6 dB. This correlation holds true if hearing loss in the three measured frequencies is relatively similar. If one threshold within the three frequencies is significantly higher than the others, the SRT will usually be considerably better than the three-frequency average. Other clinical uses of the SRT include establishing the sound level to present suprathreshold measures and determining appropriate gain during hearing aid selection.

In our clinic, we may choose to obtain the SRT from a young child as our first procedure and as a means to "break the ice." The SRT is an easy test, it gives the child a chance to become comfortable in the sound room, and it teaches the concept of listening while developing a friendly relationship. Depending on the child's acceptance of the audiometric testing situation, we may quickly set the child up on the parent's lap, and disappear into the instrument room to begin the hearing evaluation of the 2- to 4-year-old with behavioral speech testing, seeking to establish a speech reception threshold (SRT) for each ear to obtain an initial impression of the hearing levels of the child. This is done because it incorporates the child immediately into the test activity, thereby reducing any apprehension the child has about the test environment. Although the SRT task can be accomplished easily with most 3- and 4-year-olds through insert earphones, we may start with the reluctant 2-year-old by speaking through the soundfield loudspeaker system to determine a binaural SRT. Once it has been shown that the 2- to 3-year-old can perform the required tasks, an attempt is made to replicate the activity with insert earphones so that an SRT can be established for each ear. Determining binaural SRTs should take no longer than 3 to 5 minutes.

In the test side of the sound-treated room, the armamentarium of the audiologist should include a carefully selected array of toys, the names of which approach spondaic principles as closely as possible. Spondaic words are two syllable words spoken with equal emphasis on each syllable (e.g., hot dog, baseball, ice cream). Spondees are used because they are easily understandable and recognizable to young children. However, to present children with easily recognizable toys, some compromise may be necessary. It is far more important for the child to know and recognize the toy than for the clinician to worry if the toy name conforms to the equal-stress-on-each-syllable principle. Typical "spondaic" toys might include an airplane, baseball, toothbrush, hot dog, cowboy, and fire truck. Suggestions for nonspondaic toys include a baby (small doll), kitty, doggie, horsie, car, and truck. We have found that toys from pet departments are more durable than variety store items.

Of course, all procedures utilizing toys and other test items in the sound suite must adhere to universal health precautions (e.g., prevention of bodily injury and transmission of infectious disease). Decontamination, cleaning, disinfection, and sterilization of repeat and multiple use toys and equipment must be conducted before reuse according to facility-specific infection control policies and procedures (Centers for Disease Control, 1988). For children with typical kindergarten or first-grade language skills, the Children's Spondee Word List can be used.

A favorite and familiar task for the young child is to point to body parts at softer and softer speech levels until threshold is reached. Direct the child through the soundfield system or ear phones to, "Show me your nose, Billie," followed by, "Show me your ears," "Show me your eyes," each spoken at a softer intensity level. Of course, our goal is to establish an accurate hearing level SRT for each ear, but this is a useful procedure for obtaining the child's cooperation in listening, performing appropriate responses, and accepting the authority of the pediatric audiologist without apprehension. The SRT speech audiometry task should be a light and fun experience for the child, and prepare him or her for the additional hearing test tasks to be conducted.

No more than four or five correctly identified toys need be used to determine the SRT for the 2- or 3-year-old; the 4- or 5-year-old can select from among six or eight items. Responses can be made orally or by picture pointing (Figure 6–8). Picture pointing is the choice if the child's speech production is difficult to understand. If picture cards are used, the audiologist should have the child point to each picture upon request prior to starting the test to be sure the child is familiar with the names of the pictured objects. The toys can be presented via picture boards, but it is much more interesting to the child if actual toys are involved. The actual toys may be wired to a perforated board; the parent should hold the board while the child responds with a pointing response. Sometimes, very confident and mature 3- to 4-year-olds will repeat the SRT words verbally back to the audiologist.

To conduct the measurement of the SRT, the speech circuit of the audiometer is set at 50 or 60 dB HL (or as high as necessary to be sure the child can hear instructions), and the audiologist begins the procedure by saying, "Hello there, Shelby. Can you hear me talking to you? Let's have some fun. Show me the airplane." When the child makes the correct response, social reinforcement with exaggerated praise should be given through the earphone or loudspeaker, and if the child can see you through the booth window, reinforce the correct response with a big smile, and enthusiastic hand-clapping that the child can view. Then begin the traditional bracketing procedure by descending in 10 dB steps, directing the child at each intensity level to identify a different toy. When the child no longer responds, the audiologist should ascend 5 dB steps but set the carrier phrase, "Show me . . . " at a 10 or 15 dB higher level and switch quickly to the

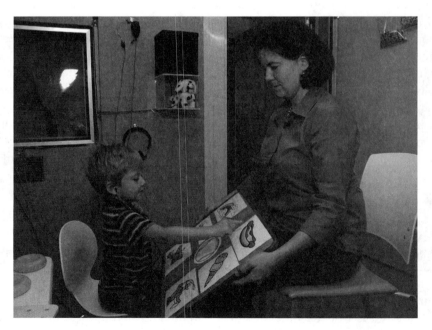

Figure 6–8. Establishing speech reception threshold (SRT) with a pediatric picture board. Photo courtesy of Colorado Children's Hospital, Aurora, CO.

lower level for the test word. Too long a silent period will lose the child, so when bracketing for the speech threshold, be sure that the louder carrier phrase should be given. Two valid responses on the ascending presentation should be accepted, and the SRT bracketing should then quickly switch to the opposite ear. Listening at low levels is not easy for a child, and one must work quickly for the sake of holding the child's attention. If discrepancies appear later, a recheck can always be easily and quickly done. It need hardly be said that the audiologist's mouth should not be visible to the child while saying the test words.

Under certain conditions it may be helpful to conduct the SRT procedure by directing the audiometer's speech circuit through the bone-oscillator placed on the forehead or mastoid of the child. This procedure might be used with a 2- to 4-year-old child who has bilateral ear canal atresia or microtia in order to determine the hearing status of the cochleas. However, it is difficult to know which ear is being tested by the speech audiometry bone-conduction technique, so masking the opposite ear through the insert earphone is necessary if the child will tolerate and respond appropriately. The bone-conduction SRT technique can be used without masking for the child with a unilateral conductive hearing loss as the Weber phenomenon will lateralize the bone-conducted speech to the involved ear.

SPEECH PERCEPTION TESTING

The purpose of evaluating speech perception in children is to determine a child's auditory recognition of words presented at conversational and suprathreshold levels. This type of testing is also referred to as word recognition, word discrimination testing, or speech intelligibility testing. According to Boothroyd (1991), speech perception is "the process by which a perceiver internally generates linguistic structures believed to correspond with those generated by a talker." This information is helpful to determine the extent to which hearing loss affects the ability to perceive, recognize, and discriminate speech stimuli. Speech intelligibility scores are useful in diagnosis of the hearing loss as well as predictive of habilitative prognosis with possible amplification devices (Diefendorf, 2011).

Evaluating speech perception in children is an area that continues to be developed with the advent of new test materials. As Olsen and Matkin (1979) point out that the selection of receptive vocabulary competency, the designation of an appropriate response task, and the utilization of reinforcement are primary factors that may affect the reliability and validity of pediatric measurements (Table 6–4). The results obtained during speech intelligibility measures may actually be more a reflection of the child's interest and motivation for the task than an accurate indication of higher auditory speech recognition abilities.

There is no standard technique or test of speech intelligibility in children. Although numerous tests have been developed over the years for this purpose, apparently none of them "fits the bill" well enough for all clinicians to agree generally on which is most suitable for clinical work. One major problem with most current speech perception procedures is that the database underlying the development of each test has not been standardized sufficiently to provide an evidence base with a broad spectrum of children of varying ages and backgrounds, and few implications can be generalized between children with normal hearing and children with hearing loss.

Table 6–4. Selected Pediatric Speech Audiometric Procedures

Test	Materials	Message set; response mode	Task domain	Minimum age (year)
SERT	30 environmental sounds (train, telephone)	Closed; picture identification	Unrestricted: 4 alternatives	3
ANT	Numbers 1 through 5	Closed; picture identification	Restricted: 5 alternatives	3
NU-CHIPS	50 monosyllabic words (food, school)	Closed; picture identification	Unrestricted: 4 alternatives	3
PSI	20 monosyllabic words (dog, spoon)	Closed; picture identification	Restricted: 5 alternatives	3
PSI	10 sentences, 2 syntactic constructions (Show me a bear brushing his teeth. A bear is brushing his teeth.)	Closed; picture identification	Restricted: 5 alternatives	3

Note: SERT, Sound Effects Recognition Test (Finitzo-Hieber, Gerling, Matkin, & Cherow-Skalka, 1980); *ANT,* Audio Numbers Test (Erber, 1980); *NU-CHIPS,* Northwestern University Children's Perception of Speech (Elliott & Katz, 1980); *PSI,* Pediatric Speech Intelligibility (Jerger, Hayes, & Jordon, 1980; Jerger, Jerger, & Lewis, 1981). From "Speech Audiometry," by S. Jerger, 1984: in J. Jerger, Ed., *Pediatric Audiology*, San Diego, CA: College-Hill Press.

Many children are too shy or inhibited to speak in the test room environment, and, of course, articulation problems are common in children, so it may be difficult for the audiologist to score speech perception tests as is done with adults. The most practical method of testing auditory perception in children has been to use some form of picture identification pointing response to a picture board. The child hears the test word and attempts to identify the correct picture representing the test word. If the young child does not hear the word correctly, there is a tendency for the child to guess at the correct picture, sometimes jumping between several pictures seeking a correct affirmation from the audiologist or parent.

Speech perception testing for children can be classified as open-message response testing or closed-response testing. Closed-response testing uses a picture-pointing technique and a picture board with photos of the test words. A number of important factors must be taken into consideration when assessing speech perception in children. These include a combination of child, task, tester, and environmental influences on test outcomes (Boothroyd, 2004). Child factors include the state of the child during testing, such as their attentiveness to the task. Moreover, children must demonstrate the requisite motor skills to perform the response task being asked of them (e.g., head turn, manipulation of objects, picture pointing, pushing a button), as well as the phonological, receptive, and expressive language skills needed to participate in speech perception testing. Tester and environmental factors include the audiologist's aptitude to work with the pediatric hearing-impaired population, the general feel of the facility, and caregiver attitudes and behaviors

(Eisenberg, Johnson, & Martinez, 2005). Jerger (1983) described two basic principles important in the history of speech testing in children: (a) basic vocabulary restriction in the selection of test material and (b) a limited response set definition. To these basic tenets she added two more important considerations necessary in pediatric speech test development and administration: (a) the need to control the influence of receptive language ability on test performance and (b) the need to consider the effect of extra-auditory (cognitive) factors on children's performance.

For nearly 50 years the most widely used speech perception test for children has been an open-ended set of stimulus words known as the Phonetically Balanced Kindergarten (PBK-50) word lists (Haskins, 1949). The PBK-50 word lists compiled for word-recognition testing with children were carefully phonetically balanced (PB). This term indicates that the phonetic composition of the lists is equivalent and representative of connected English discourse. The PBK is usually administered via live voice and is composed of three lists of phonetically balanced words selected from the spoken vocabulary of kindergartners. Thus, children younger than 5 years of age may not do well with the PBK-50 words because of limitations in their vocabulary. Olsen and Matkin (1979) recommend that clinicians use caution with the PBK-50 word lists unless there is relatively good assurance that the receptive vocabulary age of the youngster under evaluation approaches at least that of a kindergartner with normal hearing. Smith and Hodgson (1970) did show that tangible reinforcement (i.e., candies, toys, pennies) was an effective method of maintaining the interest of young children in the PBK-50 test. In fact, token reinforcement created significant improvement in speech discrim-

ination scores from children aged 4 through 8 years. Meyer and Pisoni (1999) concluded that young children and children with profound hearing loss may score poorly on the PBK test because the specific words used on the test are simply too difficult and not within the vocabulary of these children.

Another early pediatric speech perception test was the Discrimination by Identification of Pictures (DIP) test developed by Siegenthaler and Haspiel in 1966. Their test consists of 48 cards with two pictures on each card. One can quickly surmise that chance selection would produce fairly high scores, because only two choices are involved in each presentation. The investigators selected test words on the basis of contrasting acoustic dimensions rather than the traditional phonemic balance approach. The test was standardized on 295 normal-hearing children between the ages of 3 and 8 years and was administered at sensation levels of 0, 5, and 10 dB above the child's SRT.

Ross and Lerman (1970) developed a picture identification test for children with hearing loss known as the Word Intelligibility by Picture Identification (WIPI) test. They evaluated the test on 61 children 5 and 6 years old with hearing loss, and cautioned against use of the test with children younger than 5 years of age. The test consists of 25 picture plates with six pictures per plate used as test stimuli. The test is thus a closed-response set. Four of the six pictures per card have words that rhyme, and the other two words are used as distractors to decrease guessing. The lists are reported to have high reliability coefficients, and the tests are simple and rapid to administer.

Erber (1980) noted that the traditional speech perception tests developed for children are often inadequate for real diagnostic purposes or too difficult for children with severe hearing impairment. He developed a simple auditory test to determine whether a young child with hearing loss can perceive spectral aspects of speech or only gross temporal acoustic patterns. Known as the Auditory Numbers Test (ANT), this live-voice test requires the child to identify counted sequences and individual numbers. The ANT requires only that the child be able to count to five and be able to apply these number labels to sets of from one to five items. Picture cards are used that are color coded and depict groups of one to five ants with the corresponding numerals. Erber developed this simple test of speech perception for the rapid evaluation of young children with severe and profound hearing loss to aid in the planning of their auditory training and habilitation therapy programs.

The Northwestern University Children's Perception of Speech (NU-CHIPS) test developed by Elliott and Katz (1980) uses 50 monosyllabic words documented to be in the recognition vocabulary of normal children older than 3 years of age. The test includes 65 word pictures and interchanges 50 words as test items and foil items. Simple words, reflecting the most frequent phonemes of the English language, such as "food" and "school," are represented in a four-alternative picture set, and the child responds by picture pointing. In a review article regarding the effects of noise on perception of speech by children, Elliott (1982) pointed out that young children have poorer levels of performance than do adults when listening at low levels in quiet to words within their receptive vocabularies. For normal-hearing 3-year-olds to perform with nearly 100% accuracy on the NU-CHIPS test, the words had to be presented at levels more than 10 dB louder than the level at which 5-year-olds scored 100%, approximately 15 dB louder than the level at which 10-year-olds score 100%, and

nearly 25 dB louder than the level at which adults score 100%. Chermak, Pederson, and Bendel (1984) questioned the reliability of the NU-CHIPS when it is administered in a noise background.

Finitzo-Hieber et al. (1980) described the development and evaluation of a Sound Effects Recognition Test (SERT) for use in the pediatric audiologic evaluation. They point out that such a test may be the only available standardized measure of auditory discrimination in children with limited verbal abilities. The test is composed of three equivalent sets, with each containing 10 familiar environmental sounds (such as a dog barking, a toilet flushing, a mother singing, someone hammering, a cat meowing, and a baby crying). The authors indicated that the SERT is not intended to be a substitute for traditional word recognition tests but is expected to supplement them, especially for children with limited verbal abilities. By the age of 3 years a child should be able to identify 25 to 30 environmental test sounds; by the age of 5 years a child with normal hearing should be able to identify 29 of the 30 sounds.

Jerger et al. (1980) and Jerger et al. (1981) reported their use of realistic speech materials to control the receptive language factor in children by incorporating the actual responses of normal youngsters between the ages of 3 and 6 years in the Pediatric Speech Intelligibility (PSI) test. The normal children composed both monosyllabic word and sentence test items elicited by picture stimulus cards selected from lists of words and actions comprising children's early vocabularies. The PSI test is composed of 20 monosyllabic words and a 10-sentence procedure. The word lists include simple nouns such as "dog" and "spoon" and two types of sentence construction identified as Format I and Format II. An example of a Format II sentence is, "A bear is brushing his teeth." The different sentence formats represent the different speech patterns of normal children between 3 and 6 years of age. The test materials are applicable for children as young as 2.5 or 3 years old.

The Jerger group's approach to PSI test development documented information regarding the utilization of the test items in the presence of a competing message and the definition of performance-intensity functions for children of varying chronologic and receptive language age groups (Figures 6–9 and 6–10). Their results confirmed the ability of children to perform these tasks that were previously applied only to adults. They have focused attention on the importance of variables such as predetermination of receptive language ability and cognition skills, rather than considering only chronologic age.

A computer interface for scoring the PSI was developed at the House Ear Institute that computes both reaction time and accuracy scores for the PSI (Johnson et al., 2005). Mean reaction times increased systematically as the listening condition was made more difficult, even when accuracy of identification was close to ceiling. Thus, reaction time data may provide a window into the amount of effort it takes to achieve a given level of accuracy as listening conditions change from easy to difficult.

In general clinical application, in spite of the availability of a number of speech perception tests designed for use with young children, the live-voice presentation of the PBK-50 words is likely the most common in use. Many clinicians will shorten the list to 25 words, or maybe even 10 words, to shorten the procedure. Because the PBK-50 words are quite easy for children to repeat or identify, real-life application of the child's speech perception skills may

be questionable. Clearly the PBK-50s were not designed to be utilized in a shortened version. The NU-CHIPs is also a popular pediatric speech perception test, although again many clinicians shorten the original 50-word test to speed up the test. Use of live-voice allows increased flexibility with each test in terms of speed, time between word items, and so forth, but live-voice presentation of the words in these tests creates problems with test reliability when other audiologists might evaluate the child during subsequent visits. The PBK-50 and NU-CHIPs, as well as most of the other pediatric speech perception tests, are available in recorded format.

Pediatric Cochlear Implant Speech Perception Tests

With the advent of cochlear implants (CIs) and their success with young children with hearing loss, a need was identified for speech perception tests that could be used to evaluate the preimplant and postimplant status of speech recognition skills of pediatric patients. Accordingly, a number of word recognition tests were developed for children with severe and profound hearing loss who would, by definition, have extremely poor speech discrimination abilities (Figure 6–11). Decisions regarding the selection of candidates for cochlear implantation in young children require evaluation of speech perception that might lead to estimates of outcome predictions. In fact, there is an overwhelming amount of information on the large number of speech tests developed to assess speech perception in children with profound deafness as reviewed by Busby, Dettman, Altidis, Blarney, and Roberts (1990), Tyler (1993), and Plant and Spens (1995). Miyamoto and colleagues (1996, 1997)

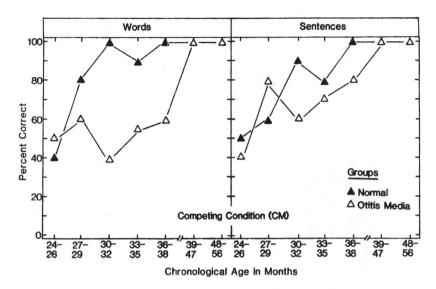

Figure 6–9. Data from the Pediatric Speech Intelligibility (PSI) test with a competing message condition for a group of normal-hearing children and a group of children with otitis media. Note the disparity between the two groups, shown with the word materials. Although the sentence materials also bring out perceptual differences between the two groups, the poorer performance by the otitis media group is especially evident with the word test. Courtesy of Susan Jerger, Baylor School of Medicine, Houston, Texas.

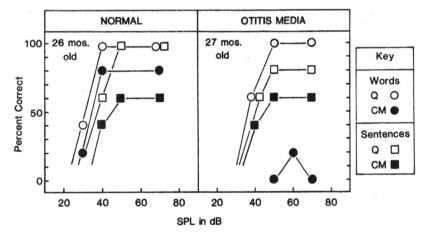

Figure 6–10. PSI data from two children of equivalent chronologic age and receptive language ability. PSI performance-intensity functions in quiet (Q) look quite similar between the two patients, but note the performance-intensity function for the child with otitis media when words are presented with a competing message (CM) background. Courtesy of Susan Jerger, Baylor School of Medicine, Houston, Texas.

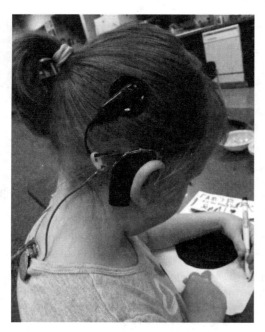

Figure 6–11. Special speech recognition tests have been developed for children with profound hearing loss and cochlear implants. Photo courtesy of H.O.P.E. Preschool, Spokane, WA.

published results from studies of the speech perception and speech production skills of children with cochlear implants. The availability of pediatric cochlear implant speech perception tests is impressive, and far too extensive to be discussed fully here. A brief overview of these special word recognition tests for children is presented below.

The Monosyllabic, Trochee, Spondee (MTS) test developed by Erber and Alencewicz (1972) consists of two presentations of 12 pictured words: four monosyllables, four trochees (two-syllable words with stress on the first syllable), and four spondees (two-syllable words with equal stress on each syllable). The pictures are placed in front of the child, who is asked to point to the correct picture requested by the examiner. Two scores are obtained that reflect the number of times the correct stress pattern

is recognized and the number of words correctly identified.

The Glendonald Auditory Screening Procedure (GASP) developed by Erber (1982) is a closed-set of 12 words and is similar to the MTS described above. The GASP uses three monosyllables, three trochees, three spondees, and three polysyllables as well as 10 common, everyday sentences, and a phoneme detection task.

The Early Speech Perception (ESP) Test was developed by Geers and Moog (1990) at the Central Institute for the Deaf to meet the needs of the very young child with profound hearing loss with limited vocabulary and language skills. The ESP is used for the 2-year-old or when the child is able to choose between two alternatives. The test is composed of three sections. Part I is a pattern perception subtest and two-word identification subtests; Part II is a 12-item spondee identification test with each word featuring a different vowel sound; Part III is a 12-item monosyllabic word identification test containing similar words. A low-verbal version of the test is the Four Choice Spondee subtest that includes four words represented by pictures or objects. Each word is presented three times in random order. The words commonly used are "baseball," "hot dog," "airplane," and "popcorn." Geers and Moog used the ESP to separate skills into categories: (a) no pattern perception, (b) consistent pattern perception, (c) inconsistent word identification, (d) consistent word identification, and (e) open-set word recognition. Performance is classified into one of four categories: detection, pattern perception, some word identification, and consistent word identification. The ESP assesses pattern perception, spondee identification, and monosyllable identification and is available in both a low verbal and standard version, based on the age and ability of the child.

The Test of Auditory Comprehension (Los Angeles County, 1980) is a closed-set, recorded test that evaluates perception of environmental sounds and speech. It has 10 subtests beginning with elementary differences between linguistic and nonlinguistic sounds, and proceeds to speech recognition within competing messages. The response mode requires the child to point to pictures.

The Minimal Auditory Capabilities Battery, widely known as the MAC (Owens, Kessler, Raggio, & Schubert, 1985), has 13 auditory tests and one speech-reading test to evaluate phonemic discrimination, sentence identification, suprasegmental features, environmental sounds, and visual enhancement with and without amplification. The test is rather demanding and cannot be used with young children.

The Lexical Neighborhood Test (LNT) and the Multisyllabic Lexical Neighborhood Test (MLNT) were developed to assess word recognition and lexical discrimination in children with hearing loss (Kirk, Pisoni, & Osberger, 1995). The words in each of the tests were selected from the vocabulary of children with profound deafness. The LNT contains two lists of "easy" and two lists of "hard" monosyllabic words; the MLNT contains one "easy" list and one "hard" list of two- and three-syllable words. The tests are in open-set response format and scored as the percentage of words correctly identified and as a function of verbal difficulty. The authors compared speech performance with the LNT and the MLNT with PB-K 50 words for a group of children with CIs. Results with the LNT and the MLNT showed better scores for the "easy" lists than obtained with the "hard" lists. Furthermore, word recognition by the children with CIs was significantly better on the lexically controlled lists than on the PB-K 50s suggesting that the PB-K 50 words were actually less familiar to the children than those of the LNT and the MLNT.

The Vowel Perception Test (Fryauf-Bertschy, Tyler, Kelsay, Gantz, and Woodworth, 1997) consists of five plates of four consonant-vowel-consonant words. On each plate the words are contrasted by medial vowel only (e.g., "bite," "boot," "boat," and "bat"). Each word is presented in the sound-only condition twice for a total of 40 test items.

Davidson, Geers, Blarney, Tobey, and Brenner (2011) conducted a longitudinal study of 112 children who received CIs between the ages of 2 and 5 years. This extensive study compared the performance of the children based on six different speech perception tests during their elementary school years (ages 8 and 9) with their performance during their high school years (ages 15 to 18). Their speech perception was measured in both optimal and demanding listening conditions (i.e., low-intensity levels and competing background noise conditions). Speech perception scores were compared based on age at test, lexical difficulty of stimuli, listening environment (optimal and demanding), input mode (visual and auditory-visual), and language age. The results showed that on average, children receiving CIs between 2 and 5 years of age exhibited significant improvement on tests of speech perception, lip-reading, speech production, and language skills measured between primary grades and adolescence. Evidence suggests that improvement in speech perception scores with age reflects increased spoken language level up to a language age of about 10 years. Speech perception performance significantly decreased with softer stimulus intensity level and with introduction of background noise.

For additional information regarding speech perception procedures and interpretations relative to children using cochlear implants, readers are referred to the comprehensive textbook written by Eisenberg (2009).

HEARING TESTING OF THE OLDER CHILD (5 YEARS AND OLDER)

By the age of 5 years and older, the child of normal intelligence can cooperate in the traditional and standard adult pure tone techniques and can repeat simple words. These youngsters will attend for fairly long periods of time to traditional hand-raising or button-pushing responses when they hear the test stimuli. Children of early school years still appreciate and benefit from praise and encouragement throughout the audiometric testing procedures. Beware of too much encouragement as the child may begin to give false responses in order to please. The pure tone audiometric technique that is chosen is a matter of preference, so long as it fulfills the requirements of the descending-ascending bracketing technique in the determination of hearing thresholds (Carhart & Jerger, 1959).

A method proposed by Berlin and Catlin (1965) has some advantages over traditional threshold bracketing procedures. The initial tone presentation is given at 0 dB HL and ascends in 10 dB steps until the level is reached at which the subject responds. Another signal is given at 5 dB above that level to confirm its validity, and then another presentation is given at 10 dB below the previous one. A second ascent is then made. If a response is given, the next tone is presented at 10 dB below that level, and the next tone ascends 5 dB. Two or three responses must be seen at "threshold." Advantages to this method are as follows: (a) it structures the bracketing of threshold; (b) it confirms the first response at a higher level; (c) it eliminates the taking of false responses as the threshold, by confirming the lowest response level through a 5 dB higher level; (d) it accustoms the child

immediately to listen for softer tones rather than louder tones; and (e) in the case of a functional hearing loss, it minimizes the "measuring stick" of the child by the presentation of lower hearing levels at the start.

The younger child in the 5- to 10-year age group may require some form of motivation to keep his or her attention on the test. This can usually be done by social approval (e.g., smiling, nodding the head, clapping the hands). The time spent in gaining rapport with this age child prior to beginning the hearing test is well worth the effort. The audiologist should talk to the child briefly about clothes, interests, toys, or activities, displaying a real interest in each youngster. During this time, useful observations are made about voice quality, articulation, extent of vocabulary, and degree of cooperation. The audiologist can then explain to the child exactly what is going to happen, telling the child what he or she is going to do—while carefully avoiding saying, "Will you do this for me?" It must also be explained to children that they need to raise their hand (or finger) or press the button even when the tone sounds very faint and far away. It should also be stressed to the young child to "listen hard for these little tiny sounds because they are a long way off."

The child and teenager between 10 and 16 years of age can be treated very much like an adult patient (Figure 6–12). Very few modifications of standard audiometric procedures are ever required for this age group. The development of rapport, the complete explanation of the test procedure, and the use of mild motivational techniques are usually sufficient for a valid test. If the clinician has been presented with an audiogram from elsewhere showing a 30 to 60 dB loss, yet the youngster responds perfectly well to soft speech levels, the audiologist should be prepared to conduct the hearing tests very carefully with concern for exaggerated hear-

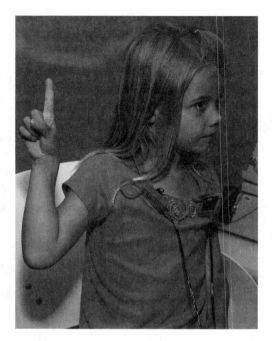

Figure 6–12. Testing the older school-aged child: "Raise your finger when you hear a tone—even if the tone is very, very soft." Photo courtesy of Colorado Children's Hospital, Aurora, CO.

ing loss responses. In this case, the testing should start with a slow, ascending presentation of both pure tones and speech stimuli. Time will be saved in arriving at an accurate understanding of the hearing problem.

The child with hearing loss may eagerly overrespond when no sound is actually heard in an attempt to appear to have more favorable hearing than really exists. It is best not to let such children see the audiologist during the test presentation. The child should face completely away from the clinician. Such children are so visually alert that they can catch even a raised eyebrow out of the corners of their eyes. During the test, there should occasionally be long periods of silence. If the child responds falsely, he or she should be gently reprimanded which is generally useful to counteract this enthusiastic response behavior.

At this and younger ages, the child has a right to understand what it means to have a hearing loss, providing the child has any receptive language at all. Too often, professionals tend to "talk over" the child to the parents, in words that the child does not understand. In the meantime, the child is sitting there, wondering what is wrong. The audiologist should take time to explain in words that the child can understand about the hearing loss, how severe it is, what are the common problems associated with it, and what is going to be done about it. Often the clinician's explanation of the problem will ease the way toward accepting the amplification and habilitation that will follow. Parents may be unable to explain these things to the child or may try to gloss over the facts, leaving the child bewildered and sometimes antagonistic. The child may be worried about what the other children will think and say in school. It should be explained that the hearing loss does create special problems but that the audiologist is going to be sure that the child can do everything "other kids" can do and that the child will now be able to hear friends, schoolmates, and the teacher better.

EVALUATING HEARING OF DIFFICULT-TO-TEST CHILDREN

The work of the pediatric audiologist would be so much simpler if all children were easy to test. But, alas, that is not to be the case. The difficult-to-test child is a child with special needs. The child's behavior or level of functioning may be so erratic that standard techniques of audiometry cannot be used. To apply appropriate tests for hearing, the pediatric audiologist must be able to recognize the dysfunction and to adjust the hearing tests to accommodate it. The classic disorders to be differentiated are the children with multiple handicaps, intellectual disability, brain injury, and pervasive developmental delay. More than one of these dysfunctions may be present in one child. In discussing the entities that must be recognized, it is necessary to reiterate an important fact, that is, cerebral dysfunction, central auditory disorders, mental retardation, and autism do not result in a decrease of auditory acuity as represented by the audiogram. At the very least, the audiologist has the responsibility of recognizing the disorder that exists, being able to apply the proper tests to complete the hearing evaluation, and making an appropriate referral for diagnosis and treatment of the disorder if needed.

The responses that can be elicited from the difficult-to-test child certainly require more ingenuity from the pediatric audiologist. The clinical audiologist's task is to choose the appropriate test procedures that will reveal the presence or absence of peripheral hearing loss and central auditory disorder. It is not always a simple task to make this distinction.

It is the audiologist's responsibility to inform and guide parents helping them reach decisions regarding their child's hearing abilities. It must, perforce, be a knowledgeable and tactful conversation without equivocation to be beneficial to family and the child. The conservative hearing aid trial with careful observations by all concerned during a diagnostic therapy period may be helpful. Consideration of a cochlear implant when appropriate should be discussed with the parents. Hesitation and undue delay in the decision-making process may deprive the child of critical time for learning auditory skills. There is little textbook information or standardized developmental scales available regarding techniques for evaluating the hearing response in these children with special needs. It is often useful to the audiologist to discuss the hearing potential of the difficult-to-test child with the parents and teachers who are with the child for long periods of time and who can, therefore, report accurately the auditory behaviors of the child.

Children With Multiple Handicaps

Children with multiple handicaps present difficult testing problems for the pediatric audiologist. By definition, profoundly multihandicapped children cannot function independently at the most basic skill levels including self-presentation, self-care, mobility, and communication (Baker, 1979). To be sure, children with multiple disabilities present themselves with handicaps that range between minimal or mild to severe. Of course it is possible to have a mild learning disability or a severe one, just as it is possible to have mild or severe autism, without a clear-cut diagnosis of intellectual disability. Multiple disabilities, by its very name, mean that an individual usually has more than one significant disability, such as movement difficulties, sensory loss, or a behavior or emotional disorder.

The greater the severity or impact on an individual, the greater likelihood for increased need for supports. Often, individuals with a severe disability require ongoing, extensive support in more than one major life activity in order to enjoy the quality of life available to people with fewer or no disabilities. Ongoing support may also be necessary to help individuals with severe or multiple disabilities to participate in integrated community settings.

In the 2002 to 2003 school years, the states reported to the U.S. Department of Education that they were providing services to 140,209 students with multiple disabilities (Twenty-Sixth Annual Report to Congress, U.S. Department of Education, 2006). Children with severe or multiple disabilities may exhibit a wide range of characteristics, depending on the combination and severity of disabilities, and the child's age. There are, however, some traits they may share, including limited speech or communication; difficulty in basic physical mobility; trouble generalizing skills from one situation to another; and a need for support in major life activities (e.g., domestic, leisure, community use, vocational). However, when viewed within the context of developmental theory, the child with multiple disabilities responds to the same stimulation parameters as the normal child of the same developmental age (Kamhi, 1982).

The evaluation of hearing in children with multiple disabilities requires the utmost in audiologic skills and application of the cross-check hearing test battery. The audiologist must observe the child's arrival in the sound suite and make initial judgments about the motor skills and possible response capabilities of the patient. It will be helpful to question the parents, caregivers, or hospital transport team about the child's communication skills, activities, motor control, and play preferences in determining how to proceed with the hearing test. Our experience is that you may often be surprised that the child can be more cooperative than you expect from your initial observations, so do not give up too soon or too easily. Although the ABR procedure may be required for definitive hearing assessment, the child with multiple disabilities cannot always be successfully tested with ABR because central nervous system damage and neurologic abnormalities often confound their problems. Accordingly, behavioral measurement of hearing must be included as a basic component of the auditory evaluation (Table 6–5). On occasion, the uncontrollable behavior of the child with multiple disabilities requires that the testing situation

be altered to accommodate and provide ample space for the involved child.

In the most severe and profound cases of multiple modality involvement (including blindness and major developmental delay), we have found it useful to rely on the simplest of behavioral commands, presented through the soundfield speaker system, of "sit down," "stand up," and observing nonintentional responses to the presence or sudden absence of sound. It may be possible to present various orienting stimuli to determine a speech awareness threshold (SAT) and visual reinforcement audiometry (VRA). Be prepared to observe quieting or listening behavior responses to specific novel stimuli presentations. With the less-involved child, slow and careful play conditioning may be possible. At the most rudimentary level, these response behaviors may suggest the presence of near-normal hearing, although the absence of consistent responses can, in no way, be interpreted as hearing loss.

Flexer and Gans (1982, 1985, 1986) studied the auditory responsiveness of children with profound multiple handicaps and supported the practice of determining auditory maturation function of these children in relation to their development age. These researchers noted that narrow bandwidth auditory signals are simply not as effective in eliciting responses from multihandicapped children as are broader bandwidth stimuli, including speech stimuli.

Accurate assessment of hearing level in children with developmental delay is crucial to optimize their rehabilitation, intervention, and follow-up. A comparative study of audiometric testing techniques with 61 moderately and 103 children with profoundly mental challenges at a large institution was conducted by Benham-Dunster and Dunster (1985). These clinicians compared behavioral observation responses with VRA, Sensitivity Prediction with the

Table 6–5. Suggestions for Audiologic Testing of the Multihandicapped Child

Concern	Adaptation
These children vary in their capabilities for selective attention	May need to reduce extraneous visual or auditory distraction to avoid "overload" (e.g., reduce demands for motoric or visual activity when eliciting auditory response)
State of arousal may vary during interaction	If child becomes lethargic, change in positioning may heighten arousal (e.g., rock from supine to sitting position); parent or teacher may suggest strategy
Child often requires more than the usual amount of response time	Careful pacing of stimulation to allow for latent responses
Interfering self-stimulatory behaviors	Provide alternative action; ask parent and teacher for input regarding methods for reducing these behaviors
Tactile defensiveness may affect interaction with examiner	Inquire and observe for incidence of this behavior; approach the child carefully if touch is nonreinforcing
VRA response requires many prerequisites that may not be in the child's repertoire	Note if the child has self-regulated looking, sufficient head-neck control, cognitive prerequisites; explore adaptive positioning (can the child lie on the floor and roll to a sound source? While in standing board, can the child shift eye gaze to light stimulus?) Are the visual and auditory stimuli reinforcing enough?
Child may exhibit subdued or noncharacteristic behavior in new environment	Observe the child in a natural setting (school or home) if possible; allow "visits" to the suite before testing; provide warm-up/exploration time and sufficient practice trials

Source: Adapted from *Sensory Organizational Issues: Multi-handicapped Child*, by M. R. Moeller, 1988, Omaha, NE: Boys Town National Institute, Coordinator for Aural Rehabilitation.

Acoustic Reflex (SPAR) test technique, and ABR. For ABR evaluation, sedation was required for 66% of moderately delayed and 91% of profoundly delayed children. The behavioral observation of auditory maturation was more reflective of developmental capabilities than of hearing loss, especially among the profoundly delayed. The acoustic reflex SPAR procedure overpredicted hearing loss and was problematic because of uncooperative behavior from the children.

The physiological audiology procedures described in the next chapter are the most likely to be successful for children with serious or multiple handicaps. Again, the crosscheck procedures are necessary to complete the hearing evaluation and to confirm normal hearing in these children or the presence of hearing loss. Some of these children will be so involved that success with any of the hearing test procedures will provide helpful information for the management of the child. The skill and experience of the pediatric audiologist will be fully called upon in meeting the challenge presented by the child with severe-to-profound multiple modality involvement. A thorough discussion of the audiological considerations of children with multiple modality involvement has been published by Diefendorf et al. (2011).

Children With Intellectual Disability (ID)

Intellectual disability (ID), once called mental retardation, is characterized by impaired cognitive functioning, below-average intelligence, and a lack of skills necessary for day-to-day living. People with intellectual disabilities can and do learn new skills, but they learn them more slowly. There are varying degrees of intellectual disability, from mild to profound. Children with intellectual disability have limitations in two general areas: (a) intellectual functioning, also known as IQ, which refers to an individual's ability to learn, reason, make decisions, and solve problems; and (b) adaptive behaviors that are skills necessary for day-to-day life, such as being able to communicate effectively, interact with others, and take care of oneself.

There are many different signs of intellectual disability in children. Signs may appear during infancy, or they may not be noticeable until a child reaches school age. It often depends on the severity of the disability. Some of the most common signs associated with intellectual disability include delayed motor development milestones, delayed speech and language development, slow to master personal care operatives such as toilet training, dressing, and feeding oneself, learning difficulties in problem solving or logical thinking, inability to connect actions with consequences, difficulties learning and remembering social skills, a lack of social inhibitions and behavior problems such as explosive tantrums. In children with severe or profound intellectual disability, there may be other health problems as well. These problems may include seizures, mental disorders, motor handicaps, vision problems, or hearing problems. The most common causes of ID are genetic, problems during pregnancy, problems during childbirth, or trauma or injury. Although there is no treatment for intellectual disability, many of these children will be on behavior control medications for mood stabilization or antipsychotics to help with behavior problems.

The key principle to be kept in mind when dealing with the children with severe developmental or intellectual limitations is that the child will behave in all areas at the level of his or her mental age. This principle will hold up in all cases except those in which autistic behavior or cerebral dysfunction is superimposed on the general retardation. Then the testing problem is further compounded, although not insoluble. Of course, this group of difficult-to-test children must absolutely be cross-checked with acoustic immittance measures, otoacoustic emissions tests, and auditory brainstem response (ABR). Dahle and McCollister (1983) summarized the procedures for evaluating children with ID. They point out that normal ABR tracings in this group of children give valuable information about their auditory peripheral sensitivity and degree of hearing loss. However, when the ABR is abnormal and ambiguous, no conclusions can be reached about the child's hearing status.

It is helpful to the audiologist to know what to expect when developmental scales or IQ test results are available prior to the child's hearing evaluation. The pediatric audiologist should be able to apply behavioral auditory tests (i.e., SAT, VRA or play conditioning) to meet the child's mental age. It is when the intellectual status is unknown that the clinician must be prepared and flexible in conducting the hearing test to match the child's behavior and skills. It may be that the only auditory responses available will be the early nonintentional behavioral responses. Accordingly, judgments about the child's hearing must be observed in the same manner as testing a normal-hearing baby of 4 to 6 months of age. The child with severe ID limitations will respond in the auditory maturation levels as described by Murphy (1962, 1979) in terms of localization development. One should expect auditory localization on a lateral plane by a mental age of 5 months; by 7 to 9 months of age, the child with ID should localize to the side and downward to find a sound source; and by 12 months, direct and brisk localization should be seen for sounds at all angles. If all behaviors are consistent for a certain age level and the auditory indices are within the normal limits listed for that age level, the hearing level is judged to be normal. These findings can be confirmed through acoustic immittance and otoacoustic emissions measurements.

Wilson, Folson, and Widen (1982) evaluated VRA in testing infants who had Down syndrome and reported poor success until the developmentally delayed infants reached at least 10 months equivalent age. Werner, Mancl, and Folsom (1996) reported success in testing the hearing of infants with Down syndrome using an observer-based procedure for babies as young as 2 months of age. Stein et al. (1987) evaluated 122 children with profound mental limitations from a single residential institution over a 4-year period. Most of the children were nonambulatory and had multiple handicapping conditions. The children ranged in age from infants to 18 years, with a mean age of 7.8 years. By definition, this group represented the most profoundly involved and generally described as untestable or difficult to test by behavioral audiometry. Stein et al. reported that 32% of the population showed hearing loss (by ABR testing) of 20 dB or greater in one or both ears, with 12% conductive loss and 20% sensorineural hearing loss; 8% of the study sample showed bilateral severe-to-profound hearing loss. Although the authors caution that the data reported are limited in generalization to the institutionalized profoundly retarded, this study confirms the presence of a high incidence of hearing loss in such populations. Six of nine children in this group were successfully fitted with hearing aids and appeared to benefit from the use of personal amplification.

A period of pretest observation will reveal to the aware audiologist what can be expected from these children. The child should be presented with toys and observed to see how familiar he or she is with them. Can the child hand them to the clinician on command? If the child recognizes most of the toys and can give them to someone on command, the audiologist can probably expect to obtain both a SRT and obtain play-conditioned hearing thresholds. Depending on the degree of accuracy required during the hearing test, the audiologist must be prepared to spend the necessary time to obtain accurate hearing thresholds by pursuing VRA, play conditioning (a low- and a high-frequency threshold in each ear may suffice), and ABR, when possible, should be conducted.

Children With Brain Injury

Brain injuries in children can be the result of a wide range of internal and external factors. A common cause is traumatic brain injury (TBI) following physical trauma or head injury from an outside source; acquired brain injury (ABI) is used to differentiate brain injuries occurring after birth from injury due to a disorder or congenital malady. Brain injuries often create impairments or disability which can vary greatly in severity. The likelihood of areas with permanent disability is great, including neurocognitive deficits, speech or movement problems, and mental handicap. The nature of the injury and the course of recovery is difficult to predict for any given child. With early diagnosis and ongoing therapeutic intervention, the severity of symptoms may decrease in varying degrees. Symptoms can vary greatly depending on the extent and location of the brain injury. Impairments in one or more areas (such as cognitive functioning, physical abilities, communication, or social/behavioral disruption) are common. Traumatic brain injury is the leading cause of disability and death in children and adolescents in the United States. According to the Centers for Disease Control and Prevention, the two age groups at greatest risk for TBI are age 0 to 4 and 15 to 19. Among those aged 0 to 19, an average of 62,000 children sustain brain injuries each year requiring hospitalization as a result of motor vehicle crashes, falls, sports injuries, physical abuse, and other causes.

A brain injury actually has a more devastating impact on a child than an injury of the same severity has on a mature adult. The cognitive impairments of children may not be immediately obvious after the injury but may become apparent as the child gets older and faces increased cognitive and social expectations for new learning and more complex, socially appropriate behavior. These delayed effects can create lifetime challenges for living and learning for children, their families, schools, and communities. Some children may have lifelong physical challenges. However, the greatest challenges many children with brain injury face are changes in their abilities to think, learn, and develop socially appropriate behaviors.

The presence of hearing loss in the child with brain injury is dependent upon the location and magnitude of the damage. Because there is such duplicity in the complex auditory pathways, hearing loss is not always a symptom of brain injury. Reduction in auditory sensitivity for pure tones, or decreased acuity for speech recognition, may be due to damage in the peripheral auditory system, not necessarily in the midbrain or higher pathways. Likewise, one can have normal peripheral hearing with impairments in the higher central pathways creating significant auditory processing problems. Only in the extremely severe centrally damaged child with gross motoric involvement will one see the complete absence of all of the four basic auditory reflexes: head turn, eye blink, startle response, and arousal from sleep.

The first guideline in testing such a child with brain injury is to determine the level of behavior through some means of informal pretesting. The audiologist should sit and talk quietly and play with the youngster in the sound room. Can the child attend for any length of time to anything that is said or done? Can the child give his or her name, age, or other appropriate information? Can the child hand the audiologist toys or repeat words on request? In the case of a very young child, as well as an older one, is eye contact steady and does it have integrity? Can the child sit still for any length of time? Is the child hyperactive? Does the child throw things around?

The child who has auditory perceptual dysfunction may be able to sit quietly and attend to visual stimuli but not be able to repeat words or to pick up objects on command. Such a child may, however, be perfectly able to participate in play-conditioned audiometry with pure tones and speech signals. If it is evident that formal testing techniques will not be successful, it is best to start at the lowest level of testing procedure, as has been described for infants. The entire battery of behavioral observations to controlled sound presentations should be made, from localization procedures to startle reactions. The child with brain injury may be inconsistent in responses to various stimuli and at various times. It is rare, however, for the entire array of behavioral auditory reflexive responses to be absent in these children. The basic and early auditory behavioral reflexive responses are mediated at the level of the brainstem and are usually intact in the presence of higher cortical dysfunction. Auditory reflexes only tell us about the integrity of the peripheral auditory system and the central auditory system through the brainstem. They tell us nothing about the higher orders of auditory perception and integration.

Only in the presence of degeneration of the brainstem at the olivary complex can the absence of the head turn and eye blink be expected. Even then the startle reflex, mediated at a low brainstem level, should be active, unless there is widespread motoric damage that prevents the muscular system from coordinating. Although the startle or eye-blink reflexes to a 65 dB HL voice signal do not eliminate the presence of a sensorineural loss, it is likely that the hearing loss is not of a degree that would produce the severe degree of symptoms found in a child with profound or total deafness. Tympanometry and otoacoustic emissions testing should be possible with this group of children, and acoustic reflex measurements, when present, may shed light on the level of brainstem injury. Success with ABR measurements may be limited and will depend on the location and extent of the brain injury. It is difficult to describe the auditory manifestations of children with brain injury as a homogeneous group because their symptoms and hearing differ widely as a function of location and degree of brain damage.

Children With Pervasive Developmental Disorders (PDDs)

Pervasive developmental disorders (PDDs) represent a range of severe developmental impairments manifested as extreme distortions in a child's socialization; delayed or disordered verbal and nonverbal communication; and rigid or stereotypical routines, interests, imaginative play, and sensory and motor behaviors (Wetherby, Prizant, & Hutchinson, 1998). The PPD classification may include five disorders: (a) pervasive developmental disorder not otherwise specified (PDD); (b) autism spectrum disorder (ASD); (c) Asperger syndrome; (d) Rett syndrome; and (e) childhood disintegrative disorder. The first three of these disorders are commonly included in the autism spectrum category; the last two disorders are much rarer and are not always included in the autism spectrum descriptions. Asperger disorder is an autism spectrum disorder (ASD) characterized by significant difficulties in social interaction and nonverbal communication, alongside restricted and repetitive patterns of behavior and interests. It differs from other autism spectrum disorders by its relative preservation of linguistic and cognitive development. Children with PDD vary widely in abilities, intelligence, and behaviors. Some children do not speak at all, others speak in limited phrases or conversations, and some have relatively normal language development. Repetitive play skills and limited social skills are generally evident. Of special interests to pediatric audiologists, children with PDD may demonstrate unusual or exaggerated responses to sensory information such as loud noises, unexpected or unfamiliar sights, sounds, and bright or moving lights.

Children within the autism spectrum may present mild, easy to deal with problems to the audiologist or more severe problems accompanied by bizarre behavior. Severely involved children with ASD may refuse to communicate, make eye contact, and demonstrate a tendency to shut off outside stimuli, stare with long-term fixation on some object, and refuse any physical contact with humans. They may inhibit responses to auditory sounds or show preference to attend only to specific sounds that they like. The child with ASD might ignore speech and pure tone signals through ear inserts or free field presentations and yet respond violently to novel or unexpected auditory stimuli. The audiologist might do well to ask the parent or caregiver, prior to the test situation, about specific sounds to which the child will attend or recognize or any specific sounds that will definitely disturb the child. There may be the heightened activity and they may physically strike out at the onset of certain sounds.

This child with ASD may consistently fail to attend to any speech stimulus, and yet will attend with awareness to other acoustic signals. One such child will localize to pure tone signals at low intensities, another will search or try to localize a novel sound or free field speech, and another may suddenly and unexpectedly localize to a white or a complex noise signal. All will startle or eye-blink to a 65 dB HL voice in a structured sound room situation if hearing is normal, although this procedure should be saved in reserve or used as the last test in case the child overreacts or becomes frightened. All the stimuli described for behavioral observation with infants should be tried when nothing else works. Some stimulus will likely produce a response if the hearing is normal, even if it is only a startle response.

Although the child with PPD presents more objectionable behaviors such as refusing to enter the sound suite, physically lashing out at the parents or the audiologist, screaming "no" or throwing the earphones or pulling out the insert phones, the test-

ing procedures described for children with intellectual disability and multiple modality disabilities are applicable with the child with ASD. It should be kept in mind that autistic symptoms are sometimes found in the deaf child. The cross-check principle is especially important in the evaluation of hearing in these children. The physiologic tests, such as ABR and immittance measurements, with special attention to acoustic reflex thresholds, are extremely valuable.

Downs, Schmidt, and Stephens (2005) conducted a study of the auditory behaviors of 106 children with PPD including 59 with ASD, 15 with Asperger disorder, and 13 with nonspecific PPD. Of importance, it is reported that the children with ASD responded well or better to speech than to nonspeech stimuli, and although they were sometimes difficult to test with behavioral audiometry, they were rarely impossible to test. Downs et al. recommend the use of the Children's Auditory Performance Scale, a parental interview format, to ascertain their child's listening habits. The most common parental complaint was that their child was bothered by loud sounds such as sirens, and environmental noises such as hair dryers. Most parents rated their child with PPD as having more listening difficulties than their peers. In their clinical approach, the Downs et al. group started each subject in a parent's lap rather than alone in a chair; utilized freefield loudspeaker presentations rather than earphones; established a speech awareness threshold, speech reception threshold, and pure tone thresholds using VRA. However, the report indicated that the audiologist choice of testing protocol was flexible depending on the child's mood, responsiveness, and parental suggestion.

The pediatric audiologist would do well to heed the suggestions from Davis and Stiegler (2005) who discuss effective audiological assessment of children with ASD. Among their advice is the recommendation to not give up too easily, or in their words, "A high level of persistence is a desirable component during the audiological assessment of children with ASD." The hearing test task may be better attempted in little steps across several trial periods separated by recesses during a single session or perhaps with multiple exposures to the clinic, the sound suite, and the audiologist, the child with ASD may become more familiar and comfortable with the various hearing test activities. Sensorineural hearing loss is not uncommon in this ASD population and conductive loss due to otitis media is a significant medical problem. Once again, this population of children with special needs deserves the very best audiological considerations possible.

Children With Deafness and Blindness

The descriptor deaf-blindness may seem initially as if the individual has total hearing loss and complete blindness. However, the term typically refers to a person who has some degree of loss in both vision and hearing. The amount of loss in either vision or hearing will vary from person to person. Our nation's special education law, the IDEA, defines "deaf-blindness" as "concomitant [simultaneous] hearing and visual impairments, the combination of which causes such severe communication and other developmental and educational needs that they cannot be accommodated in special education programs solely for children with deafness or children with blindness" [§300.8(c) (2)]. The National Consortium on Deaf-Blindness observes that the "key feature of deaf-blindness is that the combination of losses limits access to auditory and visual information." There are numerous causes of deaf-blindness including congenital problems such as maternal rubella, genetic syndromes, and so forth, as well as being acquired or developed later in life from accident, disease, or brain injury. Adventitiously deaf-blind individuals are born with both sight and hearing but lose some or all of these senses as a result of accident or illness such as Usher syndrome. Deaf-blindness is often accompanied by additional problems including cognitive disabilities or physical disabilities.

Deaf-blindness certainly limits an individual's natural opportunities to learn and communicate with others. Many children called deaf-blind have enough vision to be able to move about in their environments, recognize familiar people, or view sign language at close distances, and perhaps even read large print. Others have sufficient hearing to recognize familiar sounds, understand some speech, or develop speech themselves. The range of sensory impairments included in the term deaf-blindness is very broad. According to the 2007 National Deaf-Blind Child Count, more than 10,000 children under the age of 21 are deaf and blind.

The audiologic evaluation of a child with significant deafness and blindness may be among the most difficult tasks faced by the pediatric audiologist. These cases are often, but not always, confounded by central nervous system disorder and intellectual limitations that make it difficult to communicate with the child and structure the testing situation properly. For the young child who is profoundly deaf and totally blind, his or her experience of the world is likely extremely limited. Such children are effectively alone if no one is touching them because they cannot see or hear. Their concepts of the world depend upon what or whom they have had the opportunity to physically contact. Learning for them is extremely difficult. Pretest discussion with the parents or caregivers is mandatory to find out what auditory responses the child might have demonstrated so that the audiology testing approach might be most effectively conducted.

In severe cases of multiple modality involvement, we have found it most expedient to rely again on the auditory reflexive responses, behavioral orientation responses, and on quieting responses with the onset of sound. In the absence of speech and language, one must apply the tests as for the birth to 6-month-old infant, proceeding to the upper limits of the auditory abilities present including speech awareness threshold, speech reception threshold, and perhaps even play conditioning to ascertain hearing levels in each ear. Application of the cross-check principle using the independent measures of acoustic immittance including tympanometry and acoustic reflex measurement, otoacoustic emissions, and ABR will most likely be required with these children.

Stein, Ozdamar, and Schnabel (1981) published an excellent report on the neurologic handicaps, degree of hearing and visual disability, and the level of language and developmental characteristics of a young deaf-blind population. These authors reviewed data from 141 deaf-blind children evaluated at their clinic. Of these children seen for diagnostic hearing evaluation, 38 were found to have normal or near-normal hearing and, therefore, were technically not "deaf." The diagnosis of normal hearing in most of these difficult-to-test children was accomplished only through the use of the ABR technique. The previous diagnosis of deafness given these children was based largely on inaccurate behavioral testing. Stein et al. summarized the findings in their study as follows:

- A high incidence of neurologic handicapping conditions, including neuromuscular disorders, is associated with congenitally deaf-blind children.
- Severe hearing disability was more common than severe vision disability in this sample of deaf-blind children; 68% of the children studied had so little usable hearing that the potential benefit of wearable amplification was minimal at best.
- Many of the "deaf-blind" children referred for evaluation proved to have normal peripheral hearing without normal behavioral responses to sound. The use of the ABR as part of the audiologic evaluation is an absolute necessity with these children.
- The combination of hearing and visual problems together with neurologic handicapping conditions has a profound effect on the language level, cognitive skills, and general development of these children.
- The severe hearing loss and neurologic problems of these children will require that most, if not all, will need supervised care for the rest of their lives.

FUNCTIONAL HEARING LOSS IN CHILDREN

The pediatric audiologist will inevitably run into a child who responds as though a hearing loss is present when no problem really exists. This child is feigned a hearing loss for some consciously desired purpose. The child who makes a pretense of having a hearing loss is quite different from the malingering adult. The child is typically much less sophisticated with the deception of poor hearing than the adult. More importantly, the underlying motives and the impelling factor are usually more obscure. The needs that drive the child to give an inaccurate hearing test are probably more honest, and certainly engender more sympathy, than those that drive the adult. Furthermore, it is often the last thought for the audiologist that some cute youngster is actually exaggerating an existing hearing loss or pretending to have a hearing loss in one or both ears.

Any child who presents with a functional hearing loss has a problem, perhaps a minor transient difficulty or a deep-seated permanent issue, and likely has some sort of personal need that is not being met. Feigning a hearing loss by a child is commonly a displayed symptom of some other problem. It should never be disregarded or passed off as a temporary foible or just a mistake made by the child. It may represent a cry for attention, an apology for poor performance, or a rebuff to a hostile world.

Children who have some unfulfilled basic needs may choose from a variety of symptoms that are available to them, ranging from the conscious to the psychosomatic. They may complain of stomachaches, headaches, poor vision, poor hearing, or specific pains. They may act out their needs in aggressive behavior or withdrawal. Their symptoms may enter the psychosomatic realm, with disorders such as eczema or chronic stomach problems. Childhood psychosis may even be present. When their behavior becomes outwardly aggressive and approaches delinquency, their disturbance becomes a threat to their families and to society.

The majority of children who present to the pediatric audiologist in the clinic with such problems are referred because of failure on the hearing screening test in school. Johnny sees that Joe, who failed the hearing screening test, is given special treatment; Joe might be excused from school to have further examinations and is given special seating and attention in school. It is

like having headaches or stomachache, as it gives an excuse for poor performance and a chance to bid for sympathy. Be aware that this discussion of feigned hearing loss does not include those children who simply do not understand the instructions given them by the audiologist during the hearing test. However, this is also a primitive strategy used by the malingerer, so care should be taken to ensure that the child completely understands the directions.

The pediatric audiologist must be vigilant to recognize the child feigning hearing loss in the sound suite through exaggerated behaviors such as verbosity, brashness, withdrawal, lack of personal affect, exaggerated straining to hear the test tones, and inconsistent test-retest results. The quickest and most obvious clue is poor agreement between the pure tone average of thresholds at 500, 1000, and 2000 Hz and speech reception threshold (SRT). The naiveté of young children in responding at normal hearing levels to speech audiometry and exaggerated threshold levels with pure tones usually makes identification of the feigned hearing problem easy. Another common clue is wild audiometric threshold variation of 15 to 35 dB at the same test frequency. In the final analysis, otoacoustic emission tests, acoustic immittance, audiometric techniques, and ABR measurement may be required to reveal the true levels of hearing in these sometimes difficult-to-test children. Normal otoacoustic emissions and normal tympanograms and the presence of bilateral acoustic reflexes clearly rule out any possible conductive hearing problem. The ABR threshold exploration procedure can be used to validate hearing thresholds. It is rare that any of the classic auditory tests for functional hearing loss used with adults need to be used on children. Occasionally, in the case of a monaural feigned hearing loss, the Stenger test can be used to estimate the level of hearing in the supposedly "bad" ear (Stach, 1998). Most children feigning unilateral hearing loss are easily "caught" with the Stenger test.

Alpin and Rowson (1986, 1990) described a cohort of 30 children seen for psychological assessment following diagnosis of functional hearing loss. There were twice as many girls as boys in the sample. A large proportion of the children had experienced middle ear problems. Nine children showed serious educational delay. The children were assigned to one of three psychological problem groups depending on whether they had minor, school-based, or deeper, psychological problems. Those with deeper psychological problems tended to show greater hearing losses on pure tone audiometry. The authors concluded that functional hearing loss seemed to be related to attention factors in those with only minor or school-based problems, but not for those with deeper psychological problems.

Once the inconsistencies in the hearing test have been identified, hostility, threats, and demands from the audiologist or the family toward the child tend to make matters worse. When the child realizes that the audiologist is suspicious of the responses, "saving face" is an important step toward resolution of the problem. The use of statements such as, "Perhaps you didn't understand my instructions clearly," or "The results of this hearing test are not coming out correctly, and I would like you to listen again as carefully as you can" will be helpful in such situations. The audiologist should take his or her time in the presentation of pure tones and be prepared to wait. If normal hearing levels can be established through traditional behavioral techniques, time and effort are streamlined. The task is to establish ear- and frequency-specific thresholds. The challenge of identifying the malingering child is only half the problem —the true hearing in each ear still needs to be determined.

In terms of general management of the child with nonorganic hearing loss, it is best to discuss the situation with the parents or caregivers with perhaps a recommendation for referral to the professionals best trained to deal with abnormal behavior (Clark, 2002). The continuum of severity of emotional causes of nonorganic medical problems runs a gamut from mild, transient behaviors to severe malingering. Transient, isolated instances describe most children's attempts to feign hearing loss and, when resolved, usually cause no additional concerns. The cry for help that is inherent in the presentation of nonorganic hearing loss in a child should not be taken lightly or overlooked by the pediatric audiologist.

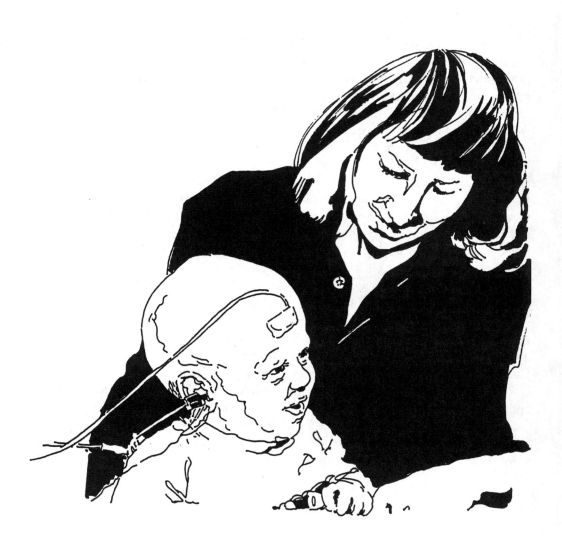

CHAPTER 7

Physiologic Hearing Tests

Nothing can be more frustrating to an audiologist than to work with a 2-year-old child who needs to have his or her hearing evaluated but who refuses to cooperate with any of the testing procedures. It seems impossible that the youngster who sat quietly and politely in the patient waiting area can suddenly turn into a crying, yelling, totally uncooperative subject in the sound-treated booth. What causes a child, who has been happily playing while waiting for his or her hearing test, to suddenly become an overly self-conscious, introverted, and unworkably shy patient? How does an audiologist establish rapport with a youngster who is hidden in mother's skirt or wrapped around father's leg? Every pediatric audiologist ultimately faces the child who cannot be tested. There are means of handling such children, but the skills necessary to evaluate the hearing in uncooperative children are gained through experience and insight.

One may expect the behavior of "normal" children occasionally to be obstinate. What about testing the hearing of a hyperactive, developmentally delayed child? How does one elicit cooperation and establish play-conditioning techniques with a youngster who displays autistic or emotionally disturbed behaviors? Play-conditioning techniques are obviously not possible with a child who will not even sit down. Just when the pediatric audiologist confidently thinks that every conceivable situation has occurred, a child shows up who baffles every hearing test approach. Audiologists continue to seek a simple and accurate objective hearing test that can be used with any uncooperative child, much like the early Spanish explorers continued to hunt for the Fountain of Youth. Almost no other aspect of audiology stimulates interest in the same manner as a new report describing a promising objective hearing test to solve problems associated with testing the hearing in difficult-to-test children.

To deal with these difficult-to-test patients, the field of audiology has worked long and hard in the development of "objective" tests of hearing. An objective hearing test is one that defines a patient's hearing ability without the patient's active participation in the test. A physiologic hearing test relies on an autonomic response not based on the child's behavioral action. In the case of children, many factors may influence or suppress the child's ability to cooperate. The child may not have the mental or physical capabilities to cooperate fully or to attend to the hearing test task required by the clinician. The child's interest span may be too short. An audiologist's success and skill in evaluating the hearing of these children often depends on the ability to establish rapport with the youngster and, at the same time, make an accurate evaluation of the child's capabilities in performing some task. A false start with these children may alienate them toward the testing situation, making additional test sessions necessary and possibly more difficult.

Many "objective" hearing tests, usually related to an autonomic physiologic response, have been suggested and reported. The Ewings of England in the early 1940s studied the "aural reflex responses" in infants described as eye blinks, squinting, involuntary jumping, and sound localization with body or head movements (Ewing & Ewing, 1944). Froeschels and Beebe (1946) evaluated the auropalpebral reflex, defined as the involuntary closing of eyelids due to acoustic stimulation in children and infants. Downs (1970) advocated use of the Moro startle reflex during infant hearing testing. Fortunately, our physiologic tests of hearing have progressed significantly since those early days.

New objective hearing tests are formulated with older children or cooperating adults, and these results are then generalized to young children. Somehow, the generalization those procedures that work well with adults should therefore also apply to children lacks credibility when the clinician comes face to face with a noncooperative 3-year-old. This chapter orients the student to a variety of physiologic, or as they are known by audiologists "objective," testing procedures commonly used in the pediatric audiology clinic. There are now complete textbooks devoted to each of the tests described in this chapter, so of course it is not necessary to describe every technical aspect of each physiologic test in the following discussions.

It needs to be made clear that the presence of some physiologic response, seemingly related to the presence of an auditory signal, does not ensure that the child does indeed "hear." Hearing, in this sense, implies meaningful interpretation of the sound so as to produce thought and language with verbal or nonverbal encoding and decoding. The challenge for a physiologic procedure to be used with children in the clinic is to prove itself to be reliable, quick, easy to administer, inexpensive, and worthwhile over a long period.

MANAGING TODDLERS FOR PHYSIOLOGIC HEARING TESTS

Most of the physiologic tests used with children require some degree of cooperation from the child in terms of remaining somewhat quiet and sitting relatively still until completion of the procedure. Unfortunately, the test booth environment often raises the young child's apprehensions and instills sufficient anxiety that the child does not want to enter or stay in the room. The enterprising pediatric audiologist anticipates these responses from the 12-month to 3-year-old and is ready to greet the child with an enticing toy in hand to take the child's mind off the strangeness of the room. It is surprising how quickly an appealing toy held out to the child can change the child's attitude from overt uncooperativeness to a smiling and cheerful disposition. There are no guarantees here, but more than likely this approach can help calm the fear of the unknown in the baby, toddler, and preschooler.

Depending on the physiologic test, it may be useful to arrange for an experienced assistant to help with the young child. It is difficult for one person to manipulate and operate the equipment while managing the child's behavior. The assistant should be kept appraised at all times as to the ongoing status and progress of the testing procedures so that he or she is aware of the remaining time needed to entertain the child. The assistant can judge when a new toy, game, or calming activity needs to be introduced to the child in terms of how much longer it will take to complete the physiologic test. Having the parent or caregiver on hand often helps calm the child, although sometimes the parents can be interfering if they take too active a role in trying to control the child. A baby or toddler may feel much more secure if actually seated in the lap of the parent during the test, while the assistant sits nearby to engage the child with a toy or activity.

The baby or toddler between the ages of 6 months and 24 months presents one of the most difficult periods in which to conduct physiologic audiometric tests. The children are not old enough to understand the test or to respond to verbal enticements, yet they are old enough to react (sometimes decisively) both to the test situation and to the insertion of a probe tip or attachment of electrodes. Often, light sleep may be the best condition in which to conduct the tests. If possible, at the time of scheduling the child, a recommendation can be made to the parent to keep the child awake as long as possible prior to the testing time, or to bring the child in at the child's nap time, so that the child arrives in a sleepy state. Sometimes providing feeding prior to the appointment when the child is tired will help the child to fall into a natural sleep in a darkened and quiet sound room.

If the child will not sleep, it may be effective to employ a distractive technique to redirect the youngster's attention from the activities of the test. The form of distraction is relatively unimportant so long as it is sufficiently novel to compel the infant to disregard the tester and remain calm and quiet. The external stimuli can be visual, tactile, auditory, or a combination of these. Frequently, the child may be comfortable and curious about the test and games are not necessary. In the case of acoustic immittance measurements or otoacoustic emissions testing, the tests can be completed before the child really has time to react or respond; however, at the first hint of rejection reaction from the child, the audiologists should be prepared to present a visual distraction. If habituation to one toy, game, or mode of distraction occurs, the audiologist must be prepared to introduce other diversionary tactics instantly. If the diversions fail, it may be possible to apply simple passive restraint of the child's body, head, or hands to complete the test. On the other hand, the audiologist should beware of a too-elaborate array of toys or gadgets because the child may want to play with the toys and not cooperate with the test procedures. It can be the case that the child has such a good time in the sound room that the child does not want to leave when the test session has been completed.

Children unable to cooperate with conventional audiometric techniques may not object to the immittance test battery if they can be focused on some diversionary activity for even a slight bit of time. The following are examples of the many possible distractive techniques that can be used with children younger than 3 years of age. The number and type of distractors, toys, games, and activities should be age appropriate and are limited only by the ingenuity of the responsible audiologist (Figure 7–1).

- *Animated toys.* Animated toys can be handed to the older child or displayed by the test assistant in front of the younger child. Movement by the child playing with the toy may interfere with the test and can be avoided by simply displaying the animated toy well out of the reach of the child.
- *Cotton ball or tissue.* A cotton ball can facilitate passive attention by balancing the cotton on the hand, arm, or knee of the child or on the hand of the assistant. It can be squeezed, blown, or allowed to fall repeatedly from one hand to

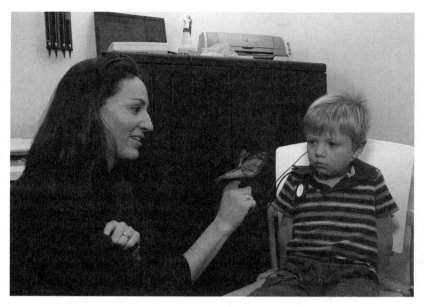

Figure 7–1. Distraction techniques are essential for diverting the attention of pediatric patients Photo courtesy of Colorado Children's Hospital, Aurora, CO.

the other or into the child's hand. A tissue can be used as a parachute, torn slowly into strips, rolled into small balls, and be placed in the child's hand, waved, and punctured. The back of the child's hand, arm, cheek, or leg can be brushed gently in a slow, even motion with a cotton swab or ball. The distraction can be made visual and tactile by making oscillatory or exaggerated movements of the cotton or tissue.

- *Hand puppets.* Hand or finger puppets can be very engaging to a young child. The puppets are soft, quiet, and colorful and may represent characters familiar to the child.

- *Pendulum.* Especially good with infants and young babies, using a bright and unusually shaped object make a pendulum with an 18-inch string. The pendulum is dangled in front of the child and swung around in various motions within the infant's vision.

- *Mirror.* To an infant around 12 months of age who is capable of reacting and attending to faces, a large mirror is sometimes irresistible.

- *Toys that produce sounds.* Toys or other devices that elicit loud sounds should be avoided. Toys that produce softer sounds or mellow music typically do not interfere with the physiologic test and can be used effectively to hold the child's attention.

- *Wristwatch.* In front of the child, simply remove one's wristwatch, pretend to put it on the child or parent's wrist; manipulate it slowly and well out of reach of the child to draw out the activity long enough until completion of the test.

- *Shoe.* Show unexpected attention to the child's shoe while talking about it. A simple yet effective technique is to begin lacing and unlacing a child's shoe. The clinician should move slowly and methodically and not appear to have any objective in mind except to dramatically lace and unlace the shoe.

- *Familiar action toys.* Superheroes, soldiers, dolls, or animals and other toys are available that perform repetitive wind-up actions.
- *Sticky tape.* One of the most effective child distractors is a roll of adhesive or paper surgical tape. Children cannot avoid the attraction of playing with sticky tape. Bits of tape can be torn off and stuck on various parts of the child's or examiner's anatomy. The child can be allowed to pull the tape off; objects can be picked up by tape or taped together with the adhesive side of the tape; fingers can be bound together; links can be made with small strips; rings can be formed, fingernails covered, and innumerable other totally nonmeaningful but time-consuming manipulations can be performed with a simple roll of tape.
- *Handheld computer games.* If possible, have the parents or caregivers encourage the child to play with their own computer-based games. This is especially useful for keeping the older child busy while testing is completed.
- *Videos.* Many pediatric sound booths are equipped with monitors that can be used to show animated cartoons or other interesting DVDs. The older child is especially vulnerable and attentive to video presentations.
- *Miscellaneous devices.* Childhood picture books, tongue blades, crayons and coloring books, colored yarn, pennies, marbles, blocks, remote controlled toys and the infamous Etch-a-Sketch can all be used as effective as distractive devices. They are best used when controlled, manipulated, or "played with" by the test assistant. If the child insists, he or she can be allowed to manipulate the toy or game, but care must be taken to permit only passive actions so as to reduce movement artifact while the physiologic test is proceeding.

There is no way to predict the behavior or reaction of children between 1 and 3 years of age. Their reaction to the test situation is influenced by past exposure to other tests, by past exposure to other health professionals, by their age, by their personalities, and by their general evaluation of what they see is about to happen to them. In many instances they are concerned about whether the procedure will be painful. For these reasons some general rules apply when testing children in this age group: the audiologist should never ask a child for permission to conduct the physiologic tests; it is way too easy for the child to respond with a bullish "No," which then requires the audiologist and parents to begin negotiating and pleading with the child to cooperate, thereby putting the child in control of the situation. Second, do not even bring up the word or the topic of "hurt"; the mere mention of the word brings the possibility of "hurt" to the child's mind. The audiologist should calmly assume that the test is going to be administered and proceed to do so; and third, avoid undue explanation to the child regarding the test procedure. Instructions to the child contribute nothing to the test results unless they help reduce physical movement. Besides, the baby or toddler would not understand explanations even if given. It is sufficient to say something like, "Here, listen to this," or "Hold still for me," or "Listen to this little radio," and then proceed with the test. Most often it is better to say nothing unless the child reacts to the placement of the headset or probe tips. Explanations usually take longer than the test itself.

For most children older than 3 years of age, no special distraction is required for the physiologic tests unless the child is particularly apprehensive in an unfamiliar clinical situation. Only a few children in this age category will demonstrate adverse reactions to the physiologic hearing testing. Where necessary, reduce the child's anxiety by saying simply, "We are going to test your hearing, so just hold still; this will just take a second or two," or some other friendly and uncomplicated statements of reassurance. Most 3-year-olds can be tested by a single audiologist. Allowing the child to observe other children or adults being tested may help allay fears or apprehensions. Perhaps an intriguing child's book will be sufficient to divert the child's attention at this age. Even with the child of 3 or older, remember the cardinal rule to refrain from asking permission to perform the test because too obvious distractive techniques may be viewed with suspicion by children 3 years or older. Children in this age category may be treated essentially as if they were school-aged, with occasional simple instructions or words encouragement.

On occasion, the pediatric audiologist must be willing to compromise the entire battery of tests with less than optimal information. Although it is desirable to complete the physiologic test battery whenever possible, with some difficult-to-manage children the audiologist may have to settle for otoacoustic emissions (OAEs), a quick tympanogram, and a single stapedial acoustic reflex measurement in each ear. Clinicians must be prepared to work rapidly and effi-

ciently; it happens, often almost unexpectedly, that a smooth, effective initial effort is often surprisingly successful.

The main limitation of our physiologic testing in young children is that the test battery cannot be completed while the youngster is vocalizing (i.e., speaking, crying, yelling, or making any combination of these unwanted noises). Acoustic stapedial reflex contraction and eustachian tube opening and closing during these vociferous vocalizations make immittance and OAE measurements nearly impossible. The pediatric audiologist's most challenging task is to find a way to distract the youngster in a way to stop, or at least to interrupt, the vocalizing for just the few necessary moments to obtain the required test data. Each clinician must devise his or her own techniques to momentarily distract the screaming child.

When the audiometric testing of the difficult-to-test child becomes problematic with questionable or limited test results, or because of behavior problems, it is an easy conclusion to turn to the array of "objective" physiologic audiology tests as a final answer. The evaluation of hearing in the developmentally delayed patient presents a most difficult task. Depending on the severity of the delay, many of these children do not condition well to pure tone play audiometry. They may not have sufficient maturation to perform auditory localization tasks or may even lack a consistent startle response. They may be too hyperactive to cooperate or too lethargic to be aware of changes in the environment. Jordan (1972) pointed out, however, that even a mild degree of hearing loss might have a disproportional impact on a child with developmental delay because he or she is less capable of compensating cerebrally with the aid of other senses. The challenge for the pediatric audiologist is to determine the hearing level in each ear and ensure that the middle ear function is normal.

Central nervous system damage in children often makes physiologic auditory responses unreliable. Yet, accurate assessment of hearing function or middle ear status of difficult-to-test children may be critical for educational placement or medical/surgical treatment. Sometimes even an OAE or tympanogram can be valuable, because the audiologist can then make reasonably accurate assumptions regarding the presence or absence of middle ear problems and the need for medical referral. Acoustic immittance and OAE measures are valuable in the evaluation of nonmobile children with severe developmental delay, who might be virtually impossible to test with any other testing procedure. These youngsters are certainly at high risk for developing chronic middle ear disease.

In summary, it can be stated that a prime requisite for pediatric audiologists confronted with a difficult youngster who appears impossible to test is professional confidence. Certainly confidence grows with each successful pediatric experience while recognizing that not every child is testable on his or her first visit. Persistence has its reward when working with children, so the audiologist should not give up easily if difficulty is encountered—a second, third, or fourth effort may yield important results. The pediatric audiologist, who manages each child with empathy, knowledge, skills, and with a matter-of-fact attitude of self-assurance, will often triumph.

ACOUSTIC IMMITTANCE MEASURES

Quite frankly, acoustic immittance measurements in children may be the pediatric audiologists' best clinical tool. Quick and easy to administer and interpret, the results can serve to help predict what can be expected during the audiometric testing or help confirm behavioral audiometric outcomes. Comparisons of audiograms and acoustic immittance measures are the basis of the cross-check principle so often referred to in this textbook. Although acoustic immittance measures are not actually hearing tests, per se, they identify normal middle ear physiology or confirm the presence of conductive hearing loss as well as provide diagnostic information about the status of the middle ear, and supply useful information about sensorineural hearing loss. Each test in the acoustic immittance battery used together and in conjunction with audiometric results contributes a huge component to the overall pediatric hearing evaluation. As James Jerger once stated, "I wonder how we ever got along without it."

The acoustic immittance testing techniques are especially well suited for children, because they are objective, accurate, quick, and easy to administer and with little or no discomfort to the child. Early publications by Brooks (1968, 1971), Jerger (1970), and Northern (1977, 1978b, 1981, 1988) validated the important benefits of acoustic immittance measures in children. Vast numbers of children have been tested with the immittance technique, and a wide variety of normative immittance test values are available.

Acoustic immittance measurement is an objective means of assessing the integrity and function of the peripheral auditory mechanism. Acoustic immittance, known in its early history as acoustic impedance, provides a number of important measures that can be used to evaluate and help diagnose a number of clinical otologic problems. The mechanic/acoustic middle ear system consists of anatomic structures that increase the force of the incoming sound wave vibrations to match the impedance and transfer the sound efficiently into the fluid medium of the cochlea. Under optimal conditions for hearing and sound transfer through the peripheral hearing mechanisms, little sound energy is reflected back from the tympanic membrane. However, under less favorable conditions of the external and middle ear, a greater portion of a delivered probe tone is reflected back into the ear canal. During immittance monitoring, some well-defined alterations are made, either an air pressure sweep (tympanometry) or presentations of stapedius reflex-eliciting stimuli (acoustic reflex measurements). The resulting probe tone reflections are compared with normal middle ear responses to such pressure sweeps or reflex stimuli. The resulting amplitude and phase of the reflected probe tone depend on the extent to which the different parts and properties of the middle ear contribute to the transfer or reflection of the particular sound (Lantz, Petrakk, & Prigge, 2004).

Immittance measurement results may be of importance to the physician who is unable to perform adequate otoscopic examination on a squirming youngster. The audiologist who has difficulty in establishing valid hearing thresholds on an uncooperative child can still get some idea of the child's middle ear status with immittance measures. Reviews on the use of immittance measurements in populations of special needs children, including those with hearing disabilities, the developmentally delayed, emotionally disturbed, the deaf-blind, those with cleft lip and palate, those with Down syndrome, and those with craniofacial disorders were published by Northern (1978b, 1980b, 1986, 1992).

The acoustic immittance (or impedance as it was then known) technique in the evaluation of the auditory mechanism was originally developed by Metz in 1946 and has been used routinely around the world since that time. North Americans, however, were slow to accept the clinical utility of this testing procedure until Alberti and Kristensen (1970) and Jerger (1970) independently utilized a new clinical instrument and published articles exalting immittance measurements as a valuable technique for assessing the nature of hearing loss. Acoustic immittance measurements are now an essential component in the evaluation of children's hearing.

The early impedance meters presented results in arbitrary compliance units ranging between 0 and 10. However, with the publication of the ANSI S3.39-1987 standard for acoustic immittance instruments, which recommended standard terminology and recording formats, equipment manufacturers changed over to quantitative physical measurements rather than arbitrary units. Immittance is a generic term that encompasses impedance, admittance, and their components.

The immittance of any mechanical system involves a complex relationship between three factors—the mass, friction, and stiffness of the system. Physical systems resist or facilitate the passage of energy through their components of stiffness, mass, and resistance. In the middle ear mechanical system, mass is represented primarily by the weight of the tympanic membrane and the three ossicles. The combined weight of the three ossicles, however, as is immediately obvious to one who has ever held the ossicles in his or her hand, constitutes very little mass. Friction in the middle ear is due primarily to the suspensory seven ligaments and two muscles that support the ossicular chain that hangs in the space of the middle ear. This intricate suspension of the ossicles in the middle ear, however, lends to ease of mobility; thus, friction as a factor in mechanical immittance constitutes meager influence in the immittance of the middle ear. The third element of immittance, stiffness, has a much more prominent role in the middle ear. The stiffness element has been identified as occurring at the footplate of the stapes, where a large resistant component must be overcome to move the fluids of the cochlear ducts. The middle ear system is dominated by stiffness, with little contribution from mass or resistance (Zwislocki, 1963).

Current immittance instruments automatically measure admittance through an immittance probe system inserted into the child's ear canal. An airtight seal is obtained in the child's ear with an appropriate sized soft rubber tip placed around a small probe. The probe is then inserted into the external auditory canal as shown in Figure 7–2. A stimulus tone is emitted from the probe, and an automated air pressure pump quickly sweeps smoothly through positive, atmospheric level and negative air pressure in the ear canal. The probe system also includes a microphone that measures the SPL of the probe tone in the canal cavity. Specifically, the SPL of the ambient probe signal is an indirect measure of the acoustic immittance of the middle ear system. The middle ear is a stiffness-dominated mechanical system that is sensitive to low-frequency tones. Thus, most electroacoustic immittance instruments use a low-frequency probe tone of 226 Hz. Some instruments have the capability to emit higher frequency probe tones, or to produce multifrequency measurements.

The immittance meter probe has three channels that serve to pass the probe tone, vary the air pressure, and measure the acoustic energy in the ear canal. Hunter and Margolis (2011) provide a clear description of the clinical immittance measurement system. The instrument measures the voltage that it takes to produce a constant sound pressure level (SPL) in the closed ear canal. As the ear canal is pressurized with air, it takes less voltage to produce the required SPL because some of the energy is reflected

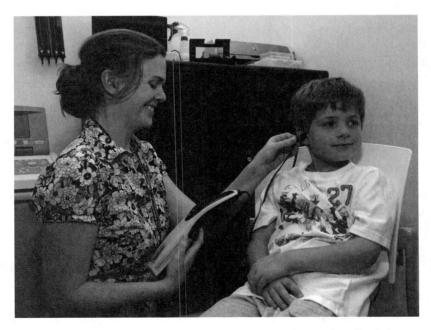

Figure 7–2. Immittance measures are an integral part of pediatric hearing tests. Photo courtesy of Colorado Children's Hospital, Aurora, CO.

from the stiffened tympanic membrane. Thus, when air pressure is high in the closed ear canal, the admittance is low. As the air pump changes toward the ambient air pressure, the admittance of the middle ear increases as the tympanic membrane becomes more mobile. The increase in flexibility of the tympanic membrane causes the voltage needed to maintain constant SPL in the enclosed ear cavity to increase until it reaches its maximum admittance (tympanogram peak pressure, TPP) that is approximately equal to the middle ear pressure. As the air pump decreases the enclosed air pressure below atmospheric pressure, the tympanic membrane stiffens again, thereby causing the voltage to maintain the constant SPL value to increase. It should be recognized that the "tails" at the positive and negative air pressures of the tympanogram represent the minimal admittance of the middle ear system.

The common immittance battery tests include tympanometry, middle ear pressure, the ear canal volume, and acoustic reflex threshold measurements. Although each of the test procedures can provide significant information, their diagnostic capabilities are strengthened when results from all three procedures are considered together as shown in Table 7–1.

For example, although tympanometry by itself is useful, interpretation of the physical volume measurement adds valuable information about the middle ear, and the threshold of the acoustic reflex, or the absence of the acoustic reflex, adds much to the final outcome decisions from the audiometric evaluation. An experienced audiologist should be able to administer the entire battery of tests, including acoustic reflex measures, in approximately 90 seconds per ear.

Audiologists using admittance measurements must follow three general rules:

Table 7–1. Summary of Immittance Measurements in Children

Tympanometry
Objectively measures tympanic membrane mobility
Measures middle ear pressure
Confirms patency of ventilation tubes in tympanic membrane
Estimate of static admittance
Static admittance
Differentiates middle ear fixation from ossicular disarticulation
Acoustic reflex threshold
Objectively measures cochlear pathology
Validates functional hearing loss
Validates conductive hearing loss
Aids in the differential diagnosis of conductive hearing loss
Provides objective inference of hearing sensitivity
Equivalent ear canal volume test
Identifies TM perforation
Validates ventilation tube patency

(a) recognize overall patterns in the tests of the immittance measurements battery, (b) pay little attention to the absolute value of any of the immittance test battery results, and (c) beware of the implicit diagnostic conclusions based only on the immittance test battery (Jerger & Hayes, 1980; Northern, 1996). Wiley and Fowler (1997) pointed out that audiograms and acoustic immittance measures can be used together to determine the cause of middle ear pathology, particularly when either measure alone does not provide adequate differential information. Similar conductive losses noted on audiograms may be differentiated by appropriate interpretations of acoustic immittance test results.

Tympanometry

Tympanometry is a dynamic and objective measurement of the acoustic immittance of the middle ear as a function of ear canal air pressure. For clinical purposes, acoustic admittance of the middle ear is determined by measuring the acoustic energy that is transmitted through the middle ear system. Clinical tympanometry is performed using a low probe tone frequency, usually 226 Hz, and measures the admittance as a function of ear canal air pressure. The result is a graphic display called a tympanogram. The low-frequency probe tone frequency used in tympanometry is sensitive to the stiffness dominated middle ear. The susceptance component (the stiffness element) contributes more to overall admittance than conductance (the frictional element).

The general term *tympanometry* refers to methods and techniques for measuring, recording, and evaluating changes in acoustic admittance created by systematic changes in air pressure contained within the external ear canal. Tympanometry varies air pressure changes ranging from positive (plus) 200 daPa to negative (minus) 400 daPa. Traditional parameters obtained from low-frequency tympanometry include static admittance (SA), tympanometric shapes and tympanometric peak pressure (TPP), ear canal volume (Veq), and tympanometric gradient or width (TW). Middle ear mobility is of particular interest, because almost any pathology located on or medial to the tympanic membrane will influence its movement.

Physicians typically identify children with middle ear effusions through visual and otoscopic examination. Physicians may not agree with each other as to what they see through the otoscope, as otoscopic diagnosis is a matter of experience, lighting, and visibility of the tympanic membrane. Although otologists teach that pneumatic otoscopy is absolutely necessary to identify the presence of middle ear effusion, not all physicians use the pneumatic otoscope. Tympanometry, however, is certainly more "objective" than the otolaryngologist's eye through an otoscope. The air pressures used in the tympanometry technique are very small compared with the heavy air pressures created with a pneumatic otoscope. Tympanic membranes noted to have normal mobility by pneumatic otoscopy examination can be shown to have abnormal mobility with tympanometry.

Otoscopy is most often accepted as the criterion test against which to compare tympanometry, although the accuracy of otoscopy varies as a function of the person behind the otoscope (Paradise, Smith, & Bluestone, 1976; Roeser, Glorig, Gerken, & Kessinger, 1977). Physicians, of course, regard pneumatic otoscopy as the primary diagnostic method for middle ear examination. However, a child's resistance to examination or the presence of cerumen that obscures the tympanic membrane may make accurate diagnosis a considerable challenge, especially in a busy office setting, in children younger than 2 years. Even when the tympanic membrane is readily visualized, findings that distinguish the diseased from the effusion-free middle ear can often be subtle (Chianese et al., 2007). Otoscopy is so subjective that it can be argued that tympanometry should be the criterion procedure because of its objectivity and test-retest reliability. Generally, the use of otoscopy as the criterion produces higher sensitivity agreement, because fewer subjects "fail" otoscopy, while many subjects may "fail" screening. The sensitivity score with tympanometry using otoscopy as the criterion measure approximately 95% with a low specificity value of about 50%. The amount of pathology in the sample population affects the sensitivity rate in research studies, because it is easy to obtain high agreement between tympanometry and otoscopy when many normal subjects are examined. The low specificity rate of immittance audiometry is likely due to the use of a too-rigid failure criterion for peaked negative pressure curves. Adherence to middle ear pressure failure criterion of −250 daPa or greater would possibly alleviate the overreferral and low-specificity problems.

The ultimate validation technique for middle ear effusion is myringotomy (surgical incision of the tympanic membrane). Studies reported by Orchik, Dunn, and McNutt (1978a) and Orchik, Morff, and Dunn (1978b) comparing acoustic immittance measures and myringotomy have shown that the combined use of tympanometry and acoustic reflex measurement showed a statistically significant correlation with the presence of middle ear fluid. The studies showed the correlation between "flat" or wide tympanometry curves, and the presence of effusion proven by myringotomy is high at 82% to 90% accurate.

The static admittance (height or TPP) of the tympanic membrane is at its maximum when air pressures on both sides of the eardrum are equal. That is, the eardrum is most mobile when the air pressure in the external auditory canal is the same as the air pressure in the middle ear as shown in Figure 7–3. Tympanometry can thereby provide an indirect measure of middle ear pressure through the determination of the air pressure in the external auditory canal at which the eardrum shows maximum mobility (low admittance). Animal research has shown the accuracy of tympanometric measurement of middle ear pressure to be within plus or minus 15 daPa of the actual middle ear pressure (Eliachar, Sando, & Northern, 1974).

Middle ear pressure is important clinical information. When the process of aeration in the middle ear is halted, as in closure of the eustachian tube, the static air in the middle ear space is absorbed in the mucosal lining. This situation produces negative air pressure in the middle ear space, causing transudation of fluid and retraction of the tympanic membrane. If the aeration process of the middle ear cavity is blocked for

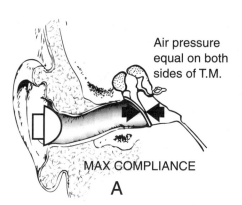

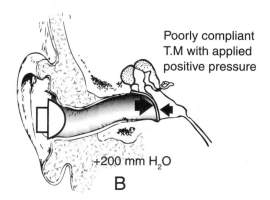

Figure 7–3. The mobility of the tympanic membrane is at its maximum when air pressure is equal on both sides of the tympanic membrane (TPP). When the air pressure on either side of the eardrum is unequal, the tympanic membrane does not move well (low admittance) and is often associated with conductive-type hearing loss.

an extended period, serous (noninfected) fluid may totally fill the middle ear space and ultimately become infected. Bluestone, Beery, and Paradise (1973) indicated that use of the middle ear pressure value is an effective tool to evaluate eustachian tube function but that it should not be used as a medical referral criterion because of its transient nature and the large variability of normal values which create unnecessary medical office visits.

The presence of unequal pressures on either side of the tympanic membrane typically occurs when negative pressure develops in the middle ear space due to eustachian tube dysfunction. This may be sufficient to cause a retraction of the eardrum accompanied by mild conductive hearing loss, although no fluid may be observed in the patient's middle ear. The most explicit example of this occurs when air pressures are changed in the passenger cabins of commercial aircraft. Passengers will first experience mild ear discomfort as the air pressure in the cabin is changed, thus creating a positive ear canal pressure relative to the passenger's middle ear air pressure. When the passenger forces open the eustachian tube to alleviate this discomfort (i.e., to equalize the pressure on both sides of the eardrum), the environmental sounds in the aircraft become suddenly louder along with relief of the mild ear discomfort. This is a practical explanation of the numbers of children who have negative middle ear pressure as noted by tympanometry, accompanied by mild conductive hearing loss.

Jerger (1970) described a simple system of basic tympanogram patterns and related them to conditions of the middle ear. Jerger's classification system of tympanometry curves is summarized in Figure 7–4. For simplicity, Jerger ascribed alphabetical letters to each type of curve. This classification is convenient, but it may be more explicit to describe each tympanogram in terms of its gradient (or width) and the air pressure at which maximal static admittance (or middle ear pressure) is noted. A drawback to the use of such categories to classify tympanograms is that there are no specific definitions to fit the curves, and the clinician inevitably comes across a tympanogram that does not clearly fit into one of the expected categories.

Type A. The Type A tympanogram is noted with normal middle ear function. The curve shows adequate static admittance and normal middle ear pressure at the point of maximal height. Some question exists concerning the limits of normal middle ear pressure values which can vary from 0 daPa to −250 daPa. Decisions regarding "limits of normal" in terms of middle ear pressure may depend on the clinical situation and circumstances.

Type A_s. This tympanogram shape is characterized by normal middle ear pressure and less than normal static admittance (height). This curve may be seen in cases of ossicular abnormality or fixation, thickened or heavily scarred tympanic membranes, with severe tympanosclerosis. The normal tympanogram width ranges between 80 and 160 daPa for children 3 to 10 years of age.

Type A_D. This tympanometic curve, also with normal middle ear pressure, represents a large change in static admittance with small changes of air pressure. The A_D curve is suggestive of middle ears with discontinuity of the ossicular chain or an extremely flaccid eardrum

Type B. The type B tympanogram is characterized by little or no change in the admittance of the middle ear as air pressure in the external ear canal is varied as low as −400 daPa. Described as a flat or very wide tympanogram, this function is seen in patients with serous and adhesive otitis media, perforations, patent ventilation

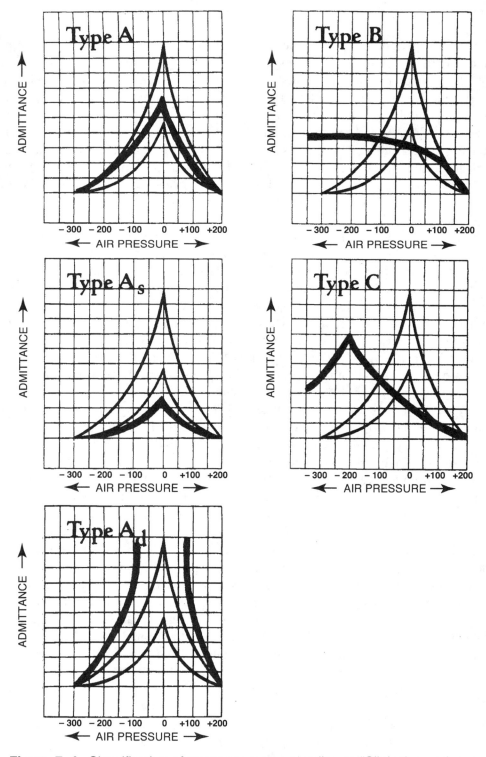

Figure 7–4. Classification of tympanograms according to "Clinical experience with impedance audiometry," by J. Jerger, 1970, *Archives of Otolaryngology, 92*, pp. 311–324. See text for clinical significance of each type of tympanogram.

tubes, and some cases of congenital middle ear malformations.

Type C. This classification of tympanogram shows near-normal static admittance (height) and middle ear pressure of −250 mm daPa or worse. This curve may or may not be related to the presence of fluid in the middle ear, but it infers poor eustachian tube function. In fact, Bluestone et al. (1973), as well as Paradise et al. (1976), reported a low incidence of middle ear effusion in a large sample of children with type C tympanograms upon whom they performed myringotomy.

Tympanometry evaluation is a useful technique to monitor the progression and resolution of serous otitis media in children. Figure 7–5 shows hypothetical results from a child who demonstrates a type A tympanogram under normal healthy conditions. As the otologic disease process begins with a closed eustachian tube, negative pressure is created in the middle ear space which retracts the eardrum and produces a type C tympanogram. As fluid develops in the middle ear, the admittance of the eardrum is decreased, resulting in wide (flat) or type B. Finally, the normal type A tympanogram is recorded when the middle ear is back in its healthy condition.

Brooks (1968) was the first to describe tympanograms in terms of "gradient." An alternative descriptor of tympanograms was suggested by Paradise and Smith (1976) who proposed describing tympanograms by use of width and gradient. Gradient is defined as the distance in dekapascals (daPa) between the sides of the tympanogram at one half of the peak admittance. Thus, the gradient measure takes into account both the height and width of the tympanogram. There is a viewpoint that the describing tympanograms by gradient and width provide a more scientific description than the traditional Jerger alphabetical classification system. Tompkins and Hall (1990) studied tympanograms in a large group of children and found no clinical significant difference in the detection of otitis media in children when the gradient measure was calculated and compared with conventional tympanometry analysis. They reported that flat tympanograms (type B) have no real gradient, and the pattern is most likely associated with otitis media. Nozza (1995) and Roush, Bryant, Mundy, Zeisel, and Roberts (1995) concluded in their studies that tympanogram width is the single best measure for separating middle ears with fluid from middle ears without fluid in children. But Hall & Swanepoel (2010) concluded that the gradient measure itself does not offer any compelling advantage in interpreting tympanograms.

An extensive study of the accuracy of tympanometry to identify middle ear effusion in children under the age of 3 years was reported by Smith et al. (2006). They compared the tympanometric and otoscopic findings of 3,686 children under 36 months of age. In their analysis, they derived an algorithm for children that predict the probability of middle ear effusion based on any combination of individual values for tympanometric height, pressure, and width. More to our purposes, however, Smith et al. concluded that normally shaped tympanograms have a high probability that middle ear effusion is not present and that flat tympanograms are likely to be associated with middle ear effusion.

In Finland, Helenius, Laine, Tähtinen, Laht, and Ruohola (2012) enrolled and followed 515 children aged 6 to 35 months at primary care level through 2,206 symptomatic visits and 1,006 asymptomatic follow-up visits with tympanometry and pneumatic otoscopy. Tympanometry was

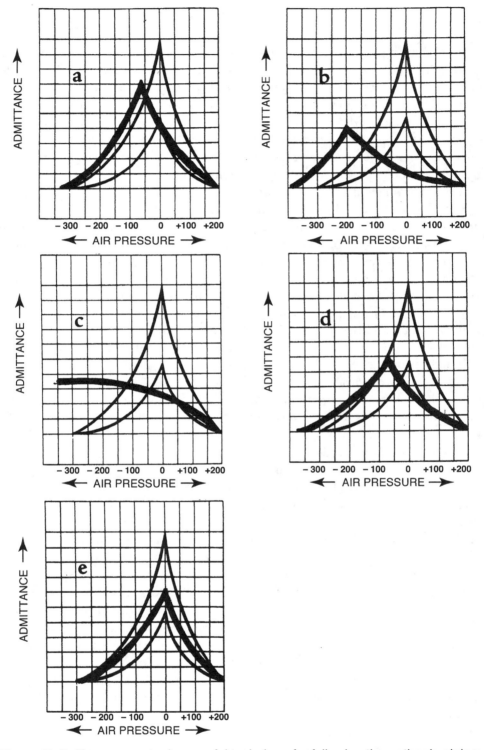

Figure 7–5. Tympanometry is a useful technique for following the pathophysiology of a middle ear effusion: **A.** A near-normal tympanogram. **B.** Negative middle ear pressure and reduced compliance often accompany an upper respiratory problem. **C.** Middle ear effusion. **D.** Improved compliance due to reduced negative middle ear pressure. **E.** Return of the middle ear to its proper normal control condition.

not helpful in detecting specific otoscopic diagnoses because it did not distinguish between otitis media with effusion and acute otitis media. However, all peaked tympanograms suggested a healthy middle ear, and a flat tympanogram was consistently useful in detecting any middle ear effusion. Thus, they concluded that tympanometry is a useful adjunctive tool, but accurate otologic diagnosis requires careful pneumatic otoscopy.

Another area of research in the arena of attempting to make tympanometry more accurate in identifying middle ear pathology has been the utilization of multifrequency and multicomponent probe tones. Multiple-frequency tympanometry is a method in which the probe tone is swept through a series of frequencies (e.g., from 250 to 2000 Hz; Hunter & Margolis, 1992). Researchers using these complex probe tones have concluded that multifrequency and multicomponent tympanogram techniques do in fact identify more accurately in high admittance pathologies of the tympanic membrane and ossicular chain. Critics of single probe tone tympanometry argue that tympanometry, per se, does not accurately identify middle ear pathology. That point of view is correct, resulting in the obligation to perform an immittance test battery in children to include equivalent ear volume and acoustic reflex tests prior to reaching any diagnostic conclusions. In spite of nearly 30 years of research with multifrequency and multicomponent probe tones, the overwhelming majority of pediatric audiologists still conduct tympanometry with the single low-frequency probe tone. Hall and Swanepoel (2010) attribute this fact to the simplicity of the technique and interpretation of results which contribute to the high clinical acumen of the single-frequency probe tone immittance battery, along with pure tone audiometry, to apparently meet the diagnostic needs of the pediatric audiologist.

Negative middle ear pressure may elevate hearing thresholds, thereby creating hearing loss. Cooper, Langley, Meyerhoff, and Gates (1977) examined 1,133 children with middle ear pressures between −150 and −400 daPa and found hearing thresholds to be elevated as much as 25 dB with severe negative middle ear pressure. They suggested that an orderly relationship exists between the degrees of negative middle ear pressure and hearing threshold shift (i.e., an 8 dB change in hearing thresholds in the speech frequency range with a middle ear pressure of −100 daPa to at least a 20 dB shift or more when middle ear pressure is −400 daPa).

Paradise (1982) published a retrospective review of tympanometry which stands true today in which he suggested that tympanometry has three major useful clinical purposes for physicians: (a) tympanometry separates infants and children into two subgroups, those with suspected or nearly certain middle ear disease who require careful examination and treatment and those who are virtually certain to be free of middle ear disorders; (b) tympanometry refines and clarifies questionable otoscopic diagnoses; and (c) tympanometry objectifies the follow-up evaluations of pediatric patients with diagnosed middle ear disease.

Static Admittance

Static admittance is a measure of middle ear mobility that represents the transmission of energy through tympanic membrane and the middle ear in its resting state (AAA, 2011a). When the tympanogram is completed, the static or resting admittance is determined automatically through subtraction of the compliance value obtained at 200 daPa from the compliance value determined at the tympanometric peak (TPP). Obviously, low static admittance values are associated with poor middle ear mobility. Roush et al. (1995) studied static admittance in 3-year-old children with normal tympanograms and established normal values to be within the range of 0.2 and 0.7 mmhos. The contribution of the static admittance measurement to the immittance test battery has limited use because of the wide variability and overlapping values specific to pathologies of the ear. Jerger et al. (1974) found the static measure to be the least informative test of the immittance battery in children younger than 6 years of age. Stach and Jerger (1990) stated that the usefulness of static admittance is limited to differentiate only between normal and extreme pathologic conditions. The static admittance measure can be used to support and confirm the other measurements in the immittance test battery but is often not reported in pediatric immittance measurements, nor considered a vital component of the immittance test battery.

Equivalent Ear Canal Volume (Veq)

Information about the relative cavity size of the ear canal medial to the probe tip can be quite important to the audiologist. This measurement is known as the equivalent ear canal volume (Veq) and is measured in cubic centimeters (cm^3). The acoustic immittance instrumentation relies on the physical principle that the intensity of a sound in a closed cavity is a direct function of the cavity size. Thus, a signal of fixed intensity introduced into a large cavity and into a small cavity will produce different SPL values in each cavity. The larger cavity will have a lower SPL, the smaller cavity will have a higher SPL, and thus the immittance instrument must increase the voltage delivered to the probe tube to maintain a con-

stant SPL when the sealed ear canal volume also includes an opening to the middle ear space. The middle ear space will contribute a larger space to the equivalent ear canal volume measurement when the tympanic membrane is perforated or contains a patent ventilating tube as shown in Figure 7–6.

In the presence of an intact eardrum, the typical enclosed ear canal cavity between the probe tip and the tympanic membrane

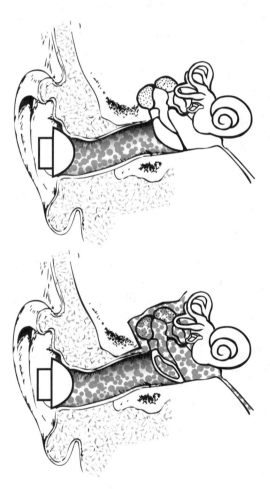

Figure 7–6. Measurement of equivalent ear canal volume (Veq). *Top:* Volume between probe tip and intact eardrum. *Bottom:* Larger Veq measurement when eardrum is perforated or has a patent ventilating tube in place.

in children between 1 and 7 years of age is between 0.3 and 0.9 cm³ (5th and 95th percentile). In infants the normal Veq value may be as low as 0.3 cc³. This value may vary depending on how far the probe tip cuff is inserted into the ear canal or the diameter of the external canal. Equivalent ear canal volume is a routine component of most current commercially available immittance instruments.

When the ear canal equivalent volume is considerably greater than the expected norms values in light of a hermetically sealed probe tip and cuff, the audiologist can reasonably assume that the "cavity" includes the external ear canal, middle ear space, and possibly even the mastoid air cells and entrance to the eustachian tube orifice. In circumstances of a nonintact tympanic membrane (TM perforation or with tympanostomy tube in place), the Veq value may be three or four times greater than normal volume values, 1.0 and 5.5 cc³ (5th and 95th percentile) according to ASHA (1990). The Veq measurement has been useful to otologists in forecasting the presence of a hidden perforation behind an exaggerated anterior external ear canal wall overhang or beneath an adherent crust on the eardrum. The Veq can be used to identify obstruction of ventilation tubes and blind attic retraction pocket perforations.

Knowledge of the equivalent ear canal volume will help clarify the etiology responsible for flat or type B tympanograms: (a) nonmobile tympanic membranes with volumes larger than 2.0 cc³ children are usually indicative of a perforation or patent ventilation tube; (b) flat or type B tympanograms with a normal volume measurement are indicative of an intact but nonmobile tympanic membrane; and (c) flat or type B tympanograms with smaller than normal volumes may be related to an occluded external canal or probe tip, or the probe tip may be closed off by pressing against the external ear canal wall as shown in Table 7–2.

Acoustic Reflex Thresholds

The stapedius is the smallest skeletal muscle in the human body. At just over 1 mm in length, its purpose is to stabilize the smallest bone in the body, the stapes. The acoustic reflex (more specifically known as the acoustic stapedius reflex) is an involuntary muscle contraction that occurs in the middle ear of mammals in response to high-intensity sound stimuli. The function of the

Table 7–2. Tympanometry and Equivalent Ear Canal Volume (Veq) in Children

Tympanogram	Equivalent ear canal volume in cc³	Etiology
Type A	0.8–1.0	Normal middle ear
Type B	<0.3	Cerumen or canal wall
	0.8–1.0	Serous otitis; middle ear congenital anomaly
	>2.5	Tympanic membrane perforation; Patent ventilation tube in TM
Type C	0.8–1.0	Inadequate eustachian tube function

stapedial muscle is still open to debate, but the classic interpretation offered by Wever and Lawrence (1954) is that the stapedial muscle reflex is responsible for protection of the inner ear from loud sounds. The stapedius contraction stiffens the ossicular chain by pulling the stapes away from the oval window of the cochlea, thereby decreasing the transmission of vibrational energy to the cochlea. The stapedius reflex is also invoked during vocalization to reduce sound intensities reaching the inner ear by approximately 20 dB (Moller, 2000). In normal middle ears, the acoustic stapedial reflex is a bilateral phenomenon—even if only one ear is stimulated with a loud sound.

The pathways involved in the acoustic reflex are complex with transmission routes that are both ipsilateral and contralateral. The ipsilateral (or uncrossed acoustic reflex pathway) involves the cochlea, ventral cochlear nucleus, cranial nerve VIII and the motor nucleus of VII, and the stapedius muscle—all on the same side as the eliciting acoustic stimulus. The contralateral (or crossed acoustic stapedial reflex) occurs when the acoustic stimulus is presented to the ear opposite the ear that is monitored for response. The contralateral pathway involves the ipsilateral cochlea, ventral cochlear nucleus, and CN VIII; the pathway crosses through the trapezoid body and then involves the contralateral medial superior olive, CN VII and its motor nucleus, and the stapedius muscle.

The acoustic reflex test is based on the presentation of a sound of sufficient intensity at which the stapedial muscles will involuntarily contract. The classic monograph published by Otto Metz (1952) showed that in normal hearing persons a bilateral acoustic muscle reflex can be elicited with pure tone signals between 70 and 100 dB hearing threshold level (HTL) and at a lower intensity of 65 dB HTL for a broadband

noise stimulus. The lowest signal intensity capable of eliciting the acoustic reflex is the acoustic reflex threshold for the stimulated ear. Acoustic stapedial reflex thresholds vary according to individual hearing sensitivity and actually are elicited by loudness. Thus, for persons with sensorineural hearing loss, acoustic stapedial reflex thresholds may be within the normal range in hearing level decibels but less than 60 dB sensation level (SL) (i.e., above their auditory threshold at the test frequency). In persons with compromised middle ear mobility due to conductive hearing loss associated with flat or B type tympanograms, it is likely that the stapedial acoustic stapedial reflex will not be observed when the probe is in the conductive-loss ear (Jerger et al., 1974a).

Because the stapedial muscles contract bilaterally in response to an appropriate acoustic stimulus presented to either ear, both an ipsilateral (uncrossed) and a contralateral (crossed) acoustic reflex may be measured (Figure 7–7). Most immittance meters will measure the acoustic reflex in ipsilateral or contralateral mode. In ipsilateral reflex measurement mode, the eliciting acoustic stimulus is presented through the probe tip, and the change in admittance is monitored in the same ear. During contralateral acoustic reflex measurement, the acoustic stimulus is presented through an earphone to the test ear with the probe tip in the opposite ear. The opposite ear probe measurement verifies the resultant change in admittance caused by stimulation of the test ear. Regardless of whether measuring ipsilateral or contralateral (crossed or uncrossed) acoustic reflexes, it is necessary to record the acoustic reflex for the stimulated ear—noting on the audiogram, of course, which mode (contralateral or ipsilateral) was used for the measurement.

The major advantage of ipsilateral stapedial reflex measurement is that confu-

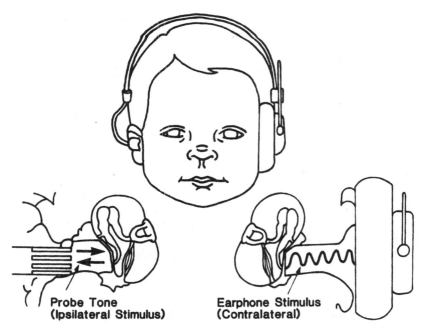

Probe Tone
(Ipsilateral Stimulus)

Earphone Stimulus
(Contralateral)

Figure 7–7. Acoustic reflex measurements may be made with a contralateral stimulus from an earphone or with an ipsilateral stimulus presented through probe tip.

sion is eliminated regarding which ear is being tested. Utilization of handheld ipsilateral reflex techniques virtually eliminates the need for the cumbersome headband-earphone arrangement used in contralateral reflex measurement. Ipsilateral reflex measurement is especially useful with pediatric patients. Research reports that compare acoustic reflex threshold sensitivity between contralateral and ipsilateral stimuli have been published, indicating that ipsilateral thresholds are 3 to 6 dB more sensitive than contralateral thresholds (Fria, LeBlanc, Kristensen, & Alberti, 1975; Moller, 1962).

Acoustic stapedial reflex threshold testing is carried out at frequencies of 500, 1000, 2000, and 4000 Hz in each ear. However, as stapedial acoustic reflex responses at 4000 Hz are often absent for no apparent reason even in normal-hearing patients, pathologic conclusions may not be valid if only the 4000 Hz reflex is not present.

Acoustic reflex thresholds are difficult to interpret in isolation, because absent or elevated acoustic reflex thresholds may occur because of a wide variety of conditions. Comparison of contralateral (crossed) and ipsilateral (uncrossed) acoustic reflexes increases confidence in interpreting the audiogram and immittance measurements results (Table 7–3) and provides powerful diagnostic information for higher level auditory dysfunction (Hall & Swanepoel, 2010).

Much emphasis has been placed on the clinical value of the acoustic reflex measurement. Because the acoustic reflex is mediated by loudness, it is a sensitive indicator of cochlear pathology. The acoustic reflex threshold level in patients with sensorineural hearing loss due to cochlear pathology usually occurs at sensation levels less than 60 dB above the auditory pure tone threshold. The patient with cochlear pathology hears the test signal as though it were much

Table 7–3. Interpreting Crossed and Uncrossed Acoustic Reflexes With the Audiogram to Identify Site of Lesion of Hearing Impairment

Reflex pattern	Audiogram	Predicted site
Neither crossed or uncrossed can be elicited from either ear	Bilateral air-bone gap	Middle ear
Neither crossed or uncrossed can be elicited from either ear	Bilateral severe sensory loss	Cochlea
Neither crossed or uncrossed can be elicited from either ear	Normal	Brainstem

Source: Reproduced with permission from "Immittance Measures in Auditory Disorders," by B. Stach and J. Jerger, 1990, in J. Jacobson and J. Northern, Eds., *Diagnostic audiology*, p. 118, Boston, MA: College-Hill Press.

louder, as a result of abnormal appreciation of loudness. Thus, the acoustic stapedial reflex threshold provides an objective, simple technique to confirm the site of auditory pathology to the cochlea.

The admittance measurement system is very sensitive in the identification of conductive-type hearing loss when the probe is in the ear with the middle ear involvement. In ears with mild-to-moderate conductive hearing loss in one ear and a normal ear on the opposite side, the stapedial reflex may be noted (although perhaps at an elevated dB level) with the probe in the ear with normal middle ear function (i.e., no conductive loss). However, whenever the probe is in the ear with conductive impairment, it is very unlikely that the stapedial reflex will be noted. In cases of bilateral conductive-type dysfunction, no acoustic reflex will be measureable from either ear.

The informed audiologist can achieve considerable diagnostic information through the subtleties of acoustic stapedial reflex interpretation. For example, the acoustic reflex sensation level (SL) shows an inverse relation to the degree of sensorineural hearing loss. The acoustic reflex threshold is approximately 50 dB SL for patients with a 20 dB sensorineural hearing loss and perhaps 25 or 30 dB SL for patients with an 85 dB sensorineural hearing loss. Jerger, Jerger, and Mauldin (1972) concluded that when the cochlear hearing loss is less than 60 dB HL, there is 90% likelihood for the presence of the acoustic reflex being observed. As the sensorineural loss increases above 60 dB HL, chances of observing the acoustic stapedial reflex is less. With an 85 dB HL hearing loss, the chances are only 50% of observing the acoustic reflex; if the loss is 100 dB HL, only a 5% to 10% chance exists of the reflex being present. Thus, the presence of acoustic reflex thresholds, in light of hearing loss, provides a powerful indication for sensorineural diagnosis. In patients with unilateral cochlear hearing loss less than 85 dB HL, the acoustic reflex should be easily observable bilaterally.

In patients with conductive hearing problems, the contralateral acoustic reflex can be observed only in mild unilateral conductive hearing loss. When the unilateral conductive hearing loss exceeds 30 dB HL, the acoustic reflex is typically obscured bilaterally. Thus, when the stimulating sound is presented to the conductive hearing loss ear, the 30 dB+ hearing loss is sufficient to prevent the signal from being perceived loudly enough to elicit the acoustic reflex from the contralateral normal ear. When the earphone is on the normal ear and the probe is in the unilateral conductive loss ear, the pathology causing the conductive loss prevents the eardrum from showing a change in admittance. Naturally, in a bilateral conductive loss, the acoustic reflexes will be absent bilaterally because the pathology in *each* ear prohibits the probe from noting an admittance change in the middle ear when the opposite ear is stimulated with sound. The ipsilateral acoustic reflex will also be absent bilaterally.

The presence of a small air-bone gap of only 10 dB is sufficient to obscure the reflex to the probe ear 80% of the time (Jerger, Burney, Mauldin, & Crump, 1974b). Conversely, if acoustic reflexes can be noted in the probe ear, it is virtually impossible for a conductive hearing loss to exist in that ear. Thus, even a very mild conductive hearing loss will obscure the acoustic reflex. Interpretation of acoustic reflexes in hearing loss can be diagnostically important and of particular value when the patient is a youngster in whom audiometric testing (with contralateral masking) is impractical or not possible.

CLINICAL APPLICATIONS OF THE IMMITTANCE BATTERY WITH CHILDREN

Acoustic immittance measurements provide quick and easy means of evaluating the middle ears of children with sensorineural hearing loss (Northern, 1980b). Whereas tympanometry, static admittance, the equivalent ear canal volume measurement, and the acoustic stapedial reflex threshold each provide some information about the function of the auditory system, their results be-come more meaningful when relationships between the tests are considered. Diagnostic judgments and patient referrals for medical treatment are made with greater authority and assurance when the overall pattern is considered. Tympanometry alone is useful to only a limited degree, static admittance norms are too variable for accurate diagnosis, and the absence of the acoustic stapedial reflex (ASR) may occur from any of several undeterminable factors. When considered together, however, the limitations of each test are reduced while their combined implications are enhanced (Table 7–4). Unfortunately, many pediatric audiologists fail to make use of the valuable information provided by acoustic stapedial reflex measurements. The additional diagnostic data provided by the extra minute or two it takes to evaluate the bilateral ASR can be a valuable and important addition to the cross-check principle of pediatric audiology.

Immittance findings from a case of negative middle ear pressure in a youngster's right ear are demonstrated in Figure 7–8. The audiogram shows a mild hearing loss with a 20 dB air-bone gap in the patient's right ear and normal hearing in the left ear. The audiogram gives no clue as to the etiology of the unilateral conductive hearing loss. The tympanogram for the left ear is superimposed within the normal pattern, while the tympanogram for the right ear shows slightly increased admittance and middle ear pressure (TPP) of −200 daPa. The contralateral acoustic reflexes are present but show elevated thresholds when the stimulating earphone is on the involved ear. The 20 dB air-conduction hearing loss in the right ear is not sufficiently severe to prohibit loudness from eliciting the acoustic reflex when the earphone is on this ear. When the earphone is placed over the normal-hearing

Table 7–4. Use of Immittance to Help Confirm Audiometric Impression in Evaluation of Young Children

Tympanometry	Static compliance	Acoustic reflex	Confirm behavioral audiometric impression
Type A bilaterally	Within normal range bilaterally	Normal bilaterally	Bilateral normal hearing or bilateral mild-to-moderate sensorineural hearing loss or unilateral mild-to-moderate sensorineural hearing loss
Type A in one ear; type B or C in other ear	Normal in A ear, low in B or C ear	Absent bilaterally	Unilateral conductive loss
Type B or C bilaterally	Low bilaterally	Absent bilaterally	Bilateral conductive loss

Source: From "Clinical Experience with Impedance Audiometry," by J. Jerger, 1970, *Archives of Otolaryngology, 92*, pp. 311–324.

left ear, the acoustic reflexes are absent. The probe tip is now in the involved conductive loss ear, and the conductive loss element prohibits admittance change in the right tympanic membrane. Knowledge of only the immittance test battery results, accompanied by experience in test interpretation, would permit a close estimation of this child's audiogram if a complete audiogram could not be accomplished successfully.

Figure 7–9 demonstrates findings in a patient with unilateral otitis media. The audiometric results show a conductive hearing loss with an approximate 30 dB air-bone gap in the right ear. Hearing in the left ear is normal. The tympanogram of the involved right ear shows a type B or flat pattern. That the contralateral stapedius reflex is absent bilaterally, in view of a unilateral hearing loss, confirms that the loss must be conductive in nature of at least 30 dB HL. This overall pattern could also represent cerumen packed in the right ear canal, a perforation of the right tympanic membrane, or otitis media. The final diagnosis is in the realm of the physician, but these immittance test findings, even without the audiogram, might suggest an appropriate referral of this child to a physician.

Bluestone et al. (1973) compared air conduction audiometry and tympanometry in 84 youngsters with concurrent or recent middle ear disease to determine which procedure could better predict the presence of middle ear effusion. They concluded that tympanometry is far more sensitive than air conduction audiometry for detecting common conduction defects in children. They caution, however, that tympanometry cannot detect sensorineural hearing loss and thus cannot be substituted for pure tone audiometry as a screening technique. They suggest that tympanometry in combination with air conduction audiometry appears to constitute the best method for detecting middle ear disease and hearing impairment in large groups of children.

Children attending schools for the hard-of-hearing and deaf tend to be evaluated on an annual basis. These children with severe-to-profound hearing loss seldom complain about their ears or of changes

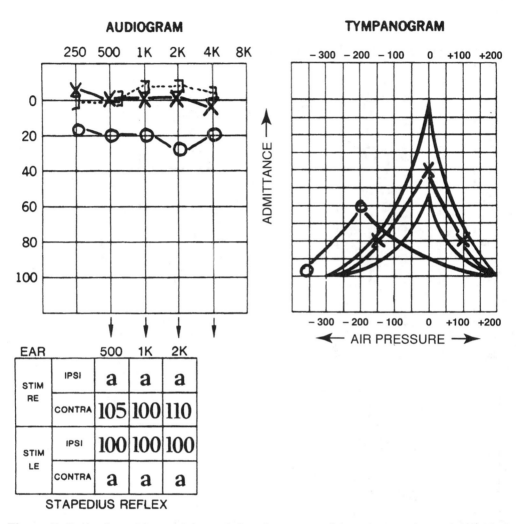

Figure 7–8. Audiometrics and acoustic immittance results accompanying a right-sided unilateral conductive hearing loss caused by negative middle ear pressure. Note contralateral and ipsilateral acoustic reflex findings. See text for full explanation.

in their hearing sensitivity due to otologic pathology. Bone-conduction measurements are of limited usefulness in this special population making tympanometry and OAEs important tests to identify middle ear pathology. Interestingly, Rossi and Sims (1977) evaluated acoustic reflex measurements in children with deafness in an effort to verify suspicious air-bone audiometric gaps. Their acoustic immittance studies on 85 students with severe-to-profound hearing loss showed that 80% of the "air-bone gaps" produced

by audiometry were, in fact, invalid likely due to tactile-vibratory stimulation with the audiometric bone oscillator. For children with hearing loss, the additional hearing loss created by the conductive component may have deleterious effects on hearing with their hearing aids. If the child is mature enough to recognize the need to turn up the hearing aid gain, problems may be created with distortion and feedback; if the child is too young to note the change in hearing, poor performance with the hearing aid may

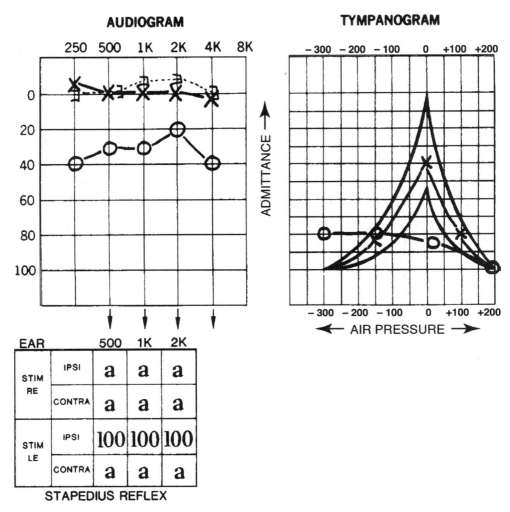

Figure 7–9. Audiometrics and acoustic immittance result in a right-sided unilateral conductive hearing loss caused by otitis media. Note contralateral and ipsilateral acoustic reflex findings. See text for full explanation.

result. OAEs and acoustic immittance measurements should, by all means, be a routine procedure for children attending schools for the deaf and the hard-of-hearing.

Acoustic Immittance Measurements With Infants

Numerous studies of tympanometry in newborn infants were published in the early and mid-1970s with conflicting and puzzling results, or as described by Margolis (1978), "results that are both promising and perplexing." Subsequent research has indicated that the problem of tympanometry in infants was related to the use of a single-frequency 220 or 226 Hz probe tone. Although there were some contrasting research reports published about the use of low-frequency probe tone tympanometry in infants, once again the problem was the focus on making tympanometry a stand-alone diagnostic test.

Several early studies showed that infants below 4 months of age not uncommonly demonstrated a normal 220 Hz tympanogram even with confirmed middle ear effusion (Hunter & Margolis, 1992; Meyer, Jardine, & Deverson, 1997; Paradise et al., 1976; Shurin, Pelton, & Klein, 1976). Furthermore, abnormal 220 Hz tympanograms in normal infant ears were reported (Keefe & Levi, 1996). It was originally hypothesized that the baby's ear canal walls were so compliant that a movement of the entire canal wall occurred creating a type A tympanogram (Paradise et al., 1976). The infant ear has a bony region that is not yet completely formed which results in a highly compliant ear canal. During development of the infant ear, several changes take place, which may influence the mechanical properties of the ear canal (Keefe & Levi, 1996). However, using video otomicroscopy, Holte et al. (1991) found no correlation between infant ear canal wall movement and tympanometric patterns.

Additional research began to produce evidence that there may be a better correlation between the presence of middle ear effusion and the shape of the tympanogram when a high-frequency probe tone is used in neonates. Studies have concluded that the higher probe tone frequency (1000 Hz) tympanometry can better identify middle ear effusion in infants less than 4 to 6 months of age than the 226 Hz probe tone (Marchant, McMillan, & Shurin, 1984; Shurin et al., 1979). Normative data for 1000 Hz tympanometry are now available for neonates and young infants (Margolis, Bass-Ringdahl, Hanks, Hotte, & Zapala, 2003). In view of the questionable accuracy of tympanograms from infants tested with a 226 Hz probe tone, most guidelines now recommend that a 1000 Hz probe tone be used in tympanometry testing of babies less than 6 to 7 months of age, but that results should be interpreted with caution. Furthermore, tympanometry should not be used as a single diagnostic test with newborns and infants, but conclusions must be based with supportive information from acoustic reflex measures, OAEs, and ABRs when necessary.

Keith (1973, 1975) examined stapedial reflex measurements in 40 infants, using a 220 Hz probe tone with stimulus presentations of 100 dB HTL at 500 and 2000 Hz. He reported that behavioral movement of the infants often contaminated acoustic stapedial reflex responses. In fact, from 160 stimulus presentations, only 33% resulted in clear stapedial reflex responses. No acoustic reflex responses were noted in 26% of the stimulus presentations, and 4 of the 40 infants showed no acoustic reflex in either ear initially although all 4 infants were later confirmed to have normal hearing responses. Keith warned that infant immittance measures cannot stand alone and should only be interpreted in combination with some independent assessment of hearing sensitivity level.

Paradise et al. (1976) found poor correlations between tympanometry and otoscopy in infants younger than 7 months of age. In fact, of 43 infants younger than 7 months of age, 40 of 81 ears had confirmed middle ear effusion (determined by myringotomy), yet 24 of the 40 abnormal ears displayed normal tympanograms. The authors concluded that although the use of tympanometry had much to offer in the diagnosis of middle ear effusion, its use (tympanometry) was not recommended in infants younger than 7 months of age.

Reichert et al. (1978) examined 878 3-month-old infants with otoscopy and tympanometry. All infants were examined tympanometrically while being held in their mothers' arms and being comforted with a pacifier or bottle. The authors concluded that tympanometry produced a low diagnostic specificity (accuracy in identifying nondiseased individuals) with a high number of false-positive results—16 flat tympanograms were found in ears that were otoscopically normal. In their discussion, Reichert et al. (1978) recognized that inclusion of the measurement of the acoustic reflex may have provided different results than were obtained only with the use of tympanometry. Studies published by Orchik et al. (1978a, 1978b) clearly show that prediction of middle ear effusion on the basis of tympanometric data alone is difficult at best, unless the tympanogram is a flat, non-mobile pattern where a 90% occurrence of effusion is present.

Schwartz and Schwartz (1978, 1980) published data that also supported the combined use of tympanometry and acoustic reflex measurement to identify middle ear effusion in infants. They concluded that while a normal tympanogram cannot be considered evidence of a mobile tympanic membrane or effusion-free middle ear, the presence of an acoustic reflex with a normal tympanogram supports normal middle ear function. Keith (1978) agreed by stating that it is imperative that tympanometry and stapedial reflex testing always be performed together. Admittedly these early studies made their measures with a 220 or 226 Hz probe tone, but each of the investigators reached the important conclusion that use of multiple immittance tests added to the accuracy of the diagnostic decision. However, they all agreed that it is prudent to use caution when performing acoustic immittance measurements with infants younger than 6 months of age.

An intriguing finding concerning infant acoustic reflexes was reported by McCandless and Allred (1978), who showed that with a 220 Hz probe tone only 4% of 53 infants younger than 48 hours of age demonstrated a measurable acoustic reflex. When the probe tone was increased to a frequency of 660 Hz, an astounding 89% of the same infants had an acoustic reflex. At about the same time, a series of studies of acoustic reflexes in infants was reported by Bennett and Weatherby (1979, 1982) and Weatherby and Bennett (1980) using a two-component variable probe tone immittance meter to record contralateral acoustic reflexes in newborns. Their studies showed that as the probe tone frequency is increased, the prevalence of the reflex increases and the threshold of the acoustic reflex decreases. With a maximum intensity of 96 dB SPL, no reflexes were detected with a 220 Hz probe, whereas with probe tones above 8000 Hz all newborns exhibited acoustic reflexes. Bennett (1984) pointed out that calibration of the contralateral earphone stimulus in infants is important because of the smaller volume of newborn ear canals and those differences in SPLs between the ear canals of adults and infants can easily exceed 6 dB. Bennett found the optimal probe tone frequency for detecting acoustic reflexes in neonates to be 1400 Hz.

Sprague, Wiley, and Goldstein (1985) reported 80% observable reflexes with the 660 Hz probe tone and only 50% observable reflexes with a 220 Hz probe tone with ipsilateral and contralateral activating stimuli. Instead of a standard earphone cushion for the contralateral stimulus, these researchers used insert receivers and found lower acoustic reflex thresholds than previously reported in other studies. McMillan, Bennett, Marchant, and Shurin (1985) investigated acoustic reflexes in neonates with probe tones of 220 and 660 Hz. Their results confirmed that ipsilateral and contralateral reflexes to pure tone activators occurred three times more frequently with a 660 Hz probe tone (76%) than with the

220 Hz probe tone (24%). In their review of research articles dealing with acoustic reflex measurements in infants, Hodges and Ruth (1987) concluded that the acoustic reflex mechanism is functional for infants as young as 9 hours after birth, and both crossed and uncrossed acoustic reflex thresholds can be measured with higher probe tone frequencies.

Hearing Loss Prediction by the Acoustic Reflex

Niemeyer and Sesterhenn (1972) developed a procedure to determine air-conduction hearing thresholds from stapedial reflex measurements. They noted that the acoustic stapedial reflex (ASR) threshold for white noise was lower than the (ASR) threshold for pure tones, and that the difference in decibels between the two thresholds is related to the degree of sensorineural hearing impairment. Jerger et al. (1974b) simplified the procedure into a test he called sensitivity prediction with the acoustic reflex (SPAR). SPAR is a technique to ascertain sensorineural hearing loss within four categories of impairment: normal hearing, mild loss, severe loss, and profound loss. The Jerger technique calls for establishment of pure tone ASRs at 500, 1000, and 2000 Hz and subtracting the ASR broadband noise threshold, using the difference in dB to predict the degree of hearing loss. In a series of more than 1,000 patients, Jerger et al. (1974b) reported that the predictive error of SPAR was clinically insignificant in 63% of the group, was moderate in 33%, and was serious in only 4% of the cohort.

Hearing loss prediction from the acoustic stapedial reflex is apparently influenced by a number of variables including chronologic age, minor middle ear abnormalities, and audiometric configuration. Jerger, Hayes, Anthony, and Mauldin (1978) concluded that predicting the presence of hearing loss of any degree can be accomplished by relying on the broadband noise and pure tone acoustic reflex difference, whereas the absolute acoustic reflex threshold level for broadband noise stimuli may be used to predict the degree of hearing loss. In the Jerger et al. (1978) study, 100% of children predicted to have normal hearing did, indeed, show normal audiograms; severe hearing loss was accurately predicted in children 85% of the time. Prediction of moderate hearing loss in children was somewhat less accurate (54%). Hall (1978) reported a revised SPAR technique, known as the 1977 SPAR which simplified, while increasing, the accuracy of the technique. Hall suggested that when the difference between the ASR thresholds at 1000 Hz and broadband noise was less than 20 dB, the prediction for the hearing loss is mild-to-moderate; when the ASR thresholds differed by more than 20 dB, the likelihood was the presence of a severe degree hearing loss. Clearly, the prediction of hearing loss with the acoustic stapedial reflex SPAR technique can be a useful tool in hearing evaluations with difficult-to-test children. This physiologic and objective prediction of hearing loss in the pediatric population, and especially as a tool for estimating the hearing of the difficult-to-test child, should be a useful test in the armamentarium of the pediatric audiologist.

OTOACOUSTIC EMISSIONS

Otoacoustic emissions (OAEs) are an important and clinically useful adjunct to physiologic-based auditory response measurements. Evoked otoacoustic emissions (OAE) are minute acoustic signals generated within the cochlea that travel in a "reverse direction" through the middle ear space and tympanic membrane out to the external ear canal. These signals are generated in response to clicks or tone bursts delivered through a probe inserted into the external ear canal. The OAE evaluation is not a test of hearing and does not quantify hearing loss or hearing threshold level. As the OAE is directly emitted from the cochlea, the testing procedure does not assess the integrity of the neural transmission of sound beyond the inner ear.

OAEs are low-level "leakage" of acoustic energy associated with the normal hearing process that can be detected with specialized equipment from the external ear canal. A probe microphone system, similar to that used in acoustic immittance measurements, is placed into the external ear canal to detect low-level, inaudible sounds reflected back by vibratory motion in the cochlea. Individuals with hearing loss greater than 30 dB HL typically do not emit OAEs. The hair cells of the cochlea are miniature biologic amplifiers that act as transducers converting mechanical energy into electrochemical energy. Otoacoustic emissions are actually a by-product of sensory outer hair cell transduction and are reflected as "echoes" into the external auditory canal. OAEs are preneural in origin and are directly dependent on outer hair cell integrity (Jacobson, 1996). These audio frequencies are transmitted from the outer hair cells in the cochlea as a release of sound energy that in some cases is spontaneous, but most likely is evoked in response to external acoustic stimulation. Thomas Gold, an English physicist, theorized the concept of extraneous acoustic energy reflected externally from the cochlea as early as 1948 and hypothesized a "cochlear amplifier" system based on an "active" process originating within the cochlea. However, it was some 30 years later when David Kemp (1978) was able to verify the presence of OAEs in the human external ear canal.

Brownell, Bader, Bertrend, and Ribaupierre (1985) demonstrated through dramatic single cell recordings that the outer hair cells are mechanically active; that is, they shorten when depolarized and lengthen when hyperpolarized. This electromotility is extremely fast and occurs at frequencies up to the limit of human hearing. This active process of length change of the outer hair cells, although miniscule in each hair cell, can be summed sufficiently to influence the mechanical responses within the organ of Corti. This finding is consistent with the cochlear amplifier concept and describes a mechanism for acoustic energy being generated and emitted from within the cochlea. This outer hair cell motility is generally accepted as the source for otoacoustic emissions.

Kemp (1980) developed a computerized system that used a sound source and a miniaturized microphone mounted in a probe tip and sealed in the external ear canal to measure otoacoustic emissions. Kemp used acoustic transients (clicks) as the stimulus and then recorded an acoustic response beginning 5 msec following the onset of the presentation of the rapidly repeating clicks. This discovery was especially important to hearing theories because of the long-held belief that the cochlear vibrations transmitted energy only upward through the auditory system. It was Brownell's research findings (1983, 1985) of the outer hair cell's active electromotile response that helped explain the mechanics of how OAEs are generated within the cochlea and reflected back into the ear canal (Hall, 2000). Somewhat amazingly then, the normal cochlea does not just receive sound; it also produces low-intensity sounds. These sounds are produced specifically by the cochlea and, most probably, by the cochlear outer hair cells as they expand and contract.

The OAE test allows for individual ear assessment, is performed quickly at any age, and is not dependent on whether the child is asleep or awake. The OAE is an effective screening measure for inner and middle ear abnormalities, because at hearing thresholds of 30 dB or higher, there is no OAE response. However, the OAE tests will miss auditory neuropathy and other neuronal abnormalities unless accompanied by ABR measures. As a test of cochlear status, and specifically hair cell function, this information can be used to: (a) screen hearing in neonates, infants, or children with developmental disabilities; (b) identify those with normal hearing and those with mild-to-moderate 30 dB+ hearing loss; (c) help differentiate between the sensory and neural components of sensorineural hearing loss, and (d) test for feigned or exaggerated hearing loss. The information can be obtained from newborns, toddlers, or children who are sleeping or inattentive (even comatose) because no behavioral response is required. Common middle ear disorders and conductive hearing loss in young children quickly eliminate the reflected emission. It might therefore be prudent to perform acoustic immittance tests (tympanometry and acoustic reflex testing) before conducting OAE tests to identify those children with middle ear conductive problems (Figure 7–10).

Although for the most part OAEs are generally easy to establish in infants and young children in a matter of a few minutes, the procedures are not without problems. Obtaining a proper fit of the ear cuff for the probe tip into the ear canal can be difficult. Both external and physiologic noise are often contaminants in the testing procedures, suggesting that testing for OAEs should be conducted in a quiet set-ting. Although the various sizes of the ear canal permit external noise to interfere with the OAE test, the well-fitted probe tip will seal the ear canal, helping to eliminate the noise contamination. A poorly fitted probe tip also permits loss of the low frequencies of the stimulus. Widen (1997) suggests that the test be considered valid if the response spectrum contains 3 dB or more power than the noise spectrum in each of three 1000-Hz frequency bands at 1500, 2500, and 3500 Hz.

The OAE procedures typically take a minute or so per ear for each test. It is non-invasive, painless, and typically does not require sedation for the patient. OAE results are contaminated by motion and noise from the patient, so passive cooperation is required. Older children are likely to hold still, while distraction techniques may be necessary for the toddler. Some suggestions for testing infants with OAEs might be providing a comfortable chair in which the parent can relax and hold the infant, darkening the room to induce the child to sleep, or reserving the test to follow the infant's feeding. Often the test can be completed with the infant sitting comfortably in an infant carrier. Careful thought should be given

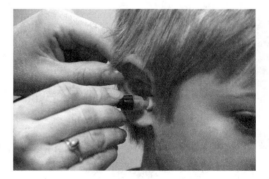

Figure 7–10. Otoacoustic emissions testing can be accomplished quickly and with ease. Photo courtesy of Colorado Children's Hospital, Aurora, CO.

when scheduling infants early in the morning or following nap times to increase success with audiometric testing. OAEs are not influenced by sedation, but seldom is such an extreme step necessary for this quick procedure. On the other hand, if a difficult-to-test child was sedated for a minor surgical intervention or some other physiologic testing, it would be prudent to perform the OAE test at the same time.

From the flurry of research activity that followed the discovery of otoacoustic emissions, two broad classes of OAEs emerged: spontaneous otoacoustic emissions (SOAEs), which occur naturally without external stimulation, and evoked otoacoustic emissions (EOAEs), which require an evoking stimulus. SOAEs are low-intensity sound reflections that can be measured in the ear canal in approximately 40% to 60% of persons with normal hearing when there is no external sound stimulation (Martin, Probst, & Lonsbury-Martin, 1990). Bright (1997) suggested that SOAEs might be the result of some minor structural irregularities within the cochlea which are not sufficiently significant to affect audiometric thresholds, but this concept has not been confirmed. The presence of SOAEs is usually considered to be a sign of cochlear health, but the absence of SOAEs is not necessarily a sign of abnormality. Because of the inability to predict which patients might have SOAEs, there has been limited suggestion as to their clinical utility.

The second category of OAEs includes low-intensity sound emissions elicited by low to moderate levels of acoustic stimulation presented through an ear canal microphone. This category includes two types of measurements known as transient evoked otoacoustic emissions (TEOAEs) and distortion product evoked otoacoustic emissions (DPEOAEs). Each type of evoked otoacoustic emission measurement is different, and each has different advantages and disadvantages. The primary differences between the TEOAEs and DPEOAEs techniques lie in what the cochlea is doing during the measurement and which parts of the whole OAE response are captured and which parts are rejected (Kemp, 1997). Both of these evoked otoacoustic emissions, the TEOAEs and the DPEOAEs, are clinically useful measurement tools.

OAEs are measured by presenting a series of brief acoustic click stimuli to the ear through a probe that is inserted in the outer third of the ear canal. The probe contains a miniature speaker that generates clicks and a miniature microphone that measures the resulting OAEs from the ear canal. The resulting sound that is picked up by the microphone is digitized and processed by specially designed hardware and software. The very low-level OAEs are separated by the software from both the background noise and from the contamination of the evoking clicks, so consideration of the noise floor is important during clinical measurements. Otoacoustic emission instrumentation is generally automated and available as desktop or smaller sized, portable, and battery-operated handheld screeners. The clinical significance of OAEs is that they are reliable, consistent, valid evidence of the vital sensory processes arising within the cochlea. It must be understood that successful measurement of OAEs is dependent upon normally operating external, middle, and inner ear structures. As stated by Dhar and Hall (2012), although there is no question that OAEs are inextricably intertwined with the active cochlear processes found in the outer hair cells, the exact nature of these biophysical processes and mode of propagation for OAEs are still not fully understood.

TEOAEs

Transient evoked otoacoustic emissions (TEOAEs) are evoked responses obtained by stimulating the cochlea with a transient signal such as a click or tone burst acoustic signal. The level of the TEOAEs is compared to the noise floor and analyzed in narrow frequency bands to determine the physiological condition of the test ear. TEOAEs are a wide frequency response in the 500 to 4000 Hz range. They are typically measured in ears hearing better than 30 to 40 dB HL. TEOAEs are stable, frequency-dispersive responses to brief acoustic stimulation presented repeatedly (clicks or tone pips) that begin 4 to 15 msec after presentation of the stimuli (Kemp & Ryan, 1993). TEOAEs are easy to record and interpret with only a single stimulation channel that requires inexpensive synchronous averaging technology that has been readily available since the 1970s. The technique samples the noise in the ear canal synchronously with stimulus presentations, and events that are time-locked to the stimuli are preserved in the resulting averaged response (Glattke & Fujikawa, 1991). Examples of normal and absent TEOAEs are shown in Figure 7–11.

When OAEs are present, it is possible to seek more specific diagnostic information by recording a DPgram for 5 or even 8 frequencies per octave over the range from 500 to 8000 Hz. TEOAEs can be recorded for all available frequency bands covering the range from 0 to 5000 Hz, providing much more information about cochlear function than a simple pass versus fail decision. Many of the available OAE instruments capable of diagnostic evaluation protocols are automated and preprogrammed. However, it must be noted that the diagnostic OAE protocols cannot be followed in light of high levels of ambient noise in the environment or physiologic noise from the patient. In addition, the diagnostic DPgram markedly extends the test time which is not always easy to do with a squirming pediatric patient. Dhar and Hall (2012) caution that the diagnostic interpretations must include awareness that the OAE is likely the collective properties of the cochlear region stimulated and not any specific frequency or isolated hair cells.

TEOAEs are especially useful in clinical hearing evaluations because they can be recorded in all nonpathologic ears that have hearing better than approximately 30 dB HL regardless of age or gender. Most OAE screening protocols test within the frequency range of 2000 to 5000 Hz. Typically, screening OAEs are measured at four discrete frequency points (2000, 3000, 4000, and 5000 Hz). In order to pass the hearing screening, OAEs must be present and be at least 5 dB above the background noise at three out of four frequencies.

In the absence of any middle ear pathology, one should be able to elicit otoacoustic emissions from any patient with hearing better than 30 to 40 dB (Hood, 1998). TEOAEs can be measured in 60 seconds or less per ear and are present in nearly all normal-hearing ears. TEOAEs show increases in amplitude in infants between 1 and 9 months of age, whereas decreases in amplitude have been observed in older children aged 4 to 13 years (Norton & Widen, 1990; Widen, 1997). Although it is not possible to estimate the threshold of hearing from characteristics of the TEOAE response, measurement of TEOAEs provide a highly sensitive technique for separating a normal-hearing ear from an abnormal-hearing ear.

Infants tend to show OAE response patterns that are inherently physiologically "noisier" than noted with adults. OAEs have wide application in hearing screening

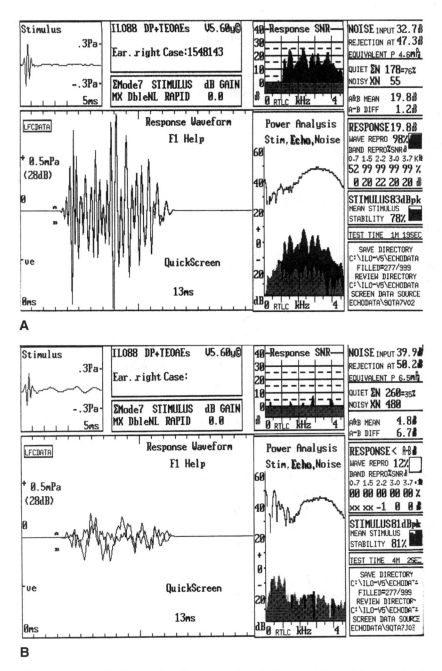

Figure 7–11. A. Example of a normal and abnormal hearing transient evoked otoacoustic emission (TEOAE) recording. **B.** Example of an absent transient evoked otoacoustic emission (TEOAE) recording.

programs as described and in the identification of children with auditory neuropathy spectrum disorder (see Chapter 8).

DPEOAEs

Distortion product evoked otoacoustic emissions (DPEOAEs) are measured in the external ear canal with two different pure tone stimuli as frequencies f_1 and f_2 are presented simultaneously. In response to the two-frequency stimulation, the healthy cochlear generates and emits additional tone signals at frequencies arithmetically related to those of the stimulus tones. DPEOAEs are tonal responses located at precise frequencies determined by the f_1 and f_2 stimulus tones; the resulting DPEOAEs occur at specific distortion product frequencies such as $2f_1-f_2$, and $2f_2-f_1$, as well as at $3f_1-2f_2$ (Lonsbury-Martin & Martin, 1990). It is generally accepted that the DPOAE energy is generated in the region of overlap between the mechanical disturbances created by the two stimulus tones (Dhar & Hall, 2012). The measurement of DPEOAEs requires specialized equipment with two separate high-quality stimulus channels and two transducers with elaborate signal and processing technology. The recorded plot of the DPOAEs is a graph level in decibel sound pressure level (dB SPL) as a function of frequency, known as a DPgram. DPOAEs are always present in ears with normal-hearing sensitivity. This type of OAE may be recorded in individuals with a greater degree of hearing loss at higher frequencies. DPOAEs are typically measured in the frequency range of 750 to 6000 Hz, although many OAE devices are capable of measuring at higher frequencies.

The primary advantage of DPOAEs is that they offer the audiologist the capability of objectively evaluating frequency-specific

regions of the cochlea. Therefore, DPEOAEs represent a method of frequency sampling along with a level of auditory sensitivity pattern related to the threshold audiogram. The primary disadvantage is that the DPEOAE is not recordable at frequency regions that show hearing loss greater than 50 dB HL (Jacobson, 1996). DPEOAEs can be used to identify frequency-specific regions that have hearing thresholds within normal limits. DPEOAEs usually take slightly longer to establish than TEOAEs and may be measured in either or both of two techniques. During one procedure, the results of the DPEOAE measurement are plotted on a DPgram as shown in Figure 7–12. The DPgram is obtained by maintaining a constant stimulus intensity level and varying the frequency response. The frequency range of the DPgram is approximately 500 to 8000 Hz, and the relatively extensive dynamic range of response amplitude (plus or minus 50 dB) allows cochlear evaluation at or near threshold and suprathreshold levels of stimulation (Lonsbury-Martin & Martin, 1990).

The second DPEOAE technique may be used to establish an input/output function where frequency is held constant and intensity is varied. The noise levels below 1000 Hz significantly affect the recording of the DPgram. The degree of separation of the noise floor levels and the actual DP emissions indicate normal outer hair cell motility. Although no standard of measurement criteria exist, it is generally agreed that the amplitude of the DPEOAE must be 3 dB or greater than the noise floor to be accepted as a true response with either of the two measurements. Collet, Gartner, Moulin, Kauffman, Disant, and Morgon (1989) confirmed, with a study of 76 subjects with sensorineural hearing loss, that OAEs are never found when hearing loss at 1000 Hz exceeds 40 dB HL or when the mean audiometric hearing

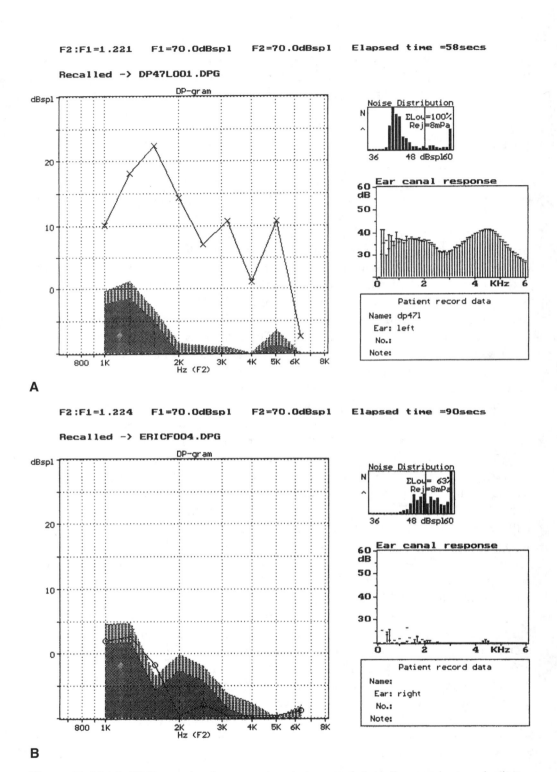

Figure 7–12. A–B. Example of a normal and abnormal distortion product evoked otoacoustic emission (DPEOAE) recording.

loss at 500, 1000, 2000, and 4000 Hz exceeds 45 dB HL. OAEs cannot be evoked by acoustic stimulation when outer hair cells are structurally damaged or nonfunctional (Norton, 1993).

EVOKED AUDITORY RESPONSES

More than 60 years ago, Davis (1939) noted that the electrical activity of the brain, as indicated by electroencephalographic recordings, showed a change when the subject heard a loud sound. This led numerous clinicians to attempt to use the standard electroencephalographic technique as a test for hearing sensitivity. Results, however, were universally disappointing. The electrical response in the cortex to auditory stimuli is so small that it is nearly impossible to see with any consistency the normal ongoing electrical activity of the brain, particularly when the stimuli are low-intensity pure tones.

In the early 1960s a number of special-purpose computers appeared on the commercial market. These signal-average computers utilize a summation technique to cancel out random ongoing background physiologic "noise" (McCandless & Best, 1964). This created an improved signal-to-noise condition to enhance specific, time-locked potentials of small magnitude. The "random" noise consists theoretically of an equal number of positive and negative electrical potentials and is averaged out. Thus, only the wanted potential activity summates in the computer. These computers store and average potentials related in time to the onset of a stimulus capable of "evoking" a response from the nervous system.

An evoked potential or evoked response is an electrical potential recorded from the nervous system of a human or other animal following presentation of a stimulus, as distinct from spontaneous potentials as detected by electroencephalography (EEG), electromyography (EMG), or other electrophysiological recording method. Evoked potential amplitudes tend to be low, ranging from less than a microvolt to several microvolts, compared to tens of microvolts for EEG, millivolts for EMG. To resolve these low-amplitude potentials against the background of ongoing spontaneous EEG, ECG, and other biological signals and ambient physiologic noise, computerized signal averaging is required. The signal is time-locked to the stimulus, and because most of the noise occurs randomly, this allows the noise to be averaged out with averaging of repeated responses. The auditory evoked potential (AEP) can be used to trace the signal generated by a sound through the ascending auditory pathway (Figure 7–13). The evoked potential is generated in the cochlea, goes through the cochlear nerve, through the cochlear nucleus, superior olivary complex, lateral lemniscus, to the inferior colliculus in the midbrain, on to the medial geniculate body, and finally to the cortex.

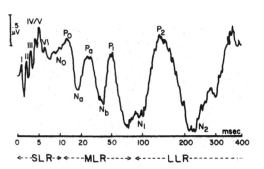

Figure 7–13. An idealized full auditory evoked potential representing the short-latency response (SLR), the middle-latency response (MLR), and the long-latency response (LLR).

The general averaged auditory evoked response is not a unitary response but rather is a composite response reflecting various activities from the auditory pathway. Davis (1976) identified these potentials in terms of their latency "epoch" as first components (0 to 2 msec: the cochlear microphonic and summating potential [CM]); fast components (2 to 10 msec: the acoustic nerve and auditory brainstem responses [ABR]); middle latency components (15 to 80 msec: thalamus and auditory cortex activity [MLR]); slow cortical components (50 to 300 msec, primary and secondary areas of the cerebral cortex); and late cortical components (300 msec and longer from the primary and association areas of the cerebral cortex).

The amplitude of these auditory evoked responses is generally related to the intensity of the stimulus; the more intense the stimulus, the larger is the average evoked response to a certain point. The growth in amplitude of the wave is accompanied by a decrease in latency of the peak components. As the stimulus signal is decreased toward threshold levels, the presence or absence of the averaged evoked response becomes difficult to separate from the biologic baseline activity. The clinical applications of evoked potential measurements are quite varied and include auditory, visual, and somatosensory evaluations. Evoked potentials are used for surgical monitoring by otolaryngologists, ophthalmologists, orthopedic surgeons, and neurosurgeons.

The evoked potential literature grew by leaps and bounds during the 1970s and 1980s. These studies were the beginning of a tremendous change in the field of physiologic evoked potential measurements. Improvements in equipment and computer technology have helped clarify the various evoked potentials in humans and, in turn, greatly influenced the field of audiology.

Although the ABR provides information regarding auditory function and hearing sensitivity, it is not a substitute for a formal hearing evaluation, and results should be used in conjunction with behavioral audiometry whenever possible.

The objective nature of this physiologic evaluation of auditory evoked response has been especially helpful in estimating hearing levels in pediatric patients and special needs populations. Stein and Kraus (1988) showed that the ABR could be the answer to evaluating hearing in many pediatric disorders including mild-to-profound cases of delayed development, deaf-blindness, hydrocephalus, meningitis, and infants and young children with autistic spectrum disorder. The authors noted, however, that although the audiologist is primarily interested in the use of the ABR as a test to estimate hearing levels, the abnormal neurologic conditions often found in these children may preclude or obviate the success of the ABR measurements. Thoughtful interpretation of AEP results must take into account not only the effect of potential peripheral hearing loss but the possibility of pathologic neurologic conditions.

Most evoked potential instrumentation now comes with software designed to automate the identification of specific wave peaks, amplitudes, and latencies. This application of automated analysis methodology facilitates the clinical use of auditory brainstem responses by reducing the time required to manually label and measure absolute and interpeak latencies (Delgato & Ozdamar, 1996). The automated systems can identify waveform thresholds and additional diagnostically significant information. In addition, automated systems have helped standardize the labeling process and nomenclature of the procedures. Most audiology and otolaryngology textbooks now include complete materials devoted to descriptions of AEPs. The task in this chapter is to present an overview of the early evoked potentials and their application in the clinical evaluation of hearing in children. The discussion has drawn from the materials of Hall (2007), Hood (1998), and Hall and Swanepoel (2010).

AUDITORY BRAINSTEM EVOKED RESPONSES (ABR)

A short history of the discovery and clinical development of the auditory brainstem evoked response (ABR) is worthy of note. In 1967, an important discovery was announced by two Israeli physicians, Sohmer and Feinmesser, who used click stimuli to evoke a new polyphasic response recorded with electrodes on the vertex of a human subject. This classic study was the first to demonstrate that ABRs recorded with surface electrodes could actually measure cochlear potentials noninvasively. This evoked potential was of very short latency, within the initial 12.5 msec poststimulus, and consisted of a specific pattern with five positive-direction waves. A few years later, Jewett and Williston (1971) provided a clear description of the human ABR and correctly interpreted the later waves as arriving from the brainstem. Jewett and Williston described the seven positive peak waveforms that occur within the initial 10 msec poststimulus that showed remarkable stability and consistent waveform latencies. An idealized auditory evoked potential is presented in Figure 7–14 that shows the component potentials (peaks) as they are commonly described with Roman numerals. Hecox, Squires, and Galambox (1976) and Starr, Arnlie, Martin, and Sanders (1977) showed that the ABR could be used for threshold estimation in adults and infants.

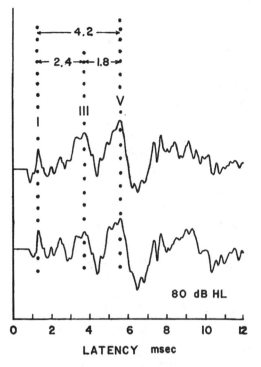

Figure 7–14. Typical latency measurements and interwave latency measurements for a high-intensity ABR. Courtesy of Laszlo Stein, PhD.

Jewett and Williston (1971) systematically recorded the early ABR human responses to varying stimulus and recording parameters. They labeled their seven positive peaks in Roman numerals from I to VII. Waves VI and VII of the ABR are not always readily apparent, so general clinical interpretation has focused on waves I through V. Wave V has proven to be the most prominent component of the response pattern and is often seen combined with wave IV to form what is termed the IV-V complex. The normal latency of each wave is about 1 msec longer than its designated number, so wave I has a latency of about 2 msec, whereas wave V has a latency of about 6 msec, as shown in Figure 7–14. Although the amplitude of the waves is easily influenced by numerous variables, the latency of the peaks is very stable.

The neural generators for the ABR are the peripheral acoustic nerve and the various nuclei of the ascending auditory brainstem pathway. Experimental studies in animals and studies of ABR in humans with confirmed lesions have led to the general conclusion that wave I represents the auditory nerve site and that waves II and III are associated with the medulla and pons, specifically the cochlear nucleus and superior olivary complex. Changes in the waveforms of IV and V are associated with lesions affecting midbrain auditory structures, the lateral lemniscus, and the inferior colliculus (Figure 7–15). Although controversy exists over the exact specification of origin sites for each wave of the ABR, Picton, Hillyard, Krausz, and Galambos (1974) suggested that waves I through IV represent activity from the auditory nerve and brainstem auditory nuclei, but that the total wave pattern is influenced by the composite contribution of multiple generators. Jerger et al. (1981) pointed out that with such a "farfield" recording technique with electrodes on the scalp, it is too simple to assume site specification of each wave to a unique generator. It is more reasonable to assume the ABR represents a complex interplay and interaction of evoked potential activity from multiple overlapping dipoles involving all the structures of the auditory system.

The clinical attributes of the ABR were summarized initially by Davis (1976) to include waveform consistency, easy recordability with proper equipment and technique, and optimal latency, yet slow enough to avoid confusion with the cochlear microphonic, yet fast enough to avoid being masked by muscle reflexes. The ABR is widely known for its freedom from the effects of central nervous system state and the replicability of the waveform pattern. In fact, the validity of an ABR tracing is usu-

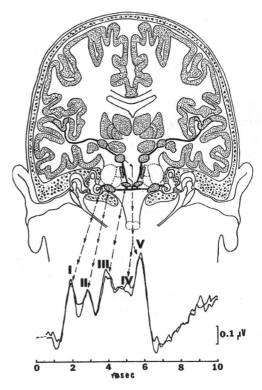

Figure 7–15. The auditory brainstem response waves and their generator sites: Wave I is associated with the auditory nerve, wave II comes from the cochlear nucleus, wave III comes from the superior olivary complex, wave IV is thought to come from the area of the lateral lemniscus, and wave V is from the inferior colliculus. Courtesy of Laszlo Stein, PhD.

ally verified by repeating the test and comparing both runs. Because ABR is relatively unaffected by the physiologic state of the patient, the measurement is accomplished with excellent results in both awake and sleep stages, thereby making the technique especially valuable with children.

The ABR recording is interpreted by evaluating several parameters including the peak amplitude (the number of neurons firing), latency (the speed of transmission), interpeak latency (the time between peaks), and interaural latency (the difference in wave V latency between ears). The ABR represents initiated activity beginning at the base of the cochlea and moving toward the apex. The amplitude peaks largely reflect activity from the most basal regions on the cochlea because the disturbance hits the basal end first and by the time it gets to the apex, a significant amount of phase cancellation occurs.

ABR measurements provide information regarding the identification of the site of a lesion in the auditory brainstem pathways (including acoustic nerve tumors), assessment of auditory function in patients with stroke or trauma, assessment of infant hearing, prediction of hearing sensitivity in difficult-to-test children, evaluation of aided versus unaided auditory performance, evaluation of neurologic disease and dysfunction, and provision of central auditory processing information. Nowadays, ABR applications are so widespread in use that evoked potentials are used by numerous other professional specialties including hearing scientists, psychologists and psycoacousticians, neurologists, ophthalmologists, neurosurgeons, and anesthesiologists.

ABR Parameters

The ABR is optimally recorded differentially from the vertex scalp to the ipsilateral mastoid or earlobe with an electrode on the contralateral mastoid serving as ground. The ABR is usually evoked with click stimuli, repetitively presented ($n = 2000$) at 30 clicks per second and summated by computer analysis. Click stimuli provide a sufficiently short rise time to ensure a synchronous neural burst from the auditory system (Hecox et al., 1976). Therein, however, is the main shortcoming of the ABR technique:

the lack of frequency-specific information about the hearing of the patient. The spectral energy of the transient click stimulus is shaped by the earphone resonant characteristics and the duration of the click. Because clicks fail to allow frequency specificity in the auditory system, the ABR reflects predominantly the basal turn of the cochlea or hearing information between 1000 and 4000 Hz.

Several techniques have been developed with stimuli other than clicks to enable ABR results to be more frequency specific. Tone pips, filtered clicks, or the subtractive masking procedure can be used as frequency-specific stimuli, although there is some question about the spread of energy around each of these transient sudden onset signals. The use of these frequency-specific stimulus techniques is typically more demanding and time consuming than the use of unmasked tone bursts or filtered clicks. A thorough tutorial describing how stimulus, masking, and recording parameters affect the frequency and place specificity of auditory brainstem responses (ABRs) to air- and bone-conducted stimuli was published by Stapells and Oats (1997).

Stimulus factors have an interactive influence on the ABR waveform which can be demonstrated by varying individual parameters of the stimulus and observing modifications of the wave pattern (Stockard & Stockard, 1979). Increasing stimulus intensity influences the ABR waveform by increasing the amplitude and decreasing wave latencies. The relationship between stimulus intensity and wave peak latencies is used to plot latency-intensity functions for each of the waves. Typical latency-intensity functions are demonstrated in Figure 7–16 as used in differential diagnosis of hearing losses compared with the normal range of latency-intensity responses.

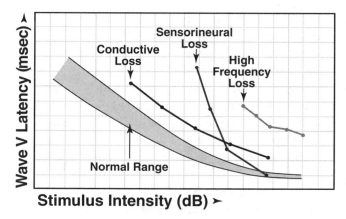

Figure 7–16. Characteristic latency-intensity functions obtained from normal-hearing patients and patients with various types of hearing loss. Courtesy of Nicolet Biomedical, Madison, WI.

The latency-intensity function is usually plotted for waves I, III, and V, and the patterns of all three functions are approximately parallel. This indicates that the interpeak intervals (sometimes called interwave latency intervals) are relatively constant over the entire intensity range. Thus, the interpeak intervals (i.e., peak I to peak III, III to V, or I to V as shown in Figure 7–14) can be measured at any intensity level without concern that the measurement will be affected. In older children and adults, the I to III interpeak interval is about 2 msec, the III to IV interpeak interval is approximately 2 msec, and thus, the I to V interval is about 4 msec.

At high stimulus intensity (80 dB HL or greater), all five waves are usually seen with clarity in normal persons. As stimulus intensity is decreased, below 60 dB HL for example, waves I, II, and IV tend to become difficult to identify with certainty. When stimulus intensity nears auditory threshold, wave V is often the only remaining landmark in the response tracing. In this fashion, as shown in Figure 7–17, ABR is used to estimate auditory threshold. The tester must keep in mind the lack of information provided from traditional audiometric test frequencies below 1000 Hz. Likewise, the ABR is very sensitive to peripheral high-frequency hearing loss and central auditory pathway disorders. These conditions, either singularly or together, can make the ABR waveform difficult to interpret.

ABRs to tonal stimuli can be successfully recorded in most clinical environments and can provide reasonably accurate estimates of 500 to 4000 Hz pure-tone behavioral thresholds in infants and children (Stapells & Oats, 1997). Gorga, Worthington, Reiland, Beauchaine, and Goldgar (1985) compared ABR responses with pure tone audiograms obtained from patients with cochlear hearing loss. The click-evoked ABR thresholds were most closely related to behavioral audiometric thresholds at 2000 and 4000 Hz, with poor agreement at 1000 and 8000 Hz. The ABR latency-intensity function slope was related to the configuration of the hearing loss so that patients with high-frequency sensorineural hearing losses had steeper slopes than patients with flat hearing losses or normal hearing.

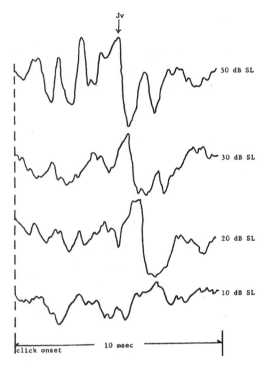

Figure 7–17. Summed brainstem evoked responses at decreasing intensities. Each response represents 2,048 click presentations.

An increase in the stimulus click rate increases the latency and reduces the amplitude of the ABR waves. The amplitude of wave V is constant up to 30 clicks per second, although the peak latency of wave V may change about 1.0 msec as the stimulus click rate is increased from 10 to 100 clicks per second. These technical considerations make it mandatory that all clinical facilities that wish to perform ABR establish their own norms for their particular test parameters and procedures before testing patients.

Maturation of the ABR

Starr et al. (1977) reported the results of ABR studies on infants as young as 28 weeks of gestational age and believed that the brainstem response wave complexes could be identified if the stimuli were sufficiently loud. However, an important variable in the interpretation of ABR tracings, especially in premature infants, is the effect of maturation on the waveforms. The effect of maturation in infant populations is significant, and without proper normative standards, misinterpretation of peak wave latencies can easily occur. Several leading laboratories have evaluated both neonatal normal and high-risk populations with ABR techniques in an attempt to determine the reliability, sensitivity, and accuracy of the procedures. Gorga, Kaminski, and Beauchaine (1988) recommended the use of insert earphones for use with infants to prevent erroneous conductive hearing loss due to collapse of the external ear canals, a common occurrence when circumaural earphones are used.

Stockard and Westmoreland (1981) identified several limitations of ABR evaluations in a neonatal population. A heightened vulnerability of the neonatal wave potentials to certain technical and subject factors should be of concern. Stimulus intensity calibration can be a major source of variability in peak and interpeak latencies. Uncertainty about the conceptual age versus gestational age of the infant may confuse the interpretation because of the rapid change of maturational levels in auditory transmission time. Between the ages of 18 months and 25 years of age, ABR shows little change in latency or amplitude.

Many waveform criteria of AEPs, including the absolute latency of waves I and V, the latency-intensity function, the wave I to V interwave interval, and the amplitude ratio of wave V to wave I, are used to identify infants with hearing loss and to distinguish peripheral hearing loss from intracranial pathology (Finitzo-Hieber, 1982). Accurate infant assessment requires age-specific norms for each of the measurements. These waveforms are first visible in a premature infant at 28 to 30 weeks after conception (or 28 to 30 weeks; gestational age), not after birth. However, latencies are prolonged and thresholds are elevated when compared with those of a full-term newborn. The maturation of the ABR is not complete until 12 to 18 months post-term (with term being 38 to 40 weeks' gestational age). Figure 7–18 illustrates the maturation of wave V and wave I over time. Note that the critical time is expressed in time after conception rather than in time after birth.

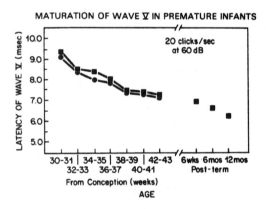

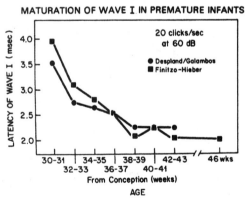

Figure 7–18. Maturation of wave V and wave I over time. Used with permission, "Auditory Brainstem Response: Its Place in Infant Audiological Evaluations," by T. Finitzo-Hieber, 1982, *Seminars in Speech, Language and Hearing, 3,* 76–87.

Finitzo-Hieber (1982) made the following recommendations for conducting ABR in premature infants. First, if a premature infant is tested far in advance of hospital discharge, the baby can present with a significant, but transient, impairment that may show partial or complete recovery at the time of discharge. If ABR is to be effective, assessment should take place near discharge time, when the infant is in an open crib and is not less than 37 weeks of gestational age. Second, a single ABR assessment is not sufficient in premature infants. Both improvement and deterioration in auditory function have been documented on follow-up testing. Therefore, at-risk infants should be monitored with ABR every 3 months in the first year of life.

Figure 7–19 shows the general maturation of the ABR from newborn to adulthood (Hecox & Jacobson, 1984). Gorga, Reiland, Beauchaine, Worthington, and Jesteadr (1987) contributed substantially to the establishment of ABR normative standards in infants and young children. Their comprehensive study of 585 graduates of an intensive care nursery showed small systematic decreases in response component latencies occurring with increasing age. The normal distribution of results, therefore, makes it possible to identify an individual infant's wave V latency or interpeak latency difference that might fall below the 5th or 10th percentile of the respective cumulative distribution. Their results also confirmed the importance of taking chronologic age of the infant into account when evaluating ABR latencies. As an extension of the above-described study of ABR with intensive care nursery infants, Gorga, Kaminski, Beauchaine, Jesteadr, and Neely (1989) reported normative data on 535 children with normal hearing from 3 months to 3 years of age. Wave V latency decreased as age increased

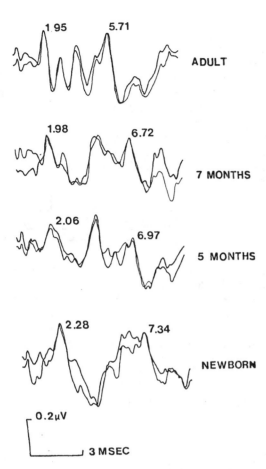

Figure 7–19. Maturation of the auditory brainstem response from postnatal newborn period to adulthood. Used with permission from "Auditory Evoked Potentials," by K. Hecox and J. Jacobson, 1984, in J. L. Northern, Ed., *Hearing Disorders,* Boston, MA: Little, Brown & Co.

at least to 18 months, whereas little or no change was noted in wave I latencies over the same age range. Interpeak wave latency differences followed the same developmental time course as wave V.

Binaural stimulation is often useful when testing children (Figure 7–20). Binaural stimulation with clicks produces waveforms that are approximately 1.5 times greater in amplitude than noted with mon-

aural stimulation of either ear. The latencies of the waves are essentially the same for monaural and binaural stimulation. The binaural stimulation technique is good for approximating auditory threshold, because the response to binaurally presented clicks is the same as the response to monaurally presented clicks in the better hearing ear. The binaural stimulation technique, however, may miss a unilateral hearing loss in one ear if the other ear has normal hearing.

A major disadvantage in ABR with children is that most children between the ages of about 6 months and 4 years must be passively quiet for the duration of the testing session. For the infant less than 12 months of age, sleep deprivation prior to arriving for the ABR procedure will be sufficient that the baby will fall asleep in a quiet and darkened room and sleep through the test duration. Somewhat older toddlers may require the use of a mild sedative to sleep through the test, but this will require professional medical staff to administer the drug and to be on hand during the session. In hospital settings, it may be easier to perform the ABR test in a surgical suite while the infant is undergoing other procedures that require anesthesia. A minimum of 1 hour for each test session is generally required for a full ABR evaluation, although it may be wise to be prepared to carry on longer if necessary to obtain adequate information about the hearing of the child. Most children older than 4.5 years can be entertained during the session or will sit fairly quietly until the test is completed.

No ABR study should be undertaken without first attempting behavioral audiometrics and immittance measurements. The ABR is only a part of the whole diagnostic process for clinicians, whose responsibility must cover history taking, traditional audiometrics, evaluation of the patient's

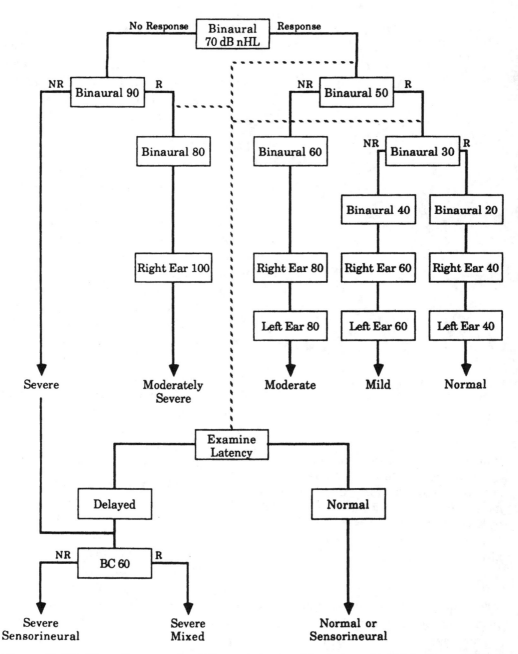

Figure 7–20. Flow diagram of a "binaural strategy" technique to obtain time-efficient ABR hearing threshold estimates in children. Used with permission from "Auditory Brainstem Response Testing Strategies," J. Jerger, T. Oliver, and B. Stach, 1985, in J. Jacobson, Ed., *The Auditory Brainstem Response*, pp. 371–388, San Diego, CA: College-Hill Press.

overall communicative abilities, parent counseling, and overall case disposition. It must be emphasized that the ABR does not test "hearing" in the perceptual sense, and it cannot identify a specific neurologic lesion at a given location; consequently, ABR results cannot stand alone and must be interpreted in the context of a cross-check with other clinical information. Jerger et al. (1980) cite overinterpretation of ABR results and failure to consider other test findings in the total clinical picture as the most common errors made by clinicians. However, the ABR has become such an integral part of the audiology armamentarium that it is widely used for newborn hearing screening, auditory threshold estimation, intraoperative monitoring, determining hearing loss type and degree, and auditory nerve and brainstem lesion detection (Figure 7–21A and B).

AUDITORY MIDDLE-LATENCY EVOKED RESPONSE (MLR)

The auditory middle-latency evoked responses (MLRs) are so called because their latency lies between that of the early ABR evoked responses and the late cortical evoked responses. The latencies of the MLR peaks are found between 10 and 50 msec post-stimulus presentations. Although latency of the MLR response is important in interpretation, the presence of the response is determined by a comparison of the amplitude of the three major wave components (Na, Pa, and Pb). There is a mix of opinion among professionals relative to the value of the middle-latency evoked response in the evaluation of hearing and hearing loss in children. Although most agree that the MLR can be used to estimate hearing sensitivity, the response is greatly influenced by the subject's age, alertness state, as well as numerous measurement parameters such as stimulus rate and filter settings. Jerger, Chmiel, Frost, and Coker (1986) and Jerger, Oliver, and Chmiel (1988) concluded that the MLR requires a large number of averages to formulate the response, thereby causing a slow rate of data acquisition, and along with the variability created by the influence of stimulus rate, the clinical value of this evoked potential is questionable.

The discovery and the major investigation of auditory middle-latency evoked potential are associated with studies by

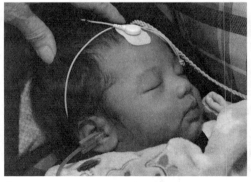
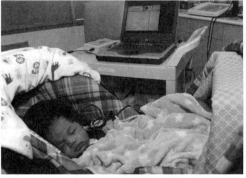

A　　　　　　　　　　　　**B**

Figure 7–21. A–B. ABR testing is an important component in the evaluation of hearing in infants. Photos courtesy of Colorado Children's Hospital, Aurora, CO.

Goldstein and Rodman (1967), Mendel and Goldstein (1969), and Mendel (1980). The sites of generation have been discussed for years, but so far there is no specific evidence to identify them precisely. It is generally accepted that the MLR is, as proposed by Beagley and Fisch (1981), situated in the auditory radiations in the thalamic region and in the primary auditory cortex in the temporal lobe.

The MLR is a very small signal embedded in high levels of background noise, so it can take a long time to acquire. The auditory middle latency response (MLR) seems to have a relatively long developmental time course, extending through the first decade of life. Characteristics of each MLR component change developmentally not only with respect to waveform morphology but also

with respect to response reliability, dependence on awareness state, and stimulus rate (McGee & Kraus, 1996). Hood (1975) described the nature of the MLR to be two major positive peaks (P_o with a latency of 12 msec, and P_a with a latency of 32 msec) and three negative troughs, N_o, N_a, and N_b, occurring at 8, 18, and 52 msec, respectively, as shown in Figure 7–22. Hood suggested that the close agreement between MLR thresholds and behavioral thresholds for the same stimuli supports the view that the MLR can be an indicator of auditory sensitivity.

Mendel and Goldstein (1971) showed that the amplitude of the MLR is influenced dramatically through various sleep stages and wakefulness. Subsequent studies have verified the sleep effect on the MLR. Work

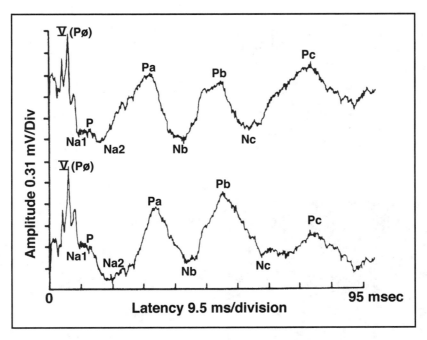

Figure 7–22. Normal MLR curves. The upper waveform was recorded with standard-phase shift settings, whereas the lower waveform was recorded with zero-phase shift (filter setting = 15 Hz, 24 dB/octave). Used with permission from "High Pass Digital and Analog Filtering of the Middle Latency Response," by K. T. Kavanagh and W. D. Domico, 1987, *Ear and Hearing, 8*(2), 102.

by Kraus, McGee, and Comperatore (1989) shows that wave P_a detectability is especially poor during certain stages of sleep. Because of the length of time required to collect the MRL data, it would be helpful for young children to be sedated; however, the effects of natural or induced sleep are crucial factors in interpreting the MLR in pediatric applications. Although early investigations reported MLRs in babies, attempts to use the MLR for infant hearing screening have been unsuccessful. Jerger et al. (1988) point out that the MLR is observed in babies only under very slow stimulus rates and is a "very fragile" response at best.

Kraus et al. (1989) stated that the occurrence of MLR in older children ages 4 to 9 years is not haphazard and that their MLR can be reliably obtained during certain states of arousal. Apparently, Kraus et al. routinely simultaneously measure the ABR and the MLR in children to obtain a measure of low-frequency hearing. When MLRs are present, they provide a useful test of auditory threshold estimation at 500 and 1000 Hz. However, because of the inconsistency of the detectability of the MLR in children, absence of the MLR cannot be interpreted as an indication of hearing loss in the low frequencies.

Kavanagh, Gould, McCormick, and Franks (1989) compared low-intensity ABR and MLR in a group of 48 persons with developmental delay. Although the ABR measurement generally showed better test-retest reliability than the MLR, several of the subjects with hearing loss were noted to have recordable MLRs when no ABR could be detected. These authors suggested that this is evidence that the ABR and MLR have different neurologic centers and that perhaps a loss of neuronal synchronization may result in the absence of the ABR but still allow identification of the low-frequency MLR.

Ozdamar and Kraus (1983) published a study of auditory MLRs and ABRs in the same persons. They found that mild sedatives did not appear to affect either MLR or ABR and that MLR differed from ABR in stimulus-related properties, implying that the neuronal mechanisms underlying their generation are not the same. In contrast to previous studies (Mendel et al., 1975), they found that MLR wave components were not as readily identifiable at low stimulus levels as the ABR wave V. They concluded that although the ABR is the test of choice when hearing threshold is in question, the MLR is likely to be most clinically useful in patients with neurologic or central auditory processing disorders as demonstrated in Figure 7–23.

Hall, Bantwal, Ramkumar, and Chhabria (2011) published a comprehensive review of the middle latency response with numerous suggestions for pediatric applications. In addition to threshold estimation, Hall et al. point out that the MRL can be used to document cochlear implant and hearing aid performance because it arises from higher auditory areas. Various studies conducted by researchers from around the world of the MRL are reviewed in terms of their application of the MLR to investigate children with auditory processing disorders, language learning disabilities, brain injury, Down syndrome, developmental delay, autism spectrum disorder, and auditory neuropathy spectrum disorder.

LATE AUDITORY EVOKED POTENTIALS (AEPs)

The late AEPs have had a long and colorful history beginning in the 1960s. In fact, during the mid-1960s, the late evoked potentials were being hailed as "the answer" to audiometric testing problems and the

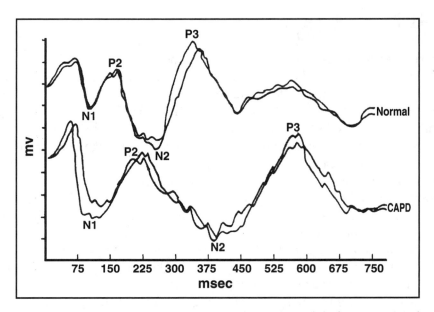

Figure 7–23. Normal long-latency auditory potentials from a normal control group (*top*) and a group of children with central auditory processing disorders (*bottom*). Note the shift in P_3 component latency. Used with permission from "Long Latency Auditory Event-Related Potentials From Children with Auditory Processing Disorders," J. Jirsa and K. Clontz, 1991, *Ear and Hearing, 11*(3), 225.

difficult-to-test patient. The success of the technique was related to the fact that under the best of conditions, auditory thresholds obtained with this "objective" procedure agreed within 20 dB of adult auditory behavioral thresholds. Unfortunately, the late potentials are extremely sensitive to even minor alterations in subject state of awareness, level of consciousness, and changes in stimulus parameters. Technical problems, equipment expense, and lack of clinical precision made routine use of auditory late potentials impractical for most clinical facilities. Thus, efforts to use late cortical potentials in clinical measurements were largely abandoned in the early 1970s.

The late cortical auditory evoked potentials (CAEPs) result from generalized electrical activity on the cortex because of the presentation of various sensory stimuli including light, vibrotactile, and sound. The CAEP is also known by a number of other terms: the N1–P2 response, slow vertex response, and the auditory cortical response. The presentation of any sensory stimulus of sufficient intensity or the abrupt change of any stimulus produces a widespread evoked potential from the human brain during the 300 msec following the stimulus presentation. Carter, Golding, Dillon, and Seymour (2010) compared an automated statistical analysis of the CAEP waveform with visual inspection from experienced audiologists to detect the presence or absence of the CAEP obtained from a group of infants. The automated analysis compared favorably with the experienced examiners, thereby helping reduce the potential errors of subjectively judging the CAEP from electrophysiologic noise.

The late cortical potentials have generated renewed interest, research, and unique applications during the recent decade. Most are easily elicited as by the onset of a tone or speech sample, in fact, the N1–P2 response results from literally any abrupt change in auditory environment such as in intensity, frequency, and so forth, or even by the offset of a sound. The N and P refer to the sign of the potential (negative and positive) at the vertex compared to the potential at the reference electrode. According to Lightfoot (http://www.corticalera.com) N1 has a latency of about 100 ms and P2 of about 200 ms at stimulus intensities well above threshold (thus sometimes described as N_{100} and P_{200}). As intensity is reduced toward threshold, the latencies increase to almost double these figures with N1 at 200 ms and P2 at 400 ms. The amplitude of the N1–P2 response may be up to about 25 µV for moderate- to high-intensity stimuli, decreasing in size to zero at or near threshold. These relationships are referred to as input-output functions, and knowledge of their characteristics helps us in evaluating an individual's hearing threshold. The generator of N1 is probably the primary auditory cortex, but P2 probably has multiple generators, perhaps within the polysensory frontal areas.

The late responses can be elicited with pure tone stimuli permitting the electrophysiologic prediction of auditory thresholds. However, these potentials are fatally confounded by subject state of consciousness, rendering them nearly unacceptable for routine hearing threshold purposes in anyone but awake, cooperating adults. The late cortical potentials are receiving renewed interest because of their presumed relationship to the perceptual attributes of sound and interhemispheric differences and because of their various neurologic and psychiatric applications. One particular wave, the P300 component, has been studied in various cognitive tasks and is thought by some to hold promise for investigating how the brain processes information (Mendel, 1985).

Because of its magnitude and relative ease in observing and recording, the N1–P2 complex has been studied extensively (Hall et al., 2011). Recently, the late auditory potentials have been creatively utilized by research groups in a number of unique clinical applications. The CAEPs as an indicator and measure of infant brain plasticity and maturation has been reported by Sharma et al. (2005a, 2005b); Lightfoot and Kennedy (2006) used the N1–N2 measure for objective cortical auditory threshold determination in adults; Sharma, Cardon, Henion, and Roland (2011) also used these late auditory potentials in the diagnosis of auditory neuropathy spectrum disorder, and as evidence of auditory processing deficits in children with reading disorder (Sharma et al., 2006). Sharma (2009) has developed a valuable clinical protocol using the peak P^1 as an indicator of benefit in infant hearing aid fittings and cochlear implants described in more detail in Chapter 9. In Australia, Dillon and colleagues have used the N1–P2 response to brief speech phonemes in an automated fashion to verify hearing aid benefit in infants (Carter et al., 2010; Dillon et al., 2005). Examples of the clinical application with late cortical potentials are shown in Figures 7–24 and 7–25. These advanced research efforts demonstrate the potential of using the N1–P2 complex for additional clinical applications in the future.

AUDITORY STEADY-STATE RESPONSE (ASSR)

The auditory steady-state response (ASSR) is an auditory evoked potential that can be used to objectively estimate hearing sensitivity

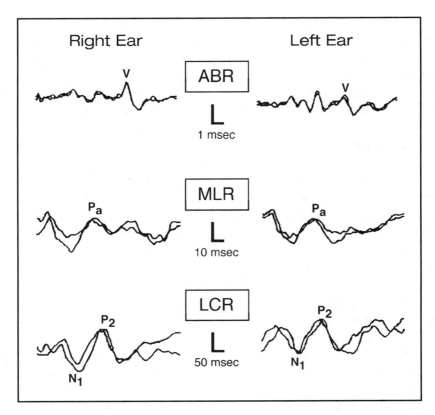

Figure 7–24. Normal auditory evoked potential series from a child with delayed speech and language development. Auditory evoked potential testing included ABR to clicks of 70 dB nHL; the MLR to clicks presented at 70 dB nHL; and the late cortical response LCR to a 500 Hz tone burst at 50 dB nHL. All auditory evoked potential components were of normal latency, amplitude, and morphology. Courtesy of Brad Stach, PhD.

in individuals with normal hearing sensitivity and individuals with various degrees and configurations of sensorineural hearing loss (Korczak, Smart, Delgado, Strobel, & Bradford, 2012). The ASSR is elicited with modulated tones that can be used to predict hearing sensitivity in patients of all ages. It is evoked by the periodic modulation, or rapid turning on and off of a tone. The ASSR neural response is a brain potential that closely follows the time course and envelope of the modulation. The response can be detected objectively at intensity levels close to behav-

ioral threshold making it a useful tool in the audiology clinic.

The ASSR was first described over 30 years ago, and independently investigated by groups of researchers in Australia (Rickards & Clark, 1982) and in Canada (Picton, 1987). Over the past two decades, it has been verified that the ASSR will yield a clinically acceptable, frequency-specific prediction of behavioral thresholds in patients, regardless of age, subject state, or degree of hearing loss (Lins et al., 1996; Rance, Rickards, Cohen, DeVidi, & Clark, 1995). Vari-

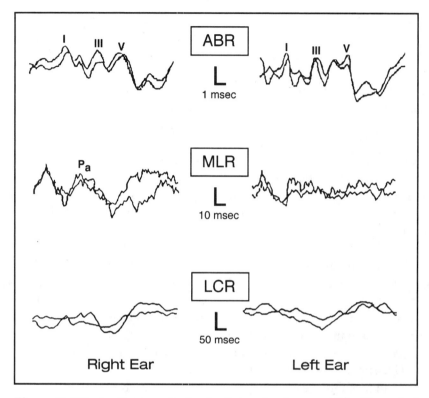

Figure 7–25. Auditory evoked potential series from a child with central auditory processing disorder: ABR to clicks presented at 70 dB nHL; MLR to clicks presented at 70 dB nHL; and the late cortical response to a 500 Hz tone burst at 60 dB nHL. Wave V is identifiable at normal latencies on the ABRs, and peak P_a is identifiable on the right-ear MLR; the P_a on the left ear is degraded in morphology. No waveform peaks were identifiable on the LCRs. Used with permission from "Clinical Experience With Personal FM Assistive Listening Devices." B. A. Stach, L. H. Loiselle, J. F. Jerger, S. L. Mintz, and C. D. Taylor, 1987, *The Hearing Journal, 40*(5), 24–30.

ous studies have shown that the ASSR can provide a reasonably accurate prediction of behavioral thresholds comparable in accuracy to the ABR (Cone-Wessen, Dowell, Tomlin, Rance, & Ming, 2002; Stach, 2002).

Rickards, Wilson, Tan, and Cohen (1990) initially noted ASSRs could be readily recorded and were particularly useful at modulation rates of greater than 60 Hz, but ultimately found that at modulation rates of around 90 Hz, robust ASSRs could be recorded from sleeping adults and infants. The ASSR is generally elicited by pure tones of 500, 1000, 2000, and 4000 Hz. The pure tone is either modulated in the amplitude domain or modulated in both the amplitude and frequency domains. That tone is modulated, or warbled, to expand the spectrum of the tone; however, the frequency spread is narrower than a tone-burst or short duration click. Because only a restricted portion of the basilar membrane is being stimulated, a more precise audiogram can be predicted (Stach, 2002). Furthermore, if the modulation rates are high enough, the ASSR seems unaffected by subject state; when the modulation rate is greater than 60 times per second (60 Hz), the auditory steady-state response can still be recorded reliably in sleeping babies (Rickards et al., 1994).

In clinical audiology, a common application of ASSR is estimation of auditory thresholds in children with severe to profound hearing loss. The maximum effective intensity level of click stimuli traditionally used to evoke the ABR is about 90 dB nHL which limits the use of the ABR as a threshold-seeking measure to those with hearing losses of 70 dB or better. The ASSR technique is able to determine hearing thresholds for individuals with severe and profound hearing loss at levels greater than 70 dB HL. Thus, infants and young children with severe and profound hearing loss will have absent ABRs, and the audiologists will be left to guess whether the loss is severe, profound, or complete. The ASSR has the potential to give an extra 50 dB worth of information about degree of loss. That is very important in determining early candidacy for amplification or implantation (Beck, Speidel, & Petrak, 2007; Stach, 2002).

Analysis of the ASSR is mathematically based and dependent on the fact that related neuronal brain potentials coincide with the stimulus repetition rate. ASSR relies on sophisticated statistics-based mathematical detection algorithms to objectively detect and define if and when an auditory threshold is present. ASSR design and functionality vary across manufacturers. The specific method of analysis is based on the equipment manufacturer's statistical detection algorithm. It occurs in the spectral domain and is composed of specific frequency components that are harmonics of the stimulus repetition rate. Currently, there is no universal standard for ASSR instrumentation. Stimulus and recording parameters and methods are designed (and may vary) by each manufacturer. As described by Stach (2002), a robust following response to the modulating tone will have a fairly consistent or coherent phase relationship; if the brain is not responding to the sound, then the phase relationship to the modulation will be totally random. A criterion level for significant phase coherence is then used to determine objectively and automatically whether or not a response occurs. Most ASSR instrumentation provides correction tables for converting ASSR thresholds to estimated hearing level audiograms and are generally found to be within 10 dB of behaviorally obtained audiometric thresholds.

Beck et al. (2007) provided a useful comparison between ASSR testing and ABR testing. ABR typically uses broad-frequency click or tone-burst stimuli in one ear at a time, but ASSR can be used binaurally while evaluating broad bands or specific frequencies (500, 1000, 2000, and 4000) simultaneously. ABR estimates thresholds basically from 1000 to 4000 Hz in typical mild-moderate-severe hearing losses; ASSR can also estimate thresholds in the same range but offers more frequency-specific information more quickly and can estimate hearing in the more severe-to-profound hearing loss ranges. ASSR looks at amplitude and phases in the spectral (frequency) domain rather than at amplitude and latency parameters as measured with ABR. ASSR is evoked using repeated sound stimuli presented at a high repetition rate rather than an abrupt sound (click) at a relatively low repetition rate. ABR depends upon a subjective analysis of the amplitude/latency function; ASSR uses a statistical analysis of the probability of a response (usually at a 95% confidence interval). ABR is measured in microvolts (millionths of a volt), and the ASSR is measured in nanovolts (billionths of a volt). Although ABR evaluation is available in most audiology clinics and facilities, ASSR currently is not as widely used, perhaps due to its complexity and redundancy to ABR results.

ELECTROCOCHLEOGRAPHY

Investigators have long been intrigued by the electrical potentials generated within the auditory system. Clinicians have made many efforts to utilize these auditory potentials in some form of clinical procedure. These measurements were termed electrocochleography (ECochG) by Lempert, Wever, and Lawrence (1947). The electrocochleogram (ECochGm) consists of more than one auditory electrical potential including the whole nerve action potential (AP), the cochlear microphonic (CM), and the summating potential (SP) as seen in Figure 7–26. The action potential is the most obvious and easily recorded component of the ECochGm.

The electrical potential from the auditory nerve is the AP, noted initially by

Derbyshire and Davis as early as 1935. The AP consists of nerve impulses in the eighth nerve triggered by the CM. The AP response consists of a well-synchronized volley of impulses called N_1 which may be followed by smaller waves known as N_2 and N_3. Although initial clinical attempts to use auditory electrical potentials focused on the CM, the compound AP response is currently proving most valuable in clinical use. The compound AP has a latency of about 2 msec when the cochlea is stimulated by an abrupt sound stimulus. Although the individual AP in each auditory nerve fiber is a diphasic spike potential, the response of the whole auditory nerve is a compound potential that gives information from the basal turn of the cochlea and, to a lesser extent, from the middle turn (Beagley & Fisch, 1981).

The CM originates from the hair cells in the organ of Corti as originally described by Wever and Bray (1930). The hair cells function as a transducer, converting the mechanical movement of the basilar membrane into electrical voltage. The CM reproduces faithfully the waveform of the stimulating auditory signal and is usually measured for

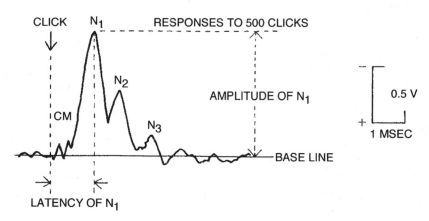

Figure 7–26. Electrocochleographic (ECochG) averaged response as recorded from an electrode in the external auditory canal. The definition of *N*, latency, and amplitude of the ECochG response.

clinical purposes by a near-field electrode on the tympanic membrane or by an electrode from the round window niche. The CM has no threshold other than the lower limits of the recording apparatus (i.e., the CM is produced to any auditory signal, no matter how slight). When the stereocilia of the outer hair cells are bent by movement of the basilar membrane, mechanically gated ion channels open and potassium (K+) and calcium (Ca^{2+}) ions enter. An AC current flows through the surface of the outer hair cells, and this increase in the flow has the same frequency as the basilar membrane movement and, hence, the acoustic stimulus frequency. This measurable AC voltage is the cochlear microphonic (CM), which mimics exactly the eliciting stimulus.

The ECochG is a powerful electrophysiologic index of cochlear integrity. Despite the lack of standardization regarding many aspects related to acquiring and recording ECochG, this tool provides useful information for a variety of clinical applications. When a response is present, one can be assured that there is at least some residual hearing; when there is no response, one can be reasonably certain that no residual hearing exists. The magnitude of the recording is dependent on the proximity of the recording electrodes to the hair cells. The CM is proportional to the displacement of the basilar membrane. Usually the recordings are generated primarily from the basal end of the cochlea which is nearest to the promontory or the electrodes. With transtympanic recording (through the tympanic membrane with the needle electrode positioned on the otic capsule), the large promontory responses require relatively few samples to obtain useful data; an entire input-output function for click stimuli can be generated very quickly. In fact, most early work with ECochG involved inserting a needle elec-

trode through the tympanic membrane, touching the promontory of the otic capsule. This "surgical" invasive procedure obviously greatly limited the clinical utilization of the technique in the United States.

It has been shown that electrodes placed in the ear canal, touching or very near to the tympanic membrane, may yield acceptable ECochG results. Placement of the electrode is crucial as there is a direct relationship, of course, between the voltage amplitude of the ECochG and the recording site; that is, the closer the electrode to the source of generation, the larger the recorded amplitude (Jacobson, 1996). Extratympanic electrodes can be used in children with appropriate sedation, and current auditory evoked potential recording systems allow for either independent or simultaneous recording of ECochG and ABR potentials

Bergholtz, Arlinger, Kyler, and Jerlvall (1977) reported interesting results from performing electrocochleography on 30 difficult-to-test children, including 11 children with severe developmental delay. When possible, informal hearing tests or free-field testing were performed to compare hearing threshold estimates. The correlation between free-field test thresholds and AP "thresholds" was reported as "good," especially in subjects with relatively good hearing. However, in spite of the Bergholtz study results, ear canal ECochG is not used often in the testing of children because it is difficult to accurately determine auditory thresholds from the technique.

In fact, ECochG has largely been replaced in the United States with widespread use of ABR. The ABR requires less technical expertise, is less expensive, is less traumatic to the patient, and offers more extensive information about the auditory system and hearing threshold estimation. With ABR, however, it is sometimes difficult to identify wave I, and under such circumstances it may prove useful to utilize ECochG measurements to demonstrate the presence of wave I. Ferraro, Beck, and Speidel (2011) suggest that using an ear canal electrocochleographic approach to record the ABR will improve the amplitude and detection of wave I in newborns and difficult-to-test patients. More recently, recording of the CM has proven valuable in the diagnosis of auditory neuropathy spectrum disorder (ANSD). Ferraro (2010) reported that patients with more than 40 to 50 dB HL hearing loss from 1000 to 4000 Hz are not good candidates for ECochG. Hall and Swanepoel (2010) published an excellent up-to-date description of ECochG techniques and clinical applications.

SEDATION

Although it is far better to test a child under natural sleep, it may occasionally be necessary to sedate a noncooperative or otherwise difficult-to-test child to conduct the necessary physiologic auditory tests. Testing the child under sedation may be the only way to determine the presence or absence of hearing or to further define a suspected hearing loss. Be fully aware, however, that the medications used for sedation and drugs used in anesthesia may have undesirable side effects that place patients at risk for adverse medical complications and reactions. Safe practice procedures for the use of sedation and topical anesthetics in audiology and speech-language pathology were developed by ASHA (1992). The guidelines urge practitioners who participate in such procedures to be fully aware of the complex factors that may expose their patients to risk or harm. Of course, administration of medi-

cations to achieve a desired patient state is a medical procedure requiring physician's prescription, monitoring, and supervision.

Every effort should be made to complete the pediatric audiologic workup with the infant and toddler in a quiet but unsedated state. This can be accomplished by directing parents and caregivers to keep the child awake as late as possible the night before the hearing test so that he or she will sleep soundly during the evaluation. A quiet, sleeping baby allows the audiologist to get better responses to each of the physiologic testing procedures. Sometimes it will help to feed the tired infant just prior to the testing to ensure a relaxed, comfortable, and sleepy baby. Perhaps the parents might bring a blanket or stuffed toy that helps make the infant calm and more comfortable during the evaluation. It may be necessary to allow for a longer block of time in the schedule, because sometimes more time is needed for the evaluation if the infant does not want to quiet down and sleep right away. Melatonin is an over-the-counter natural product that can help produce sleep and wake cycles and may be useful to help children fall sleep. Melatonin is quite mild with widely variable effect on individuals and may not have the desired effect to produce immediate sleep. Consideration might be given to mild sleep inducers such as Benadryl or melatonin with physician approval.

Audiologists should define in writing specific protocols developed in collaboration with a responsible physician for children who need to be sedated. The protocols should specify responsibility for each individual and each aspect of care and limit sedation procedures. Attention should be drawn to detail immediate access to emergency medical care. In all instances, both in development of written protocols and in actual professional practice, the comfort and safety of the patient must be paramount. In many hospital settings, sedation of children is done in an operating room at the same time of some surgical procedure, and the physiological audiology tests can be administered during that session.

Audiologists need be aware of the terminology and definitions of the various levels of sedation and anesthesia in common practice in outpatient surgery and during operative procedures, as described below:

- *Conscious sedation* describes a minimally depressed level of consciousness that retains the patient's ability to maintain a patent airway independently and continuously as well as to respond appropriately to physical stimulation and verbal commands.
- *Deep sedation* is a controlled state of depressed consciousness or unconsciousness from which the patient is not easily aroused, which may be accompanied by a partial or complete loss of protective reflexes. The patient retains the ability to maintain a patent airway independently and responds purposefully to physical stimulation and verbal command.
- *General anesthesia* is a controlled state of unconsciousness accompanied by a loss of protective reflexes, loss of the ability to maintain a patent airway, and loss of the ability to respond to physical stimulation or verbal command.

Despite the availability of newer agents, chloral hydrate remains a common choice for sedation of children for audiologic procedures. Chloral hydrate produces sedation without significant adverse effects on cardiovascular or respiratory function at therapeutic doses. Chloral hydrate produces effective sedation in 80% to 90% of patients. It is often selected because of the availability of an oral dosage form and its relatively mild adverse effect profile. Unfortunately, its unpredictable onset, long duration, and the lack of a reversal agent, make chloral hydrate less than an ideal sedative (Buck, 2005). A major disadvantage to chloral hydrate is that it is a long-acting sedative.

A number of sedatives are now available in common use in children due to their ease of administration and general effectiveness. Their action is such that drowsiness, quieting, and sometimes deep sleep are achieved within 1 hour. Following the auditory evaluation the youngster can be aroused, observed during the recovery period, and taken home. Acoustic reflexes can be observed in patients sedated with chloral hydrate or secobarbital, but researchers have suggested that the acoustic reflex thresholds may be elevated (Mitchell & Richards, 1976; Robinette, Rhodes, & Marion, 1974). Some children may already be maintained with medications for management of behavioral or convulsive disorders. Thus, the absence of acoustic reflexes in this population may be drug related. Acoustic immittance and otoacoustic emissions can be obtained under conditions of sedation but may not be successful under general anesthesia. Middle ear pressure is increased under inhalation of some gases such as nitrous oxide, thereby decreasing the compliance of the tympanic membrane and obscuring the acoustic reflex (Thomsen, Terkildsen, & Arnfred, 1965).

For the most part, sedating a child for purposes of audiologic evaluation creates complexities in scheduling, managing the patient, interpreting test results, and requiring extended appointment commitments. Accordingly, it is always preferable to find a means to test the child under natural sleep conditions as an initial effort. Clinicians and parents need to be warned that a child's reaction to sedation medication is not always as expected. Children vary considerably in their response sensitivity to sedatives, and the recommended dosages may not be sufficient to induce the desired effect. The same dosage in other children may actually increase activity and excitement levels so that the desired physiologic study is still not possible.

VESTIBULAR EVALUATION IN CHILDREN

There is a growing array of literature regarding the problems of dizziness and vestibular problems in children. Although not common, vestibular dysfunction does occur in children (O'Reilly et al., 2010). Pediatric audiologists need to be cognizant of symptoms and knowledgeable about the evaluation of children with complaints of dizziness or vertigo. Although, according to Ganz (2014), the majority of equilibrium problems that occur in infants and children manifest as delayed gross motor and balance problems, not as vertigo or dizziness.

It is important to remember that vestibular function is the primary purpose of the inner ear, and hearing can almost be considered an overlaid function. The vestibular labyrinth portion of the inner ear is the first sensory system to develop embryologically; it actually precedes cochlear development. We would not likely have survived as a species without an adequate equilibrium system. Accordingly, our vestibular system is a critical sensory component within multiple complex reflex arcs. Equilibrium requires more than just the vestibular labyrinth; it is a complex integration of the vestibular system, vision, the somatosensory system, proprioception, and the central nervous system. The vestibular labyrinth portion of the inner ear is the first sensory system to develop embryologically; it actually precedes cochlear development (Gans, 2014).

Considerable time and effort are exerted on the problem and prevention of hearing loss in children, yet we often ignore concurrent or subsequent vestibular disorders. This neglect could be due to several factors, perhaps the most common being the fact that vertiginous crises in childhood are often attributed to clumsiness or behavior problems. When a child describes vertigo, the very real possibilities for etiology include brain tumors, brainstem lesions, or epileptic seizures. In addition, because of the relatively rare incidence of childhood dizziness, one should also consider the possible presence of a functional disorder. The child with verifiable vertiginous complaints may be subjected to a series of lengthy and expensive medical tests offered in large medical centers that may not be conveniently available.

More attention should be directed to the likelihood of peripheral disturbances, rather than central etiologies, in children suffering from vertigo or disequilibrium. Basser (1964) described a syndrome called benign paroxysmal vertigo of childhood. He reported that it was common in children but differed significantly from the benign paroxysmal vertigo found in adults. The distinction rests on the childhood prevalence and on the pure paroxysmal nature of the attacks, their brevity, recurrence, absence of any prolonged disequilibrium, and the absence of the febrile illness or upper respiratory infection at the onset. Utilizing electronystagmography (ENG), Basser successfully documented vertiginous complaints from children. Koenigsberger et al.

(1970) also reported successful application of ENG testing in children with benign paroxysmal vertigo. Pediatric vestibular testing and normative data has focused primarily on school-age children with modification of adult protocols utilizing videonystagmography, rotary chair, and computerized dynamic posturography (Cyr, 1980, 1983; O'Reilly et al, 2011; Valente, 2007. Gans (2014) published an excellent up-to-date overview and discussion of the pediatric vestibular evaluation for children of all ages.

Congenital disorders by far are the leading cause of pediatric vestibular dysfunction according to Pikus (2002) who estimated that there are over 500 etiologies of deafness that are known to have an audiovestibular expressivity. Within the population of vertiginous children there are postmeningitis patients and those with combined renal dysfunction and decreased visual acuity, as in Alport's syndrome. Children displaying visual and vestibular disturbances are of particular concern because of the risk of permanent damage to two of the three systems necessary for maintenance of balance. The audiologist should be vigilant of children who have received long-term or high doses of ototoxic drugs that are particularly toxic to the vestibular portion of the inner ear (e.g., gentamicin and streptomycin).

The development of a clinically feasible battery for evaluating vestibular function in infants and preschool children has been described by Cyr, Brookhouser, Valente, and Grossman (1985), Valente (2007), and Gans (2014). Their procedures involve modifications of standard ENG testing and the use of the low-frequency rotary chair. They report that the vestibular test battery is easy to administer, takes a minimal amount of time, and is the preferred evaluation method for most children. The test battery includes pediatric ocular motor testing, positional testing, caloric testing with simultaneous binaural bithermal stimulation through a closed-loop irrigation system, and computerized rotational chair testing (harmonic acceleration). Videonystagmographic technology can also be used to provide ongoing monitoring of the child's head and eye position in a darkened test enclosure during the examination.

Gans (2014) describes the various methods for evaluation of the vestibular system in infants and young children ranging between 3 months to 3 years of age. Gans states that with a proper case history, interview of the parents, and understanding of the vestibular system's multiple reflex systems and their role in maturational motor milestones, most infants and young children can be identified as being at risk prior to comprehensive electrophysiologic examination. A thorough vestibular evaluation should be performed on any child for whom there is strong suspicion of vestibular dysfunction. The child who develops unilateral or bilateral vestibular weakness in infancy or childhood will often be asymptomatic and may adapt to the loss in a few days. However, under certain conditions (i.e., when this child is moving in total darkness), the loss of vestibular function will very quickly and suddenly become apparent. Audiologists should be able to recognize and understand the implications of vestibular dysfunction in childhood and be prepared to undertake appropriate evaluation or referral.

SUMMARY OF PHYSIOLOGIC AUDITORY TESTING

There is no question that auditory physiologic tests add an extra dimension to pediatric audiology. Today's digital technologies have contributed greatly to the evaluation of the auditory system in children. Note that we say "auditory system" and not "hearing," as it is a strong reminder that the physiologic tests are not tests of hearing, per se. The physiologic tests serve a twofold purpose: first, to provide an estimate and perhaps cross-check, of audiometric hearing thresholds, and second, as a differential diagnostic technique for otologic and auditory disorders. Although these physiologic procedures are commonly viewed and described as *objective tests*, many believe that because the interpretation of the test results depends on the skills and experience level of the audiologist, the procedures are more *subjective* than not. The physiologic tests, by no means, should be considered the audiologist's mainstay to evaluate and verify the hearing of infants and young children in place of traditional behavioral testing. The behavioral hearing test is still the gold standard of pediatric audiology. Although acoustic immittance measurements and otoacoustic emissions should be included in the routine pediatric test battery, the evoked response evaluations and procedures are usually reserved for especially difficult-to-test children or to clarify or confirm questionable diagnostic patients.

The physiological procedures have much to contribute to the auditory evaluation of children with few weaknesses. The results are "objective" in the sense that they do not require a voluntary behavioral response from the child, and they are not dependent upon the child's motivation, state of awareness, cognitive abilities, or language or verbal instructions. The various measures have the specificity to identify the site of lesion along the auditory pathway from the ear canal through the inner ear and up the ascending pathways in the brainstem to the cortex. The auditory evoked potential

measurements have added much to our understanding, and yet raised many questions, of the development and maturation of the auditory system. Using the various evoked auditory potentials, complete studies can be conducted on children under consideration for central auditory processing disorders. And yet, few of the physiologic tests can totally stand alone without additional information contributed by other auditory tests. There is little doubt that future applications of physiological auditory procedures along with the development of more sophisticated instruments and algorithms will continue to supplement today's hearing evaluation protocols.

The sensory auditory generators have been well mapped in terms of site of origin, onset, latency, and amplitude by numerous investigators. We now can figuratively follow an acoustic stimulus from its entrance into the external ear canal until it reaches the auditory cortex of the brain as summarized in Table 7–5. Audiologists have found that the early, or brainstem, potentials have the widest application because they can be easily and reliably detected in young individuals and are not affected by sedation. The MLRs may be of secondary importance and much more difficult to measure, while the late potentials that have been largely avoided because they are easily contaminated by subject state are coming to our attention with new pediatric applications. ECochG is one of the most reliable of all physiologic measures, but because of the intricate requirements for administering the procedure, it is not a routine procedure. Nonetheless, the physiological auditory tests should not be considered without behavioral and electroacoustic tests (immittance and OAEs) measurements.

The use of the array of physiologic auditory tests helps make the term *sensorineural*

Table 7–5. Evoked Auditory Response Classifications

Early response potentials	Latency (msec)	Peak amplitude (m.v.)	Source/Origin/Generators
Cochlear microphonic	1.0–5.0 ABR	0.1–10	Cochlea
Wave I	1.5–1.9		Auditory nerve
Wave II	2.6–3.0		Auditory nerve–Cochlear nucleus
Wave III	3.7–4.1		Trapezoid body–Superior olivary
Wave IV	4.8–5.4		Superior olivary–Lateral lemniscus
Wave V	5.4–6.0		Lateral lemniscus–Inferior colliculi
Wave VI	7.0–7.6		Inferior colliculi–Medial geniculate
Wave VII	8.0–9.0		Medial geniculate–Auditory cortex
Middle latency potentials	MLR	1.0–3.0	
Na	15–25		Medial geniculate–Auditory cortex
Pa (P20)	25–35		Medial Herschl's gyrus
Nb	35–45		Lateral supertemporal gyrus
Pb1	40–65		Lateral supertemporal gyrus
Pb2	60–85		Anterolateral Herschl's gyrus
Long latency potentials	**Late cortical responses**	8.0–20.0	
N100 (N1)	75–140		Auditory cortex
P200 (N2)	150–230		Auditory cortex
P300 (P3)	250–350	20.0–30.0	Auditory cortex
Very late potentials	300+		Auditory cortex

archaic. With today's procedures and tests, hearing loss can be confirmed as either *sensory* or *neural* in terms of the origins of the pathology. Knowledge of the precise ana-tomic location of a child's etiology of deafness is very important to overall management and prognosis. Future research into the prevention and treatment of deafness depends on the ability to identify accurately the anatomic location of the disorder. Hall and Swanepoel (2010) present an excellent and thorough overview article on electrophysiologic and electroacoustic assessment of hearing.

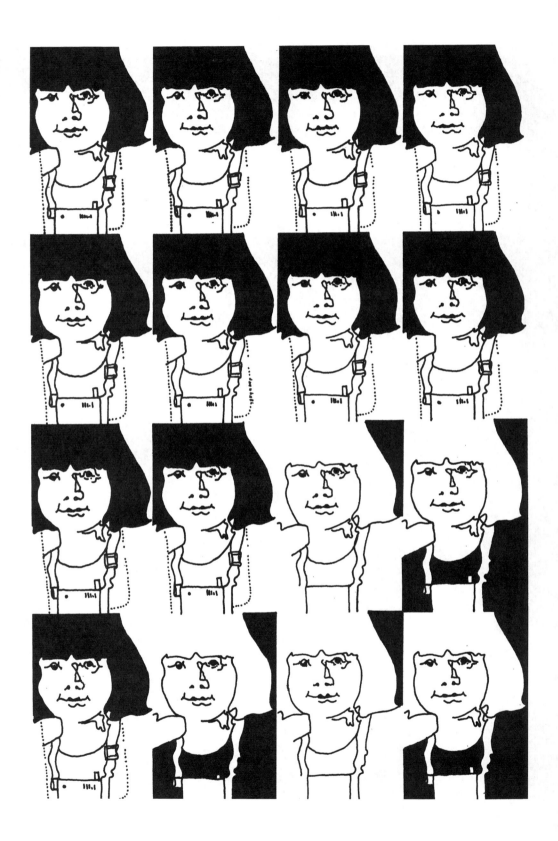

CHAPTER 8

Hearing Screening

Screening is the process of applying certain rapid and simple tests, examinations, or other procedures to generally large numbers of persons which will identify those persons with a high probability of a disorder from those who probably do not have the disorder. A criterion measurement cutoff point is always involved, below or above which the disorder is suspect. Screening is not intended as a diagnostic procedure; screening merely surveys large populations of undiagnosed and typically asymptomatic persons to identify those who are suspected of having the disorder and who require more elaborate diagnostic procedures. Persons identified with positive or suspicious findings are referred to their physician for diagnosis and, if necessary, appropriate treatment.

Screening for hearing loss in U.S. public schools has been in practice since the 1930s, and nearly every state has some sort of mandated hearing screening program to identify children with educationally handicapping hearing impairment. The early literature of audiology abounds with descriptions of various group and individual hearing tests designed for use in schools, dating from the introduction in 1927 of the Western Electric 4-C group speech test (McFarlan, 1927). Currently, either by order of legislative mandate or through some type of coordinated statewide program, hearing screening of school-aged children is conducted in nearly all U.S. states (Penn, 1999). Without mandated routine hearing screenings in schools, students with unilateral, mild, or late-onset hearing loss may not be identified or will perhaps be misdiagnosed and

ineffectively managed (Figure 8–1). Efforts to provide consistent protocols, screener training, and follow-up through school age will help ensure that children with hearing loss are identified and managed in a timely manner, and thereby minimize negative academic consequence.

Newborn screening began in the 1960s when a blood test was developed that could detect whether newborns had the metabolic

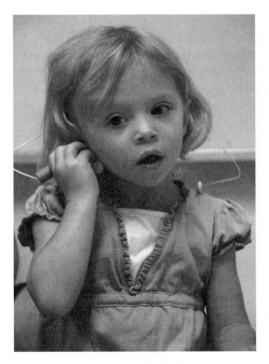

Figure 8–1. Hearing screening ensures that children with hearing loss are identified as early as possible so they can be helped with potential educational difficulties. Photo courtesy of Colorado Children's Hospital, Aurora, CO.

disorder, phenylketonuria (PKU). Since then, scientists have developed more tests to screen newborns for a variety of severe conditions. Screening tests are currently available for more than 60 disorders. However, there is variability in the number and types of conditions found on each state's newborn screening panel, which is determined by each state public health department. Newborn screening is a state public health service that reaches each of the more than four million babies born in the United States every year. It ensures that all babies are screened for certain serious conditions at birth; and for those babies with the conditions, it allows doctors to start treatment before some of the harmful effects happen. Screening for disease as early as possible in a child's life is now an accepted public health mandate.

The past six decades have seen hearing screening programs for newborns developed to identify those newborns with hearing loss so that habilitative measures can be instituted. The historical development of hearing tests for infants has evolved from early behavioral observation techniques to today's sophisticated physiologic hearing screening technologies. A great deal of effort has been expended by public health agencies and epidemiologists to analyze the performance characteristics of all types of screening procedures.

A somewhat difficult problem has been the development of simple, efficient, and accurate hearing screening techniques for young children between 2 and 4 years of age. The effect of mild-to-moderate hearing impairment in this age group has been shown to be detrimental in speech/language development, but no simple, effective, and accurate hearing screening technique has gained universal acceptance for use in Head Start Programs, primary care physician offices, or public and private preschool grades. A great deal of effort has

been expended by public health officials, agencies, and epidemiologists to analyze the performance characteristics of all types of screening procedures. This chapter examines the construction and evaluation procedures for individual screening procedures, as these are important concepts for audiologists to understand. Such discussions will help professionals to evaluate the present status of their approaches to children's hearing screening programs and specifically to provide the tools to critique yet to be developed hearing screening tests.

PRINCIPLES OF SCREENING

The following two aspects of screening philosophy are relevant to the current discussion of screening theories and how they relate to hearing conservation programs: (a) the selection of the disorder or disease, and (b) the evaluation of the screening procedures. The first question that must be asked is whether there should be a screen for a certain disease. If the answer is yes, then specific criteria described below should be applied to the selection of disorders (ASHA, 1995; Frankenburg & Camp, 1975).

Occurrence Frequent Enough or Consequence Serious Enough to Warrant Mass Screening

How prevalent is the disease in the population to be screened? Some balancing of cost with the number of children who have the disease must be made. Cunningham (1970) stated, "From the point of view of a public health program, in order to justify a mass screening program, the condition must be reasonably frequent or if rare it must have serious consequences if not detected." In the case of hearing, screening neonates for congenital deafness can be justified on the basis of its severity and resultant disastrous consequences; the screening of the young child can be justified on the basis of numbers alone and on consequences. Table 8–1 illustrates the relative status of hearing screening compared with other commonly screened newborn diseases. Hearing screening not only yields the highest returns among these diseases but also is more productive of results once the problem is identified.

Amenability to Treatment or Prevention That Will Forestall or Change the Expected Outcome

What would be the prognosis for the person if treatment is instituted or if it is not instituted? It perhaps matters little if such a disorder as color blindness is detected early, as no treatment will change it. But the tragic consequences of untreated hearing losses are all too commonly seen: the complete lack of speech or language development at ages when these functions should be well implanted; the deterioration of the parent-child relationship into subtle rejection or bewildered overprotection; and personality deviations of a wide variety, ranging from autistic-like withdrawal to hyperactivity and acting out. So long as a disease state can be accurately identified, its severity should at the very least be lessened by treatment if mandatory screening is going to be regarded as a profitable endeavor. There is no question that the sequelae of a true hearing loss can be ameliorated if the disorder is given proper treatment.

Availability of Facilities for Diagnosis and Treatment

If there is a suspicion that a child has a certain disorder, can the child be properly assessed and treated without unreasonable expenditure in money and effort? This question largely concerns the state of the art and the number of trained professionals who can be depended on to produce accurate evaluations and remediation for the child. If 1-year-old Johnny is found in a rural area to have profound deafness, there may not be a facility for his diagnosis and training for literally hundreds of miles. Even in a big city, critical fellow professionals may

Table 8–1. Yield in Infant Health Care Screen Tests

Disease screened	Yield
Phenylketonuria	7 in 100,000 births
Combined immunodeficiency disease	25 in 3 million births
Neonatal hyperthyroidism	25 in 100,000 births
Cystic fibrosis	50 in 100,000 births
Hemoglobinopathy	13 in 100,000 births
Bilateral sensorineural hearing loss	260 in 100,000 births

Source: Adapted from "Newborn Hearing Screening: The Great Omission, by A. Mehl & V. Thompson, 1998, *Pediatrics, 101*(1), p. e4.

view the facilities available with a jaundiced eye. When these situations occur—and they certainly do—can screening for the disorder in that location be justified?

Cost of Screening Reasonably Commensurate With Benefits to the Individual

Is the screening equipment costly to purchase and to maintain? Do the personnel administering the screening tests require expensive training or high-level salaries? It is very difficult to designate any costs as excessive when the health and welfare of many individuals are at stake, but there are limitations to the funds available in any area. Some equipment can continue to be used for long periods and for many thousands of tests before any repair or calibration is required. In addition, as the trend toward the use of nonprofessional aides continues, the cost of screening continues to decrease. The cost analysis of screening the infant and preschool population also varies, but in no case would it be considered exorbitant when compared with the benefits accrued.

Cooper, Gates, Owen, and Dickson (1975) published data regarding efficiency and cost of school screening programs. They reported that the ongoing practical testing rate for audiometric screening was about 5 minutes per student, or 12 students per hour. They also reported data for immittance screening to be approximately 1.1 minute per child, or 21 children per hour. Cooper et al. calculated the cost of their screening program by establishing an index of cost per accurate referral of failures. To compute the cost per accurate referral, the following formula was developed:

$$\text{Cost per Child} = \\ S + \underline{C + (M \times L)} \; R \; (N \times L)$$

$S =$ salary of person screening, in dollars per hour

$R =$ screening rate in children per hour

$C =$ cost of equipment in dollars

$M =$ annual maintenance cost of equipment in dollars

$L =$ lifetime of the equipment in years

$N =$ number of children screened per year

Mehl and Thomson (1998) calculated the cost for universal newborn hearing screening in Colorado. Their analysis can be summarized with their description that "the true cost for each infant screened is estimated to be $25 per infant, including labor costs, disposable supplies, and amortized capital equipment costs" (p. 4). They further explained that the costs of screening actually ranged from $18.30 per infant when performed by supervised volunteers, $25.60 per infant when performed by a paid technician, and to $33.30 per infant when performed by an audiologist. Considering the entire program and the number of infants identified to have significant hearing loss, Mehl and Thomson present their entire cost-analysis documentation and state that the screening costs to identify correctly one new case of congenital hearing loss equate to $9,600 in 1998 dollars.

Screening Test Performance Characteristics

The success of a screening program depends on the effectiveness of the measures used to identify those who are likely to have the target disorder and to pass over those who do not have the target disorder. It is no longer sufficient to evaluate a test procedure critically by simply reporting the percentage of positive results in patients with the "disease" and the percentage of negative results in patients without the disease (Jerger, 1983). More rigid and critical performance characteristics must be applied to each screening test to evaluate fully its effectiveness in the overall attempt to identify infants and children with hearing problems. Jacobson and Jacobson (1987) provided an excellent discussion of screening test performance characteristics, and we are grateful for their permission to use their material as the basis of the following discussion.

It must be kept in mind that the principal objective of any hearing screening program is to correctly identify hearing loss in those persons who truly have a problem, while ruling out hearing loss in normal-hearing persons. Screening tests should identify high-risk persons who are predisposed to develop disease or who are asymptomatic (undiagnosed), so that they can be effectively treated. Thus, the validity of a screening test is based on the proportion of test results that are confirmed diagnostically. If a hearing screening test too often passes infants or children who, indeed, have hearing impairment or too often mistakenly identifies normal-hearing infants or children as hearing-impaired, the screening test will not stand up to critical performance evaluation and should be considered invalid and economically unfeasible.

Decision Matrix Analysis

A decision matrix is typically a 2×2 table that describes the results of a test procedure to the actual presence or absence of the disease (i.e., hearing impairment). The four components of the matrix table are *true positive* (TP), the number of hearing-impaired persons correctly identified by the test; *true negative* (TN), the number of persons with normal hearing who are correctly identified; *false positive* (FP), the number of persons with normal hearing incorrectly labeled as hearing-impaired; and *false negative* (FN), the number of persons truly impaired but incorrectly identified as normal (Table 8–2). A screening test of choice would result in a high proportion of true-positive rates and in a low proportion of false-positive rates, because those with the disease would be identified, whereas healthy participants would pass the screen. It is the formulation of actual screening pass-fail results to this decision matrix that allows the calculation of test performance validity.

The validity of a screening test that is dependent on diagnostic confirmation for every person under consideration is determined by the relationship of three components: (a) sensitivity, the ability of a test to correctly identify patients with the disease (hearing loss); (b) specificity, the ability of a test to correctly identify those without the

Table 8–2. Matrix Analysis for Test Performance Characteristics

Test results	Impaired	Normal	Total
Positive	TP	FP	TP + FP
Negative	FN	TN	FN +TN
Totals	TP + FN	FP +TN	TP + FP + FN + TN

Note: TP, true positive; *TN*, true negative; *FN*, false negative; *FP*, false positive. From "Application of Test Performance Characteristics in Newborn Auditory Screening," J. Jacobson & C. Jacobson, 1987, *Seminars in Hearing, 8*(2), p. 133.

disease (normal hearing); and (c) disease prevalence, the total number of patients with the disease in a given population. Thus, it is the actual test results that define these terms.

Sensitivity

When a test operates at a 70% sensitivity rate, only 7 of every 10 patients who are hearing-impaired are correctly identified. The remaining three impaired patients are improperly classified. This concept is illustrated in Table 8–3, which uses a hypothetical group of 1,000 screened newborn infants. In this example, a total of 100 babies are truly hearing-impaired; however, only 70 (70%) were correctly identified as such. Thus, for this example 70% (70/100) represents the true-positive rate, whereas 30% (30/100), the misclassified (those who passed the screen), represents the false-negative rate. In hearing screening it is most desirable to use a test that gives the highest possible rate of sensitivity. For example, if a child passes a hearing screen but presents with signifi-

cant impairment, the abnormality may hold serious behavioral, developmental, and educational consequences if it goes undetected even for a short period early in the child's life.

Specificity

If all children with normal hearing passed a screening, the test would perform at a 100% specificity rate. However, as the test begins to fail normal-hearing children, the rate of specificity decreases. For example, if 8 of 10 infants were correctly identified as having normal hearing, the test would operate at 80% specificity. The remaining two incorrectly classified normal-hearing infants would be subjected to subsequent diagnostic follow-up. In Table 8–3, 720 of 900 normal-hearing babies passed the screen, resulting in 80% (720/900) test specificity. Those 180 normal-hearing newborns who were incorrectly classified rendered a 20% false-positive rate. This situation may result in parental stress and anxiety; however, misdiagnosis is usually ameliorated by further diagnostic assessment. Table 8–3 demonstrates that the terms *sensitivity* and *specificity* represent the true-positive and true-negative rates, respectively. It is evident that a reciprocal relationship exists between sensitivity and the false-negative rate and, similarly, between specificity and the false-positive rate.

Table 8–3. Matrix Analysis for Hypothetical Test Results

Test Results	Impaired	Normal	Total
Positive	70	180	250
Negative	30	720	750
Totals	100	900	1000

Note: Sensitivity, 70/100 (70.0%); specificity, 720/900 (80.0%); predictive value of positive test, 70/250 (28.0%); predictive value of negative test, 720/750 (96.0%); overall, 790/1000 (79.0%); incidence, 100/1000 (10.0%).

Source: From "Application of Test Performance Characteristics in Newborn Auditory Screening," by J. Jacobson & C. Jacobson, 1987, *Seminars in Hearing, 8*(2), pp. 133–141.

Prevalence Versus Incidence

Prevalence is distinct from incidence. Both of these characteristics describe disease frequency rate in a general population. In epidemiology, the prevalence of a disease in a statistical population is defined as the total number of cases of the disease in the population at a given time, or the total number of cases in the population, divided by the number of individuals in the population. Prevalence rate is a census measure that expresses the presence of diseased patients per 100,000 at the time of investigation. It is used as an estimate of how common a condition is within a population over a certain period of time. It helps physicians or other health professionals understand the probability of certain diagnoses and is routinely used by epidemiologists, health care providers, government agencies, and insurers. The rate of prevalence is calculated by dividing the number of diseased patients in the population at a specified time by the number of individuals in the population at that specified time. The measurement of *lifetime prevalence* is used in epidemiology as the number of individuals in a statistical population who at some point in their life (up to the time of assessment) have experienced a "case" (e.g., a disorder), compared to the total number of individuals (i.e., it is expressed as a ratio or percentage). Often, a 12-month prevalence (or some other type of *period prevalence*) is used in conjunction with lifetime prevalence. There is also *point prevalence*, which is the prevalence of disorder at a more specific (a month or less) point in time.

In contrast, incidence rate is the frequency of new outbreak of a disease condition in a population for a given period. Prevalence is a measurement of *all* individuals affected by the disease within a particular period of time, whereas incidence is a measurement of the number of *new* individuals who contract a disease during a particular period of time. To calculate incidence rate, two variables must be defined: (a) the beginning and end of the time period under study, and (b) the population at risk for developing the disorder under study. Incidence rate is calculated by dividing the number of new

diseased patients in a population during a specified period by the number of persons exposed to the risk of developing the disease during that same period.

The relationship between prevalence and incidence is clarified by the following example. The incidence of an acute disease such as middle ear effusion in high-risk infants may be high, because large numbers of neonates contract the disease during convalescence. The prevalence is usually low, however, because the disease has a relatively short duration. Conversely, the incidence of a chronic disease such as sensory hearing loss may be low in newborns, but the prevalence in the population may be high. Although only a small percentage of babies are identified as sensory-impaired each year, sensory hearing loss is irreversible and therefore cumulative. Thus, the incidence of sensory hearing loss in children increases cumulatively as the average age of the sample cohort grows older.

Predictive Value

Performance characteristics (i.e., sensitivity and specificity) define the ability of a test to estimate disease or nondisease in a given population accurately and, therefore, are of primary importance in the selection of a screening test. In contrast, predictive values, which are related to disease prevalence, examine the percentage of patients correctly labeled diseased or healthy by the test and provide information about test result interpretation. The predictive value of a positive test (PVP) is defined as the percent of all positive results that are true positive when the test is applied to a population containing both healthy and diseased subjects (TP/ (TP + FP) × 100). The predictive value of a negative test (PVN) represents the percent of all negative results that are true negatives (TN/(TN + FN) × 100).

It is important to recognize that predictive values are dependent on test performance characteristics and disease prevalence in the population under study. Once measures of sensitivity and specificity are tabulated, it is then possible to establish probability statements regarding the presence or absence of disease, because predictive values relate directly to test outcome. Predictive value measures can be derived from Table 8–3. Of the total 250 patients who failed the screen, 70 were true positive. The remaining 180 patients were false positive, leaving a PVP of 28% (70 of 250).

The PVP results mean that approximately three fourths (180 of 250) of all patients who failed the test were false positive. The PVN result was 96% (720 of 750), meaning that this test correctly identified 720 members of the normal-hearing population. Thus, for persons who were determined to have passed the screen, only 4 of every 100 negative results were false negative. Finally, the overall efficiency (i.e., a measure of the percent of all true-positive and true-negative results) was 79%.

Disease prevalence within a target population will influence predictive values. Table 8–4 presents a hypothetical example of such an effect. By decreasing the preva-

Table 8–4. Effects of Disease Prevalence on Predictive Values When Sensitivity (90%) and Specificity (90%) Remain Constant

Test results	Impaired	Normal	Total
Disease prevalence 5%			
Positive	225	475	700
Negative	25	4,275	4,300
Totals	250	4,750	5,000
PVP = 32.1%			
PVN = 99.4%			
Disease prevalence 1%			
Positive	45	495	540
Negative	5	4,455	44,560
Totals	50	4,950	5,000
PVP = 8.3%			
PVN = 99.9%			
Disease prevalence 0.1%			
Positive	4.5	499.5	504
Negative	0.5	4,495.5	4,456
Totals	5	4,995	5,000
PVP = 1.0%			
PVN = 100%			

Source: From "Application of Test Performance Characteristics in Newborn Auditory Screening," by J. Jacobson & C. Jacobson, 1987, *Seminars in Hearing, 8*(2), pp. 133–141.

lence of the disease from 5% (50/1,000) to 1% (10/1,000) to 0.1% (1/1,000) while maintaining relatively high performance characteristics (sensitivity 90%, specificity 90%), predictive values change correspondingly. The PVP result decreased from 32.1% to 8.3% to less than 1.0%, whereas the PVN result in this case remained stable. When disease prevalence is 0.1% (1/1,000), it is similar to that reported in mass auditory screening. The false-positive rate is 99.1%. This example clearly points to the importance of applying screening tests to high-prevalence populations. If not, the false-positive rate will be so great that it may be indefensible.

Pass-Fail Criteria

Given the inherent differences in biomedical investigation, it is unlikely that any test, screening, or diagnostic, will be designed that can separate all patients with disease from those without disease. The result is that there will always be those screened who are inaccurately labeled. Thorner and Remein (1967) have addressed this integration of normal and pathologic patients in the theory of overlapping distributions. The selection of a cutoff point within the overlapping distribution will directly influence the anticipated yield (incidence) of identified patients with disease as well as affect test performance characteristics. The determination of pass-fail criteria is a critical factor in the establishment of eventual test outcome.

Figure 8–2 illustrates the concept of overlapping distribution. In this hypothetical hearing screening population, a cutoff score was initially established. Using this stated pass-fail criteria (i.e., a predetermined intensity level) a certain proportion of patients passed the screen, whereas others did not. Depending on individual test outcome, measures of sensitivity and specificity, false-positive rates, and false-negative

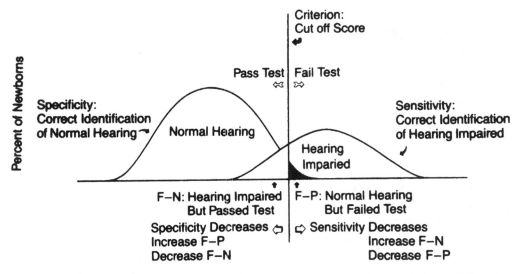

Figure 8–2. A hypothetical newborn screened population. An overlapping subject distribution and its effect on specific operating characteristics. Used with permission from "Newborn Auditory Screening," by J. Jacobson and C. Jacobson, 1987, *Seminars in Hearing, 8*(2), p. 139.

rates were established. However, if the cutoff score for hearing screening was adjusted either up (higher intensity level) or down (lower intensity level), performance values would change correspondingly. If the cutoff score was increased so that more hearing-impaired persons pass the test, sensitivity would decrease because the false-negative rate (hearing-impaired persons who pass the test) would increase. Conversely, as sensitivity decreased, specificity rate would increase as a result of the reduced number of false-positive (normal-hearing persons who fail the test) results. If, on the other hand, the cutoff point was lowered, fewer hearing-impaired persons would pass the test, and the false-negative rate would decrease. By doing so, specificity would decrease as the false-positive rate would increase. The result is a reciprocal relationship between sensitivity and specificity—as sensitivity increases, specificity decreases; and as specificity increases, sensitivity decreases.

A cutoff score is an arbitrary point that can be set to favor a specific test outcome. The PVP and PVN results also change as the pass-fail cutoff point is manipulated. Because both test performance characteristics and disease prevalence influence the predictive value, an increase in the cutoff point (e.g. using a more stringent or rigorous definition of hearing loss) will reduce the "overall incidence" of hearing impairment. Finally, the overall test efficiency will be influenced, as the cutoff point may also determine the correct identification of hearing-impaired and normal-hearing persons. The ideal hearing screening test would correctly differentiate 100% of the time between normal-hearing and hearing-impaired persons. Unfortunately, the development of such a hearing screening test that would meet the requirements of objectivity, ease of administration, rapid and simple technique, and economic feasibility is unlikely. Therefore, as each specific population targeted for hearing screening is determined, the selection and implementation of a hearing screening tool must depend heavily on the various measures of test validity and desired performance characteristics. The use of sensitivity, specificity, and their reciprocal counterparts can provide information about the number of persons correctly identified as hearing-impaired or normal-hearing as measures against predetermined pass-fail criteria. Predictive values that are dependent on the prevalence or incidence of hearing disorders describe the test's ability to separate correctly true-positive and true-negative results in those with and without hearing loss. Of course, the final validation of any screening test measure must account for the diagnostic confirmation of all individuals screened, regardless of initial test outcome.

GENETIC SCREENING

Newborn genetic screening is an area of tremendous growth in medical diagnosis and, of course, genetic counseling. In the early 1960s, the only newborn screening test required was for phenylketonuria (PKU). By the year 2000, roughly two-thirds of states in the United States screened for 10 or fewer genetic diseases in newborns. The growth in genetic screening is obvious when one considers that in 2007, 95% of states in the United States screened for more than 30 different genetic diseases in newborns. Especially as costs have come down, newborn genetic screening offers valuable return on the expenditure of health dollars. Genetic screening can provide a diagnosis of vulnerabilities to inherited diseases, paternity (genetic father), or trace a person's ancestry.

Normally, every person carries two copies of every gene (with the exception of genes related to sex-linked traits, which are only inherited from the mother by males), one inherited from their mother, one inherited from their father. The human genome contains approximately 20,000 to 25,000 genes. In addition to studying chromosomes to the level of individual genes, genetic testing in a broader sense includes biochemical tests for the possible presence of genetic diseases, or mutant forms of genes associated with increased risk of developing genetic disorders. Genetic testing identifies changes in chromosomes, genes, or proteins. Most of the times, genetic testing is used to find changes that are associated with inherited disorders. The results of a genetic test can confirm or rule out a suspected genetic condition or help determine a person's chance of developing or passing on a genetic disorder. Several hundred genetic tests are currently in use, and no doubt many more are currently being developed.

Newborn screening begins within 24 to 48 hours of a child's birth when a few drops of blood are obtained from a heel stick. The sampling, or "blood spot," is collected on a slide, a strip, or placed onto marked areas of an absorbent card. The dried blood spots are sent to a laboratory that is a part of the state or territorial public health department. The spots are analyzed by several different laboratory methods to test for biochemical and genetic markers that reveal hidden congenital (present at birth) disorders. If such markers are found, the newborn screening follow-up program notifies the parents and physicians so that the baby can receive immediate attention. Follow-up programs arrange for diagnostic tests to confirm the newborn screening results. Follow-up programs also refer the child to a treatment center to provide access to the essential medical services needed to minimize the effects of the underlying disorder.

Statistics show that one out of every 1,500 babies born will develop one of the disorders detectable through newborn screening. Because most newborns appear normal, there is no way of knowing if the child has a metabolic, or genetic, disorder until outward symptoms appear. By then, it may be too late to halt or reverse the effects. Testing is recommended also because there may be no history or knowledge of genetic disorders within a family. The fact is, most children with these disorders come from families where there is no previous history. As a precautionary measure, more than 95% of the roughly four million children born annually in the United States now undergo the heel stick test. The emphasis is on early detection, because most metabolic and endocrine illnesses respond remarkably well to pharmaceutical or nutritional treatment.

Although all states require screening for at least 21 of the 29 most debilitating endocrine and metabolic diseases, there are more than 50 disorders that can be detected through newborn screening. However, each individual state determines which disorders will be screened. Common tests for babies in the United States include those for sickle cell disease, congenital hypothyroidism, phenylketonuria, or PKU (amino acid overproduction leading to brain damage), and cystic fibrosis (CF). Undiagnosed and unattended to, these diseases can bring on liver disease, cataracts, jaundice, chronic respiratory and bacterial infections, stunted growth, mental retardation, brain damage, and diminished life expectancy.

Genetic screening can provide information about a person's genes and chromosomes throughout life. Available types of testing include:

- *Newborn screening:* Newborn screening is used just after birth to identify genetic disorders that can be treated early in life. The routine testing of infants for certain disorders is the most widespread use of genetic testing. Millions of babies are tested each year in the United States. All states currently test infants for phenylketonuria (a genetic disorder that causes mental illness if left untreated) and congenital hypothyroidism (a disorder of the thyroid gland). Most common in the field of hearing is the genetic screen for mutations of the BGJ2 Connexin 26 gene that identifies sensorineural hearing loss.

- *Diagnostic screening:* Genetic diagnostic screening is used to diagnose or rule out a specific genetic or chromosomal condition. In many cases, genetic testing is used to confirm a diagnosis when a particular condition is suspected based on physical mutations and symptoms. Diagnostic testing can be performed at any time during a person's life, but is not available for all genes or all genetic conditions. The results of a diagnostic test can influence a person's choices about health care and the management of the disease.

- *Carrier screening:* Carrier screening is used to identify people who carry one copy of a gene mutation that, when present in two copies in an individual, causes a genetic disorder. This type of testing is offered to individuals who have a family history of a genetic disorder and to people in ethnic groups with an increased risk of specific genetic conditions. If both parents are tested, the test can provide information about a couple's risk of having a child with a genetic condition.

Prevalence of Newborn Hearing Loss

Sensorineural hearing loss (SNHL) is the most common congenital sensory impairment, with an incidence of 1 to 2 per 1,000 for bilateral severe to profound losses (>70 dB) and up to 4 per 1,000 if mild to moderate and unilateral losses are included. The most frequently identified causes of pediatric SNHL are divided into three categories: infectious, anatomic, and genetic. The most common infectious cause is congenital cytomegalovirus; one of the most common anatomic findings are the presence of enlarged vestibular aqueducts and other inner-ear anomalies, some of which have a genetic basis; and the most common genetic causes are mutations in the gap junction *GJB2* (Kenna et al., 2010).

Stein (1999) asked the critical question concerning how many newborns might be expected to be found with significant hearing loss in the annual U.S. population of four million births. For many years, it was widely held that the prevalence of hearing loss in the newborn population is approximately 1 in 1,000 live births, or 4,000 infants per year. It was argued by many that this estimate was understated as it was based only on congenital, profound bilateral hearing loss. Furthermore, early surveys failed to include newborns at risk for developmental disabilities in which the prevalence of hearing loss is now known to be significantly greater than the well-birth infant population. Hearing loss of mild, moderate, or severe degree or unilateral hearing losses were not taken into account simply because of the difficulty in accurately assessing hearing in infants before the advent of otoacoustic emission (OAE) and auditory brainstem response (ABR) screening.

It has long been known that the number of babies with hearing loss identified in the newborn intensive care unit (NICU) is considerably higher than in the general well-baby population. Several studies estimated the incidence of hearing loss in this NICU-targeted population at 20 to 50 times greater than in the newborn nursery, or at least 1 in 150 babies (Davis & Wood, 1992; Schulman-Galambos & Galambos, 1979; Simmons, 1982). Although more and more research studies are underway to establish the true prevalence of hearing impairment in newborns and children, as this information is crucial for long-term planning and funding of intervention and special education programs, it is clear that the answer to the question is complex. In each study, consideration must be given to the specific description of the target population; the definition of hearing loss in terms of degree, type (sensorineural or conductive), and unilateral or bilateral presence; technique of identification and protocol followed; criteria for what degree of hearing loss constitutes pass or failure; and the success of follow-up and diagnostic confirmation of each hearing loss.

The incidence of congenital hearing loss in the general newborn population is high and is a relatively common occurrence. Mehl and Thomson (1998) compared the incidence of bilateral hearing loss in newborns in Colorado against other existing disease screening programs as shown in Table 8–1. They reported that congenital bilateral hearing loss is present in 200 of 100,000 newborns. For comparison, the incidence in galactosemia is 2 per 100,000 births; phe-

nylketonuria, 10 per 100,000 births; and hypothyroidism, 25 per 100,000 births. The prevalence of newborn and infant hearing loss has been estimated in other studies from 1.5 to 6.0 per 1,000 live births (Northern & Hayes, 1994; Parring, 1988; Watkin, 1996; White & Behrens, 1993).

HISTORY OF NEWBORN HEARING SCREENING

It is with great satisfaction that after more than five decades of controversy and debates around the need for early identification of hearing loss in newborns and the efficacy of early intervention, hearing professionals are proud that with nearly 4,000,000 births in the United States during 2010, more than 97% of newborns were screened for hearing loss prior to leaving the birthing hospital. The journey to universal newborn hearing screening was long and somewhat turbulent. Our success follows years of applying various models for identification and management of infant hearing loss, and scores of research efforts conducted by numerous clinical researchers to prove that early identification and early intervention make a difference in the outcomes of infants with hearing loss. The positive outcomes from early identification of hearing loss are due to the development of efficient, cost-effective, and accurate objective screening techniques easily applied to populations of newborn infants, research studies that have confirmed that early intervention improves speech and language outcomes, as well as the many advanced and improved features now present in hearing aids, cochlear implants, and other personal amplification systems that can be fitted to babies with hearing loss at much younger ages than in previous years.

The Early Years (Before 1970)

During the 1950s, the electrodermal response (EDR) was used as a technique for evaluating hearing in children. Electrodermal response audiometry was based on the galvanic skin response and grew out of experimental psychology. The testing technique was based on a conditioning paradigm during which the clinician paired a pure tone and mild electric shock so as to elicit an autonomic change in the sweat glands of the skin. The change in the state of the sweat glands is measured as a reduction in resistance to a small electric current flow between two electrodes taped to the patient's skin, usually between two fingers or positions on the hand. The conditioned autonomic sweat reflex, which involuntarily occurs when the patient "hears" the pure tone stimulus, is easily noted on a single-channel strip chart recorder. Auditory thresholds could be detected at single test frequencies in one ear at a time by reinforcing the autonomic galvanic skin response with mild electric shock. Fortunately, use of the EDR as a hearing testing technique with infants and young children was set aside as less invasive and more humane testing techniques were developed.

The origins of newborn screening can be traced to Sweden. In 1956, Wedenberg reported that "the most easily observable response of an infant to sound is the auropalpebral reflex" (i.e., a rapid and instinctive closing of the eyelids when they are open and squinting them closed). Wedenberg performed hearing tests on 20 infants between 1 and 10 months of age to pure tone stimuli 105 to 115 dB SPL. Wedenberg reported difficulties in the determination of the auropalpebral reflex threshold and questioned the reliability of the response in both sleeping and awake infants. (In fact, questions concerning reliability of subjec-tive hearing screening with infants was to be the focus of researchers for the next 30 years.) A few years later, Froding (1960) also from Sweden, evaluated the hearing of 2,000 newborns using a small gong and mallet that produced a sound of 126 to 133 dB SPL to observe the auropalpebral reflex. Froding was also puzzled by the lack of reliability of the infant responses, stating that "Even if the baby is awake, it might sometime occur that the reflex cannot be produced at the first stroke but only after some minutes; and it is not always possible to produce another reflex directly after the first one." In spite of his concerns, his success in eliciting positive auropalpebral reflex responses led him to conclude that, "Perhaps the time has come for us to discuss whether an examination of the hearing of newborn infants should be made obligatory."

The earliest comprehensive effort to screen the hearing of newborns in the United States came from a project conducted by audiologist Marion Downs and psychologist Graham Sterritt (1964). Downs and Sterritt teamed to conduct a city-wide project in Denver, Colorado, to test all babies born during a 12-month period. Using trained volunteers, and a specially designed, handheld battery-operated infant hearing "screener" with a sudden onset 90 dB SPL narrowband noise stimulus (centered around 3000 Hz), more than 17,000 babies were screened. The test protocol required the volunteers to rate the presence or absence of each infant's behavioral responses immediately following presentation of the stimulus. Recognizing the subjective nature of this rating system, Downs and Sterritt attempted to establish standard response criteria to verify that the subtle responses from the infant were indeed reaction to the onset of the auditory stimulus and not some naturally occurring movement. Their protocol required teams of at least two trained persons to agree on the presence or absence of infant hearing responses as related to the stimulus presentation. Although the Downs and Sterritt project successfully identified nine profoundly deaf babies during their year of the study, the researchers' review of their data raised the continuing question concerning the reliability and validity of newborn hearing screening based on subjective behavioral observation. They noted a number of false-negative results (i.e., babies who "passed" the hearing screening but were identified at a later age to have significant hearing impairment). Their concerns about the use of trained volunteers served as incentive to other researchers to develop specific test protocols that would provide more objective means of identifying infant behavioral responses to sound. Wedenberg (1956) concluded that the only reliable and valid auditory response from an infant should be arousal from sleep, which unfortunately often required the presentation of an extremely loud stimulus if the newborn was in deep sleep.

Despite numerous efforts from various researchers to improve on the Downs and Sterritt protocol, none produced an accepted protocol for the hearing screening of infants. The lack of confidence in behaviorally based mass infant hearing screening led to the use of high-risk factors to identify infants at risk for deafness, and only those babies would be subjected to hearing screening. Thus, there would be no need for hearing screening of the entire newborn population, and only those newborns identified through family history or physical examination to have risk factors would need to be screened for hearing loss.

The High-Risk Register for Deafness

During the formative years, the focus in infant hearing screening was on the risk factors for deafness. The Joint Committee on Infant Hearing (JCIH, 1973) established a list of five factors that would place an infant at risk for deafness. They recommended that all infants at risk for deafness should be identified by means of a medical history and physical examination. Any infant identified to have one or more of the at-risk factors should be scheduled for in-depth hearing screening:

1. History of hereditary childhood hearing impairment;
2. Rubella or other nonbacterial intrauterine fetal infections (e.g., cytomegalovirus or herpes infection);
3. Defect of the ear, nose, or throat; malformed, low-set, or absent pinnae; cleft lip or palate (including submucous cleft); any residual abnormality of the otorhinolaryngeal system;
4. Birth weight less than 1500 grams;
5. Bilirubin level greater than 20 mg/100 mL serum.

Downs and Silver (1972) turned the five risk factors into a widely used and easy-to-remember acronym known as the "ABCD'S of the High Risk Register for Deafness":

(A) Affected family

(B) Bilirubin level

(C) Congenital rubella syndrome

(D) Defects of the ear, nose, and throat

(S) Small birth weight

However, as it turned out, application of the high-risk register was not so simple. Use of the high-risk register required support from a full team of professionals including the audiologist, the neonatologist, the pediatrician, the otolaryngologist, and a wide array of nurses involved in infant care. It was necessary for the team to cooperate in the three stages of the high-risk factor program: (a) face-to-face interviews with the mother of the baby; (b) visual observation of the infant specifically looking for defects such as anatomical malformations or such as abnormal location of the pinna, cleft lip or palate, or signs of syndromes associated with deafness; and (c) review of the medical records of the baby and the mother including the labor and delivery process. Numerous studies confirmed that approximately 10% of all newborns have one risk factor for deafness, while 7% to 13% may have more than one risk factor (Galambos, Hicks, & Wilson, 1984; Mahoney, 1984; Stein, Clark, & Kraus, 1983; Stein, Jabaley, Spitz, Stoakley, & McGee, 1990). Additional research indicated that of the infants at risk for deafness, 30 to 50 of every 1,000 babies do have hearing impairment (Galambos, Hicks, & Wilson, 1982; Hosford-Dunn, Johnson, Simmons, Malachowski, & Low, 1987). Use of the high-risk factors in hearing screening for newborns was readily accepted and widely used through the 1970s and 1980s. Unfortunately, it has now been well confirmed that risk factor screening identified only 50% of infants with significant hearing loss (Elssman, Matkin, & Sabo, 1987; Mauk, White, Mortensen, & Behrens, 1991; Pappas, 1983).

Also during the 1970s and 1980s, considerable work was being conducted by a number of auditory researchers to develop new objective, physiologically based hearing screening techniques that could replace the widely used subjective behavioral observation of infant responses to acoustic stimuli. These early attempts to use autonomic reflex responses were quite innovative and worthy of review. Early publications of some of these potentially valuable screening procedures had important influences on future meetings of the JCIH.

Heart Rate Response Audiometry

Bartoshuk (1962, 1964) examined the cardiac response to sound in neonates. Bartoshuk and colleagues expanded on the earlier research of Zeaman and Wegner (1954, 1956) that showed that a brief, moderately loud pure tone would cause a temporary wave-like alteration of the electrocardiogram (EKG). In some subjects, the unconditioned heart rate response showed acceleration or deceleration following the presentation of an auditory stimulus. Although Bartoshuk's group verified that cardiac responses could be reliably observed in 1-, 2-, 3-, and 4-day-old infants, repeated stimulus presentations reached response habituation quickly. Other researchers evaluated heart rate response audiometry with infants and children, but with the advent of auditory brainstem response audiometry in the 1970s, interest in the heart rate as a means to testing hearing in infants quickly disappeared.

Respiration Audiometry

It is a common observation in neonates that sleeping babies often show an increase in respiration rate and amplitude following stimulation by loud sounds. This autonomic respiratory response is easy to quantify with the use of a strain gauge system around the patient's chest. Hayes and Jerger (1978) attempted to obtain more precise results with the use of a thermistor (a heat-sensing device that changes its electrical resistance in response to differences in temperature) taped below the patient's nostrils. Bradford

(1975) used pure tone stimulation with respiration audiometry to validate normal hearing in 4- and 12-month-old infants. Although the procedure was reported to be easy to administer, the subjective interpretation of respiration responses proved troublesome for clinicians, and accordingly never really caught on as a clinical tool.

The Crib-O-Gram

The Crib-O-Gram was an ingenious automated system for detecting hearing loss in newborns utilizing a motion-sensitive transducer placed under the newborn bassinet mattress to detect any motor activity from the infant stronger than an eye blink or facial grimace (Simmons & Russ, 1974). The system, developed at Stanford University by otolaryngologist F. Blair Simmons, was a microprocessor-based self-cycling, automated program that turned itself on, performed the test, interpreted the results, and then turned off following each complete stimulus presentation and response measurement interval (Jones & Simmons, 1977; Simmons, 1976). The system monitored the infant's state by measuring crib movement before and after each narrow-band noises stimulus presentation. The Stanford research group tested more than 12,000 infants with the Crib-O-Gram between 1974 and 1984. The screening device had several unique advantages for screening infants' hearing: (a) it was easily operated by minimally trained personnel; (b) it did not interrupt normal nursery routine; and (c) it was truly an objective hearing screening system. Unfortunately, it also had several disadvantages: (a) as an automatic system it was subject to mechanical failure; (b) the initial cost of the equipment was high; (c) the screening required a high-intensity stimulus greater than 75 dB SPL presented though an earphone hanging in the bassinet; and (d) the automated test paradigm was often lengthy for each infant. Although the Crib-O-Gram offered great promise as an automated infant screening system, studies by Wright and Rybak (1983) and Durieux-Smith, Picton, Edwards, Goodman, and MacMurray (1985) showed the device to produce an unacceptably high false-positive rate as well as poor test-retest reliability in repetitive studies of the same infant.

The Auditory Response Cradle

The automated Auditory Response Cradle was developed in England as a more elaborate and advanced screener than the Crib-O-Gram (Bennett, 1980). The Auditory Response Cradle was designed to measure several infant motor responses following programmed auditory stimulus presentations including trunk and limb movements, startle reflex responses, and changes in respiratory pattern. An 85 dB SPL filtered noise stimulus was presented to the infant through insert ear receivers during programmed stimulus trials. An equal number of control trials with no stimulus presented permitted the system to calculate the probability that the infant's motor responses were, in fact, related to the stimulus presentations and not just random movements. When the processor determined a 97% probability rate, which took between 2 and 10 minutes, the infant was passed with normal hearing. More than 5,000 infants were successfully screened with the Auditory Response Cradle by 1984 with acceptable low false-positive rates (Bhattacharya, Bennett, & Tucker, 1984). Although the system was well received in England, the Auditory Response

Cradle was not widely used in the United States, perhaps due to the high expense of the equipment.

UNIVERSAL NEWBORN HEARING SCREENING

The journey to universal newborn hearing screening in the United States has had an interesting, although somewhat controversial, history along the way. In 1969, at the suggestion of Marion Downs, a national multidisciplinary committee, formed of representatives from the Academy of Pediatrics, the Academy of Ophthalmology and Otolaryngology, and the American Speech and Hearing Association, met to discuss the early hearing screen of newborns to identify those with hearing loss. They agreed to call themselves the Joint Committee on Infant Hearing Screening (JCIH). They probably had no idea in 1969 that the JCIH would have a history of more than 50 years with an enormous impact on the development and implementation of early identification and early intervention for infants with hearing loss. A voluntary multidisciplinary group, bound together by a common interest in identifying and managing newborns and young children with hearing loss, the transitional membership of the committee has met irregularly through the years to establish standards and guidelines and make recommendations to ensure an effective and efficient system to benefit children with hearing loss. Their numerous position statements developed and released have proven to be the gold standard for early identification and early intervention followed in the United States and in numerous other nations around the world.

Downs presented her data from the Denver project to that initial small group of five individuals, hoping the committee would review and approve of her behavioral observation procedure (Downs & Hemenway, 1969; Downs & Sterritt, 1964). The Joint Committee applauded her efforts but declined to endorse her procedure (JCIH, 1971). Instead the JCIH met again in about 18 months and issued a supplementary statement in 1973 discouraging routine hearing screening of infants unless research oriented.

Although this decision from the JCIH was interpreted at the time by Downs as a bit of a setback, she managed to have the committee issue recommendations that infants "at risk" should be identified by means of history and physical examination and referred for hearing testing. The committee position statement indicated that those newborns identified by risk factors should be referred for "an indepth audiological evaluation of hearing during their first two months of life, and even if hearing appears to be normal, should receive regular hearing evaluations." The 1973 JCIH Supplement Statement established the first high-risk register for deafness that identified five major criteria that would put newborn infants at risk for having severe to profound hearing impairment. The five criteria were: (a) family history; (b) intrauterine fetal infection; (c) defects of the ear, nose, or throat; (d) low birth weight; and (e) high bilirubin level. These risk factors could be identified by interviewing the birth mother or by examining the medical records of each infant to see whether there was any history or physical finding that would give a high probability of hearing loss. The high-risk register approach was widely accepted and used in an attempt to focus attention on those infants most likely to have significant hearing loss, rather than screening every newborn baby. The high-risk concept assumes that one can identify a small group of children whose history or physical condition results in a high chance of having the target handicap.

The Joint Committee on Infant Hearing met again several times over the years (1982, 1990, 1994, 2000, 2007, and 2013) to review and update new position statements, based on new knowledge and reviews of current literature relevant to practices of identifying hearing-impaired neonates and infants. The evolution of recommended infant hearing screening practices presents an interesting look at the growth and application of new technologies and knowledge in continued efforts to improve the efficiency and accuracy of early identification of infants with hearing impairments.

The decade of the 1990s will no doubt be remembered for the return to the concept of implementing hearing screening for all newborns, now known as universal newborn hearing screening. As described by Hayes (1999), during the first half of the 1990s, three important activities stimulated interest in early detection of infants with hearing loss. First, in 1990, with support of federal funding, the Rhode Island Hearing Assessment Project was developed to evaluate systematically the feasibility of using the new technique of transient evoked otoacoustic emissions to screen infants for hearing loss.

The success of the Rhode Island Project stimulated the occurrence of the second activity, the NIH-sponsored Consensus Development Conference. It was recognized that the high-risk register screening approach to the identification of infants with congenital hearing loss followed in the 1980s and early 1990s was missing nearly 50% of young children later identified with hearing loss. These children had none of the risk factors at birth. Thus, the federal government convened a special meeting of experts in 1993 to evaluate existing evidence

and to recommend improved screening protocols. After 2 days of deliberation, the panel of experts concluded that "we must dramatically change our approach to infant hearing screening." The National Institute on Deafness and Other Communication Disorders (part of the National Institutes of Health) released a *Consensus Statement on Early Identification of Hearing Impairment in Infants and Young Children* strongly recommending that "universal screening be implemented for all infants within the first three months of life." The document was met with some upheaval and provoked considerable debate regarding the feasibility of, and justification for, universal newborn hearing screening. The recommendation for universal newborn hearing screening was not received with uniform enthusiasm by all professionals. Some were loudly opposed to the concept of universal infant hearing screening as being without scientific basis, being ineffective, and not being justified (Bess & Paradise, 1994).

The third important activity was the development and release of a new position statement of the now powerful Joint Committee on Infant Hearing in follow-up to the NIH Consensus Statement. Following their 1994 meeting, the JCIH, endorsed "the goal of universal detection of infants with hearing loss as early as possible. All infants with hearing loss should be identified by three months of age, and receive intervention by six months of age." Finally, even the American Academy of Pediatrics (1999) published an independent endorsement of universal newborn hearing screening calling for pediatricians to take a more active role in pediatric hearing screening programs.

The aforementioned Rhode Island Project was the first statewide effort to meet the goal of universal newborn hearing screening (Vohr, Carty, Moore, & Letourneau, 1998). A universal infant hearing screening program was established in eight maternity hospitals in Rhode Island based on a two-tiered approach of transient otoacoustic emissions (TEOAEs) for all infants, with those failing the initial screening referred for automated ABR screening. Review of the first four years of the project, 1993 through 1996, showed steady improvement in the percentage of infants completing the two-stage screen process with reasonable compliance in the rescreening and diagnostic testing stages. The Rhode Island project resulted in significant decrease in the age of identification and age of intervention for infants with confirmed hearing loss. Results were reported for the identification and habilitation of 111 infants with permanent hearing loss identified from more than 53,000 total babies screened—an amazing 99% of all babies born in Rhode Island. The study showed a rate of hearing impairment of 2 per 1,000, with the mean age of hearing loss confirmation decreasing from 8.7 months to 3.5 months, and the age of initial amplification improving from 13.3 months to 5.7 months during the 4 years of the study. The data reported by the Rhode Island group certainly made a clear impression to convince the NIH Consensus Conference that universal infant hearing screening could be successful.

Following the success of the Rhode Island Project, the NIH Consensus statement recommended that all infants should be screened for hearing loss within the first 3 months of life, and the most efficient manner to accomplish this would be to screen the infants prior to hospital discharge. The NIH Consensus Conference recommended universal newborn hearing screening using a two-stage physiologic test approach of an initial TEOAE screen for all newborns and ABR screening for those infants not passing the initial screening procedure. The 1994 JCIH position statement supported the fact that infants should be screened with established physiologic testing techniques, thereby ending more than two decades of behavioral observation screening of infants. The 1994 JCIH also encouraged continuing research to evaluate existing screening techniques and to develop new protocols and expanded the role of high-risk factors (termed *deafness indicators*) associated with sensorineural and conductive hearing loss in newborns and infants.

The 1994 recommendation for universal screening of newborns generated considerable controversy. Bess and Paradise (1994) characterized universal screening for infant hearing impairment as "not simple, not risk-free, not necessarily beneficial and not presently justifiable" (p. 330). Their commentary impugned infant hearing screening and questioned the effectiveness and need for early intervention for infants with hearing loss. Northern and Hayes (1994) took exception to their presentation and published a response in favor of universal infant hearing screening. The debate stimulated a rash of Letters to the Editor (*Pediatrics, 94*(6), 948–963, 1994), with most respondents indicating that ample data exist to support infant hearing screening and the need for early intervention. Despite the controversy, the momentum for universal hearing screening of infants grew quickly to 22 states by the year 2000.

The Rhode Island Hearing Assessment Project was the first major effort at universal hearing screening of newborns and has been described extensively (Vohr et al., 1998; White, 1996; White & Behrens, 1993). Based on a two-stage protocol using otoacoustic emissions as the birth admission screening, followed by automated ABR, results were reported for more than 53,000 newborns. Referral rates following the first-stage screen were 8%, decreasing to less than 3% following the second screening procedure. Other state programs followed with their own versions and protocols in efforts to establish statewide newborn hearing screening programs. Mehl and Thomson (1998) described the Colorado experience over a 4-year period involving the screening of more than 41,000 infants. They concluded that the cost (estimated at $9,600 per case identified) and the positive predictive value (estimated at approximately 19% for two-staged automated ABR screening) of universal newborn hearing screening compared favorably with cost and predictive value of screening for other congenital conditions. Mason and Hermann (1998) reported results of a single hospital-based program in Hawaii in which 96% of infants were successfully screened, including more than 10,000 infants over a 5-year period. In the Hawaii experience, the cost of screening at that time was reported to be $17 per infant, resulting in an estimated cost to identify each case of true bilateral hearing loss to be $17,750 per infant. Finitzo and Albright (1998) and Finitzo and Crumley (1999) described the Sounds of Texas infant screening program. They reported that during a 3-year period in 11 Texas hospitals, 98% of all newborns were screened for hearing before discharge. Texas hospitals using a two-technology screening protocol (EOAE followed by AABR screening) averaged a 3% failure rate, and hospitals using a two-stage, one-technology (either EOAE or AABR) protocol showed a 5% failure rate.

A massive project was undertaken with the New York State Universal Newborn Hearing Screening effort to determine the feasibility of universal newborn screening in seven regional perinatal centers composed of eight hospitals. Their results over a 3-year period have been described in a series of articles (Dalzell et al., 2000; Gravel et al., 2000; Prieve & Stevens, 2000; Prieve et al., 2000; Spivak et al., 2000). Over the 3-year period in New York, nearly 70,000 newborns were screened at eight hospitals, representing 96.9% of all live births. The overall failure rate of 4%, combined with the miss rate of 2.6%, resulted in 6.6% of infants referred for outpatient follow-up. The New York State Project confirmed the necessity and demonstrated the feasibility of developing a complete audiologic system of care of newborn infants, and further established a standard of care benchmark of accountability for all universal screening statewide programs (Hayes, 2000).

The Early Hearing Detection and Intervention department was established following the passage of the Newborn and Infant Hearing Screening and Intervention Act of 1999. Assigned to the CDC's responsibility as an issue of public health, federal grants were made available to fund EHDI programs in each state of the United States. As of 2010, a total of 41 states, Guam, and the District of Columbia have statutes or regulatory guidance to identify infants with hearing loss. All states and U.S. territories also have established Early Hearing Detection and Intervention (EHDI) programs, which embody evidence-based public health policy for addressing infant hearing loss. EHDI programs help ensure that newborns and infants are screened and receive recommended follow-up through data collection and outreach to hospitals, providers, and families.

Since the organized collection of data by the Early Hearing Detection and Intervention group of the CDC, the reported mean percentage of infants screened for hearing loss increased from 46.5% in 1999 to 97.0% in 2010. The increase in screening is most likely due to a combination of several factors: (a) implementation of new or revised requirements to screen infants for hearing loss (within some states); (b) improvements in screening and diagnostic technology; (c) increased reporting by hospitals and other providers of hearing screening results; (d) improvements in data collection and state and territorial EHDI tracking and surveillance systems; (e) increased awareness about the importance of screening infants for hearing loss; (f) increased follow-up efforts by state EHDI programs; and (g) support by national agencies and organizations.

Although approximately 97% of all U.S. infants can be documented as having their hearing screened before 1 month of age, challenges remain including ensuring timely diagnostic evaluation for those who do not pass the screening and enrollment in early intervention for those with diagnosed hearing loss. Unfortunately, in 2005 for example, more than 60% of infants who did not pass the final or most recent screening were lost to follow-up (LTF) or lost to documentation (LTD) if they received services without the results being reported to the EHDI program. Some of those infants might have received audiologic evaluations, but the results were not reported to the EHDI program (i.e., undocumented evaluation), and their status could not be determined from available data. By 2007, LFU/LTD among infants not passing the final or most recent screening had decreased to approximately 46%. EHDI programs such as those in Massachusetts and Colorado, which actively follow up with families and providers and reported LFU/LTD statistics for 2007 of 5.6% and 6.4%, respectively, set a good example for other programs trying to improve overall follow-up rates (Gaffney, Eichwald, Grosse, & Mason, 2010).

The number of infants identified with hearing loss, as reported by EHDI in 2010, increased from an estimated 282 newborns (1.1 per 1,000 screened) reported by nine states and territories in 1999 to 3,430 newborn (1.2 per 1,000 screened) documented cases reported by 44 states and territories in

2007 (six states and territories responding to the 2007 survey were unable to provide this information). In 2007, 43 states and territories documented that 60.8% of infants with hearing loss were enrolled in early intervention by age 6 months (Gaffney et al., 2010).

It would seem that the long journey to universal newborn hearing screening has nearly arrived at its destination with appreciation to the literally hundreds of concerned individuals who have given much of their time, effort, and professional careers. The success of universal newborn hearing cannot be overstated. It has been well established now that congenital hearing loss affects two to three infants per 1,000 live births. A journey of nearly 50 years, started by one determined individual, Marion Downs, who recognized that identifying children with hearing loss early and enrolling them in intervention programs as soon as possible could lead to their intellectual success. Downs had a vision and would not be deterred until her goals were accomplished to the benefit of all children with hearing loss.

Joint Committee on Infant Hearing Statements and Guidelines

Over the years, the JCIH has carefully reviewed ongoing research efforts to ensure that their recommendations are well founded through evidence-based studies. Considerable data have been reported which support not only the feasibility of universal newborn hearing screening (UNHS) but also the benefits of early intervention for infants with hearing loss. Specifically, infants who are hard-of-hearing and deaf who receive intervention before 6 months of age maintain language development commensurate with their cognitive abilities through the age of 5 years (Yoshinaga-Itano, 1995; Yoshinaga-Itano et al., 1998). Numerous investigators have documented the validity, reliability, and effectiveness of early detection of infants who are hard-of-hearing and deaf through UNHS (Finitzo, Albright, & O'Neal, 1998; Spivak, 1998; Vohr & Maxon, 1996; Vohr et al., 1998).

The Joint Committee on Infant Hearing (JCIH) 2007 statement is a decisive document that has had a huge impact on the world in guiding programs for early identification of hearing loss and early intervention. The JCIH 2007 position statement is a masterful and thorough set of directives that should be read carefully by all pediatric audiologists. Some of the important background information, general principles, and salient elements are reviewed in the following paragraphs.

The 2007 Joint Committees on Infant Hearing (JCIH) endorsed early detection of and intervention for infants with hearing loss (Early Hearing Detection and Intervention: EHDI) through integrated, interdisciplinary state and national systems of universal newborn hearing screening, evaluation, and family-centered intervention. The goal of EHDI is to maximize communicative competence and literacy development for children who are hard-of-hearing or deaf. Without appropriate opportunities to learn language, children who are hard-of-hearing or deaf will fall behind their hearing peers in language, cognition, and social-emotional development. Such delays may result in lower educational and employment levels in adulthood (Gallaudet University Center for Assessment and Demographic Study, 1998).

The Year 2007 document called for all infants to be screened for hearing at no later than 1 month of age; infants who do not pass the initial screening should have a comprehensive audiological evaluation at no later than 3 months of age. Infants with confirmed hearing loss should receive appropriate intervention at no later than 6 months of age. Once any degree of hearing loss is diagnosed in a child, a referral should be initiated to an early intervention program within 2 days of confirmation. If the family chooses to use personal amplification for its infant with hearing loss, the hearing aid selection and fitting should occur within 1 month of initial confirmation of the hearing loss even when additional audiological assessment is ongoing. Regardless of hearing screening outcomes, all infants, or without risk factors, should receive ongoing surveillance of communicative development beginning at 2 months of age during well-child medical visits.

Risk Factors for Deafness

Since 1972, the Joint Committee on Infant Hearing (JCIH) has identified specific risk indicators associated with infant and childhood hearing loss. With each meeting of the JCIH over the years, from 1984 to 2000, the number of risk factors associated with hearing loss in infants has evolved and lengthened. With the current emphasis on hearing screening for all babies, we no longer select only certain infants for testing based on their "risk" of having hearing loss. Numerous research studies in the 1990s proved that screening only at-risk infants identifies only 40% to 50% of infants with hearing loss, thereby missing a large number of infants with asymptomatic recessive hearing loss. On the other hand, because normal hearing at birth does not preclude delayed onset or acquired hearing loss, awareness of the risk indicators should be helpful in identifying infants who might be candidates for ongoing audiological and medical surveillance. In addition, knowledge of the risk factors is a necessity for the pediatric audiologist.

The risk factors for infants with hearing loss have transitioned and changed over time as a function of improved medical technologies, rendering some of the risk factors that existed in the 1970s nearly obsolete in current birthing facilities (Table 8–5). The JCIH Position Statement of 2000 included a listing of risk indicators divided into two categories: those indicators present during the neonatal period and those indicators that may develop as a result of certain medical conditions as presented below. In addition, the JCIH 2000 guidelines recommend that all infants who pass newborn hearing screening but who have risk indicators for other auditory disorders or speech and language delay receive ongoing audiologic and medical surveillance and monitoring for communication development. Infants with indicators associated with late-onset, progressive, or fluctuating hearing loss as well as auditory neural conduction disorders or brainstem auditory pathway dysfunction should be monitored. A more complete discussion of the medical aspects of the high risk factors for deafness may be found in Chapters 2 and 4.

Risk indicators for birth through 28 days are as follows:

- An illness or condition requiring admission of 48 hours or greater to a NICU;
- Stigmata or other findings associated with a syndrome known to include sensorineural and or conductive hearing loss;
- Family history of permanent childhood sensorineural hearing loss;
- Craniofacial anomalies, including those with morphological abnormalities of the pinna and ear canal;
- In utero infection such as cytomegalovirus, herpes, toxoplasmosis, or rubella.

Risk indicators for 29 days through 2 years:

- Parental or caregiver concern regarding hearing, speech, language, and or developmental delay;
- Family history of permanent childhood hearing loss;

Table 8–5. Causes of Deafness

Prenatal (5% to 10%): Congenital infections (TORCH); teratogen exposure (alcohol, cocaine, methylmercury, thalidomide)
Perinatal (5% to 15%): Prematurity and/or low birth weight; anoxia; hyperbilirubinemia; sepsis
Postnatal (10% to 20%): Infection (meningitis, mumps); otitis media complication; ototoxic medication
Genetic: familial or sporadic (30% to 50%): Syndromic; nonsyndromic
Questionable and other (5%): High fever, infection, trauma, seizures
Unknown (20% to 30%)

Source: Adapted from "Genetic Epidemiological Studies of Early-Onset Deafness in the U.S. School-Age Population," by M. L. Marazita, L. M. Ploughman, B. Rawlings, et al., 1993, *American Journal of Medical Genetics, 46,* p. 486.

- Stigmata or other findings associated with a syndrome known to include a sensorineural or conductive hearing loss or eustachian tube dysfunction;
- Postnatal infections associated with sensorineural hearing loss including bacterial meningitis;
- In utero infections such as cytomegalovirus, herpes, rubella, syphilis, and toxoplasmosis;
- Neonatal indicators—specifically hyperbilirubinemia at a serum level requiring exchange transfusion, persistent pulmonary hypertension of the newborn associated with mechanical ventilation, and conditions requiring the use of extracorporeal membrane oxygenation (ECMO);
- Syndromes associated with progressive hearing loss such as neurofibromatosis, osteopetrosis, and Usher syndrome;
- Neurodegenerative disorders, such as Hunter syndrome, or sensory motor neuropathies, such as Friedreich ataxia and Charcot-Marie-Tooth syndrome, head trauma;
- Recurrent or persistent otitis media with effusion for at least 3 months.

Cone-Wesson et al. (2000) analyzed the prevalence of risk indicators for infants identified with hearing loss. Some 3,134 infants evaluated during their initial birth hospitalization were re-evaluated for the presence of hearing loss between 8 and 12 months of age. The majority of these infants were NICU graduates (2,847), and the remaining 287 infants had risk indicators for hearing loss that did not require intensive care, such as family history or craniofacial anomalies. Infants with history or evidence of transient middle ear dysfunc-

tion were excluded from the final analysis, revealing 56 with permanent hearing loss. Cone-Wesson et al. determined the prevalence of hearing loss for each risk factor by dividing the number of infants with the risk factor and hearing loss by the total number of infants in the sample with a given risk factor. Hearing loss was present in 11.7% of infants with syndromes associated with hearing loss—which included Trisomy 21; Pierre Robin syndrome; CHARGE syndrome; choanal atresia; Rubinstein-Taybi syndrome; Stickler syndrome; and Goldenhar syndrome. Family history of hearing loss had a prevalence of 6.6%, meningitis 5.5%, and craniofacial anomalies 4.7%. In contrast, aminoglycoside antibiotics had a prevalence of hearing loss of only 1.5%, consistent with data of Finitzo-Hieber et al. (1985). Interpretation of the Cone-Wesson et al. data indicated that 1 of 56 infants identified with permanent hearing loss revealed clear evidence of late-onset hearing loss by 1 year of age. Analyzing ototoxicity as a risk indicator brings to light that while a large number of NICU infants with hearing loss have a history of aminoglycoside treatment, only a small percentage of those receiving ototoxic antibiotics actually incurred hearing loss. In fact, as many as 45% of infants treated in the NICU receive such treatment with potentially damaging ototoxic medications (Vohr et al., 2000).

The 2007 JCIH Position Statement dismissed the two-category listing of high-risk factors, and instead combined the factors into a single list rather than grouping them by time of likely onset. The 2007 statement recommends that the timing and number of hearing reevaluations for children with risk factors should be customized and individualized depending on the relative likelihood of a subsequent delayed-onset hearing loss. Infants who pass the neonatal hearing screening but have a risk factor should have at least one diagnostic audiology assessment by 24 to 30 months of age. Early and more frequent assessment may be indicated for children with cytomegalovirus (CMV) infection, syndromes associated with progressive hearing loss, neurodegenerative disorders, trauma, or culture-positive postnatal infections associated with sensorineural hearing loss; for children who have received extracorporeal membrane oxygenation (ECMO) or chemotherapy; and when there is caregiver concern or a family history of hearing loss.

The Multidisciplinary Team

There is no question that the ongoing evaluation and assessment of an infant or neonate identified with hearing loss should be performed by a team of professionals working in conjunction with the parent/caregiver. The multidisciplinary team must include the parent/caregiver. The multidisciplinary newborn hearing team should consist of the following members:

- A primary care physician or a physician with expertise in the management of early childhood otologic disorders;
- An audiologist with expertise in the assessment of infants and young children to determine type, degree, symmetry, stability, and configuration of hearing loss and to recommend amplification devices appropriate to the child's needs (e.g., hearing aids, personal FM systems, vibrotactile aids, or cochlear implants);
- A speech-language pathologist, audiologist, sign language specialist, or teacher of children who are deaf or hard-of-hearing with expertise in the assessment and intervention of communication skills;
- Other professionals as appropriate for the individual needs of the child and family. This team should work together to develop a program of early intervention services, an Individualized Family Service Plan (IFSP) that is based on the infant's unique strengths and needs and is consistent with the family's resources, priorities, and concerns related to enhancing the child's development.

Trained Infant Screening Volunteers

Individual volunteers, or volunteers from various community service groups, can be trained by the audiologist to perform many of the functions required in an infant hearing screening program. Not all volunteers actually want to test the hearing of babies, but the personnel support from such groups can be effectively directed to interviewing mothers, reviewing hospital medical records, data management, record keeping and other administrative tasks, and telephoning parents to ensure follow-up care. When volunteers are used in hospital situations, it is suggested that appropriate steps be taken to ensure legal protection and legal clearance for these nonprofessional people to examine medical charts, move babies from the nurseries to the audiologic test area, interview new mothers, and perform other tasks. The advantage to the use of volunteers is the low cost for supportive personnel; the major disadvantage of using volunteers is often a progressive lack of interest in this particular project, changeover in the volunteer club's officers, or a change in direction of the service organization's activities. The audiologist dependent on a volunteer staff to perform the infant hearing screening program must be a master of working with people to obtain high-quality support and ingenious at maintaining the volunteer enthusiasm for the project at hand.

HEARING SCREENING: BIRTH THROUGH 6 MONTHS

The NIH 1993 Consensus Committee, and each of the subsequent JCIH Position Statements, has made it abundantly clear that all infants should be screened using a physiologic measure (e.g., auditory brainstem response [ABR] or evoked otoacoustic emission screening [EOAE]) rather than behavioral observation). The 2007 JCIH statement requires that the physiologic hearing screening for all infants be conducted prior to 1 month of age. Although neither ABR nor EOAE is a "hearing test," per se, their results correlate very highly with normal hearing, and both have procedures adapted for infant screening. Both of these physiologic techniques can be applied to infants with automated instruments that accomplish hearing screening in effective, accurate, and efficient protocols, and, in fact, can be operated by trained volunteers. Both ABR and EOAE equipment has been adapted for newborn screening by incorporating automated response detection rather than the traditional clinical procedures that require operator interpretation and decision making. Today's screening ABR and EOAE equipment utilize preprogrammed algorithms to determine "pass" and "fail" criteria, thereby eliminating the need for individual test interpretation, reducing the effects of screener bias and errors on test outcome, and ensuring test consistency for all infants.

Both types of technology are equally recommended for newborn hearing screening and are considered efficient and accurate with high sensitivity and specificity. There are pros and cons to using either technology. The ABR approach is more time consuming and expensive, while EOAE is a quicker procedure but produces more false-positives that need rescreening. Both technologies provide objective pass-refer decisions making them ideal for volunteers to use in newborn hearing screening applications. EOAE and ABR screening equipment can be used as individual devices (EOAE only or ABR only) or in the form of a combined screener with both EOAE and ABR. Newborn screening ABR equipment is commonly referred to as automated ABR (A-ABR). However, there are significant differences between the two technologies in the manner of their application and how the screening procedure is actually conducted; the portion of the auditory system being screened; time required to screen each newborn; pass, fail, and referral rates; as well as the long-term operational costs incurred for equipment and disposables.

Automated ABR (A-ABR)

The ABR is a physiologic measure of the entire auditory system from the peripheral through the brainstem to the cortex. In fact, as sound is emitted into the infant's ear, the microelectrical brain waves are picked up and amplified by electrodes taped to the baby's head. A special computer analyzes these micro-brain waves to determine if the baby heard the sound or not. Automated ABR (A-ABR) systems have been developed and used specifically for the mass hearing screening of infants aged 34 weeks to gestational age of 6 months since the mid-1980s (Figure 8–3).

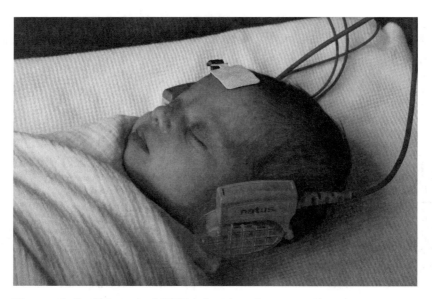

Figure 8–3. Automated ABR infant hearing screening. Image courtesy of Natus Medical Incorporated.

The A-ABR system compares the real-time responses from the infant under evaluation with a "normal" response template within the equipment that has been standardized from a large sample population of newborns. The weighted binary template matching algorithm that calculates the statistical likelihood ratio for pass/refer determination was based on the initial experiments by Herrmann and Thornton (1995) in which conventional ABR results from 451 NICU infants ranging from 30 to 58 weeks were analyzed to identify and weight the most stable points. The resulting template shifts ±1.5 msec to accommodate normal latency variations within this age range. If the test infant's responses fall within the normative latency and amplitude values of the ABR peak V, the automated ABR instrument renders a "pass" decision; if the response pattern falls outside the acceptable response template, a "refer" response is noted suggesting the need for additional testing. A-ABR systems do not rely on an individual's subjective judgments regarding the presence or absence of a wave-form or latency of a response.

The protocols and setup procedures for A-ABR include programmable screening testing techniques for screening one or both ears simultaneously, disposable electrodes, and automatic artifact rejection systems to control for both environmental ambient noise and physiologic noise from the infant. For A-ABR, the number of repetitions is ceased automatically when the response reaches statistical significance. In less than optimum conditions (e.g., excessive noise or physiologic artifact), more stimulus presentations involving longer screening time may be required. The infant passes the screening if reliable responses are present at the screening level of 35 dB nHL or lower. Automated ABR screening is especially efficient and practical because of its accuracy and the fact that a trained nonprofessional can manage the simple operation. A drawback to the automated system is the expense of replacing disposable supplies. The typical screening time required to set up and evaluate both ears in a newborn is 10 to 20 minutes.

Automated Evoked Otoacoustic Emissions (EOAE)

In contrast to the ABR hearing screen, the otoacoustic emission screening simply determines normal or abnormal peripheral auditory function. With newborn EOAE screening, a small probe is placed in the baby's ear canal, and soft tones or clicks are introduced. The sound travels through the outer ear and canal through the middle ear to the cochlea. If the cochlea is functioning normally, the outer hair cells will produce an otoacoustic emission (i.e., an "echo response") that then travels back out through the middle and outer ear canal. This reflective emission is measured by the probe and analyzed by a computer. If the emission is sufficiently robust, "pass" is displayed on the screen; if there is any dysfunction or blockage along that pathway, or if the cochlear hair cells are unable to respond, the equipment will be unable to measure the emission, and the result will be a fail or "refer" for additional testing notification. Because the OAE response is generated in the cochlea before it reaches the eighth nerve, it is referred to as a "preneural" response.

Measurement of evoked otoacoustic emissions (EOAEs) is relatively quick and easy to set up and conduct with infants requiring some 3 to 6 minutes on average. Tips for screening infants with EOAEs include testing in as quiet a location as possible; conducting a preliminary visual inspection of the baby's ear canals to be sure they are clear; and gently pulling up on the pinnae to open the ear canal for easier inser-

tion of the probe, If the baby does not pass on the first try, change the position of the infant, especially if he or she has been lying on the test ear; remove the probe and check for blockage by ear canal debris; clean the tip or replace if necessary; reposition the probe and run the test again.

Two types of EOAEs are used in infant screening programs, the transient evoked otoacoustic emissions (TEOAEs) and the distortion product evoked otoacoustic emissions (DPEOAEs), as described in Chapter 7. Both types of emissions are detected in the ear canal with a handheld probe device and are quite robust and easily measured in infants (Figure 8–4). TEOAEs are present in the normal-hearing ear canal following presentation of brief repeated click stimuli and are easy to detect, record, and interpret. The measurement of DPEOAEs requires more sophisticated equipment with two stimulus channels as described in Chapter 7.

The most common problem and cause for EOAE failure is obstruction of the tiny ear canals with vernix caseosa. Vernix can affect screening outcomes with either technology. Allowing time for the vernix to clear maximizes the opportunity for the equipment to efficiently measure an accurate response. The infant's ear canals should be examined with an otoscope prior to screening. If the EOAE response is not seen, the probe tip should be carefully inspected before it is reinserted. Another common reason for a "refer" indication with EOAEs is conductive hearing loss that can be caused by middle ear fluid present in some newborns for a few days. For best results, newborn screening should be done between 24 and 72 hours after birth, although waiting even 12 hours after birth is not always possible due to early discharge policies. If passing results are not obtained prior to the infant's discharge from the hospital, effort should be made to retest

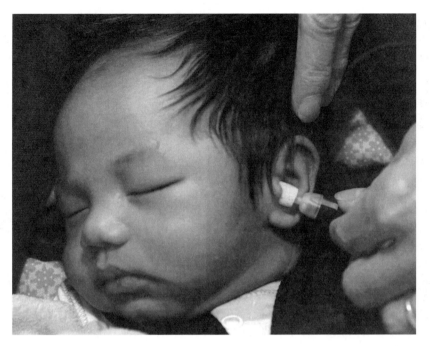

Figure 8–4. Automated OAE infant screening. Photo courtesy of Colorado Children's Hospital, Aurora, CO.

the baby within 2 weeks. The protocol in some programs requires that if the infant does not pass the first screen, the rescreen with EOAEs should be at least 12 hours later, or if the second screen is A-ABR, the retest can be done a few hours later. Because screening too early can result in high refer or false-positive rates, hospitals must implement strategies to maintain lower refer rates, such as repeating the screening prior to discharge and ensuring that all screening staff, volunteers, and professionals, are well trained to operate the equipment and to manage the infants. EOAE results were examined by Lutman, Davis, Fortnum, and Wood (1997) for a cohort of 47 children with hearing losses of 50 dB HL or greater. They reported that 11 of the 47 children passed the TEOAE screening with 9 definite false-negative results suggesting a sensitivity rate of 80% if the screening had been based on otoacoustic emissions screening alone.

The National Center for Hearing Assessment and Management (NCHAM) has suggested that infants born without complications can be screened for hearing loss as early as 6 hours old, although waiting until closer to hospital discharge is preferable; that babies screened in the NICU should be in stable condition and in an open crib or bassinet, and they may need screening more than once before discharge depending on their medical condition; and finally, home birth babies or infants born in a birthing facility should come in for screening within the first 2 weeks of life if possible.

A number of researchers have compared results obtained from both automated ABR and either or both types of EOAEs on large cohorts of well babies and infants (Chen et al., 1996; Doyle, Fuikawa, Rogers, & Newman, 1998; Freitas, Alvarenga, Bevilacqua, Martinez, & Costa, 2009; Gabbard, Northern, & Yoshinaga-Itano, 1999; Maxon, White, Behrens, & Vohr, 1995; McNellis & Klein, 1997). The studies confirm the value of A-ABR and EOAE screening in infants related to cost, time efficiency, and accuracy in identifying infants with hearing loss. Newborns and infants are easiest to test while in deep sleep or a dozing state, or following feeding. Gabbard et al. (1999) evaluated 110 infants (mean age, 15 hours) from the well-baby nursery with both automated ABR and TEOAE measures to determine pass/refer rates and recorded the time required for each of the measures. Significant difference was found for TEOAE measures in infants less than 10 hours of age from those infants between 11 and 24 hours of age and from those newborns older than 24 hours. Younger infants were less likely to pass the TEOAE screen, although age was not a factor with the automated ABR technique. A significantly greater pass rate of 97% was found for automated ABR birth admission screening compared with a 60% pass rate for TEOAE measures for these young infants. Infants who are readmitted during the first month of life for a condition associated with potential hearing loss (see risk factors for deafness) should require a repeat hearing screening or a diagnostic ABR evaluation prior to being discharged again.

A variety of hospital-based hearing screening protocols using ABR and EOAE in some format of two-stage screening methodology have been described and successfully implemented (Arehart, Yoshinaga-Itano, Thomson, Gabbard, & Stredler Brown, 1998; Finitzo et al., 1998; Mason & Hermann, 1998; Mehl & Thomson, 1998; Vohr et al., 1998). For infants born in hospitals, hearing screening should be completed close to hospital discharge allowing the infant to stabilize following the birth process. Of course, most infants pass the initial screening test or a rescreening before hospital discharge, but because the mothers are not kept in the hospital for more than a day or two, procedures must be in place to screen the infants on a 24/7 basis. Many hospital-based newborn hearing screening programs utilize sophisticated data-management systems, perhaps provided through contract with outside vendors, and likely developed as an Internet-based solution for the collection, tracking, reporting, and analysis of newborn hearing screen data. These data systems provide real-time reports of pass, fail, retest, and refer rates for individual programs analysis as well as accurate data for local, state, and federal agencies.

A number of screening protocols are available on the Internet which describe the advantages and disadvantages of two-stage screening protocols. Some protocols call for one or more repeat screenings using the same physiologic test, while others use a different physiologic test for the repeat screen. Some hospital programs use automated ABR while other programs use OAE screening protocols for the initial screening procedure, and then follow with "the other" physiologic test as the rescreen procedure for all newborns who do not pass the initial screening (Figure 8–5). Each protocol must incorporate a system for the rescreening of infants who do not pass the birth admission screening within 1 month of hospital discharge. The mechanism of rescreening is important because it minimizes the number of false-positive referrals for follow-up audiologic and medical evaluation (Eiserman et al., 2008).

The question has been raised about identification of infants with auditory neuropathy spectrum disorder in newborn screening programs. These children will pass EOAE screening and are not likely to pass the A-ABR screen because of absent or malformed brainstem wave patterns. As many hospital-based infant screening programs depend only on EOAE for their newborn

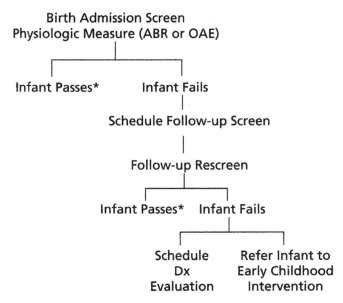

Figure 8–5. Components of a universal newborn hearing screening program. With permission from the Sounds of Texas Project, Dallas, TX.

screening test, they do not identify infant with ANSD. The combination of normal OAE responses and severely impaired ABR responses is thought to reflect normal outer hair cell (OHC) function in the cochlea and abnormal auditory nerve function. Data suggest that the incidence of ANSD in the general population may be 1 to 2 per 10,000 births (Berg, Prieve, Serpanos, & Wheaton, 2011; Foerst et al., 2006; Kirkim, Serbetcioglu, Erdag, & Ceryan, 2008). However, with OAEs being widely used as the primary screening method and the fact that infants with ANSD will pass OAEs, the exact incidence could be higher.

The choice of screening measure and screening protocol depends on many factors, and the decisions will certainly influence program outcomes (i.e., failure of the admission screen, referral percentages, and rescreening requirements). A huge multicenter study to determine how many infants

actually pass a newborn two-stage hearing screening and yet turn out to have permanent hearing loss was reported by Johnson et al. (2005). Seven birthing centers screened 86,634 infants during a 21-month period with a two-stage screening protocol utilizing EOAE as the initial screen followed by ABR for the 4% (*n* = 3,462) infants who failed the initial EOAE procedure. The results indicated that a substantial number of infants with permanent hearing loss were identified around 9 months of age, generally with a mild loss although they were not identified in the two-stage newborn screening. Although the researchers were unable to separate out babies with late-onset hearing loss from those with congenital hearing loss, the fact is the infants "passed" the follow-up A-ABR screening with click stimuli at 35 dB nHL. This conclusion draws attention to the importance of recognizing the limitations of the A-ABR procedure based on the level of the A-ABR screening stimuli and the need to continue monitoring the hearing and language development of young children.

Results from a Hawaiian population of 10,372 babies screened by A-ABR over a 5-year period were described by Mason and Herrmann (1998). Successful screening in the nursery was achieved with 96% of infants with a failure rate of 4%. The false-positive rate was 3.5% after the initial screening and decreased to 2.0% when a two-stage screening procedure was used. The incidence of bilateral congenital hearing loss in the well population was 1 in 1,000, and 5 in 1,000 in the NICU. Amplification was recommended for 15 infants; well infants who received hearing aids before the age of 6 months achieved age-appropriate speech and language development.

As of 2012, 43 states had passed legislation related to newborn hearing screening. Of those 43 states, 28 required that all babies be screened prior to hospital discharge. The National Center for Hearing Assessment and Management (NCHAM) reports that detecting and treating hearing loss at birth for one child saves $400,000 in special education costs by the time that child graduates from high school. With early intervention in mind, states have taken action to ensure children are screened and treated early for hearing loss. Screening programs are typically cost-effective at about $10 to $50 per baby.

The total infant hearing screening program requires a three-part effort: (a) parent/caregiver education to ensure that they understand the relationship between hearing, speech, and language development and that they receive information to enhance their ability to observe and monitor normal hearing, speech, and language development milestones; (b) the actual ABR and/or EOAE hearing screening; and (c) the important follow-up evaluation and management

plan to ensure that the identified infant with hearing loss receives immediate habilitation action. It is important for parents, caregivers, and those who provide primary health care to understand that "pass" on ABR screening does not rule out development of hearing impairment in infancy or early childhood. Infants who pass the ABR screen should receive audiologic follow-up as necessary for medical evaluation and management and developmental evaluation. Infants who pass the ABR screen and are at risk for progressive hearing impairment should receive audiologic monitoring on a periodic basis throughout the preschool years. A behavioral audiometric evaluation is ultimately necessary to obtain accurate ear-specific, multi-frequency-specific information and to determine the existence or extent of a transient conductive hearing loss or permanent sensorineural hearing loss.

HEARING SCREENING: INFANTS AND TODDLERS (7 MONTHS TO 3 YEARS)

All of the screening guidelines recommend to audiologists and primary health care providers the need to continue monitoring the hearing and language development of young children. Screening for children with permanent hearing loss should continue into early childhood. All programs that provide early childhood services, such as Head Start, should be vigilant in monitoring for possible hearing loss and delayed language development. In fact, Head Start Performance Standards require that an auditory screening be conducted on all new children within 45 days of their enrollment (Public Law 110-134). To this end it is important that we continue to emphasize to families and physicians that passing a hospital-based hearing screening test does not ensure normal hearing (Johnson et al., 2005). In addition to the possibilities of misidentified, late-acquired, or progressive-type permanent hearing loss, infants and toddlers are the prime candidates for transient or recurrent conductive hearing losses due to otitis media. Otitis media with effusion is the main cause of acquired hearing loss in preschool children with an estimate that 90% of them will have chronic or recurrent episodes during these early years. Often at this age, the hearing loss goes unnoticed in busy families or active day care centers, and so the parents of toddlers and preschool children might be the first to voice concern for their child's hearing.

Serous otitis media is the most widespread cause of hearing disorders in young children. Accordingly, hearing screening programs for older infants and toddlers must seek to identify both conductive and sensorineural hearing losses. In addition, it is important to identify children who have mild hearing loss or unilateral hearing loss. It is well recognized among pediatric and educational audiologists that this age group of toddlers is particularly difficult to screen. At this age, these children can be suspicious of strangers, too shy to be easily engaged, or just too young to fully cooperate with the hearing screening test. Accurate screening results are dependent on the participation of the child, experience of the tester, and involve many additional childhood factors such as maturation, motivation, attention, and intellectual abilities. Apparent, or nonapparent, developmental delays in children may limit hearing screening methods that rely on behavioral responses.

Surprisingly, there are no national or mandated standards for conducting hearing screening programs for children in the 7-months through 2-year group or for pre-school children of 3 to 5 years of age and, in general, few large sample studies have been published regarding preschool hearing screening (Serpanos & Jarmel, 2007). Unfortunately, traditional pure tone hearing screening protocols often fail to identify children who have mild hearing loss due to treatable middle ear disease. It is obvious that a screening program should include some type of pure tone hearing test as a minimum, and when possible otoscopic examination, otoacoustic emissions, and acoustic immittance (i.e., tympanometry). The screening procedures described in this section should not be confused with threshold audiology evaluations.

In some preschool screening programs, children can be brought to a sound-treated room for screening with visual reinforcement audiometry (VRA) as shown in Figure 8–6. Weber (1987) described a portable VRA system that was used extensively in a statewide program to screen infants, toddlers, and preschoolers in rural Colorado. His statistics demonstrate the effectiveness of the VRA technique. Of the nearly 25,000 children tested during the 9-year period of the report, nearly half were younger than 2 years of age. In the VRA condition, each child is screened by using conventional earphones or insert receivers at the test frequencies of 1000, 2000, and 4000 Hz. In a sound-treated room, a 20 dB HL screening intensity level can be used.

Screening With Tympanometry

Tympanometry is particularly valuable in screening this age group for identifying those children with conductive hearing loss caused by middle ear problems. Tympanometry screening is conducted with a small and portable acoustic immittance meter designed for mass screening purposes. Not

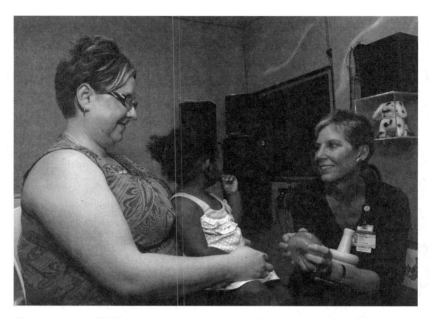

Figure 8–6. VRA screening of a toddler. Photo courtesy of Colorado Children's Hospital, Aurora, CO.

a hearing test, the tympanogram accurately measures middle ear function and identifies negative middle ear pressure that can decrease mobility of the tympanic membrane (Northern, 1980a). A small, airtight probe tip is inserted into the child's ear canal, and the instrument slowly changes air pressure in the ear canal from positive to negative values and measures the dynamic changes in the tympanic membrane mobility (Figure 8–7). The objective measurements are recorded on a graph known as a tympanogram. Tympanometry, as a screening tool, should not be used alone as it is very sensitive to middle ear problems and may result in overreferrals. The overreferral problem is reduced when tympanometry is used as an adjunct to pure tone screening and the two tests are evaluated together prior to the referral of any child for additional evaluation. For some 40 years, the combination of pure tone and tympanometry screening has improved the sensitivity and specificity resulting in accurate identifi-

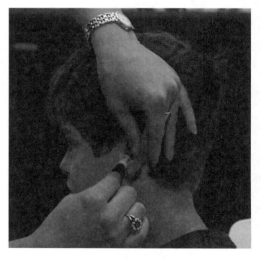

Figure 8–7. Tympanometry is often a part of school hearing screening programs. Photo courtesy of Colorado Children's Hospital, Aurora, CO.

cation and referrals of appropriate children. The pass criteria for tympanometry include the gradient (tympanometric curve width) value greater than 250 daPa in width or less than 0.2 mmhos static admittance as well as an ear canal volume (Veq) measure of 0.1 to 0.4 cc³. Larger Veq measures (greater than 1.0 cc³) are noted when an open ventilation tube is in place in the tympanic membrane (TM) observed with otoscopy (pass) or a TM perforation, possibly but not necessarily, visible with otoscopy (fail).

For those children unable to participate in behavioral procedures, some screening programs may choose to use EOAE measurements (TEOAE or DPOAE) in addition to tympanometry. Transient evoked OAEs (TEOAEs) are evoked by transient clicks and are often faster and more tolerant to noise and movement than DPOAEs, and therefore more often used in screening applications. EOAEs, of course, are not a test of hearing, but merely reflect the status of the peripheral hearing system. In order to successfully obtain an EOAE, the child's ear canal and middle ear must be in normal condition without pathology. In addition, the inner ear cochlear system must have hearing sensitivity better than 30 or 35 dB HL. A problem of interpretation arises when no EOAE can be elicited as the tester will not know if the cause is a conductive hearing loss or a mild-to-moderate sensorineural hearing loss. For most children who fail the initial EOAE procedure, a second screen is recommended. Additional testing for children who "pass" or "fail" the EOAE screen should be done with pure tone screening or tympanometry. Once again, the EOAE procedure cannot be used in screening programs alone. Accordingly, if a conductive hearing loss is present, the audiologist should be aware that conductive hearing loss obscures the EOAE response and requires referral for additional evaluation. However, a tympanogram within normal limits and normal EOAE measurements is a likely outcome for a child with normal hearing, or near-normal hearing. Pure tone results from VRA or play conditioning are essential to confirm the presence of normal hearing or the identification of hearing loss. A thorough discussion and tutorial videos of a suggested EOAE screening program are available at http://www.infanthearing.org

Results from an interesting 4-year project involved with screening of nearly 1,500 3- and 4-year-old children in Head Start programs in rural eastern North Carolina were reported by Allen, Stuart, Everett, and Elangovan (2004). The screening protocol used otoscopy, pure tone, and tympanometry to evaluate the hearing of the children. Only 54% passed the initial screening with all three screening procedures; an additional 22% passed the rescreening for an overall pass rate of 76%. Follow-up compliance in this medically underserved area was not particularly good. Slightly more than 10% of the children who failed the hearing rescreening were medically evaluated. The high referral rate was, no doubt, due to numerous factors, including the requirement to "pass" each of the three screening procedures, rigid pass-fail criteria, and the demographic characteristics of the children screened.

In a quite different demographic study, Serpanos and Jarmel (2007) provided results from a 10-year Long Island, New York, preschool hearing screening program of nearly 35,000 children between 3 and 5 years of age. Their audiologic screening program was based on pure tone and tympanometric measurement. In this large sample of preschool children, 18% were referred for further hearing and medical evaluation. In this demographic study, 93% complied with the follow-up recommendations. Of 1,316 children in the follow-up group, 37% were found to have outer and middle ear disorders in one or both ears. In total, hearing loss or otologic disorder was confirmed in 49% of the follow-up group; further analyses showed prevalence rates of 1.4%

for otologic disorder and 0.7% for previously unidentified hearing loss, revealing an overall 1.8% prevalence of hearing disorders identified by hearing screening in preschool-aged children.

HEARING SCREENING: PRESCHOOL CHILDREN (3 TO 5 YEARS)

Preschool children between the ages of 3 and 5 years usually obtain their health care with pediatricians or family practitioners during well-baby visits. At this age, the health care professional looks primarily for medically remediable hearing losses, on the assumption that the children with more severe hearing losses have already been identified. The chief pathology that is being sought is otitis media; the disease can result at this age in subtle auditory disorders or middle ear disease. The tests that are adequate to identify these disorders are hearing screening, acoustic immittance testing, EOAEs, audiometry, and otoscopic examination.

Although Head Start programs include many children who are required to have hearing screening, there are large numbers of preschool children who are not seen for health visits unless special efforts are made to reach them. Thus, nursery schools and child care centers are prime locations for preschool hearing screening programs. Although numerous efforts have been made to develop effective screening methods for the preschool child, problems arise from the definition of screening as "rapid, simple measurements applied to large numbers of children." Any test that requires a voluntary response from 3- to 5-year-olds will likely be neither rapid nor simple. The preschooler can be negativistic, apprehensive, or "eager beavers"—all attitudes that hardly make for easy screening.

The recommended hearing screening task to evaluate the preschool child is to condition the child to the desired motor response at suprathreshold levels before initiation of the screening procedure. Conditioned play audiometry is a form of operant conditioning in which the child is taught to wait and listen for a stimulus and then to perform a motor task in response to the presentation of the stimulus (Figure 8–8). Typically, the motor task itself serves as reinforcement. An example of a conditioned pure tone preschool screening test is described below:

1. Have available a pegboard, a ring tower, plain blocks, or other simple toys that are motivating to young children.
2. Take a block (or peg) and hold it up to one of your own ears as if listening. Make believe you hear a sound and say, "I hear it," and put the block on the table (or in the bucket, etc.).
3. Place the earphones or insert receivers on the child's ear and hold his or her hand with the block up to the child's ear.
4. Present a 50 dB HL tone at 1000 Hz that you can hear leaking from the earphone or insert receiver.
5. Guide the child's hand to build the block tower. Repeat twice and then see if the child can do it alone. If he or she comprehends the task, begin the hearing screen; if not, additional conditioning trials will be necessary.
6. Decrease the hearing level from 50 dB HL to 20 (or 25) dB HL and repeat the test. If the child responds, repeat the procedure at the same intensity at 2000 and 4000 Hz. Praise the child for each correct response. After each successful tone presentation, place another block in the child's hand.
7. Switch to the opposite ear and repeat the test starting at 1000 Hz, then 2000 Hz,

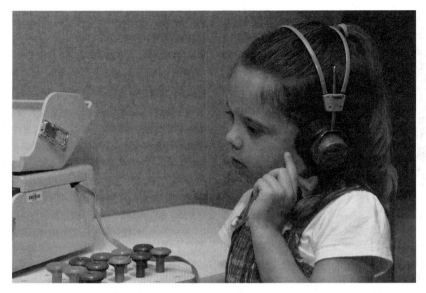

Figure 8–8. Preschool play audiometry. Photo courtesy of Colorado Children's Hospital, Aurora, CO.

and then 4000 Hz. Continue with the child holding the block to the test ear, watching to ensure the child puts the block down following presentation of the screening tone.

8. The criterion for referral is when a child does not respond at 20 (or 25) dB HL at least two of three times at any test frequency in either ear or if the child cannot be conditioned to the task. Those children between 3 and 5 years of age who cannot be conditioned for play audiometry should be screened by VRA.

HEARING SCREENING: SCHOOL-AGE CHILDREN (5 TO 18 YEARS)

The incorporation of hearing screening programs into schools was initiated during the 1920s but did not become a routine part of programs until the 1960s. The main purpose of school-based hearing screening is to keep children hearing adequately in the classroom from kindergarten through 12th grade. In addition, the goal of school hearing screening programs is to identify students who have, or who are at risk for, auditory impairment that may impact their communication abilities, health, education, and psychosocial function (Richburg & Smiley, 2012).

School hearing screening has a long and honorable history. As early as 1924, a group of dedicated otolaryngologists used a new instrument for testing the hearing of school children (McFarlan, 1927). The instrument was developed for the Western Electric Company. The Western Electric 4-A audiometer was a phonograph, connected to an assembly of 30 earphones, which would simultaneously present well-calibrated speech signals to the earphones. In the Western Electric Fading Numbers test, both a male and a female voice spoke various numbers, starting at a hearing level of 33 dB and ending at 9 dB. The reason for the change to pure tone testing was that the speech signals used in the Western Electric test did not identify children with high-frequency losses. Manual audiometric pure tone screening is the primary method for school-based hearing screening for the past 50 years, but some researchers have attempted to develop computer-based hearing screening systems for use with children (McPherson, Law, & Wong, 2010).

Although audiologists play a key role in hearing screening programs, it is generally not cost-effective for audiologists to be involved in the actual administration of the screening tests. The audiologist is the professional responsible for the oversight of the school-based screening program and most likely plans the protocol for administration of the screening tests, performs the training, and supervises the technicians or volunteer screeners who then do the actual screening of the students. The audiologist plans the implementation of follow-up procedures, sends notification letters, collects and analyzes the data, and writes up a summary of the screening project. Identification audiometry is only one part of a hearing conservation program. A well-planned program must go beyond initial hearing screening with a plan for rescreening those children who do not pass the initial screen, perhaps making arrangements for needed threshold audiometry, referral for audiologic and medical evaluations, education and counseling for parents and teachers, and commitment to follow-up procedures to ensure that adequate steps have been taken to alleviate or manage the hearing problem identified in each screening failure. Obviously, without concurrent follow-up programs, identification of hearing loss in children is a meaningless effort. Thorough descriptions of hearing screening practices

in schools have been published by Johnson et al. (1997), Roeser and Downs (2004), and Richburg and Smiley (2012).

ASHA Guidelines for Audiology Screening were published in 1997 calling for hearing screening to be conducted on initial entry into school and annually in kindergarten, first, second, and third grade; screen again in 7th and 11th grades. AAA (2011a) suggests screening in preschool, kindergarten, grades 1, 3, 5, and either grade 7 or grade 9.

Pure tone screening is the method of choice for screening the hearing of school-aged children (Figure 8–9). Of course, by school age the children should be able to respond to hearing the screening tones by a simple raising of the finger or hand (see Figure 8–8). Individualized, manual, pure tone screening under earphones at 20 dB HL (re: ANSI S3.6-1996) should be conducted for each ear of every child at test frequencies of 1000, 2000, and 4000 Hz. If it were possible to decrease the intensity of the screening level, the sensitivity of the test would be increased to identify those children with even mild hearing loss; however, it is necessary to screen at 20 dB HL (or sometimes 25 dB HL) because of the ambient noise levels in the schools where the hearing screening is conducted (Roeser & Northern, 1981). The ambient noise in the test area should be within the ANSI 1991 levels and should not exceed 49.5 dB SPL at 1000 Hz, 54.5 dB SPL at 2000 Hz, or 62 dB SPL at 4000 Hz as properly measured with a sound level meter. A lack of response from the student at any frequency in either ear constitutes failure of the hearing screen and calls for rescreening as soon as possible. Audiometric evidence of hearing loss should be substantiated by repeat screening. For the repeat hearing test, earphones should be removed and repositioned, and instructions repeated. Interval frequencies of 3000 and 6000 Hz should not

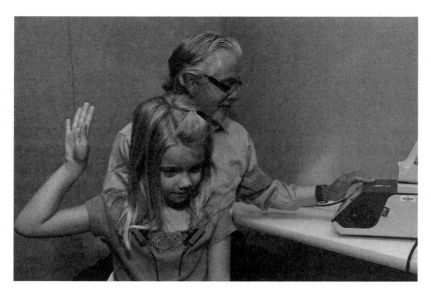

Figure 8–9. School-aged hearing screening is mandated by most state departments of education. Photo courtesy of Colorado Children's Hospital, Aurora, CO.

be included in the pure tone hearing screening protocol (Table 8–6).

Each frequency must be heard in each ear for the child to "pass" the hearing screening. Typically, following very simple instructions, earphones are put in place and two easily heard pure tones are presented to be sure the child understands and can do the required task (i.e., 1000 Hz tone at 40 dB HL). The intensity dial is then decreased and set at 20 dB HL (or 25 dB HL), and single tones are presented at each screening frequency in each ear. The screening procedure should take about 90 seconds in total. Two credible responses at each test frequency may assure good reliability. Any child who does not hear every frequency in each ear should be "tagged" and identified for additional testing. If time permits, it is acceptable to go back and present each test frequency again at the screening level to give the child a second chance to respond and pass the screening.

Tympanometry is recommended by AAA as a second-stage screening method, to be used for those students who do not pass the pure tone or otoacoustic emissions screen. The failure criteria for a tympanogram is greater than 250 daPa tympanometric width or less than 0.2 mmhos static admittance; a final choice for tympanometric failure is negative pressure of equal to or greater than −250 daPa to −400 daPa; however, the AAA guidelines caution that it is not appropriate for the negative pressure tympanogram criterion to stand alone to elicit a referral. Rescreening due to tympanometry failure should take place in 8 to 10 weeks. Only children who fail the initial pure tone screen should be retested immediately to confirm normal hearing or hearing loss.

The AAA 2011 Screening Guidelines recommend that otoacoustic emission (OAE) screening be reserved for preschool and school-age children for whom pure tone screening is not developmentally appro-

Table 8–6. Pitfalls to Avoid in Hearing Screening and Acoustic Immittance Screening

Hearing screening pitfalls
• Child observing dials. This should be avoided at all times, because children will respond to the visual cues. The most appropriate position at which to seat the child is at an oblique angle, so the tester and audiometer are out of the child's peripheral vision
• Examiner giving visual cues (facial expression, eye or head movements)
• Incorrect adjustment of the head band and earphone placement. Care must be taken to place the earphones carefully over the ears so that the protective screen mesh of the earphone diaphragm is directly over the entrance of the external auditory canal. Misplacement of the earphone by only 1 inch can cause as great as a 3035 dB threshold shift
• Vague instructions
• Noise in the test area
• Overlong test sessions. The screening should require only 35 minutes. If a child requires significantly more time than this, the routine screening should be discontinued, and a short rest should be taken. If the child continues to be difficult to test, play conditioning should be used
• Too long or too short a presentation of the test tone. The test stimulus should be presented for 12 seconds. If the stimulus is for a shorter or longer time than this, inaccurate responses may be obtained

Acoustic immittance screening pitfalls
• Clogged probe and probe tip. The probe and probe tips must be kept free from earwax
• Probe tip too large or too small. Each ear canal is different and may require a different-sized probe tip. Utilization of the correct size for each child will avoid possible errors
• Head movement, swallowing, or eye blinks. The child should be kept still during testing, as a sudden abnormal movement during testing may be interpreted as a reflex
• Probe tip against the ear canal wall. The probe tip must be inserted directly into the ear canal, and when the canal is not straight, the tip must be kept away from the canal wall
• Debris in ear canal. The ear canal should be inspected before testing to ensure that it is clear

Source: With permission from "Screening for Hearing Loss and Middle Ear Disorders," by R. J. Roeser & J. L. Northern, 1988, in R. J. Roeser and M. P. Downs, Eds., *Auditory disorders in school children*, 2nd ed., New York, NY: Thieme-Stratton.

priate (i.e., ability level of at least 3 years). Motion artifact from the student during measurement can interfere with the OAE result. The OAE screening should be conducted by an experienced audiologist familiar with this method of testing. Students with middle ear disorders or sensorineural hearing loss greater than 30 dB HL will not produce emissions. The responsible audiologist must select OAE pass-fail levels very carefully with consideration of environmental background noise interference. The OAE test does not quantify hearing loss, per se, and it does not assess the integrity of the neural transmission of sound from the VIIIth nerve to the brainstem and cortex;

accordingly, OAEs should not be used as a stand-alone hearing screening procedure.

The school-based hearing screening program should be part of a total effort that includes an educational component designed to provide parents with information on the process of hearing screening. Both sets of hearing screening guidelines also recommend obtaining informed consent before the screening procedure when appropriate.

A comprehensive review and comparison of state school-based hearing screening protocols was recently published by Sekhar and Zalewski (2013). They concluded that the prevalence of hearing loss has been on the increase among children in the United States in their study of state department of health and education websites. School-based hearing screening is currently required in 34 of 51 (67%) states including the District of Columbia. Of these 34 states, 28 (82%) mandate grades for screening, but only 20 states (59%) require screening beyond sixth grade. Pure tone audiometry is the most common screening method (33/34, 97%). A majority of states screen at 1000, 2000, and 4000 Hz usually at 20 or 25 dB hearing level. Six states recommend or require testing at 6000 or 8000 kHz to detect high-frequency hearing loss. Obviously, their results indicate that U.S. school-based hearing screens vary significantly.

There is concern, particularly considering the evolution of hazardous noise exposures, use of personal music players, and the rising prevalence of hearing loss, that the recommended hearing screening levels will not identify adolescents with high-frequency, noise-induced hearing loss. The Third National Health and Nutrition Examination Survey (NHANES III), conducted audiometric testing of 5,249 children aged 6 to 19 years at 0.5 to 8 kHz and reported that 12.5% (approximately 5.2 mil-

lion) were estimated to have a characteristic noise-induced hearing loss (NIHL) notch in one or both ears. This finding leads to the conclusion that children are being exposed to excessive amounts of hazardous levels of noise, and that children's hearing is vulnerable to these exposures (Niskar et al., 2001). According to Meinke and Dice (2007), review of state screening programs showed that more than half of the U.S. school-based hearing screening protocols will identify only 22% of the students with a high-frequency threshold notch and consequently would fail to detect a potential NIHL. These studies suggest that current school-based hearing screening guidelines are inadequate for the early identification of NIHL which further denies students the opportunity to receive early intervention to prevent further progression of NIHL. Meinke and Dice suggest that it is necessary to identify, standardize, and implement effective and efficient screening or monitoring programs for the early detection and prevention of NIHL in adolescents.

Presentation of hearing screening results to the parents of those children who do not pass the screening tests, despite repeat efforts, requires forethought and planning. It is more effective to speak directly with the parents about test results, if possible, rather than provide written notice. Some parents will become overly concerned; others will show little or no concern; and still others would like to cooperate but fear the potential expense that might be involved if your screening results are faulty. If parents believe that their child can "hear," despite the results of the hearing screening, special tact and persuasion will be required to convince them that a problem truly exists. Failures on pure tone rescreening should be referred for audiologic evaluation by an audiologist, and failures with tympanometry should be referred for medical evaluation. Follow-up audiologic evaluation should be conducted within 1 month of the screening failure and no later than 3 months after initial screening. It might be a good idea to avoid the word "fail" in reporting screening results to parents because of the negative connotation of the word. It must be remembered that many causes exist for "failing" hearing screening tests, and confirmation of the presence of hearing loss cannot be assumed until a complete audiometric evaluation is completed. Table 8–7 suggests a number of considerations that must be taken into account during any school hearing and middle ear screening program.

The data collection, reports, referral forms, and parent letters associated with a hearing screening program can be massive, although computerized database systems certainly can help track the program in a more efficient manner. Test forms, calibration data, and student records must be carefully considered and planned before the testing sessions. The language used in notices sent to parents and referral physicians about screening or rescreening results should avoid diagnostic conclusions and alarming predictions.

SCREENING FOR MIDDLE EAR DISORDERS

Middle ear disease generally refers to otitis media or middle ear effusion, one of the most common disorders of childhood. It is estimated that 35% of young children will have repeated ear infections that nearly

Table 8–7. Considerations for a School Screening Program

- What are existing state mandates for hearing screening?
- What are the purposes of the hearing screening program?
- What resources are available to the program?
- What children will be screened and how will they be referred for screening?
- What tests will be used for screening?
- How will children who cannot respond to traditional techniques be screened?
- What personnel will be necessary for the screening program?
- What equipment will be necessary, and how will it be maintained?
- What environment will be used for the screening?
- What pass/fail criteria will be used?
- How will the screening program be organized?
- What follow-up procedure will be used for failed screenings and absentees?
- What record keeping and reporting will be used in the screening program?
- What will be done to determine the effectiveness of the screening program?

Source: From *School-Based Audiology*, by Cynthia McCormick Richburg and Donna Fisher Smiley, Table 5–1, p. 71. Copyright 2013 by Plural Publishing.

always cause a temporary hearing loss capable of significantly disrupting language acquisition and other education progress (ASHA, 2011a). Controversies exist regarding the need, purpose, and techniques of screening for middle ear disease and hearing loss in children. Middle ear effusions are frequently transient and self-resolving, a situation that can lead to overreferrals and for which specific treatment may be inadvisable. Monitoring and retesting within a reasonable period of time is an essential component to minimize the potential overreferral problem.

A principal problem that accompanies all cases of otitis media is hearing loss. Although usually mild, the hearing loss in very young children may be the basis of an adverse effect on the development of speech, language, and cognition of young children (see Chapter 4). Many variables influence the outcome of otitis media and the effect it has on the development of a young child. The potential seriousness of the consequences of unidentified, and therefore untreated, asymptomatic otitis media is too important to overlook. The sequelae of otitis media with effusion that is of most concern are the suspected associations between frequent occurrences of otitis media during early childhood and delay in speech and language development. Some researchers have questioned whether this association is valid as the evidence-base is certainly lacking. Many clinicians believe that the overwhelming majority of cases of otitis media sooner or later subside spontaneously without lasting physical or developmental consequences. Nonetheless, although research continues, most speech-language specialists and audiologists believe that to wait for a definitive answer concerning the individual impact of otitis media while doing nothing is an untenable position.

Jordan and Eagles (1961) conducted otoscopic examination and audiometric thresholds for approximately 4,000 children between the ages of 5 and 10 years. When the individual pathologies were compared with the threshold audiometry, it was found that 50% of children with active ear infections had normal hearing better than 15 dB HL in each ear. Another finding was that of 30 children with nondraining perforations of the eardrum, 40% also had near normal hearing. In other words, a 20 dB HL pure tone screening criterion would have missed more than half the children with active middle ear pathologies. These facts point out that audiometric pure tone screening—and even threshold audiometry—might not identify the majority of children with significant ear pathology. This finding does not mean that there is no relationship between ear disease and hearing loss.

Because the hearing loss associated with otitis media may be episodic and mild, tympanometry is perhaps the best means to identify children with middle ear effusion. Accordingly, tympanometry can be a valuable component of school-based hearing screening programs. Critics argue that children referred from screening programs with possible middle ear disease to physicians too often are found to have normal middle ears by the time they are scheduled and seen in a medical clinic. The debate about the value of acoustic immittance screening was summarized in two points of view by Bess (1980) and Northern (1980b). However, controversy and opposing viewpoints are to be expected in light of the fact that otitis media with effusion may be fluctuant and recurrent in the same child. There is also seasonal variation in the presence and absence of the disorder, and some believe allergy plays a role in middle ear effusion. Tympanometry is an effective screening tool that is easy to use, objective, efficient, acceptable to the screening population, inexpensive, and when used in conjunction with pure tone screening, accurately identifies those children with significant negative middle ear pressure and possible effusion. Whether the child will experience serious consequences if the otitis media disorder is left untreated is not a simple or easy question, because so many other variables have influence on the final outcome (Northern, 1992).

Approximately half of U.S. states incorporate acoustic immittance as part of their recommended identification procedures (Penn, 1999). Consistent use of acoustic immittance (i.e., tympanometry) screening is also evident in local educational agencies, day care centers, Head Start programs, well-baby clinics, and private primary care medical offices. Although there is no clear-cut resolution to the many questions that surround screening, the fact is that the technique has been a positive addition to hearing screening programs when used with pure tone hearing screening. Otoacoustic emissions testing is not comparable to tympanometry as it does not provide any specific diagnostic information; therefore, children who fail OAE screening are likely to need tympanometry evaluation before a decision can be reached regarding the need for referral.

The hearing and tympanometry protocol to identify middle ear disease should be done preferably early in the school year. This is recommended because children with MEE early in the fall are more likely to have chronic, persistent effusion through the winter months. Two successive tympanometric failures should result in a letter of alert to the parents.

Guidelines for screening with tympanometry for middle ear disorders were published by ASHA in 1997. The single set of guidelines can serve for all age groups of children, including the developmentally delayed, with the following steps:

- A careful case history should be obtained, when possible, through the verbal report of a parent or guardian.
- A visual inspection of the ears should be conducted to identify risk factors for outer and middle ear disease and to ensure that no contraindications exist for performing tympanometry (e.g. drainage, foreign bodies, tympanostomy tubes).
- A lighted otoscope or video otoscope should be used to examine the external earcanal and tympanic membrane for obvious obstructions or structural defects.
- Tympanometry should be performed with a low-frequency (220 or 226 Hz) probe tone and a positive to negative air pressure sweep.
- Acoustic reflex measurements should not be used as a screenings pass/refer criteria.

Children should be referred for medical evaluation if ear drainage is observed; ear canal obstructions, impacted cerumen, or foreign objects are noted; blood or other secretions are present; stenosis or atresia are observed; otitis externa is present; or when perforations or other abnormalities of the tympanic membrane are apparent. If the tympanic equivalent ear canal volume is greater than 1.0 cm^3 and accompanied by a flat tympanogram, the child is likely to have an opening in the tympanic membrane. Referral is not necessary if a tympanostomy tube is observed and properly in place (usually visible by otoscopic examination) or if the patient is already receiving medical care for a perforation. Most investigators have concluded that the acoustic reflex measurement is too variable to be useful in acoustic immittance screening programs.

Tympanometric criteria for referral when screening for middle ear effusion vary depending on factors related to the population screened. Tympanometric peak pressure (TPP) is not recommended in the criteria for identifying children at risk for otitis media. Negative TPP associated with an otherwise normal tympanogram is a poor determinant of middle ear effusion (AAA, 2011a; ASHA, 1990). For infants and children from 1 year through school age, tympanometric width (TW) greater than 200 daPa is the recommended referral criterion. This value has been shown to have high specificity and good sensitivity for the identification of MEE in children of school age (Nozza, 1995; Roush et al., 1995). In children with a history of chronic middle ear effusion and scheduled for myringotomy and tube surgery, a more severe criterion of TW >300 daPa is recommended (Nozza, Bluestone, Kardatzke, & Bachman, 1994).

A child with a unilateral or bilateral tympanogram suggesting referral should be rescreened 4 to 6 weeks after the initial test. Because middle ear disease may resolve spontaneously, referral based on a single screening is not recommended. Various schemes for a two-stage tympanometry screening protocol have been suggested (Northern, 1992; Roush, 1990).

HEARING SCREENING OF THE DEVELOPMENTALLY DELAYED CHILD

Standards for institutions serving the developmentally delayed generally recommend that all new residents, children younger than 10 at annual intervals, and other residents at regular intervals receive hearing screenings. Appropriate behavioral procedures will depend upon the child's developmental, cognitive, and linguistic level; visual and motor development; and ability to respond appropriately. As children mature, more specific behavioral information can be obtained.

The use of a team testing approach for hearing screening with visual reinforcement audiometry (VRA) and conditioned play audiometry (CPA) may be necessary in some children who have developmental delays. The use of an appropriately trained student or test assistant may help to maintain the child's attention and ensure that proper placement of the transducers is not compromised by the child. The audiologist must be prepared to cross-check pure tone hearing screening results with acoustic immittance (tympanometry and acoustic reflex threshold tests) and otoacoustic emission (OAE) tests.

Whenever possible, conditioning techniques (VRA) are the methods of choice for hearing screening under earphones, insert phones, or in the soundfield. Modified speech audiometry using developmentally appropriate vocal commands and directions that the child is capable of following are useful screening tools. These special versions of speech audiometry at various hearing levels can help estimate hearing thresholds in each ear when necessary. Acoustic immittance and EOAEs testing should be an integral part of every hearing screening for every special needs population (Northern, 1980b). The presence of EOAEs may be used to confirm the presence of normal hearing. If the acoustic immittance battery suggests conductive hearing loss, EOAEs will likely be absent. ABR testing is not recommended as an initial screening procedure for this population because of the likely need for sedation and possible central auditory pathway dysfunction.

Hearing screening for severely and profoundly developmentally delayed children presents a difficult situation in terms of efficiency, accuracy, and required time. Limited behavioral screening may be possible for some children, seated or held in the sound suite, facing one of two speakers. Initially the noise or speech stimulus is presented through the opposite speaker so that if the child localizes, he or she must make an overt and obvious lateralization to seek the sound from the speaker furthest away. If localization to the stimulus occurs, the audiologist should quickly reinforce the head turn with a flashing light or noisy action toy. For hearing screening purposes it may be sufficient to quickly see responses at 25 or 20 dB HL which may take only a few trials. Speech is primarily used as the sound stimulus because of its strong interest to the child, but a variety of other stimuli can be employed. It is sometimes necessary to change the stimuli during testing to pure tones, warble tones, white noise, or complex noise. Obviously, the time required to achieve success in hearing screening depends on the severity of developmental disability of the patient.

Behavioral observations may include some or all of the following responses to auditory stimuli: (a) responses that indicate sound awareness such as eye opening, quieting, assuming a listening attitude, smiling, laughing, and ceasing activity; (b) preferably good localization responses; and (c) startle responses to loud sounds, which are the involuntary reflexive responses that are expected 65 to 85 dB above threshold and include eye blink, orientation reflex, tonic neck reflex, and perhaps a full-body Moro reflex.

A recommended protocol for auditory screening of developmental delayed children is presented below:

1. An ascending approach with speech or narrowband noise stimuli should be used in an attempt to obtain responses from the child at levels of 25 dB HL or better. Obvious awareness of the sound, or preferably overt localization by 25 dB HL, constitutes "passing" the observational portion of the screening.
2. If no reliable responses are obtained by 25 dB HL, the screening level should be increased in 10 dB steps in an attempt to elicit a response. If the child shows awareness or localizes by 65 dB HL, and a startle can be elicited, near-normal hearing or mild to moderate hearing loss is likely.
3. Operant play conditioning as described in Chapter 6 is recommended when possible.
4. Each screening procedure should include acoustic immittance audiometry (tympanometry and acoustic reflex testing) and EOAE measurement. These physiologic measures may rule out or establish the presence of normal hearing, confirm conductive hearing loss, as well as suggest the need for additional audiometric evaluation for possible sensorineural hearing loss.

SCREENING FOLLOW-UP ISSUES

A key point to be remembered is that the effectiveness of any screening program is only as good as the subsequent follow-up program. If experienced audiologists are unavailable or if parents have difficulty gaining access to audiologic assistance, infants and young children identified to have hearing loss may not receive the necessary follow-up and intervention. The philosophical question remains: Who is responsible for follow-up—the audiologist, the parents, or the school or institution? Who should bear the financial burden of further evaluation, the parents or the institution, when the infant or child must return for additional and possibly more expensive testing and evaluation? Audiologists responsible for hearing screening programs must also be concerned about the ever present possibility of progressive sensorineural hearing loss in infants and young children. When babies pass the admission birth screening protocols and are later determined to have hearing loss, the question always remains, did the screening test miss this baby or did the hearing loss occur after the hearing screening was applied?

An interesting case can be made by examining the reported ages of *suspicion* and *detection* of hearing loss against the age of *confirmation* of hearing loss. Parents continue to report that the chief obstacle in confirming the hearing loss is the primary care physician's unwillingness to accept the parent's opinions. In addition, there is the inability of these physicians to perform simple hearing screening tests in their offices, and finally the reluctance of the physicians to arrange for referral of the child for thorough audiologic evaluation. Detection and confirmation of a child's hearing problem depend on the astuteness and insistence of the parents as well as the alertness of the physician.

Stein et al. (1990) compared patterns of the initial identification and habilitation of infants and young children with hearing loss and found that the advantage of earlier diagnosis may easily be lost due to delays in habilitation program enrollment.

The findings revealed that advice given by managing physicians in response to parental concern, whether good or poor advice, had significant influence on the early identification (or lack thereof) of their child's hearing loss. The pattern of delays between the identification and confirmation of the hearing loss and the recommendation and the fitting of a hearing aid seemed to be threefold: (a) referral back to the physician for ear examinations and medical clearances, then long, silent intervals without action; (b) babies with multiple physical and developmental problems in which hearing was only part of the total concern of the parents; and (c) parental disbelief or avoidance of the fact that their child had an important hearing loss.

James Jerger relates that the clinical audiologist can make two mistakes when counseling parents of an infant or child suspected to have hearing loss. One of the mistakes, however, has considerably more serious consequences than the other. The lesser of the two mistakes, the false positive, is for the audiologist to initially decide that the infant or young child is deaf and then subsequently to determine that the infant has normal hearing. An embarrassing mistake for sure, but probably every experienced clinician has fallen prey to this error. In this situation, however, the final outcome of normal hearing for the infant or child is a great relief to all.

The more serious mistake, however, can be devastating to the infant or young child in question. In this grave error, the false negative, the audiologist initially informs the parent that their child has normal hearing when, in fact, the infant or young child has severe to profound hearing loss. In this situation, the parents believe the audiologist and assume with confidence that their baby hears normally. Unfortunately, by the time the mistaken diagnosis is identified and rectified, maximum habilitation for the infant or child may never be achieved.

Armed with knowledge about the potential for these two mistakes in infant hearing assessment, the pediatric audiologist must practice extreme care in pronouncing an infant or young child to have normal hearing. When in doubt, it behooves the clinician to assume that the infant has a hearing problem until proven otherwise. The pediatric audiologist is still the best professional to serve as an advocate for the child and to be the one whose ultimate responsibility is to provide maximum support for the infant under evaluation.

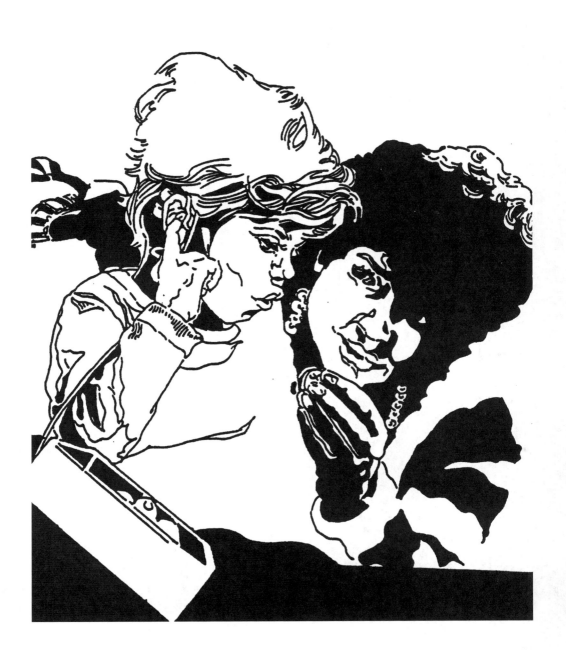

CHAPTER 9

Amplification

There is little doubt that the single most important invention to help the hearing handicapped child is the amplifying hearing aid. There is an old adage, "As we hear, so shall we speak," and it is this very close relationship between hearing, speech, and language that is so important to the hearing-impaired child. The fitting of hearing aids is the first significant step in the intervention process. Technology is now readily available to help the child with hearing impairment learn to speak through the use of voice pitch indicators, speech timing equipment, vowel indicators, voice/nonvoice meters, speech spectrum displays, and visible speech machines. None of these devices, however, is more fundamental to the hearing-impaired child's education and ability to learn speech than the properly fitted hearing aid. Hearing aids provide the hearing-impaired child with optimal use of the residual hearing so that speech and language milestones can be achieved at appropriate age levels. (Northern & Downs, *Hearing in Children*, First Edition, 1974, p. 213)

Hearing aid selection and fitting in children has made incredible progress over the last 50 years. Pediatric hearing aid fittings in the early years were largely a matter of trial and error, accompanied by the best of intentions, with no support of a scientific or evidence-based approach to the process. Of course, in those early days the only choice for a hearing aid was a body-worn device, complete with a hard-wire attachment between the processor and the button-size receiver held in the child's ear with a hard acrylic earmold. The body-type hearing aid was sufficiently large that small children had to wear a leather harness around their chest with a pocket to hold the hearing aid. The size of the device nearly precluded binaural hearing aid fittings, although occasionally it was attempted. For some years, binaural amplification was thought to be successful with a single body-aid and a Y-cord with receivers in each ear. Mark Ross (1988) of the University of Connecticut, a significant contributor to pediatric audiology, was fond of saying, "One of the most frustrating aspects of selecting a hearing aid for a young child is not being able to quantify the accuracy of our decisions."

But fortunately every subsequent decade has brought new technologies, new protocols, and vastly improved hearing aids, all of which are of immense benefit to children with hearing loss and pediatric audiologists. The assets we now have in our clinical armamentarium have provided pediatric hearing aid selection and fitting with a solid scientifically established foundation. Of course it is a more complicated process that includes audiometry, acoustic immittance, ABR and OAE hearing evaluations of the child, electroacoustic hearing aid analyzers, and real-ear probe microphone measures to determine hearing aid outputs, and hearing aid prescriptive procedures to target hearing aid performance to the optimal match for the child's hearing thresholds; all of which are followed by early intervention therapies to develop communication skills for the child and the provision of parent information and referral to family-support programs (Seewald, 2013). To be sure, these are challenging tasks for the pediatric audiologist, but when carried through to completion these tasks provide a life-changing service to the child with hearing loss and the family, as well as a great deal of self-satisfaction with a job well done.

The task of selecting and fitting hearing aids for a child with hearing loss is not to be taken lightly. The inexperienced clinician trained should not undertake the selection and fitting of hearing aids for pediatric patients. There are unique issues related to pediatric hearing aid fitting for children that are very different than fitting hearing aids on adults. The process of selecting, fitting, and management of hearing aids for a child is complex and requires numerous special considerations as described in detail in the *Clinical Guidelines for Pediatric Amplification* published by the American Academy of Audiology (2013). The pediatric evaluation and hearing aid fitting may involve many people including the otolaryngologist, pediatrician, audiologist/dispenser, speech/language pathologist, teacher of the deaf, and other auxiliary professionals such as the public health or school nurse and the social worker, and most importantly, the child's parents or caregivers. These individuals must work together closely in a coordinated effort, under direction of a pediatric audiologist, to ensure that the hearing-impaired child obtains maximal benefit from amplification.

The importance of parental involvement in the intervention and habilitation processes of their children with hearing loss is absolutely crucial to the child's success with amplification. Unfortunately, there are no specific guidelines that can be followed when dealing with parents. Just like children, parents are unique and have backgrounds, attitudes, and needs that must be dealt with on a personal basis. The audiologist may be well advised to plan on spending at least as much time talking with parents as working with the child during each appointment period. Often the parents develop a special relationship with the audiologist, as it is the audiologist who probably confirmed the presence of hearing loss in the child and is the most knowledgeable about the child's hearing aid or cochlear implant. Luterman (1979) describes different approaches for the audiologist to use in order for parents to cope with their child's special needs. The parents, not the professional, must make the decisions regarding the child's habilitation because they must accept and take the ultimate responsibility. Certainly, parents must accept and understand the need for amplification before hearing aids or cochlear implants can be placed and used successfully by the youngster with hearing loss.

Traditionally, in the hearing aid fitting process the audiologist acted as an outside expert who imparted selected information to the parents and then made decisions on behalf of the child. However, there has been an important change in the role of the parents and family in the recognition that the child cannot be viewed apart from the family. The audiologist's role is to be involved in a collaborative process with the parents to determine what is best for both the child and the family. As discussed in Chapter 5, the family-centered philosophy assumes that the child's needs are best met by meeting family needs and that families have the right to retain as much control as they desire over the intervention process (Roush & Matkin, 1994; Roush & McWilliam, 1994).

After the hearing aids have been recommended it is important for parents to observe the child's aided and unaided responses to see for themselves that their child benefits from using personal amplification. Once convinced of the need and benefits provided by amplification, the parents will likely not be embarrassed or apologetic about the hearing aids. The parents must understand that although personal amplification is absolutely necessary for the development of their child, it may require extensive auditory therapy before these newly amplified sounds will be meaningful to the child. The parents should also be made aware of the number of important assistive listening devices that are available to help the child with hearing loss gain maximum benefit and relate effectively with family, school, daily communication, and listening tasks.

The audiologist's role in parental management of their child's personal amplification and assistive listening devices has a great deal to do with the ultimate successful acceptance and utilization of these hearing instruments (Figure 9–1). That role should

include education, guidance, and counseling, because the parents' attitude regarding amplification may be the single most important factor in successful hearing aid use by the child with hearing loss.

Basic to the concept of hearing aid recommendations is a realistic understanding of what the aid can do for the child. No hearing aid will enable a youngster with impaired hearing to hear normally in all situations. The goal in providing amplification to the child with a hearing loss is to make speech audible at safe and comfortable listening levels that provide as many acoustic speech cues as possible. This goal must be accomplished while the amplification system makes soft speech audible, speech and environmental sounds comfortably loud, and loud sounds not uncomfortable (IHAFF, 1994). Of course, the amplification devices must work equally as well in a wide variety of listening situations (e.g., in

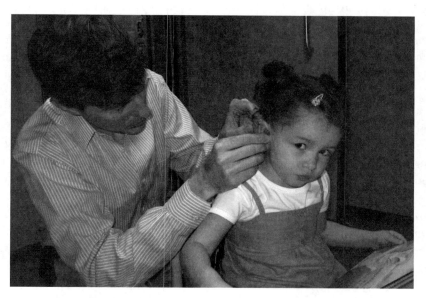

Figure 9–1. Fitting hearing aids on young children is a technically demanding task for the pediatric audiologist. Children with hearing loss have special needs and require considerable clinical attention to obtain maximum benefit from their hearing aids. Photo courtesy of H.O.P.E. Preschool, Spokane, WA.

background noise, at close distances, with multiple speakers and sounds, and amplifies sounds from far-away distances). The primary reason for recommending the use of amplification is to enable the child to communicate better with a hearing aid than without it. Ross (1969) stated that, "merely because one can 'get along' without a hearing aid is *not* an adequate reason to discourage its use."

As early as 1971, the noted auditory psychologist J.D. Harris stated that our goal in fitting personal amplification devices is to "present to the ear as faithful a representation of the acoustic world as if the hearing aid were not present." David Pascoe (1980) poignantly observed, "Although it is true that mere detection of a sound does not ensure its recognition, it's even more true that without detection, the probabilities of correct identification are greatly diminished!" The primary goal of amplification is to provide audibility across the long-term average speech spectrum (LTASS) without delivering any signal that is of an intensity that it would either be uncomfortable or unsafe (AAA, 2013).

The audiologist trained in pediatric hearing issues is recognized as the health care professional to coordinate and guide the hearing aid selection procedure by the Food and Drug Administration (FDA). The FDA regulations regarding hearing aids for children include the following rules:

Before purchase of a hearing aid, an individual with a hearing loss must have a medical evaluation of the hearing loss by a physician (preferably a physician specializing in diseases of the ear) within six months preceding the sale of the aid. Adult patients, under carefully defined circumstances, can sign a waiver of the medical clearance requirements. However, there is no waiver option of per-

sons younger than 18 years of age. The physician who examines the child must provide a written statement that the patient's hearing loss has been medically evaluated. In addition to seeing a physician for a medical evaluation, a child with a hearing loss should be directed to an audiologist for evaluation and rehabilitation since hearing loss may cause problems in language development and the educational and social growth of a child. An audiologist is qualified by training and experience to assist in the evaluation and rehabilitation of a child with hearing loss. (1977 CFR Title 21, Updated by FDA, Apr 2009)

PEDIATRIC HEARING AID FITTINGS

As required by the FDA, the pediatric audiology specialist uniquely has the skills to identify the nature and degree of the child's hearing loss, which is often a challenging task. The audiologist ensures that proper medical clearance is obtained before proceeding with the hearing aid selection procedure. The audiologist is able to evaluate the performance of hearing aids on the child, make earmold impressions, perform real-ear probe microphone measurements, and select and fit the hearing aids to obtain the maximum benefit of amplification for the child's hearing loss. As part of this process, the audiologist counsels the parents about hearing aids, their care and use, and arranges for appropriate intervention for the child and special training when necessary. Finally, the pediatric audiology specialist must be able to devote the necessary time to follow the progress of the pediatric patient and to be ever vigilant to be sure that the hearing aids are in top operating condition.

The association between habilitation success and early hearing aid fitting was officially recognized by the Joint Infant Hearing Committee (JIHC) in their 2007 guidelines. The 2007 JIHC Position Statement calls for infants who have been identified to have permanent hearing loss to be fitted with amplification *within 1 month of confirmation of the hearing impairment and before 6 months of age.* With more than 95% of the 4,000,000 babies born each year in the United States screened for hearing loss prior to discharge from the birth hospital, the pressure on audiologists to confirm the hearing loss and fit identified infants with hearing aids is quite demanding. In previous decades, pediatric patients were typically first fit with hearing aids at the age 2 to 3 years when their hearing losses were confirmed by behavioral measures. Under current physiologic hearing testing technology and standards of care requirements, the first pediatric hearing aid fitting is likely to occur as early as 2 to 3 months of age.

Certainly the JIHC 2007 guideline for early fitting of hearing aids challenged audiologists to come up with protocols and techniques to accomplish the demanding tasks on newborns identified early with hearing loss and needing to be fit with amplification within a few months of their birth. The successful fitting of hearing aids on such small infants requires exceptional skills and knowledge from an audiologist with pediatric specialty experience. No one questioned the need for such early hearing aid fittings, but at that time only a few pediatric audiologists in the United States had the knowledge and skills to deal with newborns. The subsequent years, however, have seen the publication of numerous useful how-to textbook chapters, clinical reports, and research publications describing various approaches to selecting, verifying, and validating the fitting of hearing aids on babies (Bagatto & Scollie, 2011; Bagatto et al., 2005; Beck et al., 2007; Dillon, Ching, & Golding, 2008; McCreery, 2010; Scollie & Seewald, 2002; Simmons, Beauchaine, & Eiten, 2007; Winter, 2010). Every audiology graduate study program now requires extensive study and experience with hearing aids, and we now have available a plethora of excellent textbooks detailing every aspect of the hearing aid process (Dillon, 2012; Muller et al., 2013; Taylor & Mueller, 2011; Valente, 2002a, 2002b).

The goal is to fit hearing aids on pediatric patients as soon as the presence of hearing loss is confirmed. The use of amplification must be based on evidence of hearing loss demonstrated by elevated hearing thresholds for pure tones and speech. Information regarding auditory sensitivity needs to be obtained as early as possible using a behavioral conditioned response procedure such as VRA (see Chapter 6). For the very young infant or those children with developmental delay where traditional conditioned response methods are unsuccessful, the hearing evaluation should be supported through behavioral observation of auditory behaviors or evoked potentials. Best estimates of hearing thresholds or minimum response levels obtained by these techniques can be used to set amplification targets. However, the audiologist must be aware that the child's absolute threshold values may still be in question and hearing aid fitting targets may be set on a "best estimate" plan. The hearing aids may need additional "trial-and-error" adjustments as more information is obtained about the child's hearing levels and real-ear measurements with thorough further evaluations. It is critical that ear-specific auditory thresholds be ultimately established for all test frequencies as soon as possible.

Obviously, this early fitting goal may not be achieved with every child during the first visit, or perhaps even the second or third visit. Although the audiologic information may be limited to only a few frequencies in each ear, the recommendation and provision of hearing aids should proceed as soon as reasonable. Despite everyone's best intentions, it is not uncommon for the hearing aids to take a month or more to be selected, programmed, properly fitted, and verified. It may be difficult for parents or caregivers to meet the necessary appointments in such a limited time. However, clinicians should keep in mind the important evidence presented by Yoshinaga-Itano et al. (1998), Moeller (2000), and Kennedy et al. (2006), all of whom found that significantly better language development is achieved when the child's hearing loss is identified early followed by early intervention (i.e., hearing aid fitting and speech stimulation). Sininger et al. (2009) concluded from a longitudinal study of children with hearing loss that the age of fitting amplification is the most significant factor in determining development of auditory-based outcomes.

For children who are fit "late" with hearing aids, parents may face reluctance from the child to keep using the hearing aid. The earlier a child is fit with hearing aids, acceptance without question or challenge of the devices is likely to be easier. Parents should be warned that the child's hearing aids might "accidently" end up flushed down a toilet, chewed up by the family dog, thrown out of a window, or used as a pacifier for the new baby in the family. In the final view, however, parents must accept the firm authority and responsibility of keeping the hearing aids on the child and in good working order.

The hearing aid selection and fitting process for a child with hearing loss requires extended appointment times and often supplemental visits. Pediatric hearing aid issues are not likely to be a one-stop, instant fix problem. The appointment times scheduled for hearing aid evaluations with children should include ample consideration for the hearing evaluation and the inevitable lengthy discussion, and oftentimes counseling, with parents. Real-ear measurements and electroacoustic analysis of the hearing aids are important to confirm optimal operation of the hearing instruments. Ample time for selection, programming, fitting, and verification of the new hearing aids should be scheduled; it may not be possible to accomplish all of these activities during the same appointment. Time must also be allotted for the making of earmold impressions. Additional telephone calls and letters may be required to be sent to appropriate agencies to obtain financial assistance for the purchase of the hearing aids as well as written reports for the child's clinical file and the referral source. However, the time consumed by these procedures is only fleeting seconds when compared with the long-term therapy and follow-up programs that the child will need throughout the remainder of his or her life.

THE HEARING AID

Tremendous technologic advances in the hearing aid have been made over the past three decades. Many years ago hearing aids were heavy, cumbersome units with large, unsightly battery requirements. The portable electronic hearing aid became a reality in the 1930s, and the vacuum tube became part of the system in the 1940s. Transistors permitted the hearing aid to be a much smaller unit in the 1950s. The rapid changes in hearing aid styles began with the first behind-the-ear (BTE) models introduced in the 1970s, followed by in-the-ear (ITE) aids during the 1980s, and the small in-the-canal (ITC) aids of the 1990s. Today's open-canal or receiver-in-canal (RIC) speak volumes for the engineers who design hearing instruments. Today's digital computerized circuits in the amplification devices have reduced the instrument and its power source to a miniaturized size and weight even for very young children and babies.

The operation of the hearing aid has been likened to a miniature high-fidelity set made up of a group of tiny components that picks up sound wave vibrations from the air and converts them into electrical signals and then back into "processed" sound waves. Actually, hearing aids are much more than just ultra-miniature electroacoustic amplifiers. They are sophisticated personal signal processing systems composed of the hearing instrument itself as well as technically elaborate acoustic coupling systems. The major amplification, signal limiting,

and complex controlling functions are achieved within the hearing aid itself, programmed with powerful and specialized software programs.

In simplistic terms, hearing aids have three basic components: a microphone, an amplifier, and a receiver or miniature loudspeaker as shown in Figure 9–2. The microphone and the receiver are known as transducers as they change acoustic energy into electrical energy and back again. Sounds from the environment enter the hearing aid through a tiny microphone, which converts the acoustic (sound) signals into electrical signals that are digitally processed. The electrical signal is enhanced, shaped, and increased in intensity, passed through an amplifier, and subject to various compression or expansion paradigms. The amplified electrical signal is then passed through the receiver or miniature speaker,

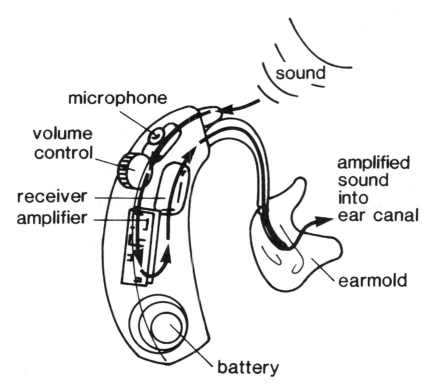

Figure 9–2. Behind-the-ear (BTE) hearing aid.

which changes the electrical signal back into amplified acoustic sound. The amplified acoustic sound is directed toward the user's ear canal through some type of earmold, ear bud, or open tube. The earmold is an important part of the system as it helps hold the hearing aid in place and ensures that the sound is appropriately amplified for the young patient. A small battery, which must be replaced at least weekly, powers the hearing aid processers.

The fact that nearly all hearing aids today are digitally-based has proven to be especially useful in fitting amplification on children. Major improvements in programming software help ensure improved and more accurate fitting protocols. Advanced digital signal processing technology has, without question, improved hearing instrument performance. These high-technology hearing aids utilize digitally programmable settings and adjustments, so that very specific prescriptive fitting can be applied to each child's individual hearing loss and audiometric configuration. Each digital hearing aid is nearly finitely adjustable to fit nearly any degree of hearing loss and almost every audiometric hearing loss configuration. Although this new technology was initially developed for adult users, the long-term benefit to children with hearing loss is very important. Digitally programmable hearing aids offer the flexibility to provide a significant range of adjustments and modifications through the fitting software programs to fit the child's changing needs for a typical instrument life of 4 to 5 years.

Digital hearing aids have provided a true revolution in hearing aid processing and given us tools for precise fitting strategies, as well as opened doors for numerous advances yet to come. Digital signal processing (DSP) can provide open architecture platforms that can process multiple incoming acoustic signals instantaneously while making adjustments to achieve faster and more transparent parallel processing actions. The earliest digital hearing aids were designed to use about 2,000 lines of code; in contrast, today's digital hearing aids might have over 4,000,000 lines of code; all the while getting smaller, faster, and smarter with more powerful chipsets.

Who could have predicted the versatility of today's digital hearing aids with nearly infinite acoustic configurations programmed through powerful software to meet the needs of nearly every person with hearing loss? Digital processing has made available a dazzling array of advanced features than would never have been possible in the old analog days. Advanced technology hearing aids now routinely include integrated systems such as adaptive directional and omnidirectional microphones, feedback cancelation with enhanced stable gain, automatic volume control, real-time acoustic environment analyzers that make simultaneous decisions and seamlessly change programs, variable noise suppression programs automatically driven by the environment, data logging, male or female voice indicators, low battery notification, self-diagnostic checks, remote adjustment capabilities, touch technology that eliminates buttons, switches, and dials, and improved direct audio input for assistive listening devices and FM microphone use.

Other innovative improvements include waterproofing the hearing aid and enabling remote programming by the use of an ordinary cell phone. And, of course, stylish new cases, tubing, and earmold in various colors and designs help make today's hearing aids a true fashion statement with special attention to please children. All of these features, along with the highest level of personal comfort and very wide dynamic range frequency responses for optimal speech clarity, reflect the dramatic change in hearing aids achieved during the past few years. Powerful computer software programs allow for personalized record keeping and fine-tuning adjustments for fitting individual hearing losses, and often include speech mapping tools and synthetic hearing loss demonstrations that are valuable applications for counseling patients, their family members, or caregivers, as well as are useful for in-service training programs.

The advent of feedback canceling algorithms has been especially valuable for reducing many of the common hearing aid problems associated with pediatric fittings. In addition to eliminating the irritating squeal of hearing aids associated with yesterday's hearing aids, complex feedback cancelation makes listening more comfortable, helps with telephone compatibility, eliminates the need for uncomfortable tight-fitting earmolds, and provides better speech understanding without sacrificing high-frequency gain. For young infants and toddlers, feedback cancellation may help reduce the period of time between earmold remakes due to growth of the external ear.

HEARING AIDS FOR CHILDREN

There may be no more challenging audiology task than the selecting and fitting of hearing aids for pediatric patients. As it is often stated, "children are not just small adults with hearing aids; they must be tested, fitted, and managed in a total different manner than adults." Scollie and Seewald (2002) point out numerous differences between the pediatric hearing aid process and the procedures used for adults. With pediatric patients, the audiologist often has to work with less-than-complete audiometric information. Thus, judgments

must necessarily come from estimates of auditory thresholds obtained through electrophysiological measures, real ear measurements of growing and changing ear canal volumes and resonances, and confronting the issue of hearing fluctuations due to transient middle ear fluid situations. Needless to say, many of the children are somewhat less than cooperative with the process or unable to contribute reliable behavioral responses.

There is no question that hearing aids used by children should meet some special requirements that are not necessarily needed by adults. Pediatric hearing aids have received considerable attention during the past decade as specific hearing aid attributes have been developed for use by young children. Today's pediatric hearing aids are manufactured to sustain all misfortunes that can come from an active youngster. Pediatric hearing aids must be rugged and reliable, waterproof, with a tamper-proof battery cover and lockable switches and controls. The pediatric hearing aid should have a wide bandwidth for optimal speech recognition, be small in size, appealing in design and color, and with direct audio input (DAI) and FM capabilities. In addition, the hearing aids should be simple for parental operation, include damage and loss coverage, as well as a loaner program for use when the child's hearing aid is away for repair, and include the manufacturer's, as well as optional extended, warranty. Many of today's pediatric hearing aids are aligned with children's favorite cartoon characters and are supplied with ample supportive materials including story books, listening stethoscopes, child-sized back packs, and carrying cases, as well as substantial product information and operational instructions for teachers and family.

The selection of children's hearing aids requires special considerations. Considerable expertise is required to select the correct amount of gain, output, and frequency response to provide optimal hearing in light of the child's degree and configuration of hearing loss. The final selection of the hearing instruments will likely be influenced by the age and motor skills of the child, cosmetic considerations including color selections of the cases and earmolds, availability of options such as direct audio input, and, of course, cost of the hearing instruments. Pediatric instruments should have a wide range of programmable adjustments such as saturated sound pressure level (OSPL90) reduction control, programmable frequency and gain possibilities, and choice of compression circuits and adjustments. The wide range of programmability is especially valuable in children's fittings because of the possible incomplete or tentative hearing threshold measurements and the fact that the child's listening skills may change over time after the hearing aids are fitted and the child learns additional communication skills.

Digital hearing instruments have exceptional sound quality, multiple frequency bands, and multiple memories for storing different prescriptive programs, plus a fully digital amplifier with or without an external volume control. Some models feature multiple microphones for improved speech understanding in the presence of background noise. Some of these requirements are not necessary for a young infant or toddler, and of course, the cost of the higher and more complex technology instruments is a factor that may preclude purchase of these options. Furthermore, experience has confirmed that more advanced and more expensive hearing aid technology does not always result in increased hearing benefit. Individual results depend on the type, severity, and duration of the hearing loss as well as the hearing instrument programming skills of the audiologist. Some parents

and families may have to make the decisions regarding whether or not to purchase spare or backup hearing aids, direct audio input features, separate FM systems, and insurance coverage for loss or breakage. The pediatric audiologist must be prepared to offer guidance about the relevance and importance of each of these features based on the needs of the child and affordability.

Today's children, with or without hearing loss, do not want to be without a personal telephone. Telecoil circuitry allows the hearing aids to amplify sounds conveyed by the magnetic signals picked up from a telephone receiver or other special assistive listening aids. The telecoil microphone picks up only the magnetic signals and does not amplify background noise. Most of today's hearing aids have an automatic sensing system to know when a magnetic signal is present and they transfer to a telephone mode. Some hearing aids may have a special microphone-telecoil two-position switch, or a memory position adjusted by the user to change from the normal microphone use to the special telecoil microphone when compatible telephone receivers are being used. The selection of hearing aids for children must have the capability for direct audio input (DAI), which allows for direct connection of the hearing aid to an assistive listening device such as a classroom amplification system, telephone receiver, radio, television, movie projector, audio stereo system, or other assistive listening system. Common wisdom requires that a child's hearing aid must be exceedingly durable; of course, consideration should also be given to an insurance protection plan for extended warranty, loss, or damage.

It is important to reemphasize that the hearing aid evaluation in newborns, infants, and young children is a long-term continuing process. The hearing aid's performance must be checked electroacoustically and with real-ear probe microphone measurements by the audiologist for every child at every clinic visit along with routine follow-up behavioral hearing tests. New hearing aid instruments should be carefully checked before they are dispensed to the patient to be sure that they meet the manufacturer's performance specifications.

Types of Hearing Aids

Hearing aids are available in a wide range of different styles, including air conduction and bone conduction models. Different styles of hearing instruments may be appropriate for children with differing type, degree, and configurations of hearing loss, as well as a function of the child's age. For younger children, the selection of hearing aid style may be influenced by the potential growth and change in the external ear size and shape. Small pinnae are likely best fitted with smaller hearing aids, while older

children with larger external ears may have more selection options. Cosmetics of the hearing aids may prove to be important to the parents, although the children themselves may be less concerned. Thoughtful counseling and guidance from the audiologist may be required to ensure that the proper fitting takes precedence over appearance of the hearing aids themselves.

As previously indicated, ear-level hearing aids are the choice for most children as shown in Figure 9–3. Ear-level aids are lightweight and provide hearing reception at the natural position of the head. Many manufacturers provide a variety of colors for the hearing aid cases. Earmolds may be selected in matching or contrasting colors to please the young pediatric patient or to be more cosmetically appropriate for the teenager. Earmolds may be fabricated in a number of sizes and styles for cosmetic and acoustic reasons for children and are typically constructed of soft silicon-based materials. Other pediatric-oriented considerations

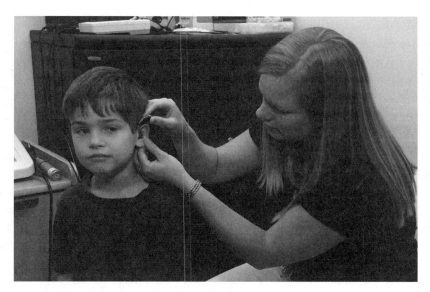

Figure 9–3. The pediatric audiologist is the professional responsible for fitting hearing aids on children with hearing loss. Photo courtesy of Colorado Children's Hospital, Aurora, CO.

include assurance that the hearing aid of choice is rugged and reliable, water resistant or waterproof, provides a wide frequency response bandwidth, with ample flexibility and programmability, size appropriate, pediatric-sized tone hooks are available, and includes an aggressive feedback suppression circuit. Older children with hearing loss will want telephone compatibility for their hearing aids and perhaps Bluetooth connectivity for personal music players. Parents will want simple and understandable operation, easy care, and reasonable battery life. Safety factors and other practical features to keep in mind in selecting a child's hearing aids are the provision of child-proof battery doors, tamper proof or volume control covers, loss and damage coverage, and a multiyear warranty opportunity.

Ear-level hearing aids may be used with all degrees of hearing loss from mild to severe, and even some profound hearing losses. These air conduction ear-level instruments include behind-the-ear (BTE) models as well as in-the-ear (ITE), in-the-canal (ITC), and completely-in-the-canal (CIC) hearing instruments. The ITE and ITC models are quite small and typically have no external wires or tubes, often without DIA input capability, and are usually less appropriate for young children.

Behind-the-Ear (BTE) Hearing Aids

The BTE hearing aid has all its components housed in a curved case that tucks neatly behind the pinna and rests against the mastoid surface. A short piece of clear plastic tubing connects the earmold to the hearing aid hook. Actually the BTE can be fixed with a sound channel of standard tubing, slim tubing, and to an open or closed ear mold. BTE hearing aids may deliver up to 85 dB SPL full-on gain and 125 to 140 dB

SPL maximum output. Because the microphone and re-ceiver of the BTE are in very close proximity to the earmold, increased opportunity exists for acoustic feedback, unless the hearing aid circuit contains an aggressive feedback cancelation system. Smaller versions of the BTE have been designed and turn out to be very practical for children because of their smaller size. Known as the mini-BTE, their smaller size may give up some features including telecoils, direct audio input for FM coupling, or locking battery doors (Figure 9–4).

In recent years, various versions of the BTE have been introduced and have become very popular. One style of the mini-BTE removes the receiver from the hearing case and places it in the ear canal. Called different names by different manufacturers, this is most commonly described as a RIC (receiver in the canal); this configuration has a wire running down the tube which connects the BTE to the receiver in the ear canal. This permits a smaller BTE case while still having the amplification power of the traditional BTE. Some select power BTEs may be appropriate for children with profound hearing loss. BTE hearing aids aimed at pediatric patients are often available in a variety of appealing colors and patterns, team logos, and familiar cartoon characters. Children frequently choose hearing aid and earmold colors and patterns that reflect their personalities and preferences.

The outer ear continues to grow and change shape well into puberty, thereby making it impractical to fit custom-shaped in-the-ear hearing aids to young children. By selecting BTE hearing aids for young children, the earmold must be replaced as the child grows and the concha and external ear canal change size and shape. The BTE hearing aid can be easily reprogrammed for more gain or different frequency response as needed by the child. As children grow

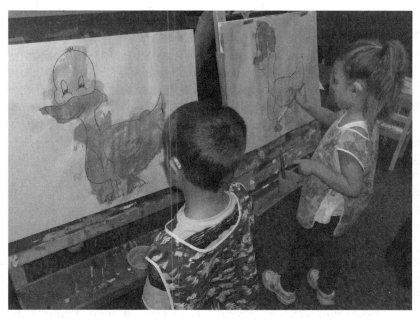

Figure 9–4. Ear level hearing aids are the preferred style for children. Photo courtesy of H.O.P.E. Preschool, Spokane, WA.

older, especially in their teen years, they may become more concerned about the cosmetic appearance of their hearing aid. As they reach those trying teen years, they often request smaller, less visible ear-level or in-the-canal hearing instruments. Parents need be apprised that the larger case of the BTE hearing aid permits inclusion of important pediatric features such as direct audio input connectivity which may not be possible with the smaller custom-style hearing aids. The changeover to in-the-ear-style hearing aids does provide a smaller device that can almost be hidden in the ear canal. However, depending on the degree and configuration of the hearing loss, the loss of pediatric features with in-the-ear style hearing aid may not be crucial. A common saying among audiologists is that "the best hearing aid is the one that is worn." For some children, the change to a smaller, less visible instrument may be the difference between wearing or rejecting the hearing aid.

Custom In-the-Ear (ITE) Hearing Aid

The custom in-the-ear (ITE) hearing aid is fabricated from an impression taken of the patient's concha, ear canal, and outer ear and submitted to the hearing aid manufacturer. The hearing aid components and circuits are embedded into the individualized earmold that is contoured to fit in the outer ear concha rather than behind the ear. Generally smaller and, by some viewpoints considered cosmetically more appealing, the ITE hearing aids tend to be not as visible as the BTE hearing aids. The family of ITE hearing devices is described by the anatomy of the outer ear where they are worn—concha or ear canal. ITE hearing aids are generally fit only to older children in whom the pinna has grown to its adult size and configuration. In some unique circumstances ITEs may be fit to younger children, but the child's growing external ear and ear canal will likely require the custom hearing aid to be remodeled periodically to assure a firm feedback-free fit. This simple recasing by the manufacturer readily solves the problem of a child outgrowing his or her custom-fitted hearing aids.

Today's ITE hearing aids can be almost as powerful as BTE hearing aids. The ITE may be fitted in a variety of forms depending on how much of the ear's anatomy the hearing aid is designed to occupy. The largest version is known as an ITE, a descriptor generally applied to a hearing aid that fits fully in the concha of the outer ear and partially extends into the external ear canal. A smaller variation is known as the half-shell ITE that fits into the lower half of the concha and outer ear canal. An even smaller version of the ITE is known as the low-profile ITE that does not extend very far out of the external ear canal into the lower portion of the concha.

A smaller version of the ITE is the in-the-canal (ITC) hearing aid. As its name suggests, it is formed primarily in the outer ear canal and extends only slightly into the concha at the entrance of the canal. And finally, the smallest style of ITE is the completely-in-the-canal (CIC) hearing aid that is built to fit entirely in the external ear canal. The ITC and the CIC are often so small that removal of the hearing aid is made easier by a thin line filament with a tiny knob at the end that extends out into the concha. These smaller hearing aids are generally not as powerful as the BTE or the full-concha ITE and are thereby fit to individuals with mild or moderate-degree hearing loss. Because of their limited size they may also lack many of the specialized features such as multiple microphones or direct audio input connections found in BTE hearing aids.

Bone Conduction Hearing Aids

Bone conduction hearing aids are used in selected children with conductive hearing loss who cannot (usually for medical or anatomical reasons) use an air conduction hearing aid. The bone conduction hearing aid is held in place by a springy headband and has a vibratory flat surface that rests on the mastoid and transduces sound waves into vibrotactile sensation. The vibrations through the skull stimulate the cochlear cells via the bone conduction auditory pathway. Bone conduction hearing aids are not commonly used today except in infants and young children with significant conductive hearing loss due to congenital anomalies such as microtia of the pinnae or atresia of the external ear canal. Bone conduction hearing aids can be fitted on infants literally at birth, although the usual fitting likely takes place at about 1 month of age. The bone oscillator can actually be placed anywhere against the skull, including the mastoid area behind the ear, the forehead, or at the back or top of the skull when the infant is placed stomach-down. Often a soft pad of some sort can be used for space filler or for comfort under the headband. The traditional bone conduction hearing aid fitting is generally not permanent. Chances are quite good that the cause of the conductive-type hearing problem will ultimately be resolved through medical or surgical intervention. Successful surgical treatment of the cause of the conductive hearing loss will permit the fitting of a traditional air conduction ear-level hearing aid if sensorineural hearing loss remains and amplification is still needed by the child.

Bone Anchored Hearing Aids (Baha). A permanent version of the bone conduction hearing aid is the surgically implanted bone anchored hearing aid (Baha). This system uses the body's natural bone conduction pathway to conduct sound through the temporal bone, bypassing the damaged parts of the external and middle ear to conduct sound to the normally functioning inner ear. Originally designed in Sweden in 1977, and approved by the U.S. FDA in 1996, the system has undergone several iterations and is now widely accepted in patients with conductive hearing loss who are unable to use conventional hearing aids. The Baha hearing aid is used in patients with significant conductive hearing loss due to malformed or absent external ears, ear canals, or middle ear structures—conditions often associated with cranial-facial malformations such as Treacher Collins syndrome or microtia of the external ear (Van der Pouw, Snik, & Cremers, 1998). The Baha hearing aid can also be used for patients with mastoidectomy cavities, chronic ear inflammation, or infections that prohibit the wearing of traditional hearing aids. The Baha has also been used successfully for patients with single-sided sensorineural deafness (Bosman, Snik, Emmanuel, Mylanus, & Cremers, 2009; Valente & Oeding, 2009).

The Baha microphone captures sound and converts it to vibrations. The hearing aid is attached to a surgically implanted abutment that has been placed behind the ear in the mastoid bone (Figure 9–5). A titanium post is surgically embedded into the skull with a small abutment exposed outside the skin. The sound processor attaches to this abutment and sound vibrations are transmitted directly through the skull to the inner ear in the same manner as a traditional bone conduction hearing aid. (Tjellstrom & Hakansson, 1995). The implanted post vibrates the skull and the cochlea, bypassing the external auditory canal and middle ear, working in the same manner as traditional bone conduction hearing aids. The vibrations, carried by the skull, stimulate the fluids and hair cells of the inner ear that then propagate signals up the auditory pathway to the auditory cortex resulting in hearing. The bone conducts the sound vibrations to

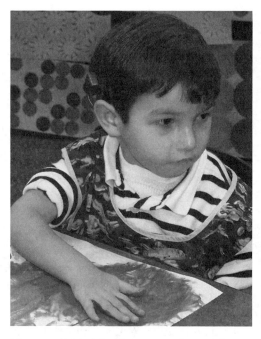

Figure 9–5. The bone anchored hearing aid (Baha) is a permanent bone conduction hearing aid that transmits sound directly to the inner ear. Photo courtesy of H.O.P.E. Preschool, Spokane, WA.

the functioning cochlea, allowing the individual to perceive sound naturally. Because of the deep direct connection to the skull, the vibrations are more effectively transmitted (Hakansson, Carlsson, Tjellstrom, & Liden, 1994). The Baha is a highly advanced sound processor that runs on batteries that must be replaced regularly.

The surgical procedure to implant the Baha is considered generally minor but requires a specially trained surgeon. The surgery may be carried out in a one-step or two-step procedure, often dependent upon the age of the patient (Portmann, Boudard, & Herman, 1997). The double-stage procedure may be considered for babies or small children waiting for the skull to continue to thicken and the process of osseointegration of the titanium screw to occur over a period of 6 to 8 months. During the second procedure the "post" is attached and skin grafted around the implanted platform that requires several more weeks for healing. This bone conduction hearing aid fitting in appropriate children can be very successful. Although in some countries the Baha unit has been surgically implanted into children as young as 13 months, the minimum age under FDA guidelines in the United States for Baha implantation is 5 years.

THE PEDIATRIC HEARING AID FITTING PROCESS

The fitting of hearing aids in children is a much more daunting task than fitting hearing aids on adults. Adults will tell you, in no uncertain terms, exactly how the hearing aid sounds to them and demand that the audiologists make adjustments until the hearing aids sound as near perfect as possible. The adjustment process is easier with adults as they can guide the audiologist with directions to achieve louder or softer amplification, better fidelity, or improved comfort. We do not have that guidance opportunity with infants and young children with hearing loss. Infants and children have to count on us to make all the settings as near perfect as possible. Therefore, we must be knowledgeable and confident with objective fitting measure protocols, designed specifically for children, so the hearing aid process with children results in the optimal amplification settings for them to hear and learn speech and language.

The goals for pediatric hearing aid fitting are for comfort and audibility of speech and environmental sounds. This requires properly programmed and adjusted ear-level hearing aids. It should be fully understood by all, especially parents, caregivers, and allied health personnel, that initial pediat-

ric hearing aid fittings are tentative and will likely need to be altered over time, perhaps more than once. The pediatric hearing aid selection and fitting is an ongoing process that is part of a complete habilitation program. The focus of routine audiologic monitoring of amplification must include not only the child's auditory status and the function of the hearing aids, but also the function of the FM auditory input system used in the school as well as the parent's understanding and cooperation in the child's habilitation program.

The ideal pediatric hearing aid fitting procedure is a patient-centered process with objective and subjective verification as the endpoint of the protocol (Beck et al., 2007). The selection of a specific hearing aid for a child with hearing loss can challenge the skills of even the most experienced audiologists. When a child has both receptive and expressive speech and language, the selection of a hearing aid is certainly easier and probably quicker. The nonverbal child poses problems because this youngster is not capable of communicating with the audiologist about the sound quality of various hearing aids. Appropriate selection of the frequency response and output characteristics must be carefully considered in fitting amplification to children. A number of techniques, both behavioral and electroacoustic, have evolved as a means to select the optimal hearing aid for each patient. None of the methods provides precise information that is valid for every hearing aid fitting, and the audiologist may have reason to make continual minor adjustments. However, each fitting procedure provides direction about the appropriate range of performance that the hearing aid must encompass. In many cases, more than one hearing aid manufacturer's instrument will meet the needed gain and output requirements, and selection is then based on other considerations such as hearing aid size, durability, cosmetics, ease of use, cost, and availability of accessories, service, and insurance.

As discussed previously, the selection and fitting of appropriate amplification devices for children must be more precise than when working with adults. This is due to the fact that children have to maximize their hearing to serve them in all activities, as this is how they continue to improve their speech and language skills. Scollie and Seewald (2002) point out that the pediatric hearing aid fitting process is a difficult task as audiologists tend to have to work with questionably accurate audiometric information further compromised by: (a) the need to estimate auditory thresholds through electrophysical measures (ABR and OAE); (b) changing ear canal volumes and resonance peaks caused by normal growth during the early years; (c) hearing fluctuations due to middle ear and inner ear pathologies; and (d) often less than cooperative infants, toddlers, and young children.

PROBE MICROPHONE MEASUREMENTS

The entire process of fitting hearing aids on infants and young children was revolutionized with the development of clinical real-ear probe-microphone equipment. The "art" of pediatric hearing aid fitting suddenly became a scientifically based procedure, and from that point on probe-microphone measurements became a required procedure for pediatric hearing aid work. Computerized probe microphone hearing aid measurement and analysis is the method of choice in fitting hearing aids on infants, toddlers, and older children (Figure 9–6). This technique utilizes a soft silicone tube that is inserted into the ear canal, under the earmold, with the hearing aid turned on and properly seated in the ear canal. The amplified sound from the hearing aid in the ear canal is picked up by the silicone tube probe-microphone, subjected to signal processing

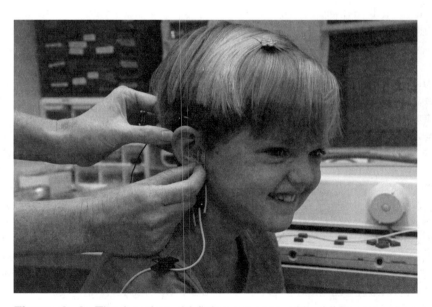

Figure 9–6. The hearing aid fitting process with children requires real-ear probe microphone measurements. Photo courtesy of Colorado Children's Hospital, Aurora, CO.

by a special-purpose computer, and visualized on a computer monitor or hard copy printout. Real-ear probe microphone measurements permit the audiologist to know precisely the aided frequency response and output levels of the amplified signal intensity at the child's eardrum. The real-ear probe microphone system can provide a wide variety of measurements to validate and verify the hearing aid fitting, especially useful in working with young children who cannot provide subjective responses about the amplified sound.

Nature provides a natural biologic sound amplifier due to the size and shape of the ear canal. This natural resonance can provide as much as 15 dB of amplification to actually help hear sounds better. This natural resonance peak is easily measured with a probe-microphone system and is described as the real-ear unaided gain (REUG) and is expressed in decibel sound pressure level (dB SPL) at the highest frequency peak in the unoccluded ear canal. It is critical to be aware that the REUG in infant ear canals occurs at a much higher frequency (6000–7200 Hz) than in adults. In fact, studies have documented that the resonance frequency of the external ear decreases gradually with age from 7200 Hz at birth until the adult resonance value of 2700 Hz is reached when the child reaches the age of 2 years (Kruger, 1987). The higher resonance in the infant is due to a smaller concha and shorter ear canal length. This information is important in selecting appropriate hearing aid frequency characteristics in babies and requires routine measurement to be sure the amplification characteristics of the hearing aid continue to match the resonance of the child's ear.

However, when an earmold or ITE hearing aid is placed into the ear canal, the biologic acoustic properties of the system are disrupted, the natural ear canal resonance is altered in frequency, and sound is diminished. The presence of the earmold or custom hearing aid in the ear canal creates an obstruction that tends to keep natural sound out of the ear canal, an effect called *insertion loss*. One must be sure that the recommended amplification has sufficient gain to overcome the insertion loss provided by the earmold or hearing instrument's obstruction of the ear canal.

The important aspect of this technique is the ability to plot hearing aid responses visually on the video screen target visible in Figure 9–7. The audiologist selects a prescriptive method of gain prediction (e.g., DSL, NAL-NL1) to achieve the best amplified responses for each child. Then, acoustic measurements are performed in the ear with probe microphone systems to provide information with minimal patient cooperation. Comparison of the probe microphone responses with the target amplification response permits an immediate comparison of the hearing instrument performance and the desired target fit. The hearing aid can be reprogrammed as often as necessary until the best fit to the target gain or output is achieved.

A major advantage of the computerized probe microphone real-ear measuring device is that the entire amplification system is evaluated so the effects of programming changes, tubing, earmold, vents, and filters can be measured precisely. Physiologic differences among children, such as the length, diameter, and shape of the ear canal, are extremely important fitting considerations and are taken into account in probe microphone measurements. Computerized probe microphone measurements provide quick, objective data regarding insertion gain, ear canal sound pressure levels, and the telemagnetic response of the hearing aid. The

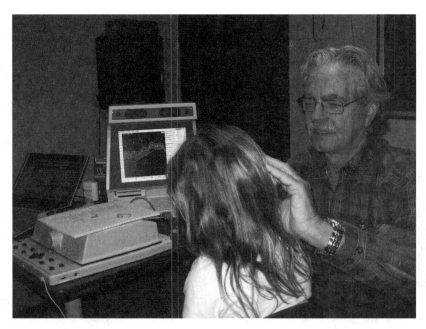

Figure 9–7. Computerized probe-microphone measurements provide objective real-ear electroacoustic information about hearing aid performance. Photo courtesy of H.O.P.E. Preschool, Spokane, WA.

measurements may be read in 1 dB intervals so that every acoustic modification or electroacoustic adjustment made with the hearing aids will be noted clearly.

Probe microphone systems have been available for at least two decades and provide the most reliable and accurate measurements you can make to ensure that the fitting of the hearing aid in the child's ear is exactly what you feel is necessary for maximum hearing benefit. Although the step-by-step procedures for each of the tests are beyond the scope of this book, the pediatric audiologist must be familiar with obtaining measurements on all ages of infants and children and all types of hearing aids fittings. Real-ear probe microphone automated tests can provide nearly all the information you need to verify your pediatric hearing aid fitting. Use of standardized prescriptive fitting formulae, selected from the equipment software, allows you to accurately determine a number of different measurements as listed by Taylor and Mueller (2011):

- Fitting targets viewed in insertion gain or ear canal SPL for a wide range of input values and signals;
- Desired settings for wide dynamic range compression (WDRC) such as knee point, compression ratio, and so forth;
- Targets for output limiting;
- Targets displayed for 2-cc coupler as well as ear canal gain and SPL;
- Corrections based on the patient's age;
- Corrections based on the number of hearing aid channels; and
- Corrections for hearing aid experience, gender, and listening in quiet versus noise.

Most probe microphone equipment includes a "listening" circuit and lightweight earphones so that the amplified sound can be heard by the child's parents and family, who can thereby gain full appreciation of exactly how their youngster's hearing aids amplify environmental and speech sounds. Another impressive demonstration for parents and caregivers is to use the probe microphone system while in place on the ear and with the hearing aid turned on, use a calibrated speech signal as the input. This procedure is known as "speech mapping" and it is possible to view "live speech" from the child or the child's parents on the monitor screen in a real-ear amplified response (REAR) format along with the various targets selected for the hearing aid performance. Although speech mapping conveys impressive information about the hearing aid's amplification, it is not sufficiently precise by which to do the actual hearing aid fitting.

Computerized probe microphone measurements have numerous distinct advantages over functional gain measurements as a method of assessing hearing aid performance, especially with children. These advantages include: (a) elimination of dependency on the behavioral threshold responses; (b) electroacoustic information across the entire frequency range of interest rather than only octave or half-octave intervals; (c) no contamination of aided threshold measures by internal hearing aid or room noise, a significant problem with functional gain measurements when hearing thresholds are in the normal or near-normal range; and (d) considerable savings in time and efficiency, with improved accuracy and reliability in the electroacoustic analysis of the hearing aid under evaluation.

An especially important concept used in pediatric hearing aid measurements is the real-ear to coupler difference (RECD).

The RECD, as it implies, is the difference in dB between the output of a hearing aid (or insert earphone) in the real ear versus a 2-cc coupler. Because there is considerable variability in children's ear canal volumes, it is best to measure the RECD for each individual child, although it is often sufficient to just make the measurement in one ear. Before probe microphone tests, there was no way to know what the actual output of a hearing aid might be in a child's small ear canal. The probe microphone technique allows the audiologist to determine the actual SPL that exists in the ear canal for each hearing instrument setting. Known as the real-ear aided response (REAR) and measured in SPL, the REAR permits easy comparisons between the patient's hearing loss, the fitting targets, the hearing aid output, and the hearing aid characteristics. This information has important implications for setting the OSPL90 of the hearing aid as well as determining the appropriate gain and frequency response.

The use of probe microphone measurements in fitting hearing aids and managing amplification for children with hearing loss provides the audiologist with objective and reliable data. The audiologist and parents must be aware, however, that these aided responses should not be misconstrued to represent what the child "hears." Hearing, of course, requires cerebral integration of speech and environmental sounds. Probe microphone evaluation gives audiologists confidence in their selection and fitting of hearing aids for this difficult-to-test population, provides objective information to resolve hearing aid problems, and permits in-office adjustments, reprogramming, and modifications to hearing instruments. We recommend that probe microphone measurements be a routine part of each child's follow-up visits so that fine-tuning adjustments can be made, or changes in auditory thresholds can be addressed with changes to the instrument gain and output as needed.

Hearing Aid Fitting Protocol

Recently, the American Academy of Audiology updated their clinical practice guidelines for pediatric amplification (2013). These guidelines provide the most extensive evidence-based overview of the hearing aid process with children, and much of the discussion below has been drawn from this thorough and complete treatise. Pediatric audiologists should be familiar with this document as it serves as a best-practices course of action when fitting hearing aids on infants and young children. Mueller and Hall (1998) described a six-step protocol for organizing the hearing aid fitting process for patients with hearing loss that can serve as a clinical model for the pediatric hearing aid process as described below.

Step 1: Assessment

The question may exist about whether or not a particular child is a candidate for hearing aids. It is our belief that any child who experiences difficulties in hearing, regardless of their hearing levels, should be considered for hearing aids. This would include those children with mild hearing losses of a sensorineural or permanent conductive nature, high-frequency hearing losses, and unilateral hearing loss. Children diagnosed with auditory neuropathy spectrum disorder (ANSD), or children who might be candidates for cochlear implants, should be given a trial session with hearing aids. Audiologists should give consideration to those children who complain that they do not hear well in the classroom, perhaps because of a mild hearing loss, who might benefit from the use of hearing aids. Some-

times a trial with loaner hearing aids, even for a brief period of time, can resolve lots of questions and problems.

During the initial assessment stage, the extent and cause of the child's hearing loss are determined as accurately as possible, using best practice clinical procedures, in order to establish candidacy for hearing aid use. Obviously, the success of hearing aid fittings depends on an accurate and in-depth hearing evaluation conducted by a pediatric audiologist familiar with amplification protocols. The decision about candidacy for hearing aids requires both auditory and nonauditory considerations, and it is agreed by most audiologists that audiometric information alone is insufficient to predict success with hearing aids. But, other factors such as parent involvement and motivation, as well as the child's personality, emotional levels, and willingness to listen through the hearing aids are considerations that also play an important role in hearing aid fitting success. Simmons et al. (2007) remind us that at this elementary stage in the hearing aid process, consideration of the family-centered, culturally sensitive aspects of the child's development is important and worthy of consideration before proceeding.

The audiologic assessment that precedes the hearing aid evaluation should be as thorough as possible given the child's age and cooperation. For newborns and infants under the developmental age of 6 months, the hearing aid fitting should be based on ear-specific physiological measures such as auditory brainstem (ABR) threshold assessment and otoacoustic emission (OAE) measures. The 2007 JCIH recommended that all children identified with hearing loss under the age of 3 be evaluated with at least one ABR session to confirm hearing levels in each ear.

Because most infants with hearing loss are being identified within a few days following their birth, there is a need for diagnostic assessment and intervention as soon as possible. In many cases, the confirmation of hearing loss in babies is determined while the infants are less than 1 month of age. In young infants where accurate and frequency-specific behavioral thresholds cannot be attained, electrophysiologic testing should be conducted to establish hearing thresholds such as the auditory brainstem response (ABR) or auditory steady-state response (ASSR). The ASSR is typically calibrated in decibels hearing level (dB HL); the ABR provides threshold estimates in decibel hearing level (e.g., referenced in decibels normalized hearing level, dB nHL). The ABR measurement of infant thresholds is more commonly utilized than the ASSR procedure. As pointed out by Bagatto (2013), ABR threshold estimates in infants are typically higher in decibel hearing level (i.e., worse) than what is ultimately obtained through behavioral testing. Accordingly, the ABR threshold estimates need to be adjusted to more accurately predict behavioral thresholds for the purposes of calculating the prescriptive hearing aid targets. Failure to apply the correction factors at each test frequency can result in inaccurate hearing aid fittings for infants. The correction is frequency specific, subtracted from the ABR threshold estimate, and recorded as decibels normalized hearing level (dB nHL) to better represent the true hearing threshold. The correction factors are based on the ABR equipment and may range from 20 dB at 500 Hz to 5 dB at 4000 Hz. Properly adjusting the ABR values prior to intervention is an important component in the assessment and fitting stages for successful fitting of hearing aids in infants (Bagatto et al., 2005; Bagatto, Scollie, Hyde, & Seewald, 2010). An advantage to the ABR fitting protocol is that hearing aids for difficult-to-test children can be fitted under sedation when necessary.

Although the initial hearing aid fitting may have been based on corrected thresholds obtained through ABR measurements, the ongoing goal should be to accurately establish behavioral thresholds as soon as possible. In the initial hearing assessments of a young child, it may be that a single, low-frequency hearing threshold and a single, high-frequency hearing threshold may have to suffice until additional frequency-specific threshold measures can be established. Although there is a positive correlation between click-ABR and pure tone thresholds average thresholds at 2000 and 4000 as shown by Baldwin and Watkin (2013), a click-ABR evaluation of a child's hearing is not sufficient for accurate hearing aid fitting. Clicks are too broadband to use for frequency-specific threshold measurements needed for hearing aid fitting, so ABR is typically conducted with tone pips.

For infants with a conductive component to their hearing loss, bone conduction threshold determination may be necessary to confirm the degree of a conductive component to the child's hearing loss. Clinicians need to be watchful because of the high incidence of middle ear pathology in young children, creating conductive hearing loss overlay on sensorineural hearing loss as this will certainly affect amplification process. It is an important principle that the pediatric hearing aid fitting process should not be delayed until a full diagnostic workup is completed or until a full behavioral audiogram can be determined.

For children with developmental age older than 6 months, behavioral thresholds should be obtained using visual reinforcement audiometry (VRA) or conditioned play audiometry (CPA) using test techniques appropriate for the child's response and understanding level. The use of physiologic test methods such as ABR, OAE, and immittance measures may be necessary for any child who is difficult to evaluate with traditional testing methods. Children have a critical need for listening and hearing, so the hearing aid fitting becomes a critical enhancement for them to hear speech better due amplification and to an improved signal-to-noise ratio over background noise. It is necessary to account for the child's personal ear canal changes so the real-ear-to-coupler difference should be routinely measured, and the hearing aid adjusted accordingly, at follow-up visits when the child is less than 2 years of age.

Step 2: Treatment Planning

This stage of the hearing aid fitting process begins at the completion of the preliminary audiological evaluation and confirmation of the child's hearing loss. The pediatric audiology specialist and family members review and discuss the results of the hearing assessment. Together, the group plans and agrees on the future steps in obtaining and fitting the hearing aids. There are numerous decisions to be made prior to the selection and fitting of a child's hearing aid. The decisions will necessarily be based on the type and degree of hearing loss, individual needs and abilities of the child and the family, the living and educational situation, and the overall understanding of the child's hearing problems and the family's motivation and commitment to help the child hear better. Certainly a topic that needs to be addressed early is the financial circumstances available for purchase of the hearing aids. Will the family apply for third-party support or deal with the financial obligations directly themselves? Too often this conversation is delayed until the fitting is completed, and

yet the financial decisions may have a great deal to do with how the treatment plan progresses (i.e., what type and how soon the hearing aids will be purchased and available for fitting on the child). It is important that the pediatric audiologist be familiar with financial support available through local and state agencies, service organizations and nonprofit foundations, or private sources that may be utilized to purchase the child's hearing aids. During this stage the audiologist needs to help guide the parents or responsible parties to obtain the hearing instruments. Again, our purpose in this pediatric hearing aid fitting is to help with communication by maximizing the child's hearing potential through appropriate amplification devices as soon as possible.

It is an easy trap for the audiologist and family members to focus attention primarily on the hearing aids, per se. But the discussion must be expanded to understand results of the hearing assessment, identify areas of the child's hearing difficulties, and for all to agree on a path of habilitative procedures of which the hearing aid fitting is just the initial step. This approach shifts the focus from being purely product oriented (i.e., focused on the hearing aids) to one that is process oriented (focused on enhancing the child's communication situation). If the child has worn hearing aids previously, the planning and assessment stage will no doubt require less time than for new candidates for hearing aids. In addition to discussions and demonstrations, the parents or caregivers should be sent home with useful printed information or be directed to online materials to help them reach the necessary decisions. This approach to a treatment plan provides opportunity for counseling about realistic expectations and should include a projected time line of when parents might expect to see results from new amplification devices (Sweetow, 2009). The family must realize that this is not a one-step, fix-it solution for their child's hearing problem, but rather the start of a long-term commitment that will ensure that their child has every opportunity to achieve the same successes of children with normal hearing.

Step 3: Hearing Aid Selection and Fitting

This step focuses on the hearing aid style, model, technology level, number of channels, special program characteristics to be entered into memories, special features, and so forth, to be recommended for the child. The audiologist needs to carefully and thoughtfully assess the lifestyle and hearing needs of the child and family prior to making hearing aid recommendations. Although the audiologist's role is to objectively present the hearing aid options available and provide guidance, the final decisions should be made, or at least the selection rational discussed and understood, by the family or caregivers. It is helpful at this stage to have samples of the various hearing aids, the color options available, as well as a discussion of earmold properties for the child and the family to see and handle.

During the selection process, the audiologist will want to consider the hearing aid's capabilities for frequency response, power output, compression circuits, direct audio input and FM compatibility, tamper-resistant features (battery door, volume control, program switches), pediatric-size BTE hooks, durability, warranty, battery life, color option availability, availability of advance features, and of course, cost of the instruments. The standard of care for children is binaural hearing aid fitting unless contraindicated.

The style of hearing aid chosen will likely depend on degree and configuration of hearing loss as well as the cosmetic considerations, battery life, and external ear geometry. Decisions might be influenced by the parent's abilities to comprehend the technology and operation of the hearing aids, as well as their manual dexterity, visual abilities, desired advanced features, and of course, their ability to pay required costs that might be expensive. There may be a divergence between the audiologist's knowledge and guidance for the parents of what styles and features are suitable for a successful fitting outcome versus the parent's desires and preferences. This situation will require the utmost tact and counseling from the audiologist in the attempt to make the parents or caregivers understand the reasons for the specific hearing aid recommendations. The parents must be reminded that the goal in hearing aid selection for their child is to provide hearing instruments that will support and ease the communication by maximizing the child's hearing abilities in different listening environments. In acceptance of their child's hearing loss, the parents or caregivers must understand that "invisibility" of the hearing aid is not a priority at this time in the child's life.

Libby (1982) provided this advice about hearing aid fittings as follows: (a) choose an amplification system with a smooth frequency response and no sharp peaks; (b) make plans to compensate for the 10 to 15 dB insertion loss at 2700 Hz created by an occluding earmold; (c) select a wide-frequency bandwidth to ensure greater fidelity for speech and music; (d) reach an appropriate balance between high-frequency amplification for speech understanding and low-frequency energy for intelligibility and preservation of sound quality; and (e) ensure that the output of the hearing aid does not exceed the patient's loudness discomfort level.

The audiologist has additional responsibilities during this stage of the hearing aid process in terms of the properties and the technology of the hearing aids under consideration. The guiding principles for pediatric hearing aids are to avoid instruments with amplification distortion, and to select instruments that have ample flexible output and frequency shaping, with adjustable compression output limiting. These general features can be programmed to provide suitable audibililty and prevent loudness discomfort (Bagatto, 2013). There are sufficient choices among manufacturers who produce pediatric-oriented hearing aids to cover nearly every fitting. Many manufacturers have special pediatric software with colorful child-oriented images or cartoon characters as well as software that automatically fills in hearing aid fitting targets based on hearing threshold values inserted by the audiologist. While the audiologist is loading the prescriptive information, the child-oriented software and monitor videos serve to hold the child's attention.

Once the hearing aids have been received, the procedure moves on to consideration of the prescriptive fitting options. Hearing aid manufacturers commonly include a proprietary fitting formula with their software which may, or may not, have a pediatric version. Nonetheless, these proprietary formulae have typically not been fully evaluated for use with children; therefore, audiologists are urged to select independently developed and evidence-based prescriptive fitting programs developed under rigid scientific protocols. A wealth of studies have been conducted to validate the use of two commonly used pediatric fitting formulae known as the Desired Sensation Level (DSL) developed at the University of Western Ontario, Canada, and the National Acoustics Laboratories (NAL) of Sydney, Australia. Multiple versions of both DSL and NAL formulae are typically available within the pediatric hearing aid manufacturer's software.

Step 4: Verification

Verification refers to the evaluation of the hearing aid fitting to determine if the hearing aid meets the desired performance for the individual child's maximum hearing benefit. Verification is the stage whereby the audiologist can confirm (i.e., verify) that the hearing aids are providing appropriate amounts of amplification throughout the frequency spectrum, including safe output limitations, and that the hearing aid actually provides the child with optimal audibility. Prior to the actual fitting, the audiologist must ensure that the instruments meet expected standards that include high electroacoustic performance, satisfactory cosmetic appearance, and comfortable fit on the child's ears. The electroacoustic hearing aid check requires 2-cc coupler measurements to ensure that the aids are performing as per the manufacturer's specifications. This analysis should be accomplished before the fitting procedure begins as it can happen that a hearing aid is delivered from the manufacture that does not meet performance standards. This is cause for returning the hearing aid and requesting a new hearing aid be sent.

The response of the hearing aids should be measured with a series of input levels to estimate the audibility of speech for the individual child's hearing, and to ensure that the maximum output levels of the instruments do not exceed prescribed levels. There are basically two methods of verification for the fitting of pediatric hearing aids described by the AAA Pediatric Guidelines (2013):

1. Real-ear aided response (REAR) probe microphone measurements: the output of the hearing aid is measured in the child's ear canal (in situ) using a probe microphone. The response of the hearing aid should be measured for a variety

of input levels including soft speech, average speech level, and maximum power output of the hearing aid. This procedure provides a direct measure of the SPL of the amplified sound in the child's ear canal at the different input levels that can then be compared to the child's threshold and uncomfortable loudness levels.

2. Simulated real-ear aided response measurements: this procedure utilizes age-appropriate average real-ear-to-coupler differences to measured 2-cc coupler electroacoustic results to verify predicted audibility and to ensure output that is below the uncomfortable loudness level (Seewald & Scollie, 1999). The response of the hearing aids should be measured with a series of input levels to estimate the audibility of speech for the individual child's hearing, and to ensure that the maximum output levels of the instruments do not exceed prescribed levels.

Obviously, verification of hearing aid performance with a real-ear probe microphone system in some infants or young children can be problematic. The 2-cc coupler in no way mimics the volume, size, and shape of the pediatric ear canal; therefore, the audiologist must account for this difference to predict the performance of the hearing aid in daily use. The RECD procedure is in common use for pediatric hearing aid fittings (RECD) and has been fully described in detail by numerous authors (Moodie, Seewald, & Sinclair, 1994; Seewald, Moodie, Scollie, & Bagatto, 2005). In simplest terms, the RECD is the difference in decibels across frequency between the SPL of a given signal measured in a 2-cc coupler and the same signal measured in the ear with an earmold in place. The SPL of the test signal is then measured in the ear

canal. The difference between the SPL of the test signal in the coupler and the SPL of the same signal in the ear is determined and applied to the coupler values as an estimate of real-ear responses (Simmons et al., 2007). These calculations are performed automatically by both DSL and NAL pediatric prescription software programs.

Verification of aided auditory function is an ongoing process designed to ensure that the child is receiving optimal speech input and that his or her own speech is adequately perceived (Pediatric Working Group, 1996). Verification of hearing aid performance should be done routinely at each audiologic visit with the child. In terms of the hearing aid performance recheck, the most accurate verification process is to confirm through probe microphone real-ear measurements that soft sounds are audible, that speech recognition (when measureable) is maintained or improved, and that loud sounds are limited to a comfortable level. The real-ear measurements are obtained with the hearing aid turned on and the earmold in place. Typically the verification real-ear measurements are conducted with advanced features such as directional microphones, feedback suppression, noise reduction, and frequency lowering turned off. However, if the child uses any of these features routinely, there are methods to verify that their performance is appropriate and meets manufacturer specifications.

Unfortunately, practice surveys confirm that less than one third of all hearing aid fittings are done with real-ear measurements (Mueller & Picou, 2010; Kochkin et al., 2010). Hopefully, these survey statistics are not representative of pediatric audiologists because the requirement for real-ear measures in pediatric patients is an absolute must in every initial fitting and follow-up evaluation. It is a concern that many audiologists apparently rely on the manufacturer's first-fit software program where it has been shown that only 12% of targets on the manufacturer's fitting software match what is actually measured in the patient's ear (Aarts & Caffee, 2005). Numerous other studies have confirmed that the manufacturer's stipulated output values, based on hard-walled coupler measures, often over- or underfit patients with amplification (Hawkins & Cook, 2003; Keidser, Brew, & Peck, 2003; Mueller, Bentler, & Wu, 2008). For children, use of adult fitting software often overestimates the high-frequency gain of the hearing aid; and with their smaller than adult ear canals, children will receive more gain than expected by the adult-averaged software. Therefore, it is important to use software with pediatric norms. Palmer (2007) warns audiologists to be aware of the broad differences between manufacturers' first-fit algorithms, and that underfitting leaves sound inaudible and overfitting can potentially create hearing damage. Palmer points out that both of these unacceptable outcomes can be avoided when the actual output of the hearing aid in the child's ear canal is determined with real-ear probe microphone measurements.

Functional Gain. Not currently recommended, it should be pointed out that functional gain measures were widely used with children to verify hearing aid fittings until the advent of probe microphone systems and development of pediatric fitting protocols using the real-ear-coupler-difference method. Functional gain measurements are the difference in dB HL between unaided and aided minimal response levels typically obtained through behavioral threshold measurements. The young child was typically seated on the parent's lap between two soundfield speakers and through visual response audiometry (VRA), minimal response levels were obtained for speech

signals and narrow bands of noise with and without the hearing aids. AAA (2003) hearing aid guidelines stated specifically that behavioral methods (i.e., functional gain) are not recommended for verifying amplification fittings in children.

Functional gain measurement to verify hearing aid benefit has been largely abandoned as we have available more accurate information that can now be supplied through real-ear probe microphone measurements. Functional gain came under a number of disadvantages pointed out by Stelmachowicz, Seewald, and Gorga (1998). Functional gain measures can be contaminated by all the variables inherent in behavioral pediatric audiometry hearing loss such as the level of language skills, and the intellectual function of the child. Aided functional gain measurements reflect performance only at minimal response or threshold levels, with no information about the input/output characteristics or the output limiting performance of the hearing aids. Thus, there is no assurance with functional gain measures that the child receives meaningful perception of speech at intensities sufficiently above threshold with appropriate output limiting to prevent overamplification. Minimal response levels established in the soundfield might underestimate functional gain when low-frequency unaided hearing levels are near normal limits. Functional gain is not recommended as a primary verification procedure and should not be used for other than basic demonstration purposes (i.e., to demonstrate to parents that the child does hear better when wearing hearing aids).

Step 5: Orientation and Counseling

Orientation and counseling refer to helping the child's family or caregivers understand the operation of the hearing aids and adjust to the changes in their daily life required by the utilization of the new hearing aids worn by their child. This is an incredibly important part of the hearing aid process and should not be taken lightly. The successful use of hearing aids by the pediatric patient may, in large part, be reflective of the audiologist's skills in conveying information during orientation and counseling. Whenever possible, the child wearing the hearing aids should be included in the orientation and counseling sessions.

The care and operation of the hearing aid is generally pretty clear, and there are a myriad of ways to provide this information. The training sessions should include hands-on practice with earmold insertion, turning the hearing aids on and off, as well as selecting alternative memory and programs. Suggestions of techniques to hold the hearing aid in place behind the child's ear may be needed. Orderly topical discussions and demonstrations are needed for cleaning the instruments, humidity and moisture concerns, overnight storage, battery life and replacement with special comment about battery toxicity if swallowed, basic troubleshooting for plugged earmold or tubing or receiver, telephone coupling, and assistive device use. Although nothing beats the personal counseling sessions and hand-on demonstrations provided by the audiologist, this information can be supplemented through online information, DVD or video presentations, handout materials, or referral to a support group composed of other adults who have children with hearing impairment. There are certainly abundant materials available to provide counseling services that do not require additional significant professional time to develop. It is helpful that parents have printed materials on hand to quickly help resolve hearing aid problems (Clark, 2007; Seaver, 2009; Waldman & Roush, 2010). In addition, most manufacturers of pediatric-oriented hearing aids include in their fitting software various innovative and sometimes interactive counseling tools and websites to supplement the audiologist's orientation and counseling sessions.

Count-the-Dots Audibility. A simple count-the-dots technique for demonstrating the improved "audibility" provided by hearing aids was developed by Mueller and Killion (1990) and updated by Killion and Mueller (2010). The count-the-dots format is easy to keep in print template form to quickly plot any child's audiogram as an instructional aid. The completed form can be used in a variety of ways, but it is especially useful to demonstrate aided versus nonaided audibility for parents, in-service presentations, or annual IEP meetings. The distribution of the 100 dots on the count-the-dots audiogram (Figures 9–8 and 9–9) represents speech at a level of 60 dB SPL (approximately 45 dB HL). The dots are distributed in a weighted manner across frequencies to represent the contribution of each frequency to speech. This method for estimating the child's Audibility Index (AI) is as simple as counting the audible dots and multiplying by 100. The count-the-dots visualization is made by marking the child's threshold hearing levels on the template and then marking the aided soundfield audiogram on the same template. This technique can be easily used to explain to parents those sounds the child can reasonably expect to hear and which sounds will be totally inaudible. The number of dots under the audiogram represents speech sounds that the patient can hear which are counted and multiplied by 100 to express the value as a percentage. Likewise, the available dots above the audiogram are sounds the child cannot hear through the hearing aid. This is an easy visual aid and estimate of the child's hearing aid benefit by frequency. Because

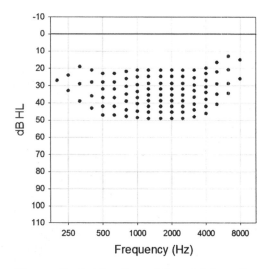

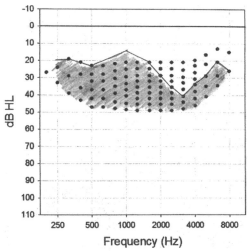

Figure 9–8. The "count-the-dots" audiogram template (2010) as developed by Mead Killion and Gus Mueller. Public domain.

Figure 9–9. The count-the-dots template overlaid with a high-frequency sensory hearing loss. The shaded area represents the speech spectrum audible to the patient. Amplification with a hearing aid would move the aided audiogram to the right on the template, allowing more of the speech spectrum to be audible.

the AI is a measure of the proportion of speech cues that are audible, it is therefore closely related to the intelligibility of speech. Most of today's probe microphone and computer hearing aid software calculates the AI automatically. Use of the 100-dot template of the speech spectrum can help make the child's aided and unaided audiogram more meaningful to the family, other medical personnel, and educators, and is valuable as a counseling and teaching aid.

Step 6: Validation

During the follow-up stage of the hearing aid process, it is critical to validate the benefits and performance of the child wearing the hearing aids in a real-world situation. This can be done through standardized subjective and objective outcome measures. This is achieved through one or more selected tools designed to evaluate the effects of amplification intervention as discerned by family members, teachers, and therapists. Validation involves determining

the impact of the hearing aid fitting through various formal and informal outcome measures. Validation is a dynamic and ongoing process with each return visit of the patient. The outcome measures can be subjective using self-assessment tests to determine the hearing aid performance in terms of patient benefits and satisfaction, or objective in terms of using standardized speech recognition measures to ascertain the patient's abilities to understand speech in standardized test conditions (Boney, 2007).

There is a wide choice of outcome measurement tools designed to evaluate the child's aided performance with various speech perception challenges. Some tools have been developed to use in the sound suite as a "functional" measure, whereas others are questionnaires designed for assessments that can be conducted in the sound suite or in the child's school environment

(AAA, 2003). Although the tools listed below can be helpful in assessing performance by individual children, many of these assessment procedures lack strong evidence-based normative statistical analyses.

Aided Speech Perception Measures:

- Northwestern University's Children's Perception of Speech Test (NUCHIPS; Katz & Elliott, 1978)
- Phonetically Balanced Kindergarten List (PBKs; Haskin, 1949)
- Pediatric Speech Intelligibility Test (PSI; Jerger et al., 1980)
- Early Speech Perception Task (Moog & Geers, 1990)
- Functional Assessment Tools
  ○ Questionnaires to be completed by educators:
- Functional Listening Evaluation (Johnson & Von Almen, 1997)
- Screening Instrument for Targeting Educational Risk (SIFTER, Anderson, 1989; preschool SIFTER, Anderson & Matkin, 1996)
- Listening Inventory for Education (LIFE; Anderson & Smaldino, 1998)
  ○ Questionnaires to be completed by parents or caregivers:
- Meaningful Auditory Integration Scale (MAIS; Robbins & Osberger, 1991a; Robbins, Renshaw, & Berry, 1991b; Robbins, Bollard, & Green, 1999)
- The Infant-Toddler MAIS (IT-MAIS; Zimmerman, Osberger, & Robbins, 1998)
- Meaningful Use of Speech Scale (MUSS; Robbins et al., 1991a, 1991b)
- Family Expectation Worksheet (Palmer & Mormer, 1999)
- Children's Home Inventory of Listening Difficulties (CHILD; Anderson & Smaldino, 2000)

- Functional Auditory Performance Indicators (FAPI; Stredler-Brown & Johnson, 2004)
- Early Listening Function (ELF; Anderson, 2002)

The validation process may lead to needed reprogramming or fine-tuning of the hearing aids to ensure the child's preferred sound quality. Reprogramming or fine-tuning will also call for new probe microphone real-ear measurements to verify the in situ hearing aid output changes. The audiologist should routinely perform a physical examination of the hearing aid and earmold to ensure patient comfort and proper aesthetics. The validation period provides opportunity for open discussions of the total and overall effects of amplification intervention on the child's daily living, communication skills, and educational achievements.

PRESCRIPTIVE FITTING METHODS

The selection of appropriate gain and output in children's hearing aids is always a challenging task, as newborns and toddlers cannot verbalize their perceptions of the amplified sound loudness or quality. Audiologists attempt to ensure optimal audibility of the speech spectrum while avoiding overamplification of the low-frequency energy found in background noise by the use of prescriptive formulae. Our goal for hearing aids in children to always be kept in mind is to provide audibility for speech as well as incidental and environmental sounds. Of concern is the prospect of overpowering an infant or toddler with hearing aid gain that is too strong. Although none of the threshold-based prescriptive procedures are guaranteed to ensure that a child will not experience discomfort or that the output levels are safe, the use of a systematic objective approach that incorporates age-dependent variables (canal volume and resonance factors) is preferred when determining gain and output functions for children. Of course, it is also possible, once the target fitting has been ascertained, to modify or adjust the frequency response of the hearing aids relative to the desired target amplified configuration if necessary.

Prescriptive formulae have been developed and normed over the years which determine frequency-specific target gains and output levels relative to the child's auditory thresholds. In infants and young children, the initial and early determined auditory thresholds may be based on ABR measurements or VRA behavioral tests. Most hearing aid manufacturers have developed propriety software algorithms that are designed apparently to fit the characteristics of their own hearing aids. Seewald, Mills, Bagatto, Scollie, and Moodie (2008) compared five different manufacturer's implementations of the same prescriptive method and found for the same hearing loss the recommended gain for average speech inputs varied by as much as 21 dB, whereas the prescriptive output limiting levels varied by as much as 30 dB.

In terms of selecting targets for pediatric patients, most audiologists chose either the Desired Sensation Level (DSLv5) developed at the National Centre for Audiology at the University of Western Ontario, Canada, or NAL-NAL$_1$ from the National Acoustic Laboratories of Sydney, Australia. Scollie et al. (2010) described differences between the two prescriptive formulae as DSL being the "habililtative audibility" approach, attempting to amplify as many sounds into audibility as possible, while the NAL approach is "effective audibility," designed to amplify only those sounds that contribute to speech intelligibility. In general, DSL targets prescribe more overall gain than the NAL for all audiometric configurations while limiting the maximum headroom to prevent loudness discomfort (Seewald, 1991). NAL provides less high-frequency gain than DSL for audiograms that demonstrate sloping high-frequency loss; DSL provides more low-frequency gain for flat audiograms than NAL. In general, however, comparative double-blind research studies of DSL and NAL prescriptive fittings have failed to show significant or major differences in the aided performances or preferences of children (Ching et al., 2006; Quar, Ching, Newall, & Sharma, 2013). Most hearing aid manufacturers incorporate the DSL and the NAL prescriptive algorithms into their fitting software making calculations and fitting targets automatically for individual pediatric hearing aid fittings.

The DSL is a method for fitting hearing aids developed specifically for determining amplified speech targets for linear and nonlinear gain hearing aids in children (Seewald et al., 1991) which has been periodically updated over the past 20 years. The DSL procedure requires a series of calculations performed with computer-assisted software and is based on a systematic protocol to provide amplified speech signals that are audible, comfortable, and undistorted across a broad frequency range. The method applies age-appropriate individual or average values for relevant acoustic characteristics that are known to vary as a function of age, specifically external ear resonance characteristics and real-ear to 2-cc coupler differences. A special advantage to the DSL method is that all measurements are made or converted to ear canal SPL. The real-ear SPL values of the residual auditory area and hearing aid targets are displayed on an SPL-o-Gram graph. It is important that auditory thresholds be established with insert receivers rather than earphones whenever possible.

The Desired Sensation Level (DSL) was developed in the early 1980s as a systematic, science-based approach to pediatric hearing instrument fitting and is widely used as the preferred fitting formula with children. Excellent overviews of the DSLv5 prescriptive method have been published by Bagatto et al. (2005), Simmons et al. (2007), and Roush and Seewald (2009). DSLv5 was developed to provide maximal audibility while maintaining comfortable loudness across all input levels. The norm values for DSLv5 were collected from 392 infants and children aged 1 month to 16 years. The DSL method includes consideration of a number of important issues relating to the assessment, selection, fitting, and verification stages of the hearing aid fitting process. DSL transforms audiometric data to dB SPL for maximum consistency and to reduce error and confusion. It provides separate prescriptive targets for adult and pediatric fittings. The algorithm prescribes corrections for conductive hearing losses (increased gain to compensate for hearing loss) and binaural hearing aid fittings (decreased gain to compensate for binaural summation). Specific prescriptions for severe and profound hearing losses are also provided. The computations of the formulae are a series of target input/output functions that define how a multichannel, multistage hearing aid should respond to speech inputs across multiple input levels (Beck, Moodie, & Speidel, 2007). Scollie et al. (2005) provide a detailed discussion of DSLv5 pointing out that it was developed to avoid loudness discomfort for the hearing aid wearer, and to ensure audibility of conversational speech by making a wide range of speech input levels audible,

along with different target values for quiet versus noise environments.

Following determination of a child's hearing thresholds, it is important to account for differences in the size and shape of the ear canals. In fact, a key feature of the DSL formula is the application of ear canal acoustics based on probe microphone real-ear measurements for older children or real-ear-to-coupler (RECD) measures in infants. If it is difficult to obtain real-ear measures in both ears of an infant, it is possible to obtain the measurement for one ear and enter those values for use with the other ear (Bagatto et al., 2005).

The DSL prescription algorithm does not use data in the HL scale in its calculations. Instead, it converts HL data to ear canal SPL and plots the results as an SPL-o-Gram for easy comparison of the patient's thresholds to the hearing aid output. As the child's ear canal grows and changes natural resonance, the HL required to generate a given SPL in the ear canal will increase. But because direct measurement of ear canal SPL thresholds is not easily accomplished, procedures for predicting the ear canal SPL for audiometric procedures were developed. These procedures require the measurement of the child's real-ear-to-coupler difference (RECD) that is used as a part of the formula that converts HL to ear canal SPL. As the child's ear canal grows over time, the changes in ear canal acoustics result in decreases in individual RECD values. The audiometric thresholds and RECD values are used to derive coupler targets using either the NAL-NAL$_1$ or the DSLv5 software. Many real-ear systems support the measurement and application of the RECD so that couple-based or simulated real-ear verification can be conducted. This involves placing the BTE hearing aid on a 2-cc coupler and applying the RECD values to view the output of the hearing aid without the need to have the hearing aid placed on an infant's ear while adjustments are being made (Bagatto, 2013).

Frequency-specific threshold measurements should be obtained prior to the hearing aid fitting, preferably with the use of insert earphones. Depending on the age of the child, these measurements might be obtained through conditioning techniques, play audiometry, or tone burst frequency-specific ABR thresholds. Audiologists must be aware that behavioral thresholds are referenced to the decibel hearing level (dB HL) scale, whereas ABR thresholds are referenced to a "normalized" scale (nHL). Therefore, a correction factor must be applied to ABR obtained thresholds prior to entering them into the DSLv5 program. It is essential

that the audiologists performing the ABR be aware of the calibration procedures used for their measurement system and that the appropriate values in "nHL" or estimated "HL" be utilized in the DSLv5 hearing instrument fitting. These threshold values are entered into the software program to generate target values for setting the hearing aid characteristics (Bagatto et al., 2005). Figure 9–10 shows a sample representation of the DSL hearing aid fitting screen.

The success of using a prescriptive fitting formula in young infants was reviewed by Roush and Seewald (2009). They reported results from 70 infants with bilateral sensory hearing loss fitted with hearing aids referred from newborn hearing screening. For those

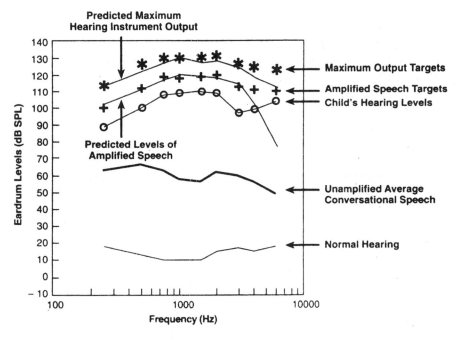

Figure 9–10. Overview of the DSL hearing aid fitting protocol displayed on a SPL-o-Gram. Note the maximum output targets and amplified speech targets. The required hearing aid gain is the difference between the average speech spectrum and the amplified speech targets. With permission from "Selecting and Verifying Hearing Aid Performance Characteristics for Children," by R. Seewald, M. Ross, and P. Stelmachowicz, 1987, *Journal of the Academy of Rehabilitative Audiology, 20,* pp. 25–38.

infants the median age at ABR testing was 2.6 months, the median age at hearing aid fitting was 3.9 months, and the median age when a frequency-specific behavioral audiogram was obtained for each ear was 8.5 months. Thus, the use of frequency-specific estimates of hearing thresholds obtained initially from ABR measures improved the age of hearing aid fitting in these infants by at least 4 months.

Lewis (1999) pointed out that: (a) children typically wear their hearing instruments at fixed settings; (b) careful consideration of the amplification characteristics selected are especially important for the child's acquisition of speech and language; (c) the amplification characteristics may be based on limited audiologic information; and (d) the age factors included in the DSL are important to consider in fitting amplification to children. It is crucial to routinely verify pediatric hearing aid fittings to determine their fit to prescribed targets for soft and conversational levels of speech as well as maximum output limits. The RECD should be remeasured routinely if possible and especially when there is an earmold change.

BINAURAL HEARING AIDS

It is not an uncommon question for parents to ask if it is really necessary for their child to use two hearing aids rather than just one. It is well recognized that there are many advantages to listening with two ears rather than one. In addition to the requirement for two hearing ears to localize sounds, listening with two ears enables better speech understanding in background noise or when there is reverberation in the environment. The critical need for optimal hearing by infants, toddlers, and children with bilateral hearing loss demands the use of binaural hearing aids. In fact, binaural fittings have become the standard of care for most pediatric patients (AAA, 2003). To be perfectly clear, all children should be fitted with binaural hearing aids whenever possible to maximize auditory potential. The fitting of binaural amplification with all children with hearing loss should prevail unless an absolute contraindication (such as total deafness in one ear) is determined. A binaural hearing aid system consists of two complete hearing aids worn simultaneously with one system in each ear. Fortunately, most third-party payers now recognize the importance of two hearing aids for hearing-impaired children to achieve their highest learning potentials.

It is generally agreed, as well as substantiated by extensive research, that two ears hear better than one; thus, two hearing aids are likewise better than one hearing aid. Despite the additional expense of two hearing aids, there are numerous advantages to using binaural hearing aids that make better listening for hearing-impaired users. In fact, there are at least three decades of overwhelming research support that two hearing aids provide better hearing performance than one hearing aid for persons with bilateral hearing loss. Mueller & Hawkins (1990) described three psychoacoustic advantages for binaural hearing aid users: binaural summation, elimination of head shadow, and binaural squelch.

When a sound is presented binaurally it is perceived louder than if the same sound is presented monaurally, a phenomenon known as *binaural summation*. Hawkins, Prosek, Walden, and Montgomery (1987) demonstrated that persons with bilateral sensorineural hearing loss have 6 to 10 dB of binaural summation. Dillon (2012) summarized that the binaural summation of loudness advantage ranges from around 3 dB at near threshold levels to a value in the range of 6 to 10 dB at higher levels. Loudness summation has significant benefit to hearing-impaired amplification users because they can have equivalent perceived loudness at lower volume control settings, thereby reducing gain distortion and feedback problems and prolonging battery life.

Head shadow, or head diffraction, describes the difference in reception of sound by both ears when the sound comes directly from one side. Thus, the head itself causes the sound waves to be diffracted as they reach the opposite ear. This head shadow effect occurs when an individual is wearing a single-side hearing aid and speech is presented from the nonaided side. Head shadow can attenuate the speech signal 6 to 12 dB as sound "bends" around the head to reach the opposite ear. According to Mueller and Hawkins (1990), the monaural hearing aid user may lose as much as 10 to 18 dB of gain compared with the binaural hearing aid wearer in the same situation due to the head shadow effect.

Binaural squelch is the term applied to the ability of the auditory system to diminish noise or reverberation more efficiently when input is received from two ears rather than one ear. The advantage provided by this phenomenon is to increase speech recognition in background noise for the binaural hearing aid user.

There are many other advantages from binaural hearing that affect our daily lives and listening situations. It is difficult to demonstrate empirically the improvement provided by binaural hearing aids versus a monaural fitting, especially in a traditional sound-treated test room environment. An array of loudspeakers must be carefully situated and calibrated, or an elaborate virtual computerized setup must be used to demonstrate binaural advantage on an individual patient. As audiologists have gained first-hand experience in dispensing, fitting, and managing patients with hearing aids, the improvement in speech recognition in noise provided by binaural hearing aids has proven the superiority of listening and the improved quality of sound (fidelity) with two ears rather than one ear.

The benefits of binaural hearing have been well documented over the years. The benefits include improved speech understanding in noise (Hawkins & Yacullo, 1984; Kobler & Rosenhall, 2002); improved localization of sound (Dreschler & Boymans, 1994); improved speech clarity and "balance" of hearing (Erdman & Sedge, 1981); and reduced listening effort (Noble, 2006). Boymans, Goverts, Kramer, Festen, and Dreschler (2008) conducted a prospective study of 214 patients in the Netherlands in an attempt to codify the benefits of bilateral hearing aids. During this study extensive testing with objective measures, functional tests of localization and speech discrimination in noise, as well as questionnaires were conducted with all subjects under unilateral and bilateral aided conditions. Their major summary was that despite the highly variable subject cohort used in this study, significant binaural benefit for speech intelligibility and sound localization was found across all subjects. Participants in the study overwhelmingly preferred the use of binaural hearing aids over a monaural hearing aid, leading the researchers to conclude that binaural fittings should be the choice for all individuals with bilateral aidable hearing loss.

Evidence from animal and human studies suggests that central auditory pathways do not develop normally in the absence of sound stimulation (Klinke, Kral, Heid, Tilleinj, & Hartmann, 1999; Kral, Hartmann, Tillein, Heide, & Klinke, 2000; Sharma et al., 2002). This premise provided another approach to understanding binaural hearing in intriguing research projects conducted by Silman, Gelfand, and Silverman (1984) and Gelfand (1987). These researchers attempted to evaluate the phenomenon of auditory deprivation in monaural and binaural aided adult subjects. The auditory performance of the subjects before their use of hearing aids was compared with their auditory performance after 4 to 5 years of hearing aid use. The most revealing finding was that the speech recognition scores remained stable in both ears of the binaurally fitted patients, whereas the unaided scores of the monaurally fitted patients showed a significant reduction over time, apparently the result of auditory deprivation. Later studies showed that the deprivation from lack of amplification could be overcome with resultant increase in speech understanding scores when amplification was added to the previously unaided ears (Boothroyd, 1993; Silverman & Emmer, 1993; Silverman & Silman, 1990). Children who experience long periods of auditory deprivation may be susceptible to large-scale reorganization of auditory cortical areas responsible for the perception of speech and language (Gilley, Sharma, Mitchell, & Dorman, 2010). These studies suggest that auditory function deteriorates in the unaided ears of patients with bilateral sensorineural hearing loss who use monaural hearing aid fittings. The results of these studies confirm the necessity of binaural hearing aids for children with bilateral hearing impairment.

In earlier decades, pediatric binaural hearing aids were limited to those children with bilaterally symmetrical hearing loss. However, with today's technologies, asymmetrical hearing loss is not a contraindication to binaural amplification. The challenge for the audiologist is to balance the performance of the two hearing aids until aided hearing symmetry is achieved. The use of computerized real-ear probe microphone measurements from each ear canal is critical to achieve symmetry in a binaural hearing aid fitting for a child with asymmetrical bilateral hearing loss.

FREQUENCY RESPONSE

Conventional hearing aids provide amplification for the frequency range between 200 and 7000 Hz depending on the quality of the components. The preferred frequency response limits for hearing aids in pediatric patients is still under discussion with only preliminary evidence-based research to provide answers. Some experts hypothesize that children need additional high-frequency gain because of the fact that speech recognition depends on perception of high-frequency phonemes; other experts argue that young children need additional low-frequency information because speech intonation and suprasegmental cues are important to the development of language.

There is no debate over the fact that children have a special need to hear high-frequency sounds as they have little experience to fill in the speech sounds that they miss with traditional amplification. Research suggests that children require audibility of a broad bandwidth of speech for optimal access to high-frequency speech cues and that hearing loss can impede normal development of affricate and fricative production (Moeller et al., 2007; Stelmachowicz, Pitman, Hoover, Lewis, & Moeller, 2004). It is recognized that high-frequency sounds are some of the most important components of spoken language; we know that children require greater audibility than adults; and that children are significantly affected by noise and reverberation (Neuman, Wroblewsi, Hajicek, & Rubinstein, 2010; Stelmachowicz, 2000). Galster, Valentine, Dundas, and Fitz (2011) pointed out that approximately 25% of the audible cures required for recognition of spoken language are above 3000 Hz (ANSI S3.5-1997). The highest frequency speech sound, the fricative /s/, is one of the most common consonant sounds in the English language. The peak energy of /s/ when spoken by a child or female talker falls between 6300 and 8300 Hz (Stelmachowicz et al., 2007) and ranges in level between 57 and 68 dB SPL (Behrens & Blumstein, 1988). For some children with sloping high-frequency hearing loss, conventional frequency amplification may not provide audibility for high-frequency speech sounds.

Efforts have been made over the years to "transpose" higher frequencies into the lower frequency spectrum with mixed results. Known as *frequency lowering* and *frequency transposition* as well as a variety of other terms, these techniques have traditionally been used with patients who have severe to profound hearing loss configurations where conventional hearing aids cannot provide enough high-frequency gain for adequate audibility. Proponents of frequency lowering hearing aids argue that it is of little value to provide amplification to areas where it is likely that no normal cochlear hair cells exist. Frequency lowering may be beneficial for improving audibility of high-frequency consonants and useful for self-monitoring of voice quality. Beyond speech recognition, frequency lowering may provide more natural perception of high-frequency environmental sounds.

Beck and Olsen (2008) suggested that improved digital processing power, along with advanced microphone and receiver technologies, can provide extended frequency bandwidth that may lead to better audibility, speech perception, and understanding, and even music appreciation.

Research evidence is emerging to support their viewpoint as Ricketts, Dittberner, and Johnson (2008) explored sound quality as it relates to degree and slope of hearing loss and hearing aid bandwidth in normal-hearing children and children with hearing loss. Their findings indicate that speech sounds up to 8000 Hz may be useful for maximal speech and language development in hearing-impaired children. Pittman (2008) found that normal-hearing and hearing-impaired children learned words significantly faster while listening to extended high-frequency bandwidths. In a convincing series of research studies, Stelmachowicz and colleagues (2001, 2004, 2007) have shown that children with hearing impairment performed better as signal bandwidth was increased to include higher frequency information. Accordingly, more hearing aid manufacturers are designing frequency lowering paradigms to shift high frequencies into lower frequency bands with applications aimed at pediatric hearing aid fittings. Certainly more research is needed to evaluate the different techniques of frequency lowering and the degrees and configurations of hearing loss in children likely to benefit from this technology (Glista et al., 2009; McCreery, 2010; Robinson, Baer, & Moore, 2007).

Developments in the microphone component of the hearing aid have extended both ends of the frequency reproduction range. Microphones are now available that are truly directional that amplify primarily sounds that are immediately in front of the hearing aid and at the same time attenuate sounds emitted from the sides or back of the listener. Directional microphones have been shown to increase the signal-to-noise relationship favorably for the listener resulting in improvement for the understanding of speech in noisy environments (Dillon, 2012).

Common wisdom supports the use of directional microphones in the hearing aids of school-aged children who are in daily classroom situations and may enjoy increased benefit from directional microphones as they face the teacher. However, consideration should be given to the importance of omnidirectional microphones in their hearing aids for picking up important incidental conversations, comments, and discussions from classmates around the classroom.

HEARING AID OUTPUT

The power output of the hearing aid is an important factor to consider in selecting hearing instruments for children with hearing loss. The maximum power output describes the decibel level of the greatest possible intensity that a hearing aid is capable of producing through amplification. The output range of the hearing aid fixes the minimum-to-maximum decibel levels of the receiver when sound enters the microphone. Nearly every modern hearing aid comes with some sort of proprietary compression circuit that may be programmed to automatically suppress loud sounds picked up by the hearing aid. In fact, many digital hearing instruments may provide more than one type of compression circuit to be selected by the audiologist.

Most of today's hearing aids are described as nonlinear; that is, they squeeze the range of amplified sounds to fit within the reduced dynamic range of an individual with sensorineural hearing loss without adding distortion. Generally, this is a good thing as it makes weak sounds audible, speech sounds comfortable, while intense sounds are loud without being uncomfortable. The term *automatic gain control* (AGC) describes certain compression circuits where the amount of gain is automatically determined by the signal level. Suffice it to say that the output limiting features of a compression program are particularly important in pediatric hearing aids to minimize loudness discomfort and prevent further damage to the auditory system while maximizing speech understanding (Dillon & Storey, 1998). Seewald, Ross, and Spiro (1985) pointed out that the selection of the hearing aid's power output must be high enough to provide adequate amplification without exceeding the saturation level frequently (which drives the hearing aid into compression mode), yet the maximum power output must not exceed the child's loudness discomfort level.

In terms of hearing aid output issues, the changing external ear canal volume in growing children presents special problems to the pediatric audiologist (Bentler, 1989). Children, from birth to the age of 9 years, experience a changing ear canal size as they mature. As the ear canals increase in volume, the output of the hearing aid may need to be increased to account for the lost intensity of the signal in the "larger" cavity. Thus, repeat real-ear-to-coupler (RECD) and probe microphone measures are necessary throughout the child's early years to evaluate hearing aid performance. The changing physical size and shape of the child's ear canals may result in underamplification in meeting target gains established within the prescription hearing aid fitting. For example, if the ear canal volume is increased by one-half, the sound pressure of the hearing aid can be decreased by as much as 6 dB.

Can Hearing Aids Damage Hearing?

Parents may worry that powerful hearing aids fitted to children may cause additional hearing damage due to overamplification.

Early studies were published showing that the use of powerful hearing aids may cause temporary and permanent threshold shift and result in further hearing loss (Macrae, 1968a, 1968b; Macrae & Farrant, 1965; Mills, 1975; Rintlemann & Bess, 1988). Of course, in those early years, there was literally no way to measure the hearing aid output in the ear canal, so audiologists had to be extremely cautious about the use of hearing aids that could provide maximal power output of 130 dB SPL. Coupled to a child's smaller ear canal, a power hearing aid could result in levels as high as 142 dB SPL. Today's real-ear probe microphone equipment easily and accurately can measure the overall sound pressure levels of the hearing aid amplification system directly in children's ear canals so that there is no excuse for "over fitting" at a level that could potentially effect the child's hearing.

Hearing aid technical specifications are reported in SPL as measured in a hard-walled 2-cc coupler. It can be expected that hearing aid sound pressures measured in a 2-cc cavity will be delivered to a child with an ear canal somewhat smaller than 2-cc. The smaller volume can create as much as 6 dB more intensity than shown on the standard hearing aid frequency response curve. A caution must be mentioned that infants with very small ear canal volumes of 0.5 cc or less may actually receive as much as 12 to 15 dB more output than shown on hearing aid technical specification sheets (Figure 9–11).

Safety for our pediatric patients must be our topmost concern. The maximum output of a hearing aid should be set within the confines of the pediatric prescriptive fitting program and measured with real-ear-to-coupler difference or directly determined with probe microphone measurement in the ear canal. The 2013 AAA Pediatric Amplification Guidelines suggest that if overamplification is suspected, monitoring of temporary threshold shift (TTS) by measuring audiometric thresholds before and after a day of hearing aid use is recommended. It is commonly accepted that recurrent TTS can lead to a permanent loss of hearing (PTS). Hearing aids fitted to children with severe-to-profound hearing impairment can potentially deliver damaging amplification to the ear; therefore, power output should be monitored routinely.

Compression circuits increase protection to the ear by limiting high-level inputs through the hearing aids. However, higher

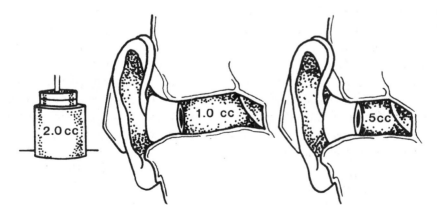

Figure 9–11. The volume of a child's ear canal is an important consideration relative to the 2-cc hearing aid specifications and the possibility of overamplification.

gain settings in excess of prescriptive targets could conceivably create additional hearing loss. Research has shown that personal amplification will not cause deterioration in hearing in the vast majority of clients if the hearing aids are set properly by the audiologist and used at safe volume settings. Parents should be warned, however, that if the hearing aids are used at volume settings higher than recommended, this increases the likelihood of TTS. Children who often use their aids during very noisy activities may be at increased risk of a noise-induced change in their hearing. In summary, a properly programmed, fitted, and maintained hearing aid will not damage hearing.

THE EARMOLD AND SOUND CHANNEL

The hearing aid sound channel consists of the ear hook, tube, and earmold through which passes the amplified sound into the child's ear canal. Hearing aid performance can be significantly enhanced or degraded with skillful application of coupling systems involving the earmold and the tubing. For example, by increasing the diameter of the end of the tube in the sound channel (known as a "horn") it increases the high-frequency response; a "reverse horn" occurs when the end of the tube becomes crimped and the high frequencies so needed by the young child will be rolled off. Today's audiologist must be cognizant of the various methods used to modify the hearing aid response without reprogramming the instrument. Gain levels and spectral modifications can be implemented to produce a uniform effect over the entire spectrum or to effect selective portions of the frequency ranges. Modifications to the hearing aid acoustic response can be influenced by a number of factors including the microphone location, frequency response adjustments, the earhook and tubing length, diameter, configuration and filter characteristics, the earmold shape and size, the seal or openness of the earmold (which can strongly influence low-frequency amplification), and the ear canal space between the tip of the earmold and the tympanic membrane. One of the most important electroacoustic characteristics of a hearing aid is the absence of "peaks and valleys" in the frequency-response curve.

The acoustic coupling of the hearing aid refers to the "plumbing" of the system (i.e., all of the external components that convey sound from the hearing aid itself into the ear canal of the user). With BTE hearing aids, the acoustic coupling refers to the earmold, tubing, and earhook. Audiologists must understand the importance of the acoustic coupling in modifying the performance of the hearing aid. Inadequate acoustic coupling efforts can essentially ruin the performance of even the best hearing aids. Today's feedback cancelation circuits permit more open ear canal couplings and some types of behind-the-ear hearing aids fitted without an earmold but with an open tube bent to fit into the external ear canal.

The earmold itself is an essential feature of the pediatric hearing aid system (Figure 9–12). It provides support for the hearing aid on or in the patient's external ear while directing the sound into the ear canal and, when properly fitted, prevents acoustic feedback. Because even minor variations in the fitting and configuration of the earmold can alter the electroacoustic parameters of the hearing aid, it is important to evaluate each hearing aid with the earmold that is to be used with it. This may require two or more sessions for fitting hearing aids on children—one session during which the earmold impression is obtained, and an additional session after the permanent cus-

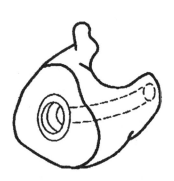

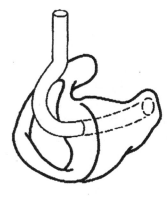

TYPICAL STANDARD MOLD   **TYPICAL SKELETON MOLD**

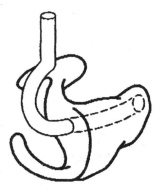

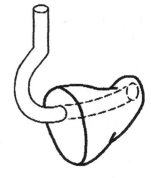

Figure 9–12. The earmold is an essential feature of the pediatric hearing aid system; basic full standard earmold, skeletal earmold, and canal earmold.

tom earmold has been fabricated. It is particularly problematic to conduct hearing aid evaluations with children using stock earmolds, because the stock earmolds often do not fit well in the child's ear canals and most certainly do not represent how the hearing aid will perform when the child has his or her own earmold. The pinna continues to grow and the concha changes shape until the child reaches approximately 9 years of age. Thus, earmolds and custom ITE hearing aids should routinely be reevaluated and remade every 3 to 6 months during the child's early years and once a year after age 5 to ensure satisfactory fit.

The earmold may be crafted in many ways (with open vents, various tubing, filters, and so on) to enhance the hearing aid. The most important factor about the earmold is that acoustic feedback must be prevented if the child is to obtain maximum benefit from the hearing aid. The material of the earmold is relatively insignificant in terms of the amplified acoustics. However, earmolds are made from a variety of different chemical compounds that dictate their properties of hardness, clarity, toxicity, water repellence, tensile strength, density, elasticity, and colors. The audiologist makes the choice of material and style for the fabricated earmold when submitting the ear impression to the manufacturer. The custom-made earmold can be ordered in hard or soft acrylic or a combination of both—hard on the external surface with a soft portion to fit in the ear canal. Soft silicone earmolds provide superior acoustic sealing properties for children and are generally nonallergenic. The choices for the style of the earmold are wide and varied, and require consideration of the degree of hearing loss, the size and shape of the pinna, and ear canal in the child. The style choices range from full-size earmolds used for children with severe and profound hearing loss, through a series of ever decreasing size earmolds, to half-shell molds and much smaller and lighter skeletal earmolds used for children with mild and moderate hearing loss. Open earmolds are also an option for children with good hearing in the low frequencies and high-frequency hearing loss. Canal earmolds are the smallest style but often cannot be securely retained in the small child's ear canal. All earmolds can be ordered with small vent holes to allow air to pass into the ear canal and to avoid discomfort from a totally occluding earmold. However, venting the earmold will likely drop the real ear sound pressure level of the amplification at the tympanic membrane.

MONITORING CHILDREN'S HEARING AIDS

Persons working with children who use hearing aids are familiar with the wide variety of occurrences and bizarre experiences that can render the hearing aid inoperable. Just because a child wears his or her hearing aid faithfully every day, the assumption cannot be made that the aid is functioning adequately. In the analysis of hearing aids in use

and worn by children, it is not uncommon to find that the hearing aids are not working to their original specifications. It is strongly recommended that each child's amplification units receive regular longitudinal electroacoustic analysis. Potts and Greenwood (1983) described a daily hearing aid monitoring program, the results of which created a significant decrease in the incidence of hearing aid malfunction in their school. The program was based on a detailed visual-auditory inspection (Table 9–1) and routine electroacoustic analysis. The Education for All Handicapped Children Act of 1975 (Public Law 94-142) states that each public agency shall ensure that those hearing aids worn by hearing-impaired students in school are functioning properly (*Federal Register,* August 23, 1977, 121a.303).

PEDIATRIC COCHLEAR IMPLANTS

One of the most dramatic and exciting developments in hearing and deafness has been the cochlear implant (CI). The idea of providing hearing to profoundly deaf patients by artificially stimulating the sensory system has progressed from a futuristic possibility to reality. A cochlear implant is a surgically implanted electronic system that provides a sense of sound to those who are profoundly deaf and cannot benefit from using hearing aids. No other development during the past century has had such an enormous impact on the habilitation of infants and young children with profound deafness. The goal of the cochlear implant in young children is to facilitate the development of spoken language and to provide sufficient hearing for better understanding of speech (AAA, 2009c). A hearing aid provides amplified sound to the ear, but the CI

Table 9–1. Total Looking/Listening Check for Hearing Aids

Component	Looking	Listening (use sounds /a/, /u/, /i/, /ʃ/, /s/)
Remove aid from child, noting "as worn" volume setting		
Earmold	Opening clear? Cracks, rough areas?	
Battery	Read voltage—compartment clean?	
Case	Cracks? Separating?	Press case gently—interruption in amplification?
Microphone	Clean? Visible damage?	
Dials	Clean? Easily rotated?	Rotate—reasonable gain variation: static?
Switches	Clean? Easy to move?	Turn on and off—static?
Tubing (ear-level aid)	Cracks? Good connection to mold and aid? Moisture? Debris?	Cover opening of earmold and turn to maximum gain—feedback?
Oscillator (bone conduction aid)	Cracks? Plug clean? Attached well to band?	Listen with oscillator on mastoid, ears plugged to block air-conducted sound
Variable controls	Proper OSPL90, frequency response, gain setting?	Speech sounds clearly amplified? Gain sounds normal for this hearing aid?
Distortion		Clear quality?
Feedback	Recheck receiver snap, tubing, earmold	Turn to maximum gain to check—external feedback? Internal?
Replace aid and check fit of the earmold to the child's ear		

Source: From "Hearing Aid Monitoring," by P. Potts & J. Greenwood, 1983, *Language, Speech and Hearing Services in Schools, 14*, p. 163.

delivers electrical stimulation to the VIIIth nerve. The quality of sound provided by the CI is somewhat different from natural hearing with less acoustic information transmitted up through the auditory pathways and processed by the brain. Many patients are able to hear and understand speech and environmental sounds, hear better in noise, enjoy television and music, and even use the telephone. The use of cochlear implants has proven to improve communication skills in children with severe to profound sensorineural hearing loss who have shown little or no auditory benefit from the use of conventional hearing aids (Figure 9–13).

The cochlear implant is a highly technical, surgically inserted device that delivers electrical stimulation directly to the VIIIth cranial nerve, sending impulses through the ascending auditory pathways directly to the cortex. A cochlear implant relies on the fact that many auditory nerve fibers remain viable in patients with sensorineural deafness. The surviving neurons of the VIIIth nerve can be stimulated to excitation by applying external electric currents of the proper strength, duration, and orientation, resulting in actively propagating neural impulses. These evoked electrical neural potentials arrive at the temporal lobes of the cortex just like the normal neural impulses generated by acoustic signals that intact cochlear

hair cells transduce. The brain interprets these artificial induced potentials as sound (Figure 9–14).

The initial single-channel CIs used in the early 1980s achieved only limited hearing success. The much improved performance of multichannel cochlear implants resulted in approval by the U.S. Food and Drug Administration (FDA) in 1984 for implantation in adults. In 1990 the FDA lowered the approved age for CIs to 2 years, then to 18 months in 1998, and finally 12 months in 2000. In 2000, the FDA also decreased the threshold degree of residual hearing for pediatric candidates for CI. This change allowed children with severe to profound hearing loss, who could correctly identify 30% to 40% of words or sentences presented in auditory-only conditions to be considered for implant technology. Gifford (2012) suggests that the FDA is overdue to establish new indicators for pediatric cochlear

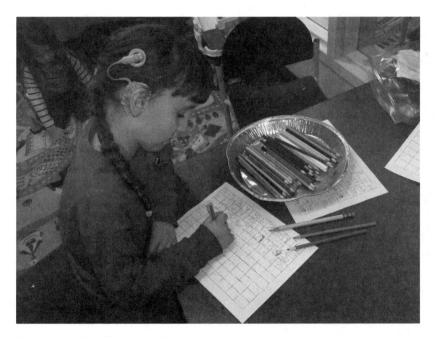

Figure 9–13. Cochlear implants have provided new and improved hearing opportunities for children with profound hearing loss. Photo courtesy of H.O.P.E. Preschool, Spokane, WA.

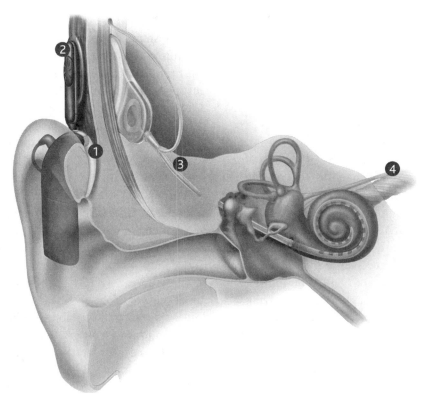

Figure 9–14. Cross section of head with internal and external cochlear implant parts in place. **1.** A sound processor worn behind the ear captures sound and turns it into digital code. The sound processor has a battery that powers the entire system. **2.** The sound processor transmits the digitally coded sound through the coil on the outside of the head to the implant. **3.** The implant converts the digitally coded sound into electrical impulses and sends them along the electrode array placed in the cochlea (the inner ear). **4.** The implant's electrodes stimulate the VIIIth nerve that then sends the impulses to the brain where they are interpreted as sound. Images courtesy of Cochlear Americas ©2013 (http://www.cochlear.com/wps/wcm/connect/intl/home/understand/hearing-and-hl/hl-treatments/cochlear-implant).

implants. Based on current research results, Gifford states that it is likely that the FDA criteria in the near future will include children as young as 9 months of age. Over time, the criteria for cochlear implant candidacy have become less stringent, and implants are being provided for individuals with greater amounts of residual hearing (Gifford, 2011). As of 2013, approximately 250,000 people worldwide have received cochlear implants with the vast majority in developed countries due to the high cost of the device, surgery, and postimplantation therapy. In the United States, approximately 50,000 adults and 30,000 children are CI recipients.

The cochlear implant devices consist of external and internal components. The external components consist of one or more microphones that pick up sound from the environment, a speech processor that selectively filters sounds to prioritize audible speech, splits the sound into channels, and sends the electrical sound signals through a thin cable to the transmitter (Figure 9–15). The transmitter is held in position by a magnet placed behind the external ear, and transmits power and the processed sound signals through the skin to the internal device by electromagnetic induction. The internal components include a receiver and stimulator that are drilled into the mastoid bone behind the pinna and placed beneath the skin. The receiver and stimulator convert the signals into electric impulses and deliver them through a thin internal cable to an array of up to 24 electrodes wound through the cochlea. These electrodes, when stimulated electrically, send the impulses to the nerves in the scala tympani and then

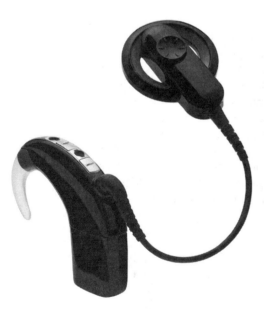

Figure 9–15. Cochlear implant processor in behind-the-ear case with magnetic transducer. Images courtesy of Cochlear Americas ©2013 (http://www.cochlear.com/wps/wcm/connect/intl/home/understand/hearing and-hl/hl-treatments/cochlear-implant).

directly to the brain through the auditory nerve system. There are a number of manufacturers of cochlear implants, and each one produces a different implant and different speech processing system coupled with a different number of electrodes. Typically, the number of channels is not a primary factor upon which a manufacturer is chosen; the signal processing algorithm is also another important block.

Throughout the 1990s, the CI external components that had been worn on the body grew smaller and smaller due to continued developments in miniaturizing electronics. Today most school-age children use a small behind-the-ear (BTE) speech processor about the size of a power hearing aid that is water-resistant and available in color preferences. As advanced programs are developed, most CI speech processors are upgradable without additional surgical intervention.

Loeb (1985a, 1985b) described the operation of the CI as follows: the loudness of the sound perceived depends roughly on the number of nerve fibers and their rates of firing as stimulated by the electrode array inserted into the cochlea. Both variables are functions of the amplitude of the stimulus current. The perceived pitch of sound is related to the place on the basilar membrane from which those nerve fibers once derived their acoustic input, in agreement with the place-pitch theory. In principle, with enough independent channels of stimulation, each controlling the activity of a small, local area and subset of the auditory nerve fibers, one could recreate the normal neural response to acoustic stimuli of any spectral composition. The brain then learns, or relearns, to process that information, and the subject "hears" the sounds.

When one ear is implanted but the other ear has sufficient residual hearing to use a hearing aid, it is called *bimodal.* The expanding FDA criteria have led to an increased number of patients who can now benefit from cochlear implantation including the use of bimodal fittings. Every child who receives a CI in one ear and has residual hearing in the opposite hear should be fitted with a hearing aid in that ear to provide bilateral stimulation. Bilateral hearing stimulation is critical whenever possible to encourage auditory development and to benefit from bilateral hearing benefits.

The "hybrid" cochlear implant uses a short electrode insertion rather than the traditional deep insertion. The hybrid cochlear implant is used to preserve hearing where possible and may also be used with a conventional hearing aid in the opposite ear. Hybrid electrode designs are being investigated to minimize trauma to the cochlea and preserve residual hearing with a short electrode array composed of six half band electrodes to ensure that the electrodes are as thin as possible. With modifications to the implant and external sound processors, successful aural rehabilitation can be provided for patients who were previously considered poor implant candidates. They can now be implanted without as much risk of loss to remaining residual hearing.

Approximately 70% of all children with cochlear implants actually use two implant devices to achieve binaural hearing (i.e., one CI for each ear). In fact, bilateral cochlear implants have become the "standard of care" for pediatric patients in the United States. For children, the binaural advantages achieved by two CIs include improved sound localization and improved understanding of speech in background noise. Perhaps more important are the effects of binaural redundancy and summation. Bilateral CIs result in signals being louder and the child "hearing" softer sounds when listening with both ears rather than one ear. When both CIs are implanted during the same surgery session, we speak of *simulta-*

neous implants; *sequential* implants occur when a second CI is implanted some time following the first implants. These surgery options depend on the preference of the surgeon or decisions made by the cochlear implant team. For children, the sequential procedures seem to be the more common and preferred surgical approach.

Of course, it is important to weigh the benefits of bilateral cochlear implants in children over the traditional unilateral implant because of the increased risk of a second surgery as well as the overall cost of two implants versus one device. Tait et al. (2010) conducted an international study of unilateral versus bilateral cochlear implantation in 69 children who received their implants prior to 3 years of age: 42 children had unilateral implants, and 27 children were bilaterally implanted. The preverbal and postverbal skills of the children were measured before implantation and 1 year after implantation by video analysis. Before implantation there was no difference in communication skills between the two groups. At 12 months following implantation, there was no significant difference in vocal autonomy; however, the bilaterally implanted group had better vocal turn-taking and nonlooking vocal turns, while the unilateral group of children showed more "gestural" autonomy. The conclusions of the study were that profoundly deafened, bilaterally implanted children are significantly more likely to use vocalization to communicate, and to use audition when communicating with adults when compared to the unilateral implanted children. These findings were independent of age of implantation and length of deafness.

The implant surgery takes between 1 and 2 hours under general anesthesia to insert the internal parts of the CI and another hour or two in the recovery suite. The surgery involves an incision in the skin behind the ear, and drilling a small depression in the mastoid bone to create a pocket for the receiver/stimulator. The drilling continues into the inner ear where the electrode array is threaded carefully into the cochlea. The patient normally goes home the same day or the day after the surgery. The operation typically destroys some or all of the residual hearing the patient may have in the implanted ear; as a result, some otologists advise single-ear implantation, saving the other for a second CI or in the event a more advanced treatment becomes available in the future.

Following 3 to 4 weeks for healing of the surgical incision, the patient is then fitted with the system's external parts (i.e., microphone(s) and speech processor). It is time to turn on and program the external equipment and initial stimulation of the device. This is a crucial and important time for the parents and the deaf child as shown in Figure 9–16. The implant creates an electrical field that directly stimulates the auditory nerve. The implanted array delivers biphasic stimulus current pulses between any pair of electrodes or between any one electrode and the remaining linked electrodes. The internal implanted electrodes and the external speech processor system need to be connected and turned on in a process known as *mapping*. This procedure is conducted to ensure that each electrode is "tuned" to fit the specific hearing loss pattern of the patient. The device is programmed through a sophisticated computerized system, usually based on audiologic behavioral hearing responses from the newly implanted patient. Mapping is conducted by an audiologist to determine how much current is required for the patient to hear sounds easily without discomfort. The mapping process can be repeated, and adjusted if necessary; during the first few

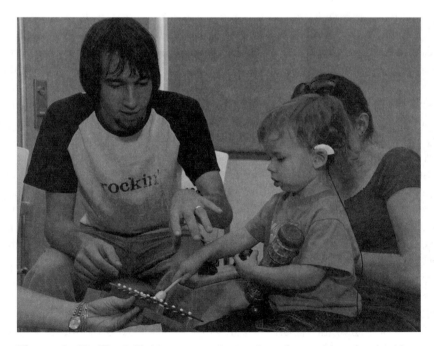

Figure 9–16. The initial turn on and mapping of a cochlear implant is a family affair. Photo courtesy of Colorado Children's Hospital, Aurora, CO.

months, repeated mapping may be desired or necessary. If changes in hearing occur over time, or as newer speech-processing algorithms are developed, the speech processor and electrodes can be reprogrammed as many times as needed with no disturbance to the implanted system or the patient. Typically, the audiologist is the cochlear implant team member responsible for programming the implant device to the individual child's needs. The audiologist sets the minimum and maximum current level outputs for each electrode in the array based on the user's reports of loudness. The audiologist also selects the appropriate speech-processing strategy and program parameters for the user.

Special procedures are taught to each child, before implant placement, to serve for initial programming and later fine-tuning of the speech processor. Preliminary to the CI surgery, training is instituted to teach the young deaf child to give reliable, time-locked behavioral responses to discrete electrical stimulation of the electrodes. It is possible to teach young children to respond to electrode threshold levels (T-levels), to establish loudness comfort levels across frequency (C-levels), and to comprehend loudness concepts to determine effective electrical dynamic range (Firszt & Reeder, 1996). Once children have experience listening to sound through the implant, they can be taught to perform loudness scaling to assess loudness growth relative to electrical current levels for each electrode. Before the initiation of the children's implant study program, concern was expressed by professionals that deaf children could not be taught to respond to such subtle differences in the acoustic stimuli necessary to program the multichannel cochlear implant. It is to the credit of the skilled audiologists involved in these early children's implant programs that techniques were successfully developed, even with the youngest of deaf

children, to measure the various psychophysical parameters necessary for the accurate programming of the cochlear implant.

Children who receive cochlear implants require ongoing audiological management and otolaryngological follow-up. Ongoing management by an audiologist includes programming the implant parameters and monitoring device performance from electrical threshold and dynamic range data. Electrically evoked auditory brainstem responses (EABR), middle latency responses (MLR), or acoustic reflexes (EART) may be needed intraoperatively with stimuli delivered to the cochlear implant prior to leaving the operating room or postoperatively on an outpatient basis to facilitate the fitting process. These objective measures can be particularly useful in children who are either difficult to condition or otherwise unable to respond consistently to the electrical stimuli used to program the speech processor. Follow-up audiological evaluations are required to assess improvement in sound and speech detection and auditory reception of speech following implantation. Medical evaluation by an otolaryngologist should be performed as needed to monitor the postoperative course and medical status of the child.

Selection of Pediatric CI Candidates

There are a number of factors that determine the degree of success to expect from the operation and the device itself. Only selected children benefit from cochlear implants, in particular those with profound deafness who have defective sensory elements (hair cells) in the cochlea with surviving intact fibers of the auditory (VIIIth) nerve. Cochlear implant centers determine implant candidacy on an individual basis and take into account a person's hearing history, cause of hearing loss, amount of residual hearing, speech recognition ability, and overall health status. There are also specific considerations from surgeons and the CI manufacturers (Gifford, 2013). In general, young children must have audiometric results that confirm severe to profound sensorineural hearing loss, demonstrate failure to reach certain defined speech-language milestones as measured on standardized age-appropriate tests, and fail to show auditory skills progress with appropriately fitted amplification accompanied with intensive therapy over a period of 3 to 6 months. These important criteria provide the evidence that if a child can successfully benefit from the use of hearing aids, he or she is not a candidate for surgical cochlear implantation. Therapy for children wearing cochlear implants is a long-term process (Figure 9–17).

The audiologist is responsible for evaluating the hearing aid benefit obtained by the candidate in terms of: (a) aided thresholds with conventional hearing aids relative to aided results reported for multichannel cochlear implant users, including aided results in the high frequencies at which important consonant cures occur; and (b) performance on word recognition tasks, administered with auditory cues only in a closed- or open-response set (American Academy of Audiology, 1995). Radiographic evidence of ossification of the inner ear may justify a shorter trial with hearing aids and therapy and a younger age for implantation.

Patients with onset of deafness from birth to 2 years of age are considered to be prelinguistically deafened; those patients with an onset of deafness from 2 to 4 years of age are considered to be perilinguistically deafened; and patients deafened after 4 years of age are considered postlinguistically deafened.

In 1995, the NIH Consensus Panel recognized that cochlear implants had been successful in meningitic pediatric patients and therefore approved implantation in younger

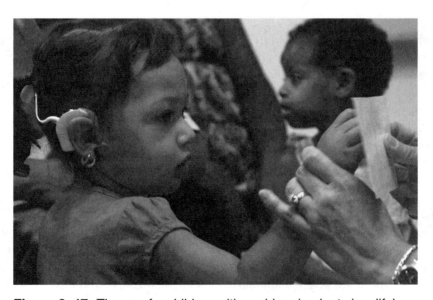

Figure 9–17. Therapy for children with cochlear implants is a lifelong process. Photo courtesy of Colorado Children's Hospital, Aurora, CO.

children in part to overcome the risk of new bone formation from postmeningitic infection that might preclude implantation at a later date. Although improvements in speech perception, speech production, and language acquisition in children are often reported as primary benefits, the NIH Panel noted that performance variability across children is substantial. Using tests of pattern perception, closed-set word identification, and open-set perception, the performance of children with implants generally increases each year after implantation.

As a part of the selection of pediatric candidates for cochlear implantation, a number of contradictors are also carefully evaluated to exclude those patients with hearing loss due to auditory nerve or central auditory pathway disorders, active external and middle ear infections, as well as those with tympanic membrane perforations, cochlear ossification that prevents electrode insertion, and allergy or intolerance of device materials. The cochlear implant team also must consider the child's cognitive ability to use auditory cues and the family's willingness to commit to an extended program of habilitation for their child as part of the preimplant evaluation program. Because of the concern and need for thorough evaluations of pediatric candidates for cochlear implants, only implant centers with an active children's cochlear implant team (composed of and experienced group including an otologist, audiologist, speech/language pathologist, auditory-verbal therapist, psychologist, deaf educator, and pediatrician) can perform the surgery and carry out the critical extensive follow-up. One of the most important components of the cochlear implant procedure is the ongoing, follow-up habilitation, with close coordination among parents, educators, therapists, and the implant center staff.

As with so many other aspects of childhood deafness, the role of the family is tantamount. Part of the pediatric candidacy evaluation includes interviews with the parents or caregivers to ensure postsurgical commitment to the necessary therapy needed by the child to ensure optimal aural habilitation. It should be apparent that the family accepts and understands the child's hearing loss, has knowledge about speech and language development, displays high motivation and willingness to be responsible for the child's educational needs, communicates well and often with the child, holds appropriate expectations relative to the cochlear implant, spends ample time with the child, and is committed to helping the child develop speech and language skills.

Although the impact of the cochlear implant in children with deafness has been lauded as exceptional, the literature on pediatric patients also notes significant individual differences in success among implanted children. Some prelinguistically deafened children do exceptionally well with their cochlear implants and progress to acquire spoken language and produce intelligible speech. Other prelinguistic children, however, develop only an awareness of sound and never appear to acquire language fully or produce intelligible speech to the same degree or proficiency as the exceptionally good users (Pisoni, 2000). The minimal criteria for pediatric patient selection for cochlear implantation are summarized in Table 9–2. The recommended minimum age constraint of 12 months is imposed not for technical surgical considerations, but rather to permit sufficient time to establish the diagnosis of deafness, with full audiologic information and hearing aid performance evaluation.

Studies of multichannel cochlear implants in the pediatric population have

Table 9–2. Minimum Requirements for Children for Cochlear Implants

Minimum 12 months of age
Bilateral, profound, sensorineural deafness
Completion of all pre-evaluation procedures
No additional handicaps that might adversely affect potential success with the implant
Strong evidence of family support
Satisfactory progress in auditory development not being made despite effective training and appropriately fitted hearing aids
Positive evaluations and agreement from cochlear implant team and child's family

shown positive postoperative speech perception and speech production results in children with congenital deafness, prelingual deafness, and acquired postlingual deafness (Eisenberg, 2009). All children, especially those implanted at a young age, demonstrated improvement in sound detection and in their auditory perception skills following implantation. Research has shown that children with multichannel cochlear implants achieved performance levels that exceeded those of their nonimplanted peers who used other sensory aids, including conventional hearing aids. Studies also have shown improvement in speech production skills and overall speech intelligibility in children with prelingual deafness. Improvements in auditory speech recognition and speech production occur over a several year time course in prelingually deafened children who have received implants. There are large individual differences in the benefit that children derive from multichannel cochlear implants due to factors such as age at onset of deafness, age at implantation, amount of cochlear implant experience, and educational training environment.

Cochlear Implant Benefits

In the early years, the use of cochlear implants in children raised concerns related to the long-term effects of the implant in the child's body. Yet it was agreed among professionals that maximum benefit afforded by these surgically implanted devices, if successful, would be most valuable to young deaf children in their quest to learn speech and develop social communication skills. In 1995, the National Institutes of Health (NIH) sponsored a national consensus conference on cochlear implants to summarize current knowledge on the benefits and limitations of the devices as well as technical and safety issues. The panel concluded that cochlear implantation definitely improves communication abilities in the majority of children, although outcomes are more variable than noted in adults. Nonetheless, gradual, steady improvement in speech perception, speech production, and language does occur following implantation throughout the educational years. The panel noted that access to optimal educational and habilitation services is critical for children to maximize the benefits available from cochlear implantation.

It is important to point out again that the amount of benefit from the cochlear implant varies greatly among children. The CI provides more high-frequency sounds to the user than most traditional hearing aids which creates improved access to speech cues. Nonetheless, children wearing cochlear implants will still have difficulties in the classroom with background noise and in understanding rapid speech communications unless the CI is equipped for FM reception. A child's ability to use the cochlear implant for communication is dependent on a variety of factors including the amount of time the device is used each day, the extent to which sound is integrated meaningfully into the child's daily life, the habilitation services the child receives, the degree of parental involvement and support, the degree of remaining auditory nerve survival, the duration of the deafness, and the age at implantation. In general, children with successful cochlear implants show a significant increase in speech intelligibility and speech perception as well as continued growth and increases in receptive and expressive language. Nonetheless, there are no preimplant predictors of outcome, as many of the child's educational abilities emerge after implantation. Different children, of course, have different styles and rates of learning. The nature of their early experience with auditory perception, if any, impacts their long-term outcomes. Most research studies have confirmed that early access to auditory information is critical to the development of spoken language, and superior results with CIs have been noted in orally trained children.

Ann Geers has conducted a masterful body of research in which she has followed 181 children with cochlear implants to document the characteristics of the children, their families, and their educational environments (Geers; 2003, 2006; Geers & Brenner, 2003). The children all received their CIs between the ages of 2 and 5 years. Prior to implantation the children demonstrated profound, bilateral hearing loss with no ability to understand speech presented in auditory-only conditions. Educational environment data included classroom placement, communication mode used, and individual intervention. Family factors included socioeconomic status, family size, education level of mother, and parental involvement in educational programs. Data on the children included age of first identification for hearing aids, preimplant residual hearing, duration of implant use, and presence of multiple disabilities.

Geers (2003) reported that by the ages of 8 and 9 years, more than 50% of the children scored within the average range for their ages on standardized reading measures. Moreover, levels of reading were associated with higher nonverbal intelligence, higher family socioeconomic status, female gender, and late onset of deafness. After accounting for these factors, reading proficiency was associated with mainstream educational placement, use of updated CI technology, and cognitive processing skills such as longer memory spans. Reading proficiency was highly predicted by level of language competence and speech production skills (Geers, 2006). Her studies concluded that a most important factor in a child's success with the CI depends on placement in an educational environment that provides a consistent emphasis on developing speech, auditory, and spoken language skills. In her studies, all performance outcomes were significantly higher for CI children in educational situations that emphasized listening and speaking.

Geers continued following this same cohort of children through their high school years, although her study sample had diminished to 112 children—albeit still a substantial study group (Geers, Tobey, & Moog, 2011). The goal of this longitudinal research effort was to learn whether the children's language and reading skills, which were close to those of age-mates with normal hearing in elementary grades, kept pace with normal development or fell further behind those of normal-hearing peers by their high school years. Results indicate that substantial development continued into adolescence for all outcomes measured. More than half of the teenagers achieved scores on language, reading, and psychosocial measures that were within 1 SD of normal-hearing age-mates. The authors note that the benefits of more recently implanted children, including advanced implant technology, auditory input from a CI before the age of 2 years, and significant amounts of preimplant amplified residual hearing, suggest that when the current population of CI children with these advantages reaches adolescence, even more of them may exhibit age-appropriate outcome scores. This body of research has shown remarkable performance outcomes for the CI children, substantiating and raising the expectation levels of what can be achieved by deaf children (Moog & Geers, 2003).

The important conclusions derived from analyzing results from this nationwide sample of adolescents with profound SNHL who used a CI since their preschool years are summarized as follows:

1. Speech perception, speech intelligibility, language, literacy, and psychosocial adjustment far exceeded that reported for similar groups before the advent of CI technology.
2. Group mean scores for language, reading, and social adjustment were generally within one standard deviation of normative samples of typically developing classmates with normal hearing.
3. Performance of children in early elementary grades (ages 8 to 9 years) was highly predictive of their relative standing in high school.
4. Children in the early elementary grades who relied on spoken language (as indicated by receiving no benefit from manual signs) exhibited better verbal rehearsal skills and higher levels of speech perception, speech intelligibility, language, and literacy in high school.

Sensitive Period for Cochlear Implantation in Children

Anu Sharma and her colleagues have studied the premise that maturation of the auditory pathways is an important factor in the development of speech and language skills in children. They use the latency and morphology of the P^1 cortical auditory evoked response, which varies as a function of chronological age, to be representative of early auditory maturation (Figure 9–18). It is well established that there are critical or sensitive periods for the neurobiological development in the brain, and Sharma's research has clearly identified the sensitive periods for cochlear implantation to achieve optimal results. One of her goals was to establish norms for the P^1 cortical auditory evoked waveform to serve as objective biomarkers to help clinicians reach decisions whether the presurgical amplification trial for children with hearing loss provides sufficient stimulation for development of auditory pathways (Sharma & Dorman, 2005; Sharma, Nash, & Dorman, 2009; Sharma et al., 2005). Using the same P^1 biomarker technique, clinicians would also be able to monitor the maturation of central auditory pathways following cochlear implantation.

Sharma and Dorman (2005b) reported P^1 response latencies from 104 congenitally deaf children who had been fit with cochlear implants at ages ranging from 1.3 years to 17.5 years of age and used them for at least 6 months. They compared the P^1 latencies in the CI children with age-matched normal-hearing peers. Their results revealed that implanted children with the longest period of auditory deprivation prior to implantation (7 or more years) had abnormal cortical response latencies to speech stimuli. In contrast to the late implanted group, the children implanted following the shortest period of auditory deprivation (approximately 3.5 years or less) showed normal P^1 latency waveforms (Figure 9–19). This important finding suggests that there is a critical period of 3.5 years during which the central auditory system is maximally plastic and that implantation prior to this time will

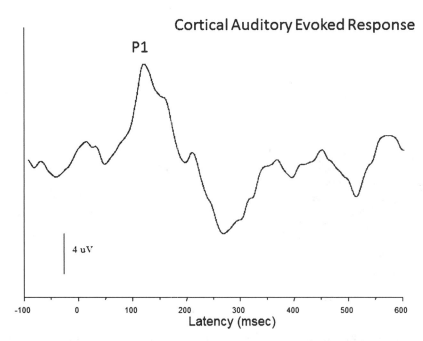

Figure 9–18. Representative waveform of the P[1] auditory cortical response with peak between 100 and 300 msec. Because the latency of the P[1] decreases with chronological age, the P[1] response can be used as a biomarker to plot the maturation of the auditory pathways (Sharma & Dorman, 2005).

result in age-appropriate cortical responses to sound within months after implantation (Sharma et al., 2002, 2009). It is of interest that this critical cutoff period coincides closely with reports from other researchers that children implanted under 3 to 4 years of age show significantly better speech perception and language skills compared to children implanted after ages 6 to 7 years (Kirk et al., 2002).

Figure 9–20 shows the 95% confidence interval for the normal development of P[1] latencies from Sharma et al. (2002). Superimposed on the normal limits boundaries is posted results from a child fitted with hearing aids at 2 months of age revealing a significantly delayed P[1] response latency. With no improvement in the P[1] latency at 13 months of age following 11 months of hearing aid use, the indications are that the use of amplification has not provided

the acoustic stimulation necessary for central auditory development. Following cochlear implantation, improvement in the P[1] latency can be seen as early as 1 month post-CI fitting. Continued rapid and large improvements in the P[1] latency are noted by 6 months of cochlear implant use, thus bringing the child's P[1] peak latency into normal limits (Sharma & Dorman, 2005).

The importance of this research cannot be overstated. We now have an objective clinical procedure for determining effectiveness of hearing aids and cochlear implants in young children. The P[1] response is a robust positive peak occurring at around 100 to 300 msec in children, and likely reflects the sum of synaptic delays throughout the peripheral and central auditory pathways (Eggermont, Ponton, Don, Waring, & Kwong, 1997). Sharma and her colleagues (2002) established a normal range for the

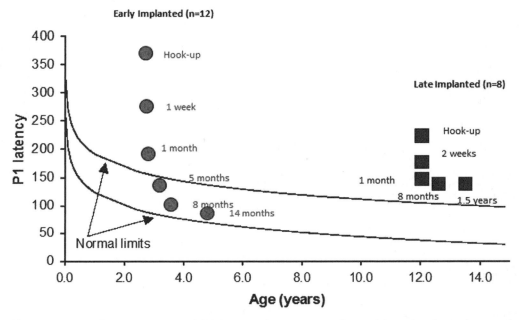

Figure 9–19. A comparison of PI latency between early cochlear implantation and late implantation in children. Note that the plasticity of the central auditory pathways is greatly reduced in the late implanted children (Sharma, Dorman, & Spahr, 2002; Sharma et al., 2005).

latency of the P^1 waveform peak at different ages: a newborn can be expected to have a P^1 peak latency of around 300 msec; by 3 years of age the P^1 peak latency has decreased to about 125 msec; adults have a P^1 latency of around 60 msec. In summary, Sharma and Dorman concluded that identification of the P^1 latency as measured through routine auditory cortical evoked potential techniques is a powerful tool of central auditory development. When combined with traditional behavioral measures of audiological speech and language assessment, P^1 latencies can provide information relative to the question of whether or not to provide a child with a cochlear implant following an appropriate hearing aid trial. Furthermore, this biomarker can be used to monitor the development of central auditory pathways after the child has been fitted with a cochlear implant (Figure 9–20).

Success With Cochlear Implants

Shortly following implantation, performance may be broadly comparable to that of some children with hearing aids. Over time, implant performance may improve to match that of children who are highly successful hearing aid users. Children who undergo implantation at younger ages are on average more accurate in their production of consonants, vowels, intonation, and rhythm. Speech produced by children with implants is more accurate than speech produced by children with comparable hearing losses using other devices. One year after implantation, speech intelligibility is twice that typically reported for children with profound hearing impairments and continues to improve with time. Oral language development in deaf children with cochlear

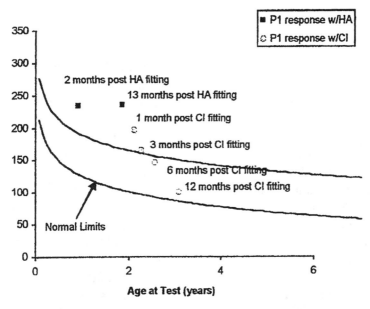

Figure 9–20. Case study showing how the cortical auditory evoked potential (P[1]) can serve as an objective clinical indicator of auditory maturation in a child who showed no auditory progress with hearing aids followed by rapid developmental progress with cochlear implant. Reprinted from "The Clinical Use of P1 Latency as a Bio-marker for Assessment of Central Auditory Development in Children With Hearing Impairment," A. Sharma and M. Dorman, 2005, *Audiology Today, 17*(3), pp. 18–19, with permission from American Academy of Audiology.

implants remains a slow, training-intensive process.

In general, children with acquired deafness are better candidates for cochlear implants than children with congenital deafness; children who have been deaf for only a short time do better with cochlear implants than children who have been deaf for an extended length of time; and deaf children from auditory-oral educational training backgrounds are more likely to achieve success with a cochlear implant than deaf children from total communication (manual) educational settings. When clinically appropriate, the poorer ear is always selected for implantation, as surgical placement of the device will result in complete loss of hearing in the implanted ear. These general guidelines have proven useful in counseling parents and educators about the relative potential for a child's success with a cochlear implant.

Pediatric cochlear implant users require training and therapy to maximize the benefits that they receive from their devices. Rehabilitation should focus on the development of a wide range of listening behaviors within meaningful communicative contexts. Ideally, there should be close interaction between the audiologist at the implant center, the clinician who provides rehabilitative services, and educators working on a day-to-day basis with the child. For a child to realize optimal benefit from a multichannel cochlear implant, school educators should have an understanding of device function and maintenance, as well as an appropriate level of expectation regarding the child's abilities, limitations, and expected progress with the implant.

Geers and Moog (1994) compared the use of traditional hearing aids, vibrotactile aids, and cochlear implants in matched triad sets of children with hearing impairment. Analysis of data showed that the children with cochlear implants outperformed their matched peers in every area of evaluation. The children with cochlear implants showed significantly faster growth in speech and language acquisition than the matched children wearing other sensory aids. The researchers reported that the children with cochlear implants were able to identify words based on spectral, rather than temporal, cues after 1 year of implant use. Following 2 years of cochlear implant use, the children showed a dramatic increase in perception and production of the suprasegmental and vowel features of spoken speech.

Parents' attitudes are especially revealing when they are asked about their children with cochlear implants. Tucker (1999) reported a survey of 176 parents. The children with cochlear implants were largely prelingually deaf (86%) and had been fit with a variety of implant devices. An amazing 100% of parents said they were glad that their children received cochlear implants, and 86% rated their children's implants as very successful, 10% as moderately successful, and 2% as mildly successful. Most of the postlingual deafened children, especially those deafened from meningitis, understood some open-set speech without visual clues with multichannel cochlear implants. The survey of parental attitudes supports the view that the earlier a child receives a cochlear implant, the more open-speech discrimination and eventual language development the child will acquire.

It has been more than 25 years since the first clinical trials began with cochlear implants in deaf children. The FDA has expanded the original rigid criteria for implant candidacy to include younger children with less profound hearing losses. The results of children's cochlear implant programs have been so encouraging that the application of the technology has now been extended to include prelingual deafened children who lost their hearing before developing speech and language. Device modifications have allowed implantation in younger children as the hardware becomes thinner and smaller with more flexible receiver/stimulators. Cohen and Waltzman (1996) were among the first to report successful cochlear implant results in children younger than 2 years of age. Surgical techniques require minimal surgical modification because the cochlea is full adult size at birth. Initial progress reviews of these children have shown positive results, and there is little doubt that more children will be candidates for cochlear implants at earlier ages.

Current results in young children with profound deafness have exceeded the expectations of most professionals. The technology and surgery are expensive, although private insurance or Medicaid may cover most costs. The future for cochlear implants in children is especially bright, and technology is continually improving in terms of better speech-processing paradigms and hardware design. It is likely that as more experience is gained with today's cochlear implants, future candidates will have lesser degrees of sensorineural loss. Excellent materials are available to describe every aspect of cochlear implants online and in textbooks by Clark, Cowan, and Dowell (1997), Eisenberg (2009), and Gifford (2013). An especially useful cochlear implant book aimed at parents was written by Loy & Roland (2009).

Cochlear implantation continues to be a viable treatment option for many children with severe to profound hearing loss. One indication of the widespread acceptance of CIs is found in *Healthy People 2010*, a national report that called for an increase in the proportion of CI users (U.S. Department of Health and Human Services, 2000); the proposed 2020 document retains this goal (Tobey, 2010). Technological advances will lead to the development of more sophisticated and improved devices. It appears inevitable that as technology for cochlear prostheses advances, candidacy criteria for implantation will continue to expand to include a wider range of the population with severe and profound hearing impairments. Audiological training programs must provide course work and clinical experience with cochlear prostheses. Audiologists with expertise in the diagnosis (including the use of electrophysiological techniques), management, and habilitation of children with hearing impairments are necessary to ensure competent provision of professional services by pediatric cochlear implant programs.

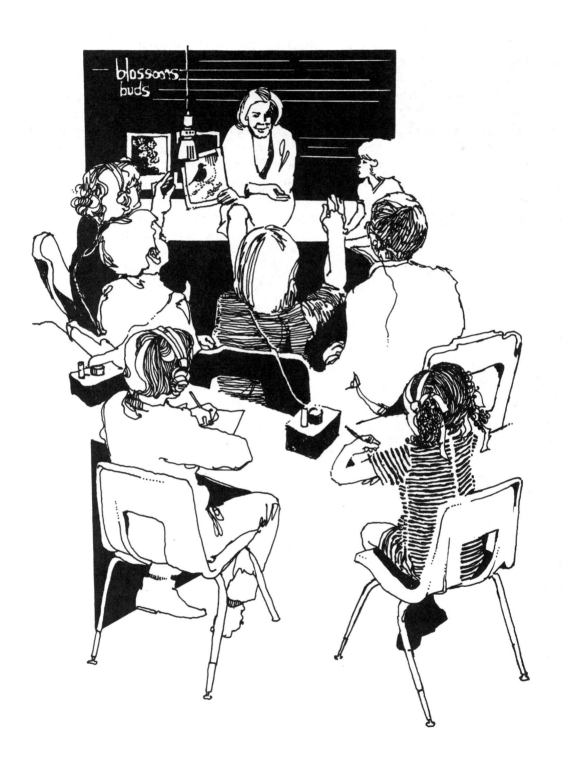

CHAPTER 10

Education

The future for children with hearing loss has reached new heights with the explosion of information and technologies for early identification, intervention, and choices of educational opportunities. As a result of successful early identification of babies with hearing loss, we are presently dealing with a vastly different population of these infants, toddlers, and children with special needs than ever before. Today's education processes begin as soon as the infant is identified and diagnosed with hearing loss. With these babies and young children in our hands at such an early age, we can now truly work from a developmental and preventive educational perspective rather than from the traditional models of remediation and corrective systems (Cole & Flexer, 2008). The audiologist, by nature of being the responsible professional to confirm the presence and degree of hearing loss, also becomes the initial resource for parents and family of the child with hearing loss.

Hearing and auditory function have significant impact on the development and use of language and communication that can affect academic progress and outcomes for students. Federal special education legislation has provided the underlying support for audiology services in the schools for more than 30 years. Education of deaf and hard-of-hearing children has undergone dramatic improvement since passage of the federal law known as the Education for All Handicapped Children of 1975 (Public Law 94-142), currently known as the Individuals with Disabilities Education Act (IDEA). This legislative mandate has undergone

several iterations (PL94-142, 1975; IDEA 1997, 2004), but maintains its basic premise that education programs must be customized to address each special student's unique needs. In 1986, the U.S. Congress reauthorized and amended Public Law 94-142 to include mandatory special education services for preschool children age 3 to 5 years. Additional education and civil rights legislation (e.g., No Child Left Behind, 2001; Section 504 of the Rehabilitation Act of 1973; Americans with Disabilities Act, 1990) require schools to provide all students with access to the educational environment and to incorporate accommodations and modifications for students who need assistance in order to access general education instruction and curricula (http://www.cde.state.co.us).

Furthermore, these legislative initiatives provided substantial incentives for states to develop comprehensive, multidisciplinary early identification and intervention services for infants and toddlers, as well as funds to support educational programs for infants age birth to 3 years with developmental disabilities and their families. These extensive resources and programs have had a huge positive impact on the education of children with deafness and hearing problems.

Our definition of "hard-of-hearing children" includes *all* children with hearing loss who are handicapped to any extent that some form of special education is required. Obviously, this broad definition includes those with profound hearing loss traditionally defined as "deaf." The Conference of Executives of American Schools for the

Deaf defines "the deaf" as having a hearing loss of 70 dB hearing level (HL) or greater in their better ear, while the "hard-of-hearing" student has a loss of 25 to 69 dB HL in the better hearing ear. In fact, the definition of "deaf" describes a hearing impairment so severe that a child experiences difficulty in processing linguistic information through hearing, with or without amplification. Although it is easy to speak in general terms about the education of students with various degrees of hearing impairment or deafness, the point must be made that these groups are by no means homogeneous. Furthermore, it must be realized that there is no single educational method, system, or approach that is uniformly applicable to all children with varying degrees of hearing impairment or deafness. This chapter is oriented toward the single most important aspect of management of the child with hearing loss—achieving the maximum potential of the child through education.

Matkin and Wilcox (1999) point out that it is a common misconception to equate the term *hearing impairment* to those children with severe to profound bilateral hearing loss. Although these children with severe hearing losses receive the largest share of attention, children with minimal hearing loss deserve equal educational opportunity. Fortunately, schools are beginning to extend support services to include children with mild to moderate bilateral sensorineural hearing losses, those with permanent unilateral hearing loss, younger children with bilateral conductive losses, and even high-frequency losses identified through screening of school-aged children. According to Matkin and Wilcox (1999), these children with mild to moderate hearing loss are best described as having *educationally significant hearing loss* (Table 10–1).

THE EDUCATIONAL AUDIOLOGIST

The educational audiologist is the appropriate intermediary trained in deafness education methodologies and management

Table 10–1. Guidelines for Educationally Significant Hearing Loss

An average pure-tone hearing loss in the speech frequency range (0.5–2 kHz) of 20 dB HL in the better ear, which is not reversible within a reasonable period

An average high-frequency pure tone hearing loss of 35 dB HL or greater in the better ear at two or more of the following frequencies: 2, 3, 4, and 6 kHz

A permanent unilateral hearing loss of 35 dB HL or greater in the speech range (0.5–2 kHz)

Any hearing impairment that significantly affects communication with others and in which the individual requires supplemental assistance or modification of instructional methods to achieve optimum performance

Source: Adapted from *Effectiveness indicators for audiological services*, by the Colorado Department of Education, 1991, Denver, CO: CDE.

of children with hearing loss. As defined by the Educational Audiology Association (EAA), an educational audiologist is a specialist who ensures that all aspects of children's hearing and learning are maximized so that their educational and real-life capabilities can be met. The Educational Audiology Association is an international organization of audiologists and related professionals who deliver a full spectrum of hearing services to all children, particularly those in educational settings (http://www.edaud.org). The educational audiologist is the person responsible for the child with hearing difficulties in the school and family environments. In many instances, the role could be the case manager. The educational audiologist is qualified in the overall ramifications of audibility, environmental sounds, hearing, hearing loss, hearing aids, cochlear implants, auditory perception (including central auditory abilities), and their impact on development, learning, and life. The educational audiologist is responsible for identification, diagnosis, assessment, amplification programming, aural rehabilitation programming (and training when feasible), and central auditory processing disorders (CAPDs) programming. In addition, this specialty area audiologist is responsible for support personnel training, parent training and support, specialist coordination, listening training, hearing conservation programming, supervision of specialized testing, otologic referral, and ongoing evaluations of the child's classroom and educational functioning. The educational audiologist is a specialist with enormous responsibilities for the management of large numbers of children with hearing loss.

The audiologist is clearly the professional best able to manage the complete hearing care in the educational environment of a child who experiences hearing loss of any

degree (Flexer, 1990). Even a "mild" hearing loss can sabotage the development of academic competencies, and there is a growing population of schoolchildren with mild to moderate hearing loss. Unfortunately, there are far too few audiologists employed in educational settings. The EAA supports a target ratio of one full-time equivalent (FTE) educational audiologist for every 10,000 students served by the local education agency (LEA) or regional cooperative. Workload factors such as extensive travel time or time-intensive services (e.g., direct intervention; services to infants, toddlers, students with multiple disabilities; service provision to regional or self-contained programs designed for multiple students who are deaf or hard-of-hearing) may result in the need for adjustment of this ratio. Educational audiologists must meet current state and federal requirements for credentialing through licensure and/or certification (http://www.edaud.org).

The audiologist is often hard-pressed to maintain the distinction between being an expert in the measurement and management of hearing and hearing disorders and the necessary role of serving as an advocate for the child with hearing impairment. When the audiologist expresses an objective statement within the field of hearing measurement, the facts are based on standardized and solid data. However, when the audiologist expresses a viewpoint or an opinion advocating a position on questions of general policy not directly related to audiology (i.e., approaches to education of hearing-impaired children), the stated opinion may be based on limited knowledge and information. In the area of education of hearing-impaired children, it behooves the audiologist to know as much as possible about all avenues, methodologies, techniques, and systems for teaching this special population. It is obligatory that the audiologist who specializes in pediatric hearing evaluation also be knowledgeable and well informed on the current status of education for hearing-impaired children.

This book has described objective tests and behavioral measures that have been adequately standardized and has also outlined subjective assessments that lend themselves to some measurable degree of judgment. Within these topics, the audiologist has a fair amount of control. However, in the field of directing children with hearing impairment into educational channels, the audiologist becomes an "advocate of a cause." Some audiologists may not have knowledge or experience with various educational training methods for deaf and hard-of-hearing students, and audiologists do not necessarily have an understanding of all the variables that will affect the child's functioning in a given training method. To rectify these inadequacies, the audiologist must, in addition to personal empirical testing, actively work with various members of the deafness management team including the child's parents, physicians, educators, psychologists, sociologists, and others. Working with the child's parents and family, and with these specialists, the audiologist should be involved with the decisions concerning the educational direction of the child—decisions that are flexible enough to change with the further accumulation of information.

The difficulty comes from the fact that few "experts" have the important ingredient of "total objectivity" when it comes to evaluating the field of deaf education. The professional groups that know most about this area are the teachers themselves or education program administrators. Yet these people may be limited in number and may be isolated from new parents of a deaf or hard-of-hearing child. The audiologist should operate as an "advocate without a cause" in the field of educational management for the child. The audiologist should not be biased in the direction of any training method or philosophy and should consider only what will best ensure the child, and the child's family, maximal ultimate development.

Of course, in the practice of family-centered services, the audiologist must work closely with the parents or caregivers of the child to ensure proper educational placement. The decision regarding placement of the child in an educational program must be the parents' prerogative. Unless the parents have made the decision, there will be second thoughts and possibly recriminations at a later date. The parents' decision should consider the following contributions from the child's deafness team: (a) information as to the type and degree of hearing loss; (b) the contributions to the child's audition from personal amplification; (c) results of the speech and language evaluations, if relevant; (d) an introduction and understanding of the various educational programs available in the community (this should include visits to each of the facilities that are offering programs for children with hearing loss); and (e) open support of their choice to the point that that they will feel comfortable should they decide to make an educational change at a later date if at any time it appears that another program will better benefit their child.

In another sense, however, the audiologist can espouse advocacy for principle or cause alone. This is in the sense of fighting for the child's right to be given a chance to show what he or she can do despite contrary information, differences in personal opinions, and even in light of questionable evidence. Audiologists must be sufficiently sensitive to let hope play a part in the judgments for the prognosis of a sensory-limited child. Audiologists would be less than human if they failed to glow with satisfaction when a child develops useful speech with hearing aids and hearing therapy, or when an infant with hearing impairment becomes in every way a hearing child with continually improving speech and language skills.

INDIVIDUALS WITH DISABILITIES EDUCATION ACT (IDEA)

The passage of the Education for All Handicapped Children Act of 1975, otherwise known as Public Law 94-142, represented a landmark in federal recognition of their responsibility to provide funding for the costs of special education that ensures a basic minimum level of program quality for handicapped children and their parents. The importance of this legislation was to assure the right of all children to be educated in the school districts in which they live. Federal legislation since 1975 has changed focus from the concept of *handicap* to that of *disability.*

The basic purposes of Public Law 94-142 were to ensure that every disabled child in the United States receives a free, appropriate public education. This free (at no cost to the child or parents) education is to be appropriately designed to fit the special needs of the child and public. The state education department has the legal responsibility to provide appropriate educational services under public auspices at public expense. The basic goals of this legislation broadened the options available to educate deaf students, recognized the diverse needs of individual children, and supported the need for early identification and diagnosis.

Although the 1970s will be remembered for this encompassing law, the economic conditions of the 1980s created challenges for the enactment and fulfillment of the law's provisions. The "education of all handicapped children" is a multibillion dollar per year undertaking for which most funding has been allocated to the state and local communities.

The Individuals with Disabilities Education Act (IDEA), so named in 1990, was developed from the Education for All Handicapped Children Act (Public Law 94-142) placed in rule in 1975. IDEA is a law that ensures services to children with disabilities and addresses their educational needs from birth to age 18 or 21 involving 13 specified categories of disability, including hearing impairment. IDEA governs how states and public agencies provide early intervention, special education, and related services to more than 6.5 million eligible infants, toddlers, children, and youth with disabilities during the year 2006. Children and youth, ages 3 to 21, receive special education and related services under IDEA Part B; infants and toddlers with disabilities, birth to 2, and their families receive early intervention services under IDEA Part C.

Prior to enactment of the Education for All Handicapped Children Act (EHA) in 1975, U.S. public schools accommodated only one out of five children with disabilities. Until that time, many states had laws that explicitly excluded children with certain types of disabilities from attending public school, including children who were blind, or deaf, and children labeled "emotionally disturbed" or "mentally retarded." At the time the EHA was enacted, more than one million children in the United States had no access to the public school system. Many of these children lived at state institutions where they received limited or no educational or rehabilitation services. Another 3.5 million children attended school but were "warehoused" in segregated facilities and received little or no effective instruction (National Council on Disability, 2000).

Eligibility for IDEA Services

Having a disability does not automatically qualify a student for special education services under the IDEA. The disability must result in the student needing additional or different services to participate in school. IDEA defines a "child with a disability" as a:

> ... child ... with an intellectual disability, hearing impairments (including deafness), speech or language impairments, visual impairments (including blindness), serious emotional disturbance ..., orthopedic impairments, autism, traumatic brain injury, other health impairments, or specific learning disabilities; and, who because of the condition needs special education and related services.

An interesting court case established the "zero reject rule" in 1989 which ruled that even if the student is completely incapable of benefiting from educational services and all efforts to educate are futile—even if the child is unconscious or in a coma—the school is still required to provide educational services to the child.

Individualized Education Program

The IDEA law requires that public schools create an Individualized Education Program (IEP) for each student who is found to be eligible under both the federal and state eligibility/disability standards. The IEP is the cornerstone of a student's educational program. It specifies the services to be provided and how often, describes the student's present levels of performance and how the student's disabilities affect academic performance, and specifies accommodations and modifications to be provided for the student. An IEP team is convened for each child to design an IEP that is formally reviewed annually. Based on the full educational evaluation results, this team collaborates to write an IEP for the individual child; a plan that will provide a free, appropriate public education.

Free Appropriate Public Education (FAPE)

In defining the purpose of special education, IDEA (2004) clarified Congress' intended outcome for each child with a disability: students must be provided a Free Appropriate Public Education (FAPE) that prepares them for further education, employment, and independent living. FAPE is defined as an educational program that is individualized to a specific child, designed to meet that child's unique needs, and from which the child receives educational benefit. To provide FAPE, schools must provide students with an "education that emphasizes special education and related services designed to meet their unique needs and prepare them for further education, employment, and independent living." The criteria specified in various sections of the IDEA statute includes requirements that schools provide each disabled student an education that is designed to meet the unique needs of that one student and provides "access to the general curriculum to meet the challenging expectations established for all children," that is, it meets the approximate grade-level standards of the state educational agency.

Least Restrictive Environment (LRE)

Simply put, the Least Restrictive Environment is the environment most like that of typical children in which the child with a disability can succeed academically (as measured by the specific goals in the student's IEP). The regulations that describe the implementation of the LRE within IDEA state: "to the maximum extent appropriate, children with disabilities including children in public or private institutions or care facilities, are educated with children who are *non*disabled; and special classes, separate schooling or other removal of children with disabilities from regular educational environment occurs only if the nature or severity of the disability is such that education in regular classes with the use of supplementary aids and services cannot be achieved satisfactorily" (U.S. Department of Education, 2005). The law itself is not a panacea, but it has served to substantially improve services and education for deaf students since its enactment. The limited numbers of deaf and hard-of-hearing students may make it difficult to group these children with other children with hearing loss in day programs in smaller school districts. The law does not necessarily mean that *least restrictive environment* and *maximal integration* are synonymous terms or concepts. Considering the ultimate objective of producing well-educated, socially adjusted, and responsible adults, the least restrictive environment is also not necessarily the one that is closest to home or the one that has maximum integration in schools.

IDEA Procedural Safeguards

IDEA includes a set of procedural safeguards designed to protect the rights of children with disabilities and their families, and to ensure that children with disabilities receive a Free Appropriate Public Education in the least restrictive environment. The procedural safeguards include the opportunity for parents to review their child's full educational records; full parent participation in identification and Individualized Education Program team meetings; parent involvement in placement decisions; prior written notice for the parents; and the right of parents to request independent educational evaluations at public expense including objective mediation funded by the state education agency and impartial due process hearings.

Legislative Growth of IDEA

IDEA has had a long legislative history, and it has grown in scope and form over the past 25 years (http://www2.ed.gov/policy/speced/leg/idea/history.pdf). IDEA has been reauthorized and amended a number of times and contains several significant amendments. Its terms are further defined by regulations of the U.S. Department of Education (Parts 300 and 301 of Title 34 of the Code of Federal Regulations):

- 1975: The Education for All Handicapped Children Act (EAHCA) became law. It was renamed the Individuals with Disabilities Education Act (IDEA) in 1990.
- 1990: IDEA first came into being on October 30, 1990, when the "Education of All Handicapped Children Act" (itself having been introduced in 1975) was renamed "Individuals with Disabilities Education Act" (Pub. L. No. 101-476, 104 Stat. 1142). IDEA received minor amendments in October 1991 (Pub. L. No. 102-119, 105 Stat. 587).
- 1997: IDEA received significant amendments. The definition of disabled children expanded to include developmentally delayed children between 3 and 9 years of age.

It also required parents to attempt to resolve disputes with schools and local educational agencies (LEAs) through mediation, and provided a process for doing so. The amendments authorized additional grants for technology, disabled infants and toddlers, parent training, and professional development (Pub. L. No. 105-17, 111 Stat. 37).

- 2004: IDEA was amended by the Individuals with Disabilities Education Improvement Act of 2004, now known as IDEIA. Several provisions aligned IDEA with the No Child Left Behind Act of 2001, signed by President George W. Bush. It authorized 15 states to implement 3-year Independent Educational Programs (IEPs) on a trial basis when parents continually agree. Drawing on the report of the President's Commission on Excellence in Special Education, the law revised the requirements for evaluating children with learning disabilities. More concrete provisions relating to discipline of special education students were also added (Pub. L. No. 108-446, 118 Stat. 2647).

- 2009: Following a campaign promise for "funding the Individuals with Disabilities Education Act," President Barack Obama signed the American Recovery and Reinvestment Act of 2009 (ARRA) on February 17, 2009, including $12.2 billion in additional funds.

These legislative mandates have resulted in the placement of special classrooms for children with hearing loss in many local schools, thereby dispersing these children away from the special schools in which they were grouped together at one location.

These circumstances may be cause for concern regarding special staffing and support services not available or available only on an itinerant basis. Educational audiologists often serve large numbers of students spread over an extensive number of schools within a huge school district. The communication and socialization limits for the children resulting from this isolation and dispersion may impact the deaf and hard-of-hearing student's emotional and behavioral development. The profound effect of a serious hearing impairment on the communication, social, and academic achievement of deaf children may not be realized by school officials, boards of education, or local lawmakers.

The requirements of IDEIA challenge professionals in the fields of audiology, speech-language pathology, and especially deaf educators to reexamine basic assumptions and develop new ranges of services for deaf and hard-of-hearing students and their families. Educational programs meeting the IDEIA spirit and requirements have opportunities to develop innovative programs and research while engaged in cooperative working relationships between related-service professionals outside the discipline of deafness.

EDUCATIONAL GOALS FOR THE CHILD WITH HEARING LOSS

Among the fundamental rights that audiologists must insist upon is a child's right to achieve his or her maximal potential communication abilities. Society should make special provisions to help the deaf and hard-of-hearing child become as "normal" as limitations will allow. The world-famous child psychologist A. L. Gesell stated, "The aim should not be to convert the deaf child into a somewhat fictitious version of a normal hearing child, but into a well-adjusted non-hearing child who is completely managing the limitations of his [or her] sensory deficit" (1956).

Obviously, there are many goals to be achieved in educating hearing-impaired and deaf children, and we highlight only the four most important as we see them. These goals, presented in order of importance, are the achievement of adequate language skills, the establishment of sound mental health, the establishment of intelligible speech, and the establishment of easy communication with peers. These goals are by no means to be interpreted as limiting the range of objectives that one might have for the hard-of-hearing or deaf child. However, other goals that might be enumerated such as high employability, job satisfaction, and enrichment of life, all depend on the success of achieving the four goals described below.

Language

The importance of language cannot be denied. Language comes so easily to normal-hearing children and is a giant stone wall for children with significant hearing impairment. Educators of hearing-impaired students realize the long-term commitment and years of diligent work needed to establish communicative competence based on adequate linguistic abilities. The process of developing language competency is very difficult for the child who has significant hearing impairment, and all children who are prelingually deaf will experience serious difficulties and delays in acquiring language skills. For some children, full language acquisition may be a feasible goal; for other children, lesser language skills will have to be acceptable. The hearing-impaired child

with limited language skills will have additional difficulties in subjects other than language studies, because each new step in education requires mastery of the previous steps. It is the role of the school or program to create an environment for learning that maximizes the language acquisition process of children with hearing impairments.

The primary goal in education of the hearing-impaired child must be to develop linguistic abilities and ensure communication development by whatever means possible. A secondary goal should be to develop intelligible oral expression of that language —a skill that depends on the acquisition of a high degree of language competence through auditory or visual input. Montgomery and Matkin (1992) stated that successful language learning for a child with a hearing loss depends on several variables: (a) the type, severity, and configuration of the hearing loss in each ear; (b) the effects of the hearing loss on the child's ability to detect and discriminate the key acoustic components of the speech signal; and (c) consistency in the use of amplification to provide optimal recognition and discrimination of auditory signals.

The Audiologists' Role in Promoting Literacy

Reading literacy has been a significant concern in the United States for the last two decades. A report from the National Assessment of Educational Progress (2007) stated that 37% of fourth graders fail to achieve basic levels of reading achievement. The incidence of reading failure is even higher within low-income families, ethnic minority groups, and English-language learners (Forget-Dubois et al., 2009; West, Denton, & Germino-Hausken, 2000). Only 48% of low socioeconomic children are ready for reading in school by age 5; it has been reported that 80% of African American and Latino public school children are unable to read at grade level in the 4th, 8th, or 12th grades (Isaacs, 2012; State of America's Children, 2011). These concerns, no doubt, also have great implications in our deaf and hard-of-hearing children who face additional literacy obstacles in their general language learning.

An enormous attainment gap emerges early in life as reported by Hart and Risley (1995) showing that socioeconomic status separates out groups quickly based on vocabulary development. By example, they state that at age 36 months, high socioeconomic children have a cumulative vocabulary of some 1,200 words, while low socioeconomic children's vocabulary is around 300 words. They cite fault with parenting because the first years of a child's life pave the way for future development. The critical factor in this disparate outcome is the parents' lack of knowledge, skills, and motivation to interact with their child in a way that enriches their language development and therefore their reading readiness (Reilly et al., 2010).

It should come as no surprise that the poor reading skills of deaf children reflect a major obstacle in their education. Deaf and hard-of-hearing students "level off" in their reading comprehension achievement at about the fourth- to fifth-grade level. Because reading ability is highly correlated with language skills, many deaf and hard-of-hearing students also have difficulty in becoming proficient readers. Language skills are fundamental for development of cognitive ability that leads to school readiness. The ability to express or comprehend language in written form is closely allied with the ability to express and comprehend language through face-to-face spoken communication. Historically, deaf education programs have not been very successful in assisting the majority of students with hearing loss to achieve age-level reading skills. Some believe that it is the inherent complexity of the English grammar that is the primary block to reading for the deaf child.

Audiologists have a role in ensuring the child's readiness for language, learning, and literacy. Of course, prompt identification of the hearing loss, followed by early intervention and appropriate amplification all help establish opportunities for the child's development of language. The audiologist is responsible for providing audibility for the child, which can be considered a precursor for achieving literacy reading skills. All children require early, consistent, real-time exposure to their native language for optimum learning opportunities as well as for social and emotional development. The foundations of literacy are laid in infancy and early childhood. As many reading precursor skills are auditory based, the application of hearing aids or cochlear implants, supplemented with FM utilization and other assistive systems, are extremely important. For children who are deaf or hard-of-hearing, ongoing monitoring of their amplification, functional auditory skills, as well as their language and speech development should be considered during every audiological assessment. Of value is the cooperative multidisciplinary approach with the deaf and hard-of-hearing child with early language specialists such as the speech-language pathologist, early interventionist, or teacher of the deaf.

Family involvement is a critical factor in the success of language and literacy development for the deaf or hard-of-hearing child. Early language exposure has profound impact on outcomes of children with hearing loss. Therefore, educating parents about communication options, working with them to improve communication skills, as well as reinforcing the importance of consistent use of amplification are important to the development of language and literacy of the child. Maternal communicative skills are predictive of language and literacy for deaf children (Calderon, 2000). High levels of family involvement correlate with positive language outcomes for deaf and hard-of-hearing children (Huttenlocher, Waterfall, Vasilyeva, Vevea, & Hedges, 2010; Moeller, 2000). Children who received early intervention and whose father was present have significantly better academic and language outcomes than those without a father present (Calderon & Low, 1998). There are many activities that parents and families can do to improve the literacy development of their deaf and hard-of-hearing child. Suggestions from teachers of the deaf might include home and parent programs of language-enhancement and oral language skills practices, oral reading, and book sharing activities that can have significant positive

effects on children's spelling and reading readiness (Figure 10–1).

The easiest facilitation the family can provide is reading to their child. Children love being read stories and learning the depth of knowledge that can come from print of all kinds. The art of reading aloud to deaf and hard-of-hearing children conditions their brains to associate reading with pleasure. Reading expands the child's vocabulary, auditory memory, attention span, and familiarity with the syntax of spoken language. And, writing grows from reading (Flexer, 2012). Conventional reading and writing skills that are developed in the years from birth to age 5 have a clear and consistently strong relationship with later conventional literacy skills (see Figure 10–1). Additionally, five variables representing early literacy skills or precursor literacy skills have positive predictive relationships with later measures of literacy

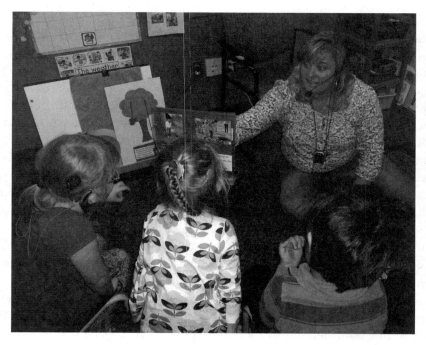

Figure 10–1. Development of language skills is the prerequisite to school readiness. Photo courtesy of H.O.P.E. Preschool, Spokane, WA.

development even when the role of other variables, such as IQ or socioeconomic status, were accounted for (National Center for Family Literacy, 2007). These five variables are as follows:

- Alphabet knowledge: knowledge of names and sounds associated with printed letter;
- Phonological awareness: the ability to detect, manipulate, or analyze the auditory aspects of spoken language;
- Random automatic naming; digits or numbers and objects or colors: the ability to rapidly name a sequence of random letters or digits and objects or colors;
- Writing or writing name: the ability to write letters in isolation or request (or to write one's own name); and
- Phonological memory: the ability to remember spoken information for a short period of time.

Osberger and Hesketh (1988) described the language difficulties experienced by hearing-impaired and deaf children in terms of language form (syntax), content (semantics), and function (pragmatics). According to these authors, hearing-impaired children may have only minor difficulties in acquiring the basic rules of English, compared with the profoundly deaf child who has a great deal of difficulty in syntax acquisition because of his or her dependence on learning language through the visual modality. Language content as reflected by word knowledge is commonly limited and delayed even in children with mild hearing losses. Hearing-impaired children have a restricted knowledge of synonyms and special difficulties in recognizing relationships between words. In terms of language function, children with hearing impairment must be directly taught the

rules that govern conversations, such as turn-taking and topic negotiation.

An important question that has been debated for years centers on whether combining signing with spoken language contributes to or interferes with the development of spoken language. Geers, Moog, and Schick (1984) attempted to answer this question by testing a nationwide sample of 327 congenital, profoundly deaf children from 13 oral/aural programs and 15 total communication programs through their own tool, the Grammatical Analysis of Elicited Language-Simple Sentence Level (GAEL-S). The GAEL-S measures production of selected English language structures in a standardized manner, so that each child's "spontaneous" language sample is evoked in precisely the same manner. In their study, Geers et al. examined their data separately for four different response modes: the oral productions of the oral/aural children, the oral productions of the total communication children, the manual productions of the total communication children, and the combined productions of the total communication children. The results showed that the percentages of correct scores for the oral productions of the total communication children were substantially below the scores for their manual productions and below scores of the oral/aural children in all grammatical categories sampled on the GAEL-S. Most of the children in the total communication programs tested in this study did not simultaneously talk and sign, and their signed productions were far superior to their spoken productions. Thus, based on this study, the children in total communication programs did not develop competence with selected simple sentence structures at a rate faster than those children trained in the oral/aural programs. The authors point out that both groups of children showed relatively poor performance in language production and urged that more emphasis on systematic instruction in English be included in all training programs regardless of the mode of communication.

In summary, there are a number of factors and complex issues that influence acquisition of language and literacy skills in deaf and hard-of-hearing children. Certainly, early exposure to natural language and communication is critical. Parents must be encouraged to talk extensively to their children; they need training to help them stimulate enriched language experiences from their child. The child's education must be individualized, and parents need information on the full range of communication options so they can make informed decisions. Parents often have limited information and resources during the early diagnostic and intervention periods. For the school-aged deaf or hard-of-hearing child, there may be a shortage of qualified teachers and interpreters, and special services may not be locally available or expensive and difficult for schools to provide. Pediatric audiologists must be aware of their responsibilities for their pediatric patients to ensure appropriate management and progress with language and literacy as well as serving as the child's advocate and a resource person for the parents and families.

Sound Mental Health

The most effective learning takes place in the context of warm, nurturing relationships within the family. This is particularly important for the very young child during the critical years for language development. Whatever type of educational program a child is receiving, the parents should be given close emotional support and guidance in their management of the child's disability. The results should be the development of the child's self-confidence, high self-esteem, and the ability to relate well to people in the environment. The warm relationship between parents and child can be fostered by helpful, supportive communications from the physician and educational personnel. The initial phase of reporting the child's deafness to the parents is crucial to the parents' attitude toward the problem. Time should be allowed for the parents to air their feelings and their sorrow over having an "imperfect" child. Grief must be expressed if acceptance of the disability is to come. These natural feelings should be shared with empathy and understanding. The physician and the audiologist can create the kind of atmosphere out of which nurturing attitudes can grow.

Together with the parents, the audiologist can help guide decisions about an educational program for the child that will allow the continuation of good parent nurturing. As Schlesinger (1973) pointed out, "Early parent-child communication is a traumatic issue between hearing parents and their deaf children. Although the hearing parents talk to and in front of the child, they can only guess at the level of understanding." Frustration results for both parents and child; thus, it is important that an educational program be chosen that minimizes this frustration. It should be noted that such problems are minimized in the relationships of deaf parents to their deaf children. Denton et al. (1974) stated, "Deaf parents, as they communicate to and in front of the child, can test the child's understanding more easily. The child can learn the symbols, the signs the parents use, and learn to understand and reproduce them more easily." It is estimated that 3% of congenitally deaf children are born to deaf parents.

Intelligible Speech

Certainly an important goal in the education of deaf children is intelligible speech. However, caution should be used when placing this skill too high in the hierarchy of educational goals. Intelligible speech without good language skills is an exercise in futility; intelligible speech in an emotionally disordered mind is a useless function. Articulate speech is greatly desired, but a program producing excellence only in this skill and not in language or emotional stability cannot be highly rated. Clear oral speech is also greatly desired but should not become the mainstay of the child's educational efforts. So-called "deaf speech" is characterized by a significantly higher fundamental frequency, a slower speaking rate than found in normal-hearing persons, and typical increased voice intensity with abnormally large amplitude fluctuations.

Oral production of speech for the deaf child is a problem that stems from inadequate control at nearly all levels of production. In addition, there is a systematic relationship between the degree of hearing impairment and the intelligibility of the child's speech so that the greater the hearing loss, the more unintelligible the child's speech is likely to be. Although exceptions to this rule do exist, for whatever unknown reasons, all audiologists have seen children with profound hearing loss and exceptionally clear oral speech.

Parents of a newly diagnosed hearing-impaired child must decide whether their child will be taught to communicate with manual signs, by speech reading and producing speech, or by some combination of methods. The choice is a difficult one. In general, parents can be advised that children with greater hearing loss will be less likely to succeed in speech reading and will most likely benefit from sign language. The disadvantages of sign language are obvious and compelling to hearing parents. Because it is not the language of society or the family, parents worry that their child will be difficult to communicate with, and they will naturally be worried about learning a new language to communicate with their own child. On the other hand, the most important advantage of sign language is that it is easily learned. Children whose parents sign acquire sign language at the same rate that hearing children acquire spoken language. For instance, they begin a "sign babble" of repetitive hand motions by 10 months, just as hearing infants begin to babble in sound at that same age (Petitto & Marentette, 1991). A hearing-impaired infant who understands and learns signs can achieve the same level of language production as the normal-hearing child at the same age milestones. The audiologist can encourage parents who feel intimidated about learning signs by assuring them that they have years to become really fluent, but that it is extremely valuable to use a limited vocabulary of "baby signs" while the child is young.

One of the major factors that opened up the education potential of children with profound deafness has been the cochlear implant (see Chapter 9). Carefully documented prospective and long-term studies of children with cochlear implants have provided a volume of information about the development of learning, speech recognition, and speech production in young children with hearing impairment. Increased awareness of the precise parameters of the speech of deaf individuals has accompanied the development of the cochlear implant. In general, the immediate effect of the cochlear implant is that the patient has an improved ability to monitor and adjust vocal output as well as an increased clarity of oral speech. Admittedly, even with the best of personal amplification or a cochlear implant, the deafened child is destined to spend long hours in speech therapy. It is to be remembered, however, that the goal of clear oral speech is secondary to the goal of developing a strong language base, so that when the deaf child speaks, something of value will have been spoken. When the desire to communicate is instilled in deaf children and the necessary language skills to do so are provided, teaching speech will become a far easier task.

The family, particularly the parents, is the most important part of the child's support system. Families need assistance in understanding the problems of deafness and in learning those skills that will, in turn, be of benefit to the hearing-impaired child. The family must be inherently involved in all decisions regarding their child and must believe positively about the child's potential. Many parents of deaf children complain that their concerns and desires were not given consideration when their child was beginning special education programs. It is essential that parents be committed to, and trained in the use of, whichever communication system is used by their child. It is likely that behind most successful deaf children will be found highly motivated and concerned parents.

For any child, disabled or not, a positive self-concept is crucial. Emotional stability and maturity are often problem areas for children who are deaf. When a child has low self-esteem, has tendencies to be withdrawn, or exhibits inappropriate behaviors, strategies must be established to improve the child's emotional well-being. Both the home and the school environment should be evaluated, and everyone concerned must be flexible to make the necessary adjustments for the good of the child. The goal of sound mental health is essential to any successful achievement that can be desired for the hearing-impaired child.

Communication With Peers

Humans have a special need for communication, and happiness and satisfaction go hand-in-hand with the ease by which we transmit and receive information. It is too often the case that without careful guidance and intervention that the child with hearing impairment or deafness can become isolated from family and friends. Interaction with peers is an important part of normal development, and it is critical that deaf children be able to communicate freely and easily with children of their own age. Peer relationships serve as models for appropriate behavior and self-identity. It is recommended that deaf children be exposed to older, same-gender role models who are also deaf, as recognition of deafness in others provides a sense of belonging for the child, rather than a feeling of pure isolation in a world of hearing people.

Deaf Culture

Children have cultural needs. Culture is knowledge that gives individuals a shared understanding of the world and accepted behaviors and values. Culture enables us to know what is expected and anticipated and permits individuals to gauge their place within the group. When not recognized, differing cultural standards can interfere with the learning process in the classroom and in the home. In recent years, there has been a strong movement among deaf adults to recognize their unique needs and their accommodation to the world around them as *deaf culture*. Dolnick (1993) wrote explicitly about the deaf culture movement. He points out that the view of deafness as a culture is held vehemently by many deaf adults. So strong is the feeling of deaf cultural solidarity that many deaf parents cheer on discovering that their newborn is also deaf. Thus, the well-meaning efforts to integrate deaf children into conventional schools and to help them learn to speak provokes fierce resistance from activists who favor sign language and argue that the world of deafness is distinctive, rewarding, and worth preserving.

The deaf child, who most of the time has two hearing parents, may experience rejection through dislike, pity, and misunderstanding from the hearing world. It is thus not surprising that the deaf child of deaf parents seems to be much happier and better adjusted than the deaf child of hearing parents. Many deaf children have social problems that complicate their language disability. Accordingly, the frustrated deaf child is noted to show outbursts of anger and rage throughout the school years. In schools and classes for the hearing impaired taught only by hearing teachers, children with hearing impairment and deafness may develop strong emotional ties and loyalties to each other as classmates, which leads them to the exclusive and excluded community of the deaf as adults. This presents a difficult position for audiologists to accept and advocate when faced with management of the future of a deaf child born into a family of "deaf culturists."

Schwartz (1987) stated that no method for teaching hearing-impaired children can completely make up for a lack of communication at home. In a classic comment, Schwartz says that "staunch advocates of oralism, of total communication, and of cued speech, alternately inspire and terrify parents with various tales of triumph and tragedy." Obviously, success in communication for the hearing-impaired child will be enhanced when the particular methodology used at home is also used at school. Cornett (1985) charged that few hearing parents of profoundly deaf children actually become competent in manual communication. Hearing parents, according to Cornett,

tend to learn a few signs and do reasonably well in communicating until the child starts school. As the child's signing sophistication increases, communication with the parents may become more and more limited. Certainly, in today's environment, ample books, videos, and classes are readily available to teach parents and other interested persons how to communicate in standard American Sign Language (ASL). It is important that when parents make a choice and commitment to communication that the choice be made for the benefit of the entire family and not just for one parent to be able to talk to the hearing-impaired youngster.

The degree to which hearing-impaired children of hearing-impaired parents demonstrate an advantage in their acquisition of signed and spoken English when compared to hearing-impaired children of hearing parents was studied by Geers and Schick (1988). Their results indicated that by ages 7 and 8, the deaf children of deaf parents demonstrated a significant linguistic advantage in both spoken and signed English over children with hearing loss of normal hearing parents. The deaf children of deaf parents appeared better able to utilize a language training program to produce linguistic structures of English in both manual and oral modes than the children with hearing loss of normal hearing parents.

The child with hearing loss must be in an environment in which communication can be accomplished successfully, without stress or censure. Because the family has a strong vested interest in placement decisions, the family's opinions and preferences must be given ample consideration whenever possible. The real world of normal-hearing, fast-talking adults and siblings is a difficult environment for the deaf child to understand and overcome without achieving some means of easy communication. At the same time, the culture of the deaf community and the possible positive role it can play in the lives of children with profound hearing loss must be taken into account.

CURRENT STATUS OF EDUCATION

The disability of hearing loss and deafness often results in significant and unique educational needs for the individual child. The major barriers to learning associated with deafness relate to language and communication, which, in turn, profoundly affect most aspects of the educational process. For example, acquiring basic English language skills is a tremendous challenge for most students who are deaf. Moores (2000) described three basic questions yet to be resolved completely: (a) How shall we teach deaf children? (b) Where should we teach deaf children? and (c) What should we teach deaf children? It is likely that the answers will be greatly influenced by the emotional factors and associated biases within the various communities of professionals and concerned consumers who care about education of the deaf. The "how shall we teach" question addresses the oral versus manual controversy (signed or spoken language). The "where shall we teach" question concerns actual academic placement (residential schools, day school programs, or mainstreamed public schools). The "what should we teach" question relates to exactly what should be taught to a deaf student on any typical day? Common wisdom would direct us to focus on language development, academic content, speech production, and auditory training while we attempt to integrate all of these areas as much as possible into every moment of the child's day in the classroom. The most important consideration in the education of these special

needs children is that the answers to these questions must lead to overcoming their difficulties in mastering language skills. For deaf children, it is that language barrier that stands between them and the full realization of their academic, intellectual, emotional, and social development.

Traditionally, residential schools have been aligned with manual-type communication in their education system, while private day schools tend to be auditory-oral in nature. Such dichotomy, however, is no longer so specific. With increased individualization of academic placement, more complex patterns of teaching and communication are available, and teachers are realizing that the use of FM amplification systems and classroom sign language interpreters has, in some locations, distorted the pure boundaries of the oralism and manualism controversy. The deinstitutionalization movement has dropped residential school enrollment considerably, while local school attendance now accounts for nearly 70% of attendance by deaf and hearing-impaired students. Special schools now enroll a higher percentage of the more seriously hearing-impaired students than did previous placement patterns (Schildroth, 1988). It can be seen that education of the deaf has undergone tremendous changes in recent years. Since 1990, classroom instruction in programs for children with hearing loss has evolved to primarily auditory-oral for the youngest children or total communication techniques at every education level, from primary grades to secondary school classes (Schildroth & Hotto, 1993).

The selection of an appropriate educational setting is not a simple decision. Parents, in fact, have the task (and the responsibility) to choose for themselves the educational setting for their deaf or hard-of-hearing child: public school education, private school education, home schooling, and so forth. Although practical considerations such as cost, geographic location, and transportation must be taken into account and may play important roles, the decisions should be based on a thorough understanding of the child's unique needs and learning modes and an awareness of the educational facilities and personnel available to meet those needs (Palmer & Yantis, 1990). If the parents lack sufficient information to make these judgments independently, the audiologist may need to provide resources or referrals to help the parents make an educational placement decision. If the parents choose public school education for their child, they are then part of the decision-making team in establishing and monitoring the IEP. The IEP will determine the services and educational goals that the teacher and school will provide for the child. If the parent chooses home schooling or a private school placement, a different set of rules apply to what they can and cannot expect from special education under the IDEA mandate (http://www.handsandvoices.org).

The IEP team is a group of persons, including the parents and other persons knowledgeable about the child (i.e., the classroom teacher, speech pathologist, audiologist, etc.), knowledgeable about placement options, and knowledgeable about evaluating the child's education and maturation processes. The following are three interrelated areas of need that the IEP must discuss on an annual basis:

1. Academic level of the student: The IEP team discusses the student's academic progress and identifies the language or communication mode through which the student best receives academic information.
2. Social needs: The IEP team considers opportunities for interaction and direct communication with peers and adult role models.
3. Communication needs: The IEP team looks at how the student communicates with others (i.e., the student's language level and preferred method of communication).

The School Environment

After the IEP teams have reviewed each of these three areas, they need to decide the best way to address problems and issues as well as decide which school environment best meets the student's needs (http://www.handsandvoices.org). Finding the right school placement for the deaf and hard-of-hearing student, and doing as much as possible to help the child succeed in school requires the IEP team to truly look at the individual needs of the child in making each of their decisions.

In urban communities, consultation for parents is normally provided by state and government agencies serving the needs of communicatively impaired children. Internet website searches are often the basis of information gathering, although parents should be advised to consider website information with care and consideration for accuracy and nonbiased statements. Because of the growth of choices in local educational options, schools use different approaches to provide educational services to students with hearing loss.

Residential Schools

Residential schools for deaf and hard-of-hearing children provide total living accommodations in addition to their required educational needs. Historically, each state in the United States supported at least one residential school, and larger states such as California and New York have several residential schools. In many situations, the residential school has evolved to accommodate day students who live within commuting distance or weekday residents who return home for weekends and holidays. The effect of Public Law 94-142 was to change the scope of the residential school with the LRE requirement and the current model of mainstreaming. The result is that the residential school programs are generally smaller in total attendees with more day students than actual resident students.

Day Schools

Day schools are generally located in larger metropolitan areas. These educational programs are typically established in separate and special school facilities. Special schools may be specifically designed, staffed, and resourced to provide the appropriate special education for children with additional needs. Students attending special schools generally do not attend any classes in mainstream schools. Special schools provide individualized education, addressing specific needs. Student-teacher ratios are kept low, often 6:1 or lower depending on the needs of the children. Special schools will also have other facilities for the development of children with special needs, such as soft play areas, sensory rooms, or swimming pools, which are vital for the therapy of certain conditions. Placements in special schools are declining as more children with special needs are educated in mainstream schools. There will always be some children, however, whose learning needs are not appropriately met in a regular classroom setting and will require specialized education and resources to provide the level of support they require. Children commute

to these programs daily, and there may or may not be peer normal-hearing students included in classes.

Resource Rooms

Most resource room programs are planned so that children spend most of their day in the regular classroom with normal-hearing classmates, returning to the resource room for special or supplemental education activities. Special skills teacher(s) in the resource room are expected to provide individualized services to students varying in age, hearing loss, and academic achievement.

Self-Contained Classrooms

In this educational setting, students with special needs spend no time in ordinary classes or with nondisabled students. Segregated students may attend the same larger school where regular classes are provided, but they spend their time exclusively in a separate classroom for students with special needs. The self-contained classroom typically is staffed by specially trained teachers who provide instruction one-on-one to students or individualized teaching to small groups. If their special class is located in an ordinary school, they may be provided opportunities for social integration (e.g., eating meals with nondisabled students, gym class, or other group activities).

Itinerant Programs

In this setting, children with hearing disabilities attend regular classes full time and receive support services from an "itinerant" teacher who travels to work with children from several schools. The support education services may vary from daily to weekly lessons, depending on the child's needs and the teacher's availability as well as travel distances.

Exclusion Programs

A student who cannot receive instructions in any school is prohibited from attending school. Exclusion may still occur in some places as long as there is no legal mandate for special education services, such as in developing countries. It may also occur when a student is in the hospital, housebound, or detained by the criminal justice system. These students are candidates for one-on-one instruction or group instruction.

The total U.S. economic cost (Table 10–2) for children with hearing loss and deafness in special education programs during the 1999–2000 school year was $652 million or $11,006 per child. The lifetime educational cost (year 2007 base value) of a student with moderate hearing loss, without other disabilities, was estimated at $11,560 (http://www.cdc.gov/ncbddd/hearingloss/data

Table 10–2. Comparison of Education Costs

Placement	Annual cost
Regular education (no special services)	$4,064
Itinerant/consultant (up to 5 hours/week)	$5,767
Resource teacher (usually 20 hours/week)	$6,397
Self-contained classroom (more than 20 hours/week)	$12,389
Preschool (special education 3 days/week)	$8,193
Residential (Room and board)	$31,139
Early home intervention program (90 minutes/week)	$2,600

Source: From "Educational Audiology Association [Letters to the Editor], Von Almen et al., 1994, *Pediatrics, 94*(6), p. 957.

.html). On average, it costs $10,615 to send a normal-hearing child to public school for a year based on costs of federal, state, and local government spending combined (http://www.npr.org). Approximately 20 years ago it was reported that educating deaf and hard-of-hearing students in state residential programs cost $32,397 per child per year more than children educated in regular classrooms (Von Almen et al., 1994). It is an interesting point that our current programs of early identification and mainstreaming have resulted in an economic bargain. Children with mild-to-moderate degrees of hearing impairment have the potential to be educated in regular classrooms with minimal extra support (Grosse, 2007). Looking back to 1994, the Educational Audiology Association suggested that taxpayers should be willing to pay a little more for hearing services earlier in a child's life (i.e., cost of hearing screening and early intervention) rather than paying a lot more later due to the specialized educational requirements for children identified with hearing loss at an older age (Von Almen et al., 1994).

CHALLENGES IN TEACHING DEAF AND HEARING-IMPAIRED STUDENTS

All educators would agree that the most vital aspect of any child's intellectual development is language. For the deaf child, language is the facilitating system for acquiring knowledge. The child's successful learning of language skills paves the road of progress in school and throughout life. The ability to communicate thoughts, wants, and needs to others and, in turn, the understanding of thoughts and feelings of others depends on crucial language skills. The deaf child's problem is that hearing plays a vital role in language development to build concepts and clarify them. The deaf child lacks this valuable input channel and accordingly throughout life has trouble developing and clarifying concepts. The entire process is slowed down and becomes laborious. Although deafness itself has no effect on intellectual potential, it may lead to impoverished communication skills that can limit development severely, unless the children are provided with some compensatory tools (Moores, 2000).

Language and concept developments are tied closely with successful communication. For the normal-hearing child, the early stages of communication are primarily via speech and hearing and may be categorized into five components:

- *Reception:* Sensory data fed into the brain via the senses;
- *Symbols:* Words, signs, gestures that are used in reception;
- *Encoding:* Meaningful arrangement of symbols;
- *Transmission:* Meaningful sending of encoded material to someone else; and
- *Decoding:* Receiver's mind processes the message and extracts meaning from it.

For smooth, free-flowing communication, all five components must be operating efficiently. There must be a sufficient number of symbols to represent the message (vocabulary). There must be sufficient skill to encode the symbols (grammar). There must be sufficient mechanisms for transmission, such as speech and writing. The process of decoding involves understanding the vocabulary and grammar that form the very basis of the most important factor, the substance or content of the message itself. Incomplete communication and frustration result from a breakdown anywhere along the line.

The teacher of the deaf faces the problem with every deaf and hard-of-hearing child who may be stuck at the very first element of the communication process. The deaf child's mind is deprived of the rich sensory data supplied normally through the auditory mechanism and depends only on a meager supply of symbols to use for labeling, categorizing, and storing. New symbols are difficult to come by. The deaf or hard-of-hearing child functions initially on the concrete level of mental operations; thus, abstract operations are most difficult because they are performed with words—the very commodity of which the deaf child never has enough. Abstract operations demand precise encoding and decoding and mastery of "word" concepts. Deaf children seldom attain sufficient language skills to master abstract operations even after arduous effort.

The usual process of trial-and-error learning, or teaching, is seriously hampered for the deaf child. The deaf child cannot hear errors of vocabulary or grammar. Attempts to correct the deaf child's errors are chancy undertakings. Because of the often indistinct transmissions (speech), the listener cannot be certain that the child made an error in the use of words or grammar or whether the listener just did not understand the spoken phrase. Suppose the listener thinks an error was indeed committed; imagine the task of trying to correct the error. Or suppose an error was committed but the listener is unsure and, because of the problems in trying to correct the error situation, is content to deduce an answer and let the error go. Thus, the child's error is reinforced and will surely be perpetuated.

One is never really sure what the child with hearing loss is thinking because of difficulties in communication. Consider this example relayed to the authors by a teacher of the deaf. In her classroom of preschoolers with hearing loss, when some object would drop accidentally on the floor with a loud noise, the concept was conveyed to the children by the teacher who quickly held her hands over her ears and showed exaggerated facial expression of disdain. The children could see the situation clearly and quickly followed example, with similar behavior each time an object was dropped. A few days after this lesson, a pencil was dropped on a soft carpet accidentally. As expected, the preschoolers clapped their hands over their ears and made exaggerated faces! To what were they reacting? Surely not "noise" as the teacher thought she was teaching a few days previously. And so every concept must be carefully considered by the deaf educator from the eyes and mind of the hearing-impaired child.

Today, the problems of teaching the children who are hard-of-hearing and deaf are further complicated by the fact that a greater proportion of these young people are born deaf or lose their hearing before the acquisition of language than was the case 25 years ago. In fact, today, with medical achievements over the various etiologies of deafness, there are fewer children with acquired hearing loss (who might have some language acquisition before their deafness) entering special education programs. Today's child with hearing loss is likely to be congenitally deaf (or at least, loses his or her hearing during the prelinguistic stage) and accordingly may exhibit more difficulties in meeting language needs and speech skills than the child who lost hearing after the critical language acquisition age of 2 years. Furthermore, many of today's profoundly deaf or hard-of-hearing children, if born decades ago, might not have survived to enter school. Today they are in our school systems, but perhaps exhibiting additional disabilities, significantly adding to the complexity of the education issue (Roush et al., 2004).

Legislation has influenced, and been influenced by, public perceptions of deafness and deaf individuals. It is an important sign that increasing numbers of deaf adults are entering the professions and taking advantage of more and more business opportunities. Deaf teachers, psychologists, counselors, researchers, and administrators are now having great influence on the education of deaf children. However, the irony of a field of communication specialists locked in seemingly intractable problems and conflicts cannot be overlooked. Despite overall documented improvements in education of the deaf, the academic achievement of deaf children remains unacceptably low. Limitations on literacy (i.e., reading and writing) continue to block achievement of reaching full potential for many deaf students. Opportunities for economically deprived deaf children, with less than adequate family environments, are still woefully inadequate. It is hoped that increased emphasis on early detection of hearing loss in newborns and early intervention will positively influence successful outcomes for children with severe to profound hearing impairments.

Deafness and Visual Acuity

As the education of children with hearing loss depends a great deal on vision, concern for visual acuity in deaf children is critical. It is vitally important that information concerning the importance of visual assessment for children with hearing loss be brought to the attention of the parents of children with hearing loss (Kimberling & Pieke-Dahl, 1998). The combination of hearing loss and visual impairment in children may be congenital or occur later in life. There are numerous genetic and chromosomal syndromes that include hearing and visual impairment such as Goldenhar syndrome, CHARGE syndrome, cytomegalovirus, toxoplasmosis, meningitis, trisomy 13, and fetal alcohol syndrome, to name just a few.

The combination of retinitis pigmentosa and deafness is known as Usher syndrome (see Appendix A: Pediatric Hearing Disorders). Children with Usher syndrome type 1 are born profoundly deaf and begin to lose their vision in the first decade of life. They may also exhibit balance difficulties and learn to walk slowly as children, due to problems in their vestibular system. Individuals with Usher syndrome type 2 are not born deaf but do have hearing loss that tends to begin during the second decade of life (Kimmerling & Moller, 1995). Of the adult deaf-blind individuals in the United States, more than half are believed to have Usher syndrome.

Understandably, severe deafness and blindness require unique educational approaches and specially trained teachers. The obstacles in teaching these children to communicate are significant, and learning language may be a lifelong pursuit. The prognosis for pediatric deaf-blind patients is certainly looking more favorable as they are approved for cochlear implantation. It is vitally important that information concerning the importance of visual assessment for persons with hearing loss be provided to parents of hearing-impaired children and to professionals (Roush et al., 2004). The concern for identification of Usher syndrome in the congenitally deaf child is very important, because the child and family will need extensive special education, counseling, social-emotional support, and vocational consideration. It is recommended that every child with hearing loss undergo routine ophthalmologic and optometry examination to ensure that the child's vision is corrected with eyeglasses when necessary.

IMPLEMENTING THE INDIVIDUALIZED EDUCATIONAL PLAN (IEP)

Education of deaf and hard-of-hearing children is the teaching of students with various degrees of hearing loss in a way that addresses the students' individual differences and needs. Ideally, this process involves the individually planned and systematically monitored arrangement of teaching procedures, adapted equipment and materials, accessible settings, and other interventions designed to help learners of various hearing levels achieve a higher level of personal self-sufficiency and success in school and community than would be available if the students were only given access to a typical classroom education. Deaf educators provide a continuum of services in which deaf students receive in varying degrees based on their individual needs. It is essential for deaf education programs to be individualized to address the unique combination of needs for each student.

All deaf students receive an Individualized Education Program (IEP) that outlines how the school will meet the student's individual needs. The Individuals with Disabilities Education Act (IDEA) requires that students with special needs be provided with a Free Appropriate Public Education (FAPE) in the Least Restrictive Environment (LRE) that is appropriate to the student's needs. School districts provide education for deaf and hard-of-hearing students in varying degrees from the least restrictive settings (i.e., mainstreaming) to the most restrictive settings, such as segregation in a deaf school. The education offered by the school must be appropriate to the student's individual needs. Schools are not required to maximize the student's potential or to provide the "best" possible services. Schools are required to provide other services, such as speech and occupational therapy, if the student needs these services. In addition to the child's parents, the IEP team must include at least one of the child's regular education teachers, a special education teacher, someone who can interpret the educational implications of the child's evaluation, such as a school psychologist, any related service personnel deemed appropriate or necessary, and an administrator or Committee of Special Education (CSE) representative who has adequate knowledge of the availability of services in the district and the authority to commit those services on behalf of the child. Parents are considered to be equal members of the IEP team along with the school staff.

A key factor in successful mainstreaming is the guarantee that deaf and hard-of-hearing students will not be "dumped and forgotten" into the regular classroom. This proviso is covered by the requirement in Public Law 94-142 for all handicapped children to receive personalized instruction and supportive services they need to benefit from an individualized educational program. The IEP is confirmation for hearing-impaired children that a more objective and scientific educational decision-making process will be followed. Through the use of IEPs, educators no longer rely on their own personal biases and preconceived ideas of what is best for the hearing-impaired child.

The team IEP written statement for each disabled child will include: (a) a statement of the present level of educational performance of such a child, (b) a statement of annual goals including short-term instructional objectives, (c) a statement of the specific educational services to be provided to such child, and the extent to which such child will be able to participate in regular educational programs, and (d) the projected date for initiation and anticipated duration of

such services, and appropriate objective criteria and evaluation procedures and schedules for determining, on at least an annual basis, whether instructional objectives are being achieved (Johnson et al., 1997).

Flexer (1990) points out that it is the school audiologist's role to actively integrate hearing services into the overall educational program of the child with hearing loss in a manner consistent with the philosophy, goals, and objectives of the child's IEP. If the provision of hearing services or auditory pieces of equipment is not mentioned in the IEP, there is no assurance that the child's hearing needs will be met. When the audiologist is included as an IEP team member and a signatory of the IEP, there is greater probability that the hearing needs will be noted, understood, and appropriately managed.

No one is more important to the success of today's mainstreamed hearing-impaired student than well-informed and assertive parents who are intimately involved in their child's mainstreamed program on a regular basis and are serving as IEP team members. Hearing-impaired children must have strong advocates if they are to be educated successfully in public schools. Most regular teachers, special educators, and administrators receive little training in the effects of hearing loss. Moreover, administrators are responsible for a wide variety of students and programs under their jurisdiction. Their problem is to stretch inadequate resources to cover many programs, and they cannot serve as effective advocates for individual or small groups of special needs children.

Data regarding the psychoeducational status of children with mild and moderate hearing loss are scarce. Despite the limited database, audiologists and speech-language pathologists might counsel parents regarding the possible deleterious effects of mild-to-moderate hearing loss and must help establish IEPs to enhance communication with these children and thus enrich their academic achievement. A project conducted by the University of Iowa (Davis et al., 1986) attempted to evaluate the psychoeducational performance of 40 hearing-impaired children to study the effects of degree of hearing loss, age, and other factors on intellectual, social, academic, and language behavior. Their data did not predict the children's language or educational performance on the basis of the degree of hearing impairment alone. Although some children evaluated in this study were performing exceptionally well, as a group the children fell into three major categories of significant delay: verbal skills, academic achievement, and social development. Some of these deficits did not manifest themselves until the child was in school for several years. The differences exhibited by the hearing-impaired children on the personality inventories suggest that these children are more likely to show aggressive tendencies, to express physical complaints, and to show significant behavior difficulties, especially social problems involving isolation and adjustment to school. It must be pointed out, however, that the individual results of this study confirmed the heterogeneity of hearing-impaired children and that the effects of hearing loss vary from child to child. The study concluded that children with any degree of hearing loss appear to be at risk for delayed development of verbal skills and reduced academic achievement.

EDUCATIONAL METHODOLOGIES

Deaf and hard-of-hearing children begin their educational journey as soon as possible following the confirmation of their hearing loss. The communication nature for children with hearing loss can be isolating but can be overcome through interaction with parents, peers, and teachers, all of whom contribute to the educational process. This interaction, for the purpose of transmitting knowledge and developing the child's self-esteem and identity, is dependent on direct one-to-one communication. Yet, communication is the area most hampered between a deaf child and his or her hearing siblings and parents, peers, and teachers. Certainly applications of hearing aids, cochlear implants, and other amplifying systems have brightened the communication arena. Because deafness is a low incidence disability, there is not widespread understanding of its educational implications, and it is somewhat beyond the general training of the classroom teacher. This lack of knowledge and skills in our education system contributes to the already substantial barriers to deaf and hard-of-hearing students in receiving appropriate educational services.

Many claims have been made about success of education of the deaf and hard-of-hearing children. Many claims, however, are from educators who have a strong personal belief in their own teaching techniques. Most claims, furthermore, are testimonials supported by a demonstration from one or two children with hearing loss who have performed exceedingly well under the advocated, or advertised, educational method. During the past decade, more and better research efforts have been conducted to evaluate various methodologies used to teach deaf children. However, knowledgeable professionals agree that no single methodology works for all deaf children. Although virtually volumes of material have been written on the methodologies through the years regarding education of hearing-impaired students, only a basic synopsis is provided in these pages.

The terms *auditory-oral* and *auditory-verbal* are used to describe programs that depend on the use of the child's residual hearing with teaching achieved mainly through spoken language. These auditory emphasis approaches are based on the expectation that young children who are deaf or hard-of-hearing can be educated through use of their own residual hearing, however slight. The descriptor *manual communication* is used to refer to programs that incorporate signs and fingerspelling. The term *total communication* is used to describe programs in which communication is accomplished by incorporating all means including the simultaneous use of auditory input, speech, and signs with fingerspelling along with natural gestures.

Although an enormous amount of research effort has been expended to determine the "best" communication mode for hearing-impaired children, the overall results have been, frankly, somewhat inconsistent. Contrary to the expectations of proponents for each of the deaf education methods, there are no widespread and consistent interactions between the degree of a child's hearing loss and communication mode or between the child's intelligence and preferred communication mode. Some studies have shown the superiority of auditory/verbal programs in specific education areas, whereas other studies favor total communication systems. Obviously a number of factors, which may or may not be interrelated, influence the results as well as the interpretation of the results among these many studies.

Auditory-Oral and Auditory-Verbal Methods

The auditory-oral (A-O) and auditory-verbal (A-V) methods, collectively sometimes termed listening and spoken language (LSL), are forms of oral education for deaf and hard-of-hearing children. These methods are based on the belief that a deaf child can learn to listen and speak so that his or her family does not need to learn sign language or cued speech (Harrison & Hutsell, 2009). Success with these methods relies, to a large degree, on parental involvement. Toddlers and preschoolers are typically taught through an auditory-verbal method utilizing personal amplification, with teachers who may be certified as Auditory-Verbal Therapists. The goal for these children is that they enter the mainstream school program after they have had time to develop their language, social, and cognitive development in an auditory-verbal classroom. Natural gestures used in typical conversation are utilized and encouraged. This approach can be used with all children regardless of hearing levels, including those with severe to profound hearing loss. Children who use this option may be placed in a continuum of educational placements including oral-oriented schools, self-contained classrooms for deaf students in public schools, or mainstream classrooms with hearing students.

The fundamental assumption of auditory-oral (also termed *oral-aural*) teaching programs is that every deaf child should be given an opportunity to communicate by speech. In addition to maximizing use of their residual hearing and personal amplification systems, speechreading is taught as a skill. Advocates of the A-O method believe that children who are deaf or hard-of-hearing should be educated in regular learning and living environments, and that this will enable them to become independent, participating, and contributing adults. Within the spirit of this philosophy, the thought is that a future employer is more inclined to hire a deaf or hard-of-hearing individual capable of understanding oral instructions rather than an equally capable deaf person to whom the employer must communicate in gestures and writing. Proponents of these auditory-emphasis approaches believe that auditory-oral (A-O) trained children do well in life, and that training in speech and speechreading permits an earlier adjustment to a world in which speech is the chief means of communication.

Today's popular listening and spoken language (LSL) programs combine the elements of the auditory-verbal approach (A-V) and the auditory-oral approach (A-O). As a result of advances in newborn hearing screening, hearing technologies, early intervention programs, and the specialty skills of professionals, the LSL approach has captured most of the toddler and preschool children with hearing loss. There has been a significant shift from the number of children in total communication programs to more children in auditory/oral programs in recent years. This shift has, no doubt, been a by-product of successful utilization of hearing aids and cochlear implants in young hard-of-hearing and deaf children. Furthermore, the success of legislative mandates in terms of early identification of children with hearing loss has been largely responsible for the decrease in the age of intervention for younger and younger children with hearing losses. Clearly there has been an increase in the number of school-aged children with hearing loss who are integrated (mainstreamed) with normal-hearing student peers and an increased emphasis on parental involvement.

The auditory/verbal systems teach that children who are to become good listeners also must use their vision to become good speechreaders. Because the two events do not happen simultaneously, it is necessary to establish the acoustic channel as the primary input means whenever possible. The use and development of the visual channel then seems to come naturally as needed. Conversely, auditory/verbal proponents would suggest that if the visual channel is established first as the main source of the child's perceptions and information, then the use of hearing will not come naturally but only laboriously and slowly and with much intensive training.

Researchers studied 139 preschool children with severe to profound hearing loss to investigate the relationship of several background and educational variables with the linguistic, academic, and social aspects of the children over a 4-year period (Musselman, Lindsay, & Wilson, 1988). Despite their careful analysis, they concluded that unequivocal statements about the value of particular approaches or the consequences of not following one approach or another were unwarranted. They did state strongly, however, that no approach succeeded in reversing the devastating effects on language of severe to profound hearing loss. As they tracked the children's movement among programs, it was found that auditory/oral programs with IEPs were the programs of choice, whereas the children in total communication programs and group education programs tended to do less well.

Musselman et al. (1988) noted that language itself is not a unitary ability but consists of a number of skills that respond differently to different interventions. In particular, it is necessary to distinguish among spoken language, receptive language, and mother-child communication. Despite the placement factors that operated in their study, these researchers found those children in total communication programs scored higher on measures of receptive language and mother-child communication, whereas children in auditory/verbal programs had better spoken language.

Historically, in the United States, the auditory/oral approach in education for deaf and hard-of-hearing children has undergone significant changes. All auditory/oral methods share the commonality that they depend on speechreading and audition and, generally, wholly exclude the use of sign language. The commonality between auditory-oral approaches over the years makes it difficult to separate these auditory-based methods, and elements of all seem to have evolved into today's LSL programs. In the early years, the auditory-oral approaches were most successful with those children who had lesser degrees of hearing loss (i.e., good residual hearing and good listening skills), while children with profound hearing loss were directed into manual or total communication education programs. The common goal in all of the auditory-oral programs is to make the youngsters with hearing loss or deafness an integral part of the hearing society through good speechreading and hearing aid use. With today's amplification technologies, degree of hearing loss is less of a factor in directing children with hearing loss into educational programs, and most deaf and hard-of-hearing infants, toddlers, and preschoolers are initially entered into the LSL arena.

An early oral method, known as *pure oralism/auditory stimulation* was developed at the Clarke School for the Deaf during the late 19th century. All sign language was discouraged, and the children were fitted with hearing aids and exposed to sounds and spoken language at every opportunity. In theory, the deaf youngster was to "hear" everything that a youngster with normal hearing might hear; only the auditory stimulation was presented with more deliberate action and intensity than usual circumstances might dictate. The method included ample visual attention to speechreading and included training with isolated sound elements, sound combinations, words, and finally connected speech. Much of the work was done at home with the parents.

When auditory stimulation or speechreading was perhaps not sufficient to initiate satisfactory speech and language development in the auditory-oral child, an oral method known as the *multisensory/ syllable unit method* was used. It is essentially the same as the pure oral procedure with speechreading, except that reading and writing of orthographic forms of English were included. Sight and touch therapies were used to formulate the multisensory approach. Pieces of this auditory-oral teaching system are still widely used in special classrooms and one-to-one programs. Everything in the hard-of-hearing or deaf child's environment is labeled, and his or her attention is drawn to the relation between the written form and the object, as well as the relation between the written form and the spoken word. The teacher may use the motokinesthetic and tactile methods to supplement speech learning, where the child mimics speech production by feeling the teacher's face and reproducing the same breathing and vibration effects.

Another important historical oral method was the *language association-element method* or *natural language method*. It was developed at the Lexington School for the Deaf in New York City with the premise that the deaf child should learn to speak through normal living and daily activities. This type of program is developed around ordinary learning activities, the classroom might include a kitchen and normal household accessories, and the teachers continually talk to the children and encourage them to ask questions through vocalized speech. Activities, of course, are supplemented with specialized instruction in speechreading and speech production as well as the written form of the activity or object.

Not to be overlooked or forgotten is the well-recognized variant of the auditory/oral method called the *unisensory* or *aural approach* to education of the deaf developed by Doreen Pollack at the University of Denver in the early 1970s. Doreen Pollack (1982) felt that audition is the most suitable perceptual modality by which a child learns speech and language; therefore, her unisensory approach develops the impaired hearing modality to its fullest by focusing attention on auditory activities including speech. As with all auditory-oral approaches, the unisensory approach is dependent on very early identification, early parental guidance and participation, early amplification, and total exposure to normal language stimulation. The principles of the Pollack approach have been incorporated into what is known as the *auditory-verbal practice method*. Luterman (1976) agreed that through the auditory-verbal practice method approach, speechreading or visual awareness of the face need not be taught; rather, the impaired auditory modality must be trained while allowing the child to use supplemental visual information.

Today's natural auditory oral programs, supported through today's numerous technology advances, are quite different from the old oral programs (Clark, 2007). The auditory-verbal practice method (now also known as Listening and Spoken Language) has achieved increased popularity in recent years from the need for cochlear implant recipients to receive an intensive auditory therapy program in order to maximize their newly acquired auditory potential. Listening and Spoken Language focuses on audition and listening as the major forces in nurturing the development of the child's personal, social, and academic life. It is based on the belief that the use of amplified residual hearing permits children who are deaf or hard-of-hearing to learn to listen, process verbal language, and speak within their family and community constellations (Estabrooks, 2000). Verbal-auditory training goals and activities are tied to the developmental stages of each child and incorporated into ordinary daily routines, in song, educational activities, and play. An active international nonprofit organization, with stringent certification requirements for teachers, has been established as Auditory-Verbal International, Inc., to support professionals, parents, and persons who are deaf or hard-of-hearing.

Opponents argue against the auditory/verbal methods, citing several objections to the approach. In general, the complainants are opposed to teaching speechreading as a basic skill and the dependence on the impaired residual hearing to pick up auditory cues. They cite the fact that the auditory-oral methods depend too heavily on the development of speechreading skills that are difficult for many to achieve at any level of proficiency. Speechreading is notoriously ambiguous because: (a) many sounds and words look alike on the lips (homophonous words such as [mat], [pan], and [bat]; (b) many sounds are not visible because they are made in the back of the throat such as /k/, /g/, and /ng/; (c) many people do not speak clearly and distinctly; and (d) speaking styles among persons vary tremendously. In fact, speechreading is an art mastered by very few. Speechreading depends on good language skills, acute vision, good lighting, and exposure of the lips, and is limited by distance between speakers. Speechreading is less useful in dimly lit environments, within groups of talkers, or for speaker-audience formats.

The practice of inclusion in mainstream classrooms has been criticized by some parents of children with special needs because some of these students require instructional methods that differ dramatically from typical classroom methods. Critics assert that it is not possible to deliver effectively two or more very different instructional methods in the same classroom. As a result, the educational progress of students who depend on different instructional methods to learn often fall even further behind their peers. Parents of typically normal developing children sometimes fear that the special needs of "fully included" students will take critical levels of attention and energy away from the rest of the class and thereby impair the academic achievements of all students.

A classic study initiated at the University of Minnesota by Weiss, Goodwin, and Moores (1975) intensively evaluated children in several well-known programs for the deaf and hard-of-hearing. The programs provided a diverse representation of approaches to deaf education, ranging from auditory/oral to visual/oral. One of the findings regarding children who were integrated into mainstream education was that these children had better hearing acuity and superior articulation before integration. It seemed conclusively evident that children do not speak better because of integration but are integrated because they speak better. Other measures in the 6-year Minnesota study compared relative communication efficiency between modes of training. Children were found to receive communication most efficiently when stimuli were presented simultaneously through speech and signs. Next were simultaneous speech and fingerspelling, followed by speechreading and sound. The least efficient means was teaching through auditory methods alone. In the area of expressive speech, the better-hearing students had better articulation scores. The training method seemed not to affect articulation scores; rather, skill in articulation was related to the emphasis on auditory training and articulation provided in a program.

Despite the best of altruistic expectations, the auditory/oral methods cannot be successful with every deaf child. For example, some deaf children have no measurable hearing for one reason or another. Temporal bone studies from children with profound deafness have been reported with total absence of the cochlear structures or eighth nerve fibers. Cochlear implants may not be recommended or some children may not do well with their implants for any one of a variety of reasons. Amplification, through personal hearing aids, may provide little or no substantive benefit. For the deaf and hearing-impaired children who fall into these categories, some other educational method may be the appropriate choice.

Visual-Oral Methods

The visual/oral methods are contrasted with the auditory/oral methods by their inclusion of manual signs and fingerspelling and, in fact, are most commonly known as *manual communication systems*. The basic philosophy behind these teaching techniques is that the visual aspect of signing and fingerspelling adds a component to the process that makes communication considerably easier. Deaf and hard-of-hearing children receive input through a standardized system of signs and fingerspelling and are taught to express themselves through speech, signs, and fingerspelling. The visual/oral methods do not exclude speechreading and auditory training and speech production, but they do not make these facets of the educational method the main focus. The primary goal in visual/oral education is to provide deaf and hard-of-hearing children with a strong knowledge base, with production and reception of speech per se as a secondary goal.

Manualists critique the auditory/oral methods that place emphasis on speechreading as a major component to the curriculum to the diminution of the basic education subjects. Manual education specialists believe that language skills are paramount to speech production or speechreading, both educationally and socially.

Speechreading

Speechreading (or lip reading) is utilized by every hard-of-hearing or deaf individual inherently, regardless of their communication system choice. Speechreading helps persons with hearing loss understand speech. It involves watching the movements of a speaker's mouth and face to help understand what the speaker is saying. It is estimated that 40% of the sounds in the English language can be seen on the lips of a speaker in good conditions, such as a well-lit room where the child can see the speaker's face. But many words look exactly the same on the lips; therefore, speechreading is seldom used in isolation. For example, "bop," "mop," and "pop," look exactly alike when spoken. Speechreading skills vary tremendously among those with hearing loss; some individuals are quite good at the task, while others are admittedly hopeless. A good speech reader might be able to see only 4 to 5 words in a 12-word sentence. Speechreading is usually used in combination with other tools, such as auditory training (listening), total communication, cued speech, and others. Babies naturally begin using this building block if they can see the speaker's mouth and face. But as a child gets older, he or she will still need some training. Sometimes, when talking with a person who is deaf or hard-of-hearing, people will exaggerate their mouth movements or talk very loudly. Exaggerated mouth movements and a loud voice can make speechreading very difficult.

American Sign Language (ASL)

Manual signing was first acknowledged as a language and incorporated into deaf education in 18th century France and brought to the United States in the early 1800s. At about that same time, Alexander Graham Bell was advocating auditory/oral education inspired by his communication success with his deaf wife. So began the often emotional and totally unresolved 200-year-old debate of which method of educating deaf children should prevail. Although strong feeling can still be elicited among educators of the deaf, and the two definitive camps still exist exhorting the value of manual communication versus auditory-oral communication, conventional wisdom prevails and supports the viewpoint that all means of communication are of value to deaf and hard-of-hearing individuals. Today, American Sign Language (ASL) is said to be the third most used bilingual language in the United States, following Spanish and Italian. ASL is the natural and cultural language of the majority of the early-onset deaf population comprising today's adult deaf (Lotke, 1995).

The beginnings of ASL are said to lie with the work of L'Abbè de L'Epèe, a French priest, who undertook the education of two deaf sisters in 1750. Fingerspelling had been used earlier to teach language to the deaf in France, but to it L'Epèe added a "natural language of gestures." He established a school to teach the deaf in Paris in 1760 and was later succeeded by his equally famous pupil, L'Abbè Sicard. In 1815, an American named Thomas Hopkins Gallaudet, a minister from Hartford, Connecticut, met a young deaf neighbor girl, Alice Cogswell. Gallaudet was deeply taken by Alice's plight of "mutism" and the fact that she had no place to go to school. He sought support from families of other deaf children and ultimately went to Europe to study methods of teaching the deaf. He visited London and was refused access to Watson's Asylum, where secret and expensive educational methods were jealously guarded. However, he met L'Abbè Sicard and was invited to Paris to learn L'Epèe's system of sign language. From this warm welcome in France, he returned to America with a young deaf teacher, Laurent Clerc, and established the first school for the deaf in the United States in 1817, the American School for the Deaf in Hartford. The school was replicated throughout the United States, and L'Epèe's sign language was fused with the natural gestures used in America and became the basis for present-day sign language.

Years later, Thomas Hopkins Gallaudet, enjoying the success of establishing schools for the deaf across the United States, was still not satisfied. As an older man he passed his vision on to his son, Edward Miner Gallaudet, and his dream was realized with the establishment of Gallaudet College in 1864, the world's first college of the deaf, in Washington, DC. The establishment of the National Technical Institute for the Deaf, associated with Rochester Institute of Technology in New York, was the second full college program for the deaf—more than 100 years following the dedication of Gallaudet College.

It is said by many, including the vast majority of deaf adults, that sign language is the common, natural language of the deaf and is the basis of the Deaf Culture movement. The signs have concrete meanings. Words can be spelled on the fingers to connect the signs into sentences. In normal conversations using ASL, the speaker combines signs and fingerspelling. Signs are generally easier to understand ("read"), and fingerspelling can be fast, rapid, and implemented to fill in gaps where signs are unavailable or unknown to the speaker. According to Ridgeway (1969), "American

Sign Language is part mime; it is beautiful to watch, highly expressive and receptive." ASL serves communication purposes with far more than just signs and fingerspelling, as facial expression and body language convey much of the content and emotion of the communication (Kelly, 2009).

The language of signs has been subjected to systematic analysis by several investigators including Tervoort (1964), Bornstein (1973, 1978, 1979), and Wilber (1987). Their conclusion is that sign language is an independent language that is not just a translation of oral language. ASL has true linguistic parameters such as morphology, phonology, and syntax in the same manner as any foreign language. Natural gestures and fingerspelling depend on situational understanding; when a sign has a tendency to become repeated and understood by more than one person, the sign is "formalized" and is no longer a natural gesture. ASL users communicate with their fingers and hands through the use of hand shapes, hand localizations and movements, and palm orientations. Users of ASL understand the importance of facial expression in effective communication. Body and facial movements with use of the eyes, head, and shoulders can convey subtle, complex, and abstract thoughts as well as many of the subtleties needed to enrich communication.

There are certainly limitations to the use of sign language and fingerspelling in communication and teaching. ASL is somewhat limited in power when compared with oral language, although it can be argued that the skill of the ASL user is paramount in this regard. For many, ASL is bound to the concrete and limited in expression of abstractions, metaphor, irony, and humor. In everyday communication, ASL does not necessarily follow the formal language use of written or oral English. For these reasons, the detractors of ASL feel that its use interferes with the learning of language. Likewise, parents or family members may not achieve the necessary skills to use ASL in natural language communication, and it becomes nonstandard "pidgin" English. Of concern in the educational system, teachers and teacher-aides working with deaf and hard-of-hearing children may lack a sufficient proficiency in ASL to be good models for their students.

On the other hand, the visual-spatial aspects of ASL make it an easy means of communication for those deaf children who cannot easily access auditory information. ASL permits parents to interact fully with their children at a very early age and certainly encourages and stimulates communication. Like any other language, ASL must be learned. Motivated parents pick up easy ASL signs and start teaching their normal-hearing babies to build early vocabulary. A baby with hearing loss can learn ASL as a first language that is used simultaneously with ASL, thereby promoting oral interactions. In fact, simultaneous use of the spoken voice along with ASL is practiced routinely by many as it provides additional communication information through lip-reading and enhances facial expression. This common approach is known as the simultaneous method and uses speech, speechreading, amplification, and finger-spelling and signing—all at the same time. Koch (2009) points out that when teachers or parents simultaneously use sign and spoken language, it is often used without natural order of English and may not include function words and word endings. Koch states that in simultaneous sign and speech, the child does not get a clear representation of either English or ASL. Given that ASL does not follow English word order, it cannot be "spoken." Spoken language is, by nature, difficult to see on the lips, so the child does not get the complete English message either. This leads some experts to believe it is more effective to use either ASL without voice, or spoken English without sign. However, studies have shown that when used appropriately and correctly, signing can effectively facilitate the development of spoken language.

The standardization of ASL has been enhanced by the availability of numerous ASL dictionaries, teaching videos and DVDs, and innumerable sign language books. The quality and expertise of interpreters for the deaf using ASL is maintained and administrated through the National Registry of Interpreters for the Deaf (RID). The Registry of Interpreters for the Deaf, Inc. (RID), a national membership organization, plays a leading role in advocating for excellence in the delivery of interpretation and transliteration services between people who use sign language and people who use spoken language. The RID has a current membership of more than 15,000 certified ASL-qualified interpreters. RID members are often seen standing beside public speakers, providing excellent interpretive services for the benefit of the deaf who might be in the audience. Today, the Internet is awash with literally thousands of postings and videos demonstrating ASL as well as many online ASL courses for those interested in learning the system (Figure 10–2).

Brief mention should be made of variants of the manual communications systems known as the combined method and the Rochester method. The combined method uses speech, speechreading, amplification, and fingerspelling but with no signing; the Rochester method uses fingerspelling and oral language only. The idea behind the Rochester Method was to make deaf communication like English print as much as possible, a sort of "writing in air" technique superimposed on normal speech. The Rochester method fell out of favor because

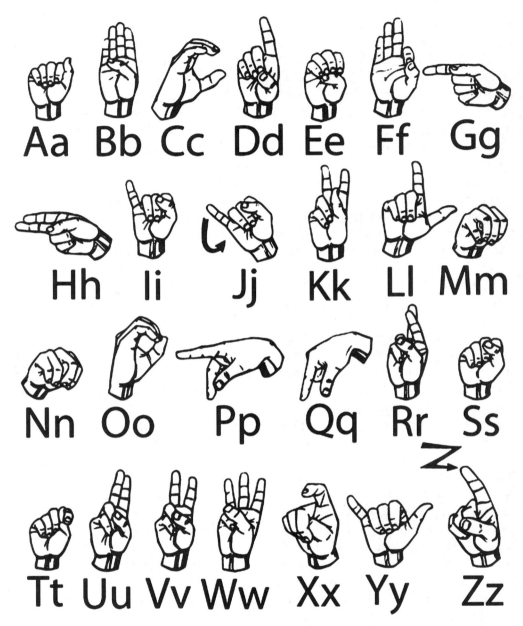

Figure 10–2. The American Sign Language (ASL) manual alphabet has been in use for nearly two centuries (user: L'Aquatique/Wikimedia Commons/CC-A-SA 3.0, GFDL 1.2).

it is a tedious and time-consuming process to fingerspell everything manually. These variant systems of visual communication have essentially disappeared due to their limited success.

Total Communication

Total communication (TC) is a philosophy of educating children with hearing loss that incorporates all means of communication including natural gestures, fingerspelling, sign language, body language, lipreading, and speech. The goal is simply to optimize language development in whatever way is most effective for the individual child, recognizing that different environments, speakers, and topics may benefit from any or all communication approaches. The proponents of total communication recognized the educational advantages of visible speech, yet they also noted certain difficulties. The manual dexterity of the preschool child limits his or her ability to fingerspell quickly, and the child's limited attention span makes it difficult to attend intensely on "flying fingers and fleeting flexible faces" for an all-day instruction session. Total communication is a philosophy that requires the incorporation of appropriate aural, manual, and oral modes of communication to ensure effective communication with and among persons with hearing loss.

Total communication, as it is stressed by its advocates, is a *philosophy* and not simply another method for teaching deaf children. The basic premise is to use all means to communicate with deaf children from infancy to school age. No particular method or system is to be omitted or stressed. The student is exposed to natural gestures, ASL, fingerspelling, facial expression, and body English, all accompanied simultaneously with speech heard through hearing aids. The idea is to use any means that works to convey vocabulary, language, and idea concepts between the deaf child and everyone to whom he or she is exposed. The important concept is to provide an easy, free, two-way communication means between the deaf child and his or her family, teacher, and schoolmates. In some environments and educational facilities, total communication is practiced continually with all pupils throughout their school years.

Opponents of total communication complain that if a teacher of the deaf really favors one method over another, the teacher will unwittingly move the students in the direction of that approach under the guise of teaching total communication. Some educators believe that it is not possible to evaluate the effectiveness of any one approach while using all the approaches at the same time. These arguments, however, seem to miss the main concept of total communication, which says that it is paramount to communicate without regard for which method is really achieving it. The total communication approach has been criticized because it is too much of a shotgun approach to education of the deaf. Critics argue that the overstimulation of the deaf child with speech and signs is actually detrimental to learning communication. On the other hand, new interest in total communication was the result of several research studies reporting the superiority of deaf children of deaf parents who were exposed to manual communication over deaf children of hearing parents in English skills, academic achievement, writing, reading, and social maturity. The two groups showed no differences in speech skills.

An interesting survey was reported by Matkin and Matkin (1985) of parents whose hearing-impaired children had initially been enrolled in an aural/oral program for a minimum of 2 years and then subsequently enrolled in a total communication class in a day school setting for at least 2 years. The parents were asked a series of questions concerning the social, emotional, and educational growth of their child as well as the impact of the change in school communication system on their speech, speechreading, and hearing aid use. The study found a significant positive correlation between parents' overall perception as to the benefits of total communication and their perception of their children's educational and emotional growth. In addition, the parents did not perceive the use of total communication as adversely affecting speechreading, speech production, or hearing aid use.

Total communication (TC) is an important concept on behalf of the deaf child. In reality, it is a philosophy of anything goes that helps communicate with the deaf and hard-of-hearing. TC teachers are encouraged to use whatever communication tools are most effective for the individual child. This is a significant change in attitude from stressing a particular "method" to an overall concern for the deaf child's needs to be immersed in two-way communication. Because TC is a philosophy, rather than a teaching method, per se, there are no particular strategies, guidelines, standards, or rules in its application.

Other Sign Systems

During the 1970s, several manual sign systems were developed as improvements to American Sign Language (ASL) such that they represent more accurately spoken or written English. Not all of these new systems survived the test of time. Known collectively as manually coded English (MCE),

they represent a variety of visual communication methods expressed through the hands which attempt to represent more precisely the English language. Unlike deaf sign languages that have evolved naturally in deaf communities, the different forms of MCE were artificially created, and generally follow the grammar of English. MCE can be used while simultaneously speaking and signing at the same time. This is not possible with, for example, ASL because it has a very different grammar (including word order) than spoken or written English. Deaf sign languages make use of spatial relationships, facial expression, and body positioning, while manually coded systems tend to be linear and purely manual communication systems, not to be construed as new languages. Comprehensibility of such simultaneously produced MCE has, however, been shown to be compromised in practice. Although experience can improve the degree to which the information coded in English (morphologically as well as syntactically) is successfully communicated manually, there appear to be limits, and attempting to code everything precisely for more than very brief messages is extremely taxing on the person communicating simultaneously.

These sign systems are described here to orient readers to the basic philosophies, approaches, nomenclature, and differences, because these approaches have been developed to overcome apparent inadequacies of the ASL. The idea of MCE systems is that they can be the visual equivalent of spoken English. Furthermore, they share the philosophy that if this type of visual communication system is introduced to the deaf or hard-of-hearing child at a very early age, their language skills, total experiences, mental health, and communicative abilities will be improved over traditional communication and educational approaches. Manual communication proponents assume that the more syntactically correct the visual symbols, the more it will aid in development of language in the deaf child.

Cued Speech

Cued speech is a method of communication developed in the late 1960s for the deaf and hard-of-hearing using the mouth and hand to visually distinguish the phonemes of spoken language. The basic concept was to develop natural language and literacy visually for those who do not receive sufficient input through listening or assistive devices (Roffe, 2009). The method sought to combat poor reading skills among deaf college students by providing deaf children with a solid linguistic background. The system uses eight hand configurations and four hand placements at locations around the speaking mouth to supplement the visible manifestations of natural speech from the lips and facial expressions. The 12 cues described above are used around the chin, cheek, and neck, drawing attention to the speaker's face and lips. The cued speech system provides a visible phonetic analog of speech in the form of lip movements supplemented by hand cues with both vowel and consonant cues, thereby making it easier for a child to differentiate sounds that look alike on the lips such as /b/ and /p/ (Waldman & Roush, 2010).

Cued speech was hailed in its early years by some as a possible answer to the oralism versus manualism controversy and is currently the choice of some parents who have children using hearing aids or cochlear implants. An advantage to cued speech is that it facilitates the acquisition of the vocabulary and the syllabic-phonemic-rhythmic patterns of the spoken language to interpolate the written form of English (Cornett, 1985). Cued speech forces the use of information on the lips without subjecting the child to the confusion of speechreading. The hand cues are not intelligible without proper mouth motions. Cued speech can be learned in 12 to 15 hours and can be used to cue accents and dialects, foreign languages, and idiomatic expressions. Cued speech has been adapted for languages and dialects around the world.

Signing Exact English (SEE)

Signing Exact English was developed in 1972 as a sign system that matches signs with the English language. The system provides a visual counterpart to match both spoken and written English. The use of SEE does not exclude the use of ASL or other sign systems. In fact, 75% of the signs used in SEE are the traditional signs that are common to all sign language systems (Stephenson, 2009). In SEE, the signs represent only one English word as well as affixes as needed. The signs are used in combinations to form any desired word. To reflect English syntax, SEE emphasizes complete English word order. Verb tense is clearly indicated and irregular verb forms have signed representation. English compound words are often made up of elements different from the single sign element often used in ASL.

SEE is quickly and easily learned as it follows the rules of spoken language. SEE has become popular to support language development in the growing number of children who use cochlear implants or hearing aids as it allows them to match what they see with what they hear and speak. Because each sign represents a spoken and written word, the transfer to the printed English form is done naturally. Additionally, the use of ASL visual features such as facial expression, body language, use of placement, and directionality support ease of communication with SEE (Stephenson & Zawolkow, 2009). Considerable information regarding SEE is available on the Internet, through DVDs or college courses.

Bilingual-Bicultural Education

In this educational method, deafness is seen as a cultural issue. The bilingual-bicultural education method advocates that children who are deaf are taught ASL as a first language, and then are taught written and spoken English as a second language. As the children learn two languages at the same time, they are considered bilingual. Bilingual-bicultural programs emphasize that English and ASL are equal languages, and they work to help children develop age-appropriate levels of fluency in both languages. The bilingual-bicultural approach holds the belief that deaf children are visual learners as opposed to auditory learners; therefore, classes should be conducted in a complete visual language. Because ASL and spoken English cannot be used simultaneously for the fear of harming the accuracy and fluency of both, ASL alone with no oral language, or voice-off ASL, is usually used. Many bilingual-bicultural schools have dormitories, and students can either commute to school every day or stay in a dormitory as part of the residential program and visit their families on weekends and holidays and school vacations. Most students trained in bilingual-bicultural method use their languages for different purposes (e.g., they may use one language at home and another at school, one with siblings or peers, and one with parents or family). Proficiency in each language depends on how and when

the language was learned and the level of skill needed in each context of use. The National Association of the Deaf advocates for a bilingual approach to best support deaf students in their education (Baker & Baker, 1997; Fish & Morford, 2012; Marschark, Lang, & Albertini, 2002).

MAINSTREAM EDUCATION

Mainstreaming may be the most important issue in education of deaf children in the past few decades. In the context of children with hearing loss, mainstreaming refers to the placement of a deaf or hard-of-hearing student alongside his or her hearing peers in a regular school classroom. Mainstreaming is an educational programming option for youth with disabilities to pursue all or a majority of their education within a regular school program with students who do not have disabilities. Mainstreaming used to be known as "integration" of the hard-of-hearing student into regular classrooms of hearing children. Mainstreaming is a procedure that is well established in the United States and is the crest of a fast-moving wave in education circles. The real push for mainstreaming children with disabilities has been the stimulation provided by the least restrictive environment (LRE) portion of the Individuals with Disabilities Education Act (IDEA) developed out of the federal law known as the Education for All Handicapped Children Act of 1975. Recognizing the cost effectiveness of removing a student from a self-contained special education model and placing that student in a typical classroom was a boon for school districts that embraced the idea of LRE and interpreted it as mainstreaming (Mathers, 2009). Although mainstreaming has become nearly synonymous with the least restrictive environment, in actuality LRE does not necessarily mean a mainstream placement.

The organization of educational programs for hearing-impaired students has undergone considerable change in most states. The change is from serving only a few students, mainly in residential schools, to serving many hard-of-hearing and deaf students in local community schools with a system that provides a variety of educational opportunities to the students and their parents. It has become commonly accepted that the student with a hearing loss in a mainstream placement will likely receive a superior education through exposure to typical peers and instruction in the typical classroom (Mathers, 2009).

It has become apparent over time, however, that partial or full-time integration for hearing-impaired students into regular classes is not a realistic goal for every child, and the policy of self-containment classes is not suitable for all hearing-impaired children. In short, mainstreaming is not for every child. It happens in some classroom situations that the child with hearing loss is not held to the same expectations as the peer children resulting in moving through the education system without becoming appropriately educated. Classroom teachers without training in the education of children with hearing loss are stymied in the classroom and not sure how to teach or what to require from these special needs students.

The child with hearing loss may have special supplementary educational needs such as a classroom interpreter or note taker to facilitate understanding the teacher. The presence of hearing aids or cochlear implants on the student may create embarrassment or difficult situations for the hard-of-hearing student. The integration of students with hearing loss into the regu-

lar classroom is a means of eliminating the deleterious effects of segregation and the stigma often attached to the "handicapped" child. Normal children are thus exposed to disabled children on a daily basis in everyday situations, hopefully resulting in positive and enlightened responses toward the integrated student. Of course, a negative response to the integrated child or disability condition is also possible, with devastating results to the integrated child.

In practice, mainstreaming has as many variations as there are schools with enrollment of students with hearing loss. Ideally, each student's mainstreaming experience should be as unique as the specific needs of the individual; a student might be placed with his peers in the normal classroom for as little as 30 minutes per day to a full-day placement. The key to success is that the student has good access to the curriculum and is consistently demonstrating understanding and mastery of the materials. Specialized services may be provided inside or outside the regular classroom. Selected students with hearing loss may occasionally leave the regular classroom to attend smaller, more intensive instructional sessions in a resource room, or to receive other related services that might require specialized equipment or might be disruptive to the rest of the class, such as speech and language therapy. However, it must be said that simply being placed in the mainstream classroom does not guarantee the student a superior education.

Birch (1976) suggested that mainstreaming deaf and hard-of-hearing children should be done only after thorough preparation, with sensitivity to the needs of all parties, and with careful monitoring and support. Birch stated that degree and onset of hearing loss are not the primary factors in selecting children for mainstreaming.

Advanced technologies, including hearing aids, cochlear implants, and FM amplification systems provide students with various degrees of hearing loss with excellent access to classroom speech at optimal signal-to-noise ratios. Most regular classroom teachers are accepting of students with hearing loss and are willing to design programs for complete or partial mainstreaming, depending on the child's capabilities, requirements, and the school's resources. The overall success of regular classroom teachers' efforts in mainstreaming deaf and hard-of-hearing students is the reason for its continued utilization and further development.

The ASL communicating child should only be put into a class with hearing children when a qualified ASL interpreter is available to translate everything said in the classroom into sign language and fingerspelling. The best scenario exists when the interpreter is a trained teacher of the deaf or a specially trained teacher's aide, so that the teacher-aide function is utilized constantly to help the student understand what is being said by the teacher and classmates. The tutor-interpreter helps the deaf and hard-of-hearing child to keep up with the rest of the class and grasp fully what is going on at all times. Acceptance of such a program in the regular school is enhanced by teaching all the normal-hearing peer classmates and the regular classroom teachers elements of ASL and fingerspelling.

Special consideration must be given when hearing aids and cochlear implants are worn by the deaf and hard-of-hearing child mainstreamed into the regular classroom without regard for the acoustic characteristics of the normal schoolroom. Poor signal-to-noise ratios can produce detrimental effects on speech discrimination and understanding by the student dependent on amplification aids. Brackett and Maxon (1986) published a useful listing of services for hearing-impaired mainstreamed children that might be provided by the educational audiologist in the public school setting (Table 10–3).

Ling (1975) likened the deaf education controversy to cyclic sunspot activity: it flared up on numerous occasions in the past and abates only when the protagonists realize that there is no one method or mixture of methods that can possibly meet all the needs of deaf and hard-of-hearing children and their parents. Davis, Shepard, Stelmachowicz, and Gorga (1981) described the population of hearing-impaired children as "vastly heterogeneous" and correctly pointed out that the best use of the residual hearing in each child will require different procedures and emphasis. These authors provide a strong summary statement for this topic by stating:

> We really must stop arguing over whether children use the auditory system alone or in conjunction with visual or tactual information during educational endeavors. If the energy spent in futile attempts to convince each other of the supremacy of one educational method over another had been spent in devising ways to maximize reception through all modalities, including hearing, it is unlikely that the educational achievement levels of hearing-impaired children would be as low as they are today.

In view of the current social climate and to meet the mandated federal laws, mainstreaming is here to stay. Nevertheless, caution must be exercised so that professionals and parents do not perceive mainstreaming as "the only way to go." The most important issue is to ensure that parents have the option of choice and that they fully understand all of the possible educational placements available for their child with hearing loss.

Table 10–3. Suggested Responsibilities for Educational Audiologists

Comprehensive audiologic and amplification evaluation:

Unaided: pure tone air and bone conduction thresholds

Unaided: speech reception and speech perception

Electroacoustic impedance measures

Aided sound field warble tone for hearing aids and FM systems thresholds

Aided (aids and FM): soundfield speech measures

Electroacoustic analysis of hearing aids, FM and cochlear implant systems

Thorough report from evaluator

Comprehensive communication evaluation

Preferred receptive mode: auditory only, visual only, auditory-visual combined

Comprehension of spoken language: vocabulary level, sentence level, connected discourse

Production of spoken language: vocabulary level, sentence level, connected discourse

Speech intelligibility

Written language

Annual reevaluation

Educational evaluation

Skill differentiation within subtests important

Test presentation and format to be considered during interpretation of results

Annual reevaluation

Psychosocial evaluation

Performance subtests used as an estimate of potential

Verbal subtests measure language ability

Triennial reevaluation

Classroom observation

Child/teacher interaction

Child/child interaction

Child participation

Classroom modifications

Learning strategies

Use of FM systems

Analysis of noise sources

Visual distractions

Use of classroom aide/interpreter

Audiologic management

Improving classroom acoustics

Recommending and using FM systems

Daily troubleshooting of personal aids and FM system

Assessing use of FM system within various settings Monitoring of middle ear problems with appropriate referrals

Speech-language management

Focus on deficit areas that affect academic performance and social interaction

Coordination with other support personnel and classroom teacher

Educational management

Favorable seating

Buddy system

Notetaker

Discussion of hearing impairment/ amplification

Improving classroom presentation: characteristics of teacher's speech, paraphrasing of content, directing classroom discussion using visual aids

Improving the use of classroom amplification

Improving classroom flexibility

Discussing teacher's expectations

Facilitating teacher/tutor exchange

Preview/review tutoring

Academic vocabulary

Academic content

Classroom aide/interpreter

Psychosocial management

Adolescent group, including career information

Parent support group

Extracurricular social activities

Parent involvement

Home support

continues

Table 10–3. *continued*

Program planning	Alternative educational placement
Regular contact with school personnel	Full mainstreaming
In-service training	Partial mainstreaming
Staff: whole school: once each year	Social mainstreaming
Direct service personnel: twice per year	Self-contained class in regular school
Individual as needed	
Peers: once per year	

Source: Adapted from "Service Delivery Alternatives for the Mainstreamed Hearing Impaired Child," by D. Brackett and A. B. Maxon, 1986, *Language, Speech and Hearing Services in Schools, 17*, pp. 115–125.

CLASSROOM ACOUSTICS

Anyone who has visited a school recently must realize what a noisy environment surrounds our children who spend most of their day in classrooms, hallways, auditoriums, and gymnasiums. The open-plan classroom is nearly the standard in today's elementary schools, along with a teacher who constantly moves about the room while talking. It has been well-recognized that these learning areas, with their poor acoustic conditions and noisy backgrounds, provide a "soundscape that is a barrier to learning" for all students, but especially for students with hearing loss (Anderson, 2004). The school acoustic environment in which students with hearing loss learn typically has high noise levels and poor acoustic conditions. Numerous studies have shown that classroom acoustics are an important consideration that can be deleterious to the student with hearing loss. The three critical factors that contribute to the poor acoustics and noise in the classroom are the level of speech from the teacher, the distance from the teacher, and the amount of room reverberation (Finitzo-Hieber, 1988).

Much of the noise that exists in the classroom could be reduced or eliminated through simple architectural modifications. Of course there is the unwanted noise from the children themselves, the teachers in the next-door classrooms who can be heard through the walls, the crowd playing outside the window enjoying recess, unnecessary public address announcements, music from the band room and cafeteria, gymnasium, and so forth. Other extraneous and unwanted noise is inherent in the building from the heating and air-conditioning systems and outside traffic patterns. Some schools are actually located under commercial air traffic lanes or near heavy traffic highways. Some of these noises could be reduced with thoughtful consideration from the school administration to effect a quieter environment for the students. It makes sense that older classrooms could be modified to improve their acoustic properties and that new classrooms be designed and built to absorb unwanted noises. However, in our current economic era, it is unlikely that schools currently strapped for finances to meet students' educational goals are not likely to expend funds to improve the acoustics of classrooms unless motivated by outside sources.

Acoustical engineers and audiologists have worked to develop standards and guidelines to reduce the noise and draw attention to the problems of acoustics in school classrooms. Currently, the ANSI standards document (ANSI S12.60-2002), ASHA (2005a, 2005b) documents, and an American Academy of Audiology statement on classroom acoustics (2008) provide excellent resource information to improve classroom listening conditions. The 2002 ANSI standards call for classroom noise levels in unoccupied core learning spaces to not exceed 35 dBA SPL, depending on room size; reverberation time should not exceed 0.6 seconds in small rooms to 0.7 seconds in larger rooms.

Reverberation time (RT) is used to determine how quickly a sound decays in a room. Reverberation time depends on the physical volume and surface materials of a room. Large spaces, such as cathedrals and gymnasiums, usually have longer reverberation times and sound "lively" or sometimes "boomy." Small rooms, such as bedrooms and recording studios, with sound-absorbing materials, are usually less reverberant and sound "dry" or "dead." Ideally, classrooms should have RTs in the range of 0.4 to 0.6 seconds, but many existing classrooms have RTs of 0.8 to 1 second or more creating "echoes" that interfere with speech intelligibility and make the teacher much more difficult to understand. Many studies have demonstrated that the higher the reverberation time (greater than 0.6), the more difficult it becomes to understand speech.

The most common complaint from adult hearing aid users is regarding the difficulty of understanding speech in the presence of background noise, so the same must be true for children wearing hearing aids. High ambient noise from mechanical equipment such as noisy heating, ventilation, and air-conditioning systems is all too common in existing schools. This is a serious problem for teachers and students alike. Teachers must raise their voices to maintain the 15 dB signal-to-noise ratio necessary for good speech intelligibility. That results in many teachers taking several sick days each year, as well as seeking alternative employment, as a result of vocal strain. At the same time, students must either struggle to hear or else become distracted and stop paying attention to tasks and activities.

The single feature that helps overcome the difficulties of hearing in noise is to hear the teacher's voice comfortably louder than the noise. Nelson and Soli (2000) found that adults are able to understand familiar speech when the speech and noise are at equal loudness levels; young children need to hear the speaker at 4 dB louder than background noise; students unfamiliar with English need a 7 dB advantage; and children with hearing loss require the greatest signal-to-noise ratio at 15 dB. The ANSI S12.60-2001 standard recommends the teacher's voice should be SNR + 15 dB (signal-to-noise ratio) to permit all the children in the classroom to hear the spoken message well enough to receive the full meaning, no matter where they are sitting (Richburg & Smiley, 2012).

The problem of poor classroom acoustics applies to students at all levels of education. Flexor (2004) describes the terms *sound-field distribution, sound field amplification,* or *classroom amplification* to mean that all sounds in the classroom are made louder to the benefit of all students. Such a system, when installed correctly, amplifies the teacher's voice to a comfortable listening level distributed evenly throughout the classroom. Vickers et al. (2013) evaluated soundfield amplification with 44 children in two classrooms and showed that test score performance was indeed higher under soundfield amplification conditions than without it. The challenge of helping children with hearing loss who wear hearing aids in the typical noisy classroom situation creates serious problems for the teacher and the educational audiologist. Anderson

(2004) has provided an excellent and thorough review of research studies dealing with classroom amplification and acoustics and their impact on students with normal hearing and students with hearing loss.

Classroom acoustics problems tend to be universal and endemic, yet the solutions are neither necessarily difficult nor expensive (Smiley & Richburg, 2012a). The main reason is not lack of funds or limited knowledge, but the lack of awareness of the problem and its possible solutions. Bess and McConnell (1981) reported the mean background noise values of normal school classrooms to be between 55 and 65 dBA SPL and sometimes as high as 69 dBA SPL. In a normal setting, the teacher's regular speaking voice is approximately 65 dBA SPL, perhaps only 5 dB louder than the background noise. For the student with a hearing loss to hear the teacher's voice adequately, the speech signal needs to be 15 louder than the background noise. Excessive noise and reverberation resulting in reduced understanding, especially for students wearing hearing aids and cochlear implants, has been reported by Crandell, Smaldino, and Flexer (1995), Smaldino and Crandell (2004), and Smiley and Richburg (2012a).

For students with hearing loss, the use of a personal FM system overcomes the problems presented by poor classroom acoustics and the inability to hear the teacher speaking over background noise. The personal FM system, as discussed more fully below, uses a frequency-modulated (FM) signal to wirelessly transmit the speaker's voice to the student. The teacher wears a wireless transmitter (a microphone) and the student wears a receiver (within his or her personal amplifying device) to receive the teacher's voice. In this scenario, the effect is as though the teacher is speaking directly into the ear of the student with hearing loss, thereby creating a favorable signal-to-noise ratio of at least 15 dB. Although this may be an expensive personal solution, the resulting improvement in audibility helps overcome the classroom acoustics problems.

A study conducted by Klatte et al. (2010) analyzed the effects of classroom reverberation on children's performance and well-being at school. Performance and questionnaire data were collected from 487 children from 21 classrooms which differed in mean reverberation time from 0.49 to 1.1 seconds. Significant effects of reverberation on speech perception and short-term memory of spoken items were found. Furthermore, the children from reverberating classrooms performed lower in a phonological processing task, reported a higher burden of indoor noise in the classrooms, and judged the relationships to their peers and teachers less positively than children from classrooms with good acoustics.

Adherence to ANSI S12.60-2002 is voluntary, but many school districts and state and local agencies have adopted the standard as part of their construction or renovation requirements for schools. Parents, teachers, audiologists, and speech-language pathologists can help promote good classroom acoustics for their schools. Architectural improvements, such as acoustically treated walls, sound-absorbent ceiling materials, and perhaps even commercial-type carpeting, can be installed in schoolrooms to help reduce unwanted noise and limit reverberation. In these days of mainstreaming children with handicaps, however, it is unlikely that all school classrooms can be modified to meet the needs of students with hearing loss. Thus, it may fall to the educational audiologist to be familiar with solutions to classroom acoustics issues and to advocate for quieter classroom environments by bringing problems to the attention of school administrators or to seek support from parent-teacher organizations.

PERSONAL FM SYSTEMS

Poor classroom acoustics is the bane of the student who wears hearing aids or cochlear implants. Personal amplifiers such as hearing aids and cochlear implants are, of course, the most common means of providing audibility in the schoolroom. However, as previously discussed, it is unlikely that the typical classroom architecture will be altered to improve classroom acoustics for the benefit of one or two children wearing personal amplification. The major drawback to hearing through these personal units is their dependence on being close to the speaker. As the speaker moves farther away from the aided listener, the signal-to-noise ratio is diminished. Unfortunately, this is difficult to control in the typical classroom. As the teacher moves around the room and turns away from the child, the increase in distance and change in speaking direction contribute quickly to the demise of signal amplification. For example, when the level of the teacher's voice is 70 dB SPL at the source, it is just 58 dB SPL at 6 feet and decreases to 52 dB SPL 12 feet away. Because the ambient noise level in the room remains the same, this causes a decrease in speech intelligibility, particularly for students with hearing loss. As the acoustic signal gets weaker (softer, or lost within the background noise), the student must turn up the gain of his or her device, which also increases the background noise, creating unavoidable distortion and masking effects. Obviously, this is not a good situation.

The best means to overcome these classroom hearing problems is the radio frequency transmission unit (FM), with a wireless microphone and receiver, known as an FM system (Lewis, 1994b). More recently the term remote microphone technology (RMT) has also been used (AAA, 2011b).

The teacher simply clips a transmitter to his or her belt or slips it into a pocket, positions the wireless microphone approximately 6 inches from the mouth, and speaks normally. An FM system basically reduces the distance between the teacher and the student to just 2 to 3 inches, the average distance of the transmitter microphone to the speaker's mouth. The student wears a receiver (as part of the hearing aid or cochlear implant) to collect the speaker's voice. Because the microphone is so close to the teacher's mouth, the system minimizes the effect of background sounds and room reverberation when the teacher faces toward or away from the class. External receivers may be coupled to personal earmolds for children with normal hearing, hearing aids (including bone-anchored hearing aids), and cochlear implants worn by the child with hearing loss. The student-worn receivers can be adjusted to make them adaptable to a wide range of individual frequency responses. It is well documented that improving the signal-to-noise ratio (SNR) for cochlear implant and hearing aid users through the use of an FM system improves speech recognition significantly in the presence of background noise. FM systems are able to overcome competing background noise problems by improving the signal-to-noise ratio by up to 20 dB. The ASHA (2005a, 2005b) and the AAA (2008) have developed and published guidelines for fitting and monitoring FM systems.

Personal FM systems are produced by numerous manufacturers, but their basic operation is similar. A personal FM radio system functions for the child wearing a hearing aid by providing a clearer signal in unfavorable listening conditions. It consists of at least one transmitter and one receiver although multiple receivers worn by several children can be integrated into the classroom. The FM transmitter sends an audio signal picked up by its microphone. This signal is coded (frequency-modulated, FM) onto a carrier radio frequency on a channel much higher than the audio frequency range. The carrier frequency is sent to the receiver, which recovers the original audio signal and transfers it to an attached hearing aid or cochlear implant. In this way, the distance between the sound source and the hearing aid user is effectively reduced, thereby providing the listener with a better signal representation of the source than with the hearing aid or cochlear implant alone. The resulting improvement in the signal (+S/N ratio) heard by the hearing aid user is called the "FM advantage," because the FM signal in the hearing aid is louder than the signal from the hearing aid microphone picking up the same sound source, only from much farther away. A 10 dB advantage in the FM signal louder than the hearing aid signal is achieved due to the shorter distance between the FM microphone and the speaker's voice compared with the distance between the speaker and the traditional hearing aid microphone. The operational range of the FM system can vary by location, but more than 500 feet can be expected if there is no interference of any kind.

The major benefit of FM soundfield amplification is that the system "amplifies" or "projects" the teacher's voice an average of 6 to 10 dB above the classroom background noise. The speech signal drops 6 dB each time the distance doubles. The FM system produces a uniform loudness level in the classroom that is unaffected by the teacher's location, while reducing the effects of noise, reverberation, and distance. FM systems can transmit through objects, so line-of-sight transmission is not necessary. Rosenberg (1995) showed that FM soundfield systems can even improve the performance and behavior of children with normal hearing in regular school classrooms while enhancing their learning skills.

Different kinds of FM receivers are available that can either be worn on the body or worn at ear level. Ear-level receivers are the most convenient and smallest in size and are most often recommended for children with hearing loss wearing behind-the-ear (BTE) hearing aids with a direct audio input feature (Figure 10–3). The advantages of an FM radio transmission through a wireless microphone attached close to the mouth of the speaker, sending high-fidelity signals to the personal amplifier of a child with hearing loss (who may be as far as 200 m [650 ft] away), are obvious. With the help of an FM system, the distance between the primary signal and the listener becomes effectively no more than 6 inches, almost as though the speaker is talking directly into the ear of the listener.

There are innumerable ways to use remote microphone FM technology to the benefit of the individual with hearing loss. In a small group or conference table condition, the speaker's microphone can be placed at the center of the table to allow the person using the FM system to hear more than one voice originating from various locations around the table. Directional microphones can be used when the listener wants to focus on one speaker (i.e., church or community center meeting) in a background of high noise. There are also remote directional microphones that can be held by the listener who points the microphone toward the speaker.

There are generally three different settings to choose from when an FM receiver is connected to the child's hearing aid: (a) hearing aid only with no signal from the FM microphone—the hearing aid operates as though no FM signal is available; (b) FM only with no signal from the hearing aid—now the listening focus is on

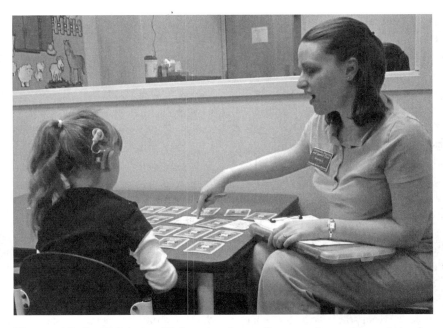

Figure 10–3. Children with hearing loss often need supplemental educational support. Photo courtesy of H.O.P.E. Preschool, Spokane, WA.

the speaker only; and (c) hearing aid and FM on together at the same time permitting the FM advantage for the speaker while still being able to hear environmental voices and sounds. In the classroom, the child would typically be listening with the hearing aid and FM system on together to hear the teacher as well as comments from other pupils. For at-home use, the FM microphone is likely turned on to hear parents and siblings talking to the child in a noisy background. The FM microphone might be utilized when the parent is speaking to the child from a distance. The hearing aid microphone usually stays on so that the child can hear other sounds and voices as well as his or her own voice.

Hawkins (1984) showed that the advantage of the FM system over the use of hearing aids alone can be substantial, equivalent to a 12 to 18 dB improvement in signal-to-noise ratio when the child is in an optimal classroom position. It is important to conduct a performance assessment of the FM

system with the individual user. Verification of the FM system is important to ascertain that the expected performance of the system is being achieved. Verification procedures have been detailed in the AAA Guidelines (2008) and may be conducted with electroacoustical analysis, real-ear measurement, or behavioral procedure (Smiley & Richburg, 2000b). The FM-cochlear implant system can only be verified through behavioral verification procedures.

The applications of the assistive personal listening system are much broader than just schoolroom use. Lewis (1994) describes the benefits and limitations of large-area induction-loop-amplification systems and sound-field amplification systems as alternatives to FM amplification. The increased cost of the FM systems as an additive expense to the assistive hearing devices is, unfortunately, the price of the advantages of the increased sound audibility and fidelity that are so incredibly helpful to the child with hearing loss. Pediatric audiologists must make parents aware of the incredible value of a personal FM system for communicating with their child at home and in daily life. These assistive listening systems are practical for at-home use, for coaching and playing sports, for automobile conversations between the front and back seats, as well as for small and large group theater, church, community center, and auditorium activities. Because a large part of learning is accomplished through incidental listening, the FM system puts the child with hearing loss into the center of family activities, whether at the grocery store, at the park, singing around the piano, on family vacations, or at social gatherings. FM systems help the child hear better when the child has constant access to a stable and clear speech signal. When children are out of sight but wearing their FM system, everyone including the parents and the child feels more secure knowing they are still in contact. The FM system as an assistive listening device should no longer be considered an accessory "special instrument" but an integral and important part of the daily life for every child with hearing loss (Figures 10–4A and 10–4B).

PARENT EDUCATION

Perhaps no calling is more important than that of being a parent, and no job is more challenging. For families whose children have permanent hearing loss, the experiences of the first few days and encounters

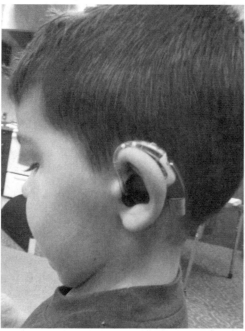

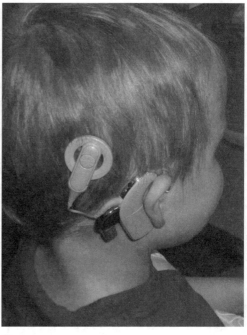

A   B

Figure 10–4. A–B. FM assistive technology is an integral part of the education program for children with hearing loss. The FM receiver can be seen as an external boot on the bottom of the BTE case and the cochlear implant processor. Photos courtesy of H.O.P.E. Preschool, Spokane, WA.

with the professional team members can be a bit overwhelming. These early experiences will mark the beginning of a lifelong relationship with audiologists, an array of physicians, speech-language pathologists, teachers of the deaf, and representatives from family-to-family support networks. Depending on the needs of the child, the family may also be dealing with physical therapists, occupational therapists, and psychologists who specialize in deaf and hard-of-hearing children with emotional or behavioral issues. Handled effectively, perhaps with navigation of the health care systems provided by the audiologist, these early interactions will hopefully set a positive tone for the successful long-term collaboration of parents and professionals (Roush & Kamo, 2008).

For most parents, raising children is a trial-and-error process. This is especially challenging for parents of children with hearing loss. When asked, most parents readily admit that they would benefit from learning more about children and parenting. Fortunately, numerous education and training programs are available through books, support groups, and online websites to help parents of hearing-impaired children. Parent support programs seek to provide basic education while striving to improve parental attitudes and behavior toward their disabled children. Researchers have found that parent training programs have consistent and persistent influence on both parental behavior and the intellectual development of the young child. Training program participants express more confidence and satisfaction with parenting. The Carnegie Task Force on Meeting the Needs of Young Children (1994) confirmed that improved interactions within the family system have a substantial and lasting influence on the family environment and the child's long-term development.

Certainly in the past, the attention of audiologists has been devoted to the hard-of-hearing or deaf child with only minor consideration given to the parents. This approach of lack of communication from the audiologist to the parents has created a backlash from parents who actually have less than positive feelings toward the audiologist. We hear remarks from parents that they did not understand the audiologist's initial counseling session about their child's hearing loss or the impact that it would have on their family. A recent survey of parents revealed that they felt the audiologist seemed rushed and did not allow sufficient time to meet with parents, resulting in parent's questions and concerns being unanswered. This is unfortunate as the parents of the hard-of-hearing or deaf child may be the most significant factor in the deaf youngster's successful development (Meadow-Orlans et al., 2003). Fortunately, during the past few years, parent-oriented and family-centered habilitation programs for children with hearing loss have become the standard of care.

The major emphasis of parent training includes emotional support for the parents by helping them recognize, realize, accept, and understand the implications of their child's hearing problem. This increased awareness should help reduce anxiety and worry often expressed by parents of hearing-disabled children. Education for the parents is important so that they might fully understand the nature of their child's hearing loss with realistic expectations of the educational future for their youngster. The parent is taught to understand child growth and development as well as the need for communication skills, social contact, and emotional expression.

There are many technologies beyond the hearing aid and cochlear implant now available that can be used to facilitate family life for the hard-of-hearing or deaf child. The audiologist is in a good position to advise the families of children with permanent hearing loss to learn about, and obtain if they are interested, special listening accessories to assist their child to hear under difficult conditions. These auditory accessories range from bed-shaking alarm clocks, TV audio amplifiers and closed captioning, illuminating smoke-fire alarms, and blinking-light doorbell systems to personal hearing assist dogs.

There are several communication approaches that can help communication within the family, each emphasizing different language learning skills. Some families rely on a single communication, while other families may use two or more communication systems to fit the environment or ongoing activity as needed. The important thing is that the parents encourage and facilitate communication with their hard-of-hearing or deaf child, regardless of the choice of the method used. As children with hearing loss mature and find themselves in different situations and circumstances, at school or college, or in a working environment, it is to their advantage to be able to use and move between any of several methods of communication including auditory-verbal, total communication, and ASL to be able to communicate wherever they might find themselves.

It is vitally important to teach the parents how to utilize and adapt daily activities of the home as experiential teaching events for the preschool child. It is hoped that the result is a stimulating home environment for the hearing-impaired child where auditory, speech, and language development is daily, ongoing, and natural. Some programs have a model home completely furnished and operational with kitchen, bathroom, bedroom, and playroom. The home is stocked with typical utensils and furnishings. Parents spend time with the parent-training supervisor to learn how to develop a repertoire of experiences and activities to stimulate interaction with their children. Videotape is used extensively to observe parent-child interaction, with immediate feedback to the parents to increase their abilities with their children. Horton (1975) summarized the objectives of parent training programs:

- To teach parents to optimize the auditory environment for their child;
- To teach parents how to talk with their child;
- To teach parents strategies of behavior management;
- To familiarize parents with the principles, stages, and sequence of normal development (including language development) and apply this frame of reference in stimulating their child to meet age norms; and
- To supply effective support to aid parents in coping with their feelings about their child and to reduce the stresses that a child with hearing loss places on the integrity of the family.

Parents must be involved in the choice of the communication system used with their child, be it hearing aids, a cochlear implant, or FM system. The communication system itself is secondary to parental agreement, enthusiasm, and commitment to the system. Professionals can provide guidance, exposure, and background to the parents, but the final choice should be made with full cooperation and agreement with the parents. Imposing the use of signs on parents who lack confidence in their ability to interact with the child is a common cause of failure. If the parents choose to use signs, the entire family must develop fluency with this means of communication.

The decision regarding placement of the child in an educational program must be the parents' prerogative. Unless the parents have made the decision, there will be second thoughts and possibly recriminations at a later date. The parents' decision is based on the following contributions from the child's deafness team: (a) information as to the degree of loss; (b) results of the speech and language evaluations, if relevant; (c) an introduction to the types of education available in the community (this would include visits to each of the facilities that are offering programs for hearing-impaired children); and (d) encouragement to choose freely and to feel comfortable with making a change at a later date if at any time it appears that another program will better benefit the child (http://www.handsandvoices.org).

Major cities and most large clinic programs have parent-centered projects underway, and it would appear that the deaf child will be the ultimate beneficiary of the support and education aimed at his or her parents during the initial stages of discovery of the hearing loss. Meadow and Trybus (1979), in a review of emotional problems of the deaf, report three family variables of importance to a deaf child's mental health: (a) degree of parental overprotectiveness, (b) development of unrealistic expectations for the child's progress, and (c) effectiveness of parent-child communication.

Greenberg (1975) published an important study that examined the attitudes and stress of hearing families with a profoundly deaf preschool child. The author studied 28 families that were equally divided into two groups: those using oral and those using simultaneous communication. These groups were further subdivided based on communicative ability (high versus low). Mothers completed questionnaires and interviews on stress concerns, parent attitudes, and their child's developmental level. Results showed few differences between families using simultaneous and oral communication. However, comparison of the four subgroups indicated that those with high-competence simultaneous communication skills had more positive attitudes and less stress than highly competent oral communication families.

The parents of children who are hard-of-hearing or deaf are likely to be bombarded with well-intended but conflicting messages from everyone, ranging from helpful friends, the Internet, to experts in various fields. Monitoring the child's development during those early years is essential, because good communication will continue to be the key to development as the child gets older. Brothers and sisters, as well as extended family members, are important components of the communication network. Support groups are available to help families be in touch with others who share similar problems, but support groups need to be selected carefully in the beginning as they often come with a strong bias for one or another point of view. Parents need exposure to various advocates of all points of view, but in the end the parent must make decisions based on what is best for the child and the family.

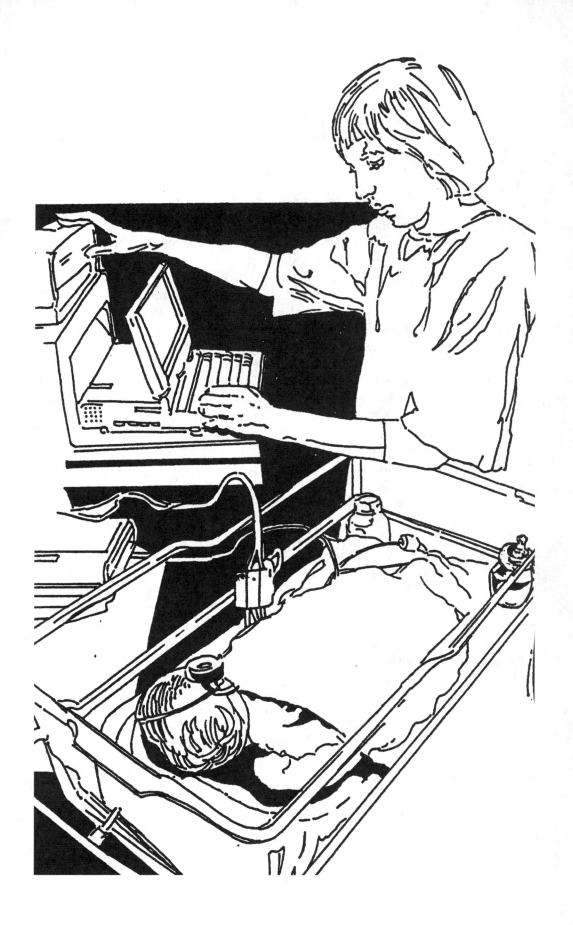

APPENDIX A

Pediatric Hearing Disorders

This appendix presents synopses of various syndromes and disorders associated with acquired and congenital pediatric hearing loss and deafness. It is recognized that many of these syndromes and disorders are rare and may never be seen by most audiologists. However, the information is published here in an attempt to be a quick and easy reference when that unexpected pediatric patient arrives at your clinic or office with unusual facial or body characteristics or perhaps is identified by a syndrome name that you do not recognize. To be sure, there are many more children with a few of these characteristics or without sufficient penetration of symptoms to be awarded a specific name. Nonetheless, this limited compendium has been compiled to provide information that will be useful to audiologists with a focus on the basic description of the disorder or syndrome along with a statement, as informative as possible, relative to the type of hearing loss that might be expected. Additional details are easily available on the Internet for most of these pediatric auditory disorders, but this appendix at least provides a starting point.

The description of a syndrome usually includes a number of essential characteristics, together with one or more minor characteristics, which when concurrent lead to diagnosis of the syndrome. A *syndrome* is a pattern of anomalies with a specific cause; a *sequence* represents a pattern of anomalies that directly result from a primary anomaly; and an *association* is a heterogeneous group of anomalies that occur together more often

than expected by chance (Toriello, 1995). Within the nearly 400 types of identified hereditary hearing loss, most occur without easily observable clinical indicators. Only one third of hereditary hearing loss disorders occur with recognizable physical characteristics.

Beginning in the 1970s, considerable effort was devoted to the classification and identification of children with syndromes and their associated disorders and manifestations. Since the first gene for deafness was identified in 1988, technological advances in human genetics have generally focused on chromosome mapping and the genetic-linkage analysis of inherited syndromes. It is estimated at this time that 70% to 80% of genetic deafness is nonsyndromic. Nance (2007) reported that at that time 58 recessive, 48 dominant, and 5 X-linked loci had been mapped, and among these, 45 of the causal genes had been identified. The search for specific genes for nonsyndromic as well as syndromic forms of deafness has met with astonishing success, resulting in the identification of more than 110 chromosomal loci and at least 65 genes (Morton & Nance, 2006).

The materials presented here provide brief summaries of information that are pertinent to the audiologist. To be sure, these are not everyday pediatric patients; their presence in the general pediatric population is relatively uncommon and rare. However, because these children are highly likely to have associated hearing disorders, it is also likely that, when identified, their treatment and management will involve audiologic evaluations and management. The information in this appendix is by no means intended to be exhaustive or even complete; the intent is to provide a concise, clear, and informative reference regarding special patients who have an inordinately high risk for hearing impairment. The authors recognize that children with symptoms that are variants from the generalized information about each disorder will be seen. Our intent is to provide an orientation or a guide to help understand those children who demonstrate these disorders and to instill a desire to learn more about the syndromes and diseases. An accurate identification and diagnosis of a specific genetic disorder in a child may be helpful in anticipation of associated complications. More knowledge regarding a specific diagnosis will aid in long-term management decisions that will benefit the patient.

During the past two decades, interest in genetic deafness burgeoned, and there is now a multitude of reference materials available in libraries and online. In fact, the Internet lists 1,048 causes of deafness (http://www.rightdiagnosis.com/symptoms/deafness/causes.htm). Clinicians may wish to consult those more complete reference sources for detailed accounts of syndromes included in this section or to pursue information on syndromes not included here (Table A–1). Such references often cover much more than individual journal articles and may touch on many aspects of the disorders not covered in these necessarily brief summaries. Accordingly, a list of recommended readings is presented at the end of this appendix that the authors have found to be immeasurably useful in reviewing and updating birth defects, syndromes, and diseases associated with hearing loss. An excellent starting point for readers interested in more information about genetic disorders is available at various websites such as those provided by the National Institutes of Health at Genetics Home Reference (http://ghr.nlm.nih.gov), Rare Diseases (http://rarediseases.info.nih.gov), PubMed Health (http://www.ncbi.nlm.nih.gov/pubmedhealth), the National Center for Biotechnology Information (http://www.ncbi.nlm.nih.gov), and the Hereditary Hearing Loss website (http://hereditaryhearingloss.org). In addition, many of the more common syndromes have support group websites that provide supplemental and family-oriented information.

Table A–1. Hearing Loss—Syndrome and Condition List for Congenital and Progressive Hearing Loss

	Title	Description	Hearing loss
A	Achondroplasia	Dwarfism, skeletal ossification disorder	Conductive and sensorineural hearing loss
	Albers-Schonberg disease of osteopetrosis	Brittle, thickened, chalky bones	Conductive and sensorineural hearing loss
	Albinism with blue irides	Pigmentation disorder eyes, skin, hair	Sensorineural hearing loss
	Alport's syndrome	Nephritis and cataracts	Progressive sensorineural hearing loss
	Apert syndrome	Craniosynostosis, midface anomalies, middle ear involvement	Conductive hearing loss
	Aplasias (errors during embryonic development)		
	Michel aplasia	Complete absence of inner ear and auditory nerve	Sensorineural hearing loss
	Mondini aplasia	Abnormal development of the structure (turns) of the cochlear membrane	Sensorineural hearing loss
	Scheibe aplasia	Abnormal formation of the cochlear membrane	Sensorineural hearing loss
	Asphyxia at birth/ neonatal period	Resuscitation required/ poor APGARs, seizures, neurological involvement	Sensorineural hearing loss, auditory neuropathy
B	Bacterial meningitis	Auditory involvement, can have sudden permanent hearing loss	Sensorineural hearing loss, central effects
	Bjornstad syndrome	Dry, brittle, flat, twisted hair	Sensorineural hearing loss
	Branchio-oto-renal syndrome (BOR)	Renal anomalies, auricular pits, pinnae malformations	Conductive, sensorineural, and mixed hearing losses
	Carraro syndrome	Absence of the tibia bone	Sensorineural hearing loss
C	Camurati-Engelmann disease	Skeletal—enlarged diaphysis of the long bones	Conductive and sensorineural hearing loss
	Chemotherapy medications (mother and baby)	Cisplatin, carboplatin— inner ear hair cells affected	Sensorineural hearing loss

continues

Table A–1. *continued*

	Title	Description	Hearing loss
	Cerebral palsy	Hypoxic episode during development or birth asphyxia	Sensorineural hearing loss
	Craniofacial abnormalities		
	Atresia of the ear canal	Atresia, stenosis of the ear channel	Conductive, sensorineural hearing loss/mixed
	Absence or malformed pinna	Atresia, stenosis, malformation of the pinnae	Conductive, sensorineural hearing loss/mixed
	Cleft palate	Malformation of the hard palate (exclude cleft lip if only feature present)	Conductive hearing loss
	CHARGE syndrome	Coloboma (eyes), heart, atresia of the nares, genital, ear (deafness)	Conductive, sensorineural hearing loss, and mixed; can have auditory neuropathy
	Cleidocranial dysostosis	Retarded ossification, narrowed auditory canal	Conductive and sensorineural hearing loss
	Cockayne's syndrome	Growth failure and neuro-logic delay, retinal atrophy	Sensorineural hearing loss
	Cornelia de Lange syndrome	Small for gestational age, limb malformations, cardiac defects, cleft palate	Conductive, sensorineural, or mixed hearing losses
	Crouzon's syndrome	Craniosynostosis, midface anomalies, outer and middle ear defects	Conductive, sensorineural, or mixed (majority are conductive)
D	Dwarfism	Skeletal anomalies, shortness, short fingers	Sensorineural hearing loss
	Down syndrome	Middle ear anomalies— ossicles, otitis media infections	Conductive, sensorineural, or mixed hearing losses
E	Encephalitis	Infection, auditory involvement	Sudden permanent sensorineural hearing loss
	Engelmann's syndrome	Bone dysplasia, increased skeletal density affecting auditory function	
F	Fanconi's anemia syndrome	Impaired renal transport, growth delay	Sensorineural hearing loss
	Family history of hearing loss	Permanent hearing loss evident in early infancy <6 years	Conductive or sensorineural

Table A–1. *continued*

	Title	Description	Hearing loss
	Fetal alcohol syndrome	Low birth weight, skeletal anomalies, cleft palate, pinnae anomalies	Conductive and sensorineural hearing loss
	Fraser syndrome	Adherent eyelids, external ear malformations, syndactyly	Conductive and sensorineural hearing loss
	Friedreich ataxia	Progressive ataxia, cataracts	Sensorineural hearing loss
G	Goldenhar's syndrome	Eye, ear, and mouth anomalies	Conductive hearing loss or sensorineural hearing loss
H	Hemifacial microsomia	Abnormal development on one side of the face, atresia/stenosis canal	Conductive hearing loss or sensorineural hearing loss
	Hermann's syndrome	Late onset of disease; epilepsy, speech, ataxia, renal disease	Sensorineural hearing loss
	Hyperbilirubinemia	Dampening of the auditory nerve function due to excessive bilirubin	Sensorineural hearing loss, may have auditory neuropathy
	Hypoxic ischaemic encephalopathy (**HIE**)	Severe asphyxia with neurological sequelae, hypotonic limbs, significant morbidity	Sensorineural hearing loss, may have auditory neuropathy
	Hydrocephalus	Intraventricular hemorrhage, grades 3 and 4, internal cranial anomalies, eighth cranial nerve involvement	Sensorineural hearing loss
	Hunter's and Hurler's syndrome	Progressive manifestation of coarse facial features	Mixed hearing loss
I	**Infections**		
	Cytomegalovirus	Herpes virus 5, microcephaly, hepatosplenomegaly, jaundice, intrauterine growth retardation	Sensorineural hearing loss
	Herpes	Congenital neonatal herpes infection HSV-1 and 2, high mortality	Sensorineural hearing loss
	Rubella	Low birth weight, purpura, jaundice, organ of Corti degeneration	Sensorineural hearing loss

continues

	Title	Description	Hearing loss
	Toxoplasmosis	Parasitic infection, chorioretinitis, cerebral calcification, convulsions	Sensorineural hearing loss
	Syphilis	Nasal discharge, rash, anemia, jaundice, osteochondritis	Sensorineural hearing loss
	Intraventricular hemorrhage (**IVH**)	Bleeding within the brain structures causing adverse neurological complications	Sensorineural hearing loss and central effects
J	Jervell and Lange-Nielsen syndrome	Cardiovascular disorder, fainting, sudden death a feature, auditory involvement	Sensorineural hearing loss
K	Keratopachyderma and digital constrictions nephrosis	Pigment disorder, may include renal disease	Sensorineural hearing loss
	Klippel-Feil syndrome	Craniofacial and skeletal disorder, short neck, cleft, poorly developed inner ear structures	Conductive and sensorineural hearing loss
L	Laurence-Moon-Biedl-Bardet syndromes	Retinitis pigmentosa, polydactyly	Sensorineural hearing loss
	LEOPARD syndrome (multiple lentigines syndrome)	Pigment disorder, café au lait spots, cardiac, ocular, genital, growth delay	Sensorineural hearing loss
	Long QT syndrome	Cardiac condition	
M	Marshall syndrome	Short stature, skeletal defects, cataracts	Sensorineural hearing loss
	Meningitis	Inner hair cells in cochlear damaged by virus	Sensorineural hearing loss
	Mitochondrial disorders	DNA—Maternal inheritance pattern	
	Moeibus (Mobius) syndrome	Connective tissue disorder, facial paralysis; cranial nerves 6 and 7, middle ear anomalies	Conductive and sensorineural hearing loss
	Muckle-Wells syndrome	Onset in teens, urticaria, renal failure	Sensorineural hearing loss
N	Neurofibromatosis type II	Intracranial tumors, eighth cranial nerve, acoustic neuroma	Sensorineural hearing loss

Table A–1. *continued*

	Title	Description	Hearing loss
	Noonan's syndrome	See Leopard syndrome, café au lait spots	Sensorineural hearing loss
	Norries syndrome	Eye disorder, auditory impairment	Sensorineural hearing loss
O	Oculo-auriculo-vertebralia spectrum (OAV)	Facial asymmetry, anomalies of external, middle ear, cranial nerve	Sensorineural hearing loss and central effects
	Optic atrophy and polyneuropathy	Progressive visual loss, polyneuropathy in childhoods	Sensorineural hearing loss(progressive)
	Ototoxic medication—affecting inner ear hair cells	Neomycin, amikacin, gentamicin, kanamycin, sisomicin, tobramycin, dibekacin, streptomycin	Sensorineural hearing loss
		Furosemide (loop diuretic used in conjunction with antibiotics); quinine-malarial treatment	Sensorineural hearing loss
	Osteogenesis imperfecta	"Brittle bones," stapes malformation	Conductive hearing loss and sensorineural hearing loss
P	Paget's disease	Juvenile skeletal disorder, bone pain, swelling	Progressive mixed hearing loss
	Persistent pulmonary hypertension of the newborn (**PPHN**)	Ventilation, progressive hypoxia, persistent fetal circulation	Sensorineural hearing loss and central effects
	Pierre Robin syndrome	Craniofacial anomaly, micrognathia, glossoptosis, may have cleft palate	Conductive and sensorineural hearing loss
	Periauricular abnormalities	Periauricular pits, tags, fistulas, ear canal atresia, facial paralysis	Conductive or sensorineural
	Periventricular leukomalacia (**PVL**)	Ischemic cystic changes in the brain matter predisposing to cerebral palsy	
	Piebaldness	Lack of pigment in hair, ataxia, blue irides	Sensorineural hearing loss
	Pendred's syndrome	Thyroid goiter—iodine imbalance in inner hair cells	Sensorineural hearing loss

continues

	Title	Description	Hearing loss
	Pyle's syndrome	Enlargement and sclerosis of the facial bones, ribs, clavicles	Sensorineural hearing loss
Q			
R	Refsum's syndrome	Organ of Corti degeneration, inner ear anomalies, eye disorder	Progressive sensorineural hearing loss
	Richards-Rundle syndrome	Central nervous system disorder, ataxia muscle wasting	Progressive sensorineural hearing loss
S	Stickler syndrome	Flattened facial profile, cleft palate, ocular changes	Conductive and sensorineural hearing loss
T	Treacher Collins syndrome	Head and neck anomalies, atresia of canal, abnormal middle ear	Conductive hearing loss
	Trisomy 21 (Down syndrome)	Recurrent middle ear infections	Conductive and sensorineural hearing loss
	Trisomy 13–15 and 18	High mortality rate	Conductive or sensorineural hearing loss
	Turner's syndrome	Gonadal dysgenesis, webbed neck and digits, micrognathia	Conductive and sensorineural hearing loss
U	Usher's syndrome	Retinitis pigmentosa, tunnel vision, vertigo, organ of Corti degeneration	Sensorineural hearing loss
V	Ventilation	Mechanical ventilation for longer than 5 days, increased neonatal risks	Sensorineural hearing loss
	Van der Hoeve's syndrome	"Brittle bone," stapes malformation	Conductive and sensorineural hearing loss
	Vohwinkel-Nockemann syndrome	See Keratopachyderma reference above	Sensorineural hearing loss (may be progressive)
	Von Reckinghausen's syndrome	Hyperkeratosis of palms, soles, knees, elbows, acoustic neuroma, renal	Sensorineural hearing loss
W	Waardenburg's syndrome (types 1 and 2)	White forelock, iris color different in one eye, prominent mandible, cleft	Sensorineural hearing loss

Table A–1. *continued*

Title	Description	Hearing loss
Wildervanck's syndrome	Dysmorphic facial features, atresia of ear canals, eyeball retraction	Sensorineural hearing loss or mixed
Winter syndrome	Renal anomalies, genital malformation, malformed ear and canals	Conductive hearing loss
XYZ		
References	*John Muir Medical Centre USA, Hearing loss indication list 2000; Patricia Gillilan, Audiologist USA; Northern and Downs Text, Hearing in Children, 5th ed., 2002; Newton, Paediatric Audiological Medicine, 2002.*	
Reviewed May 2007; amended March 2012	*Delene Thomas, RBWH, Co-ordinator HHP; Katrina Roberts, TTH, Co-ordinator HHP; Kelly Nicholls, RCH, Audiologist; Jackie Moon, MMH, Audiologist; Shree Aithal, TTH, Audiologist.*	
Reviewed August 2013; amended September 2013	*Delene Thomas, Area Co-ordinator HHP; Rachael Beswick, Audiologist Advanc, HHP.*	

Source: From "Universal Newborn Hearing Screening: Protocols and Guidelines," Healthy Hearing Program, October 2009, Brisbane, Queensland, Australia: Queensland Government (http://www.health.qld.gov.au/healthyhearing/docs/protocolap6.pdf). Used with permission.

ABSENCE OF THE TIBIA AND CONGENITAL HEARING LOSS

Carraro Syndrome; Tibial Hemimelia-Deafness Syndrome

Rare skeletal disorder; likely autosomal recessive inheritance; characterized by congenital absence of one or both tibias (lower leg bones), shortened malformed fibulas, and severe congenital sensorineural hearing loss. These may be accompanied by cleft palate, split hand/foot anomaly, and other congenital defects (Pashayan, Pruzansky, & Soloman, 1974; Richieri-Costa, DeMirander, Kamiya, & Freire-Maia, 1990).

ACHONDROPLASIA

A congenital skeletal anomaly characterized by slow growth of cartilage and endochondral ossification, with near-normal periosteal bone formation (Figure A–1). Macrocephaly and hydrocephaly may be present due to decreased foramen magnum. Those affected are short in stature with disproportionately short limbs, large heads with prominent foreheads, depressed nasal bridge, and "button" nose. Early motor development is often slow. Intelligence is usually normal, but lack of verbal comprehension may be evident. Respiratory, pulmonary, and other complications increase with age. Diagnosis

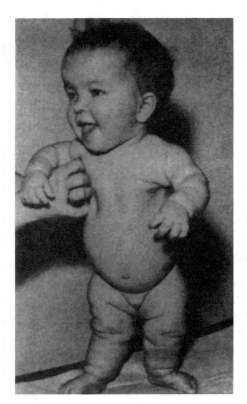

Figure A–1. Achondroplasia. Reproduced with permission from "The Congenitally Malformed: Achondroplastic Dwarfism: Diagnosis and Management," T. H. Shepard and B. Graham, 1967, *Northwest Medicine*, 66, pp. 451–456.

may be suspected by clinical examination but is confirmed by radiographic evaluation. Autosomal dominant inheritance; however, 90% of cases are due to fresh mutation, with both parents being normal. Incidence increases with increasing parental age and approximated as 1 per 15,000 births. Both conductive and sensorineural loss may be present. Middle ear anomalies include fusion of ossicles to surrounding bony structures as well as dense, thick trabeculae without islands of cartilage in the endochondral and periosteal bone. Associated anomalies of the inner ear include deformed cochlea and thickened interco-

chlear partitions. Conductive hearing losses are common due to poor eustachian tube resulting in a high incidence of otitis media. Management consists of genetic counseling, amplification, and medical and surgical treatment as indicated (American Academy of Pediatrics, Committee on Genetics, 1995; Cohen, 1967; Glass, Shapiro, Hodge, Bergstrom, & Rimoin, 1981; Mettler & Fraser, 2000; Shohat et al., 1993).

ACOUSTIC NEUROMA

See Neurofibromatosis

Acoustic tumors should be expected in all children with von Recklinghausen's disease or who have a family history of neurofibromatosis. The hearing loss is unilateral in 95% of cases (bilateral in patients with neurofibromatosis type II), progressive, and sensorineural. It appears and grows slowly and may be difficult to identify in children. The acoustic tumor diagnosis may be made from ABR wave morphology abnormalities as well as specialized radiographic techniques. Treatment requires careful monitoring and possible surgery. Acoustic neuromas, not associated with von Recklinghausen's disease, are extremely rare in children.

ALBERS-SCHÒNBERG DISEASE OF OSTEOPETROSIS

Chalk Bone Disease; Ivory Bone Disease; Marble Bone Disease

This is a rare, mild form of osteopetrosis with delayed manifestations reported to appear during the second year of life and may be associated with hearing loss, bone pain, facial palsy, and involvement of the optic and trigeminal nerves. Osteomyelitis of the mandible is common. A recessive craniofacial-skeletal disorder is evidenced with brittle, but paradoxically sclerotic, thickened bones. The head may be somewhat enlarged; delayed growth is shown in one third of cases. Visual loss is noted in approximately 80% of cases, which may lead to blindness. Mental abilities vary considerably; gross motor skills are mildly to moderately delayed during the first 2 years. Little detailed audiometric data are available, but 25% to 50% of patients are reported to have mild to moderate, progressive sensorineural or conductive hearing loss (Bollerslev, Grodum, & Grontved, 1987; Charles & Key, 1998; Johnston et al., 1968; Myers & Stool, 1969; Shapiro, 1993).

ALBINISM AND HEARING LOSS

Tietz-Smith Syndrome; Oculocutaneous Albinism

Albinism refers to a group of rare inherited disorders that are present from birth and affect the amount of pigment found in the skin, hair, and eyes. People with albinism usually have little to no pigment in their eyes, skin, and hair, but the degree of pigment loss can be quite variable. Many persons with this disorder have complete absence of pigment. Their skin, hair, and eyes lack all pigment from birth, and they do not develop freckles or moles at any time during their lifetimes. Eye problems, such as poor vision (usually cannot be fully corrected with glasses or contacts), functional

blindness, nystagmus, amblyopia (lazy eye), and photophobia (sensitivity to light) are common symptoms. Portions of the hair are often white (see Waardenberg syndrome). Certain rare types of albinism can include hearing loss, but there is no specific association of albinism and hearing loss. However, cases of severe sensorineural congenital deafness have been described in patients with albinism (Reed, Struve, & Maynard, 1967; Tietz, 1963).

ALPORT SYNDROME

Hereditary Nephritis with Sensorineural Hearing Loss

This is a genetic condition characterized by progressive kidney disease, hearing loss, and eye abnormalities. Progressive nephritis begins with hematuria and can lead to progressive renal failure and death. Alport syndrome is a genetically heterogeneous group with as many as six different specific disorders. The overall incidence is 1:10,000. Characteristics include autosomal dominant inheritance more common in men who are typically more severely affected than women. Diagnoses based on identification of progressive nephritis with uremia, ocular lens abnormalities such as cataracts, or misshapen lenses of the eyes, accompanied by progressive sensorineural hearing loss. Hearing loss with variable expressivity occurs in 40% to 60% of cases; the progressive bilateral hearing loss usually begins in preadolescence, initially showing high-frequency loss but may proceed to profound degree of hearing loss. Ocular defects appear in about 15% of this population. Hearing loss is due to abnormalities of the inner ears and develops as mild to severe, high-frequency, usually bilaterally symmetrical, and may occur alone or in combination with renal disease. Most cases are caused by mutations in the *COL4A5* gene and are inherited in an X-linked pattern. Males with the X-linked form of Alport syndrome are more severely affected than females (Johnson & Arenberg, 1981; Merchant et al., 2004; M'Rad et al., 1992; Nance, 2007; Wester, Atkin, & Gergory, 1995; http://ghr.nlm.nih.gov/condition/alport-syndrome).

AMYLOIDOSIS, NEPHRITIS, AND URTICARIA

Muckle-Wells Syndrome

This syndrome is characterized by periodic episodes of skin rash, fever, and joint pain accompanied by progressive hearing loss and kidney damage. It is a rare disorder of unknown prevalence due to mutations in the *NLRP3* gene. This autosomal dominant syndrome typically has its onset in teen years with recurrent vascular reaction of the skin with elevated patches and itching with onset of recurrent limb and joint pain. Patients have recurrent "flare-ups" that begin in infancy or early childhood. Amyloidosis (starchy-like substance in the blood) precedes nephropathy and renal failure. Progression of sensorineural hearing loss tends to parallel progression of renal failure, resulting in severe hearing impairment by third or fourth decade of life. Endocrine and metabolic disorder are seen with late progressive sensorineural hearing loss of adolescent onset (Champion, 1989; El-Darouti, Marzouk, & Abdel-Halim, 2006; Haas et al. 1978; Muckle, 1979; http://ghr.nlm.nih.gov/condition/muckle-wells-syndrome).

APERT SYNDROME

Acrocephalosyndactyly

Patients have genetic skeletal and associated skull malformations characterized by the premature fusion of certain skull bones (craniosynostosis). This early fusion prevents the skull from growing normally and affects the shape of the head and face. In addition, a varied number of toes and fingers are fused together (syndactyly). Diagnosis is based on craniofacial dysostosis, syndactyly, brachiocephaly, hypertelorism, bilateral proptosis, saddle nose, high arched palate, ankylosis of joints, spinal bifida, and mental deficiency (Figures A–2 and A–3). Syndactyly (fusion of fingers and toes) may be complete on both hands and feet. Some individuals may have extra fingers or toes (polydactyly). Other signs and symptoms can include conductive or sensorineural hearing loss with repeated bouts of oti-

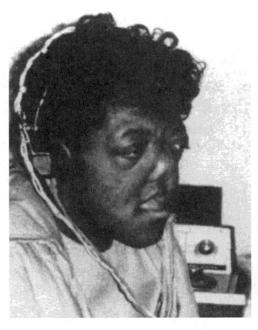

Figure A–2. Apert syndrome.

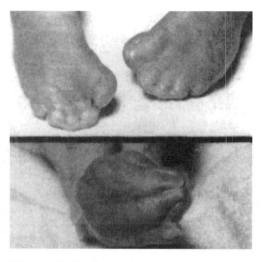

Figure A–3. Apert syndrome.

tis media. Patients may also demonstrate unusually heavy sweating, oily skin with severe acne, patches of missing hair in the eyebrows, fusion of cervical vertebrae, and hearing loss. The typical individual presenting has characteristic "tower skull," with flat forehead. Most reported cases appear sporadic caused by mutations in the *FGFR2* gene. When reproduction is possible, the disorder is apparently of autosomal dominant transmission. There appears to be a high mutation rate related to increasing parent age. Manifestations are present at birth. Surgical explorations have revealed congenital stapedial footplate fixation, abnormal patency of cochlear aqueduct, and enlarged internal auditory meatus (Bergstrom, Neblett, & Hemenway, 1972; Cohen & Kreiborg, 1993; Gould & Caldarelli, 1982; Lindsay, Black, & Donnelly, 1975; http://ghr.nlm.nih.gov/condition/apert-syndrome).

ATOPIC DERMATITIS

Atopic dermatitis is a very common, often chronic (long-lasting) skin disease that affects a large percentage of the world's population. Most commonly, it may be thought of as a type of skin allergy or sensitivity. Congenital recessive atopic dermatitis triad includes asthma, allergies (hay fever), and eczema. The hallmarks of the disease include skin rashes and itching. The skin becomes dry, itchy, and inflamed, causing redness, swelling, cracking, weeping, and crusting. It may be associated with mild-to-moderate, nonprogressive sensorineural hearing loss that may not be detected until school years. At about age 10, affected persons develop lichenified skin eruptions especially on forearms, hands, elbows, trunk, and arms. It is an integumentary and pigmentary disorder with congenital sensorineural hearing loss (Frentz et al., 1976; Konigsmark, Hollander, & Berlin, 1968; Konigsmark, Mengel, & Haskins, 1970; Schultz, Vase, & Schmidt, 1978).

BARAITSER-WINTER SYNDROME

Baraitser-Winter syndrome is extremely rare. It affects the development of many parts of the body, particularly the face and the brain. Distinctive facial features include widely spaced eyes (hypertelorism), large eyelid openings, droopy eyelids (ptosis), high-arched eyebrows, a broad nasal bridge and tip of the nose, a long space between the nose and upper lip (philtrum), full cheeks, and a pointed chin. Structural brain abnormalities are also present in Baraitser-Winter syndrome. These abnormalities are related to impaired neuronal migration, a process by which nerve cells (neurons) move to their proper positions in the developing brain. These structural changes can cause mild-to-severe intellectual disability, developmental delay, seizures, and may involve the entire brain surface. Other features of Baraitser-Winter syndrome can include ear abnormalities and hearing loss, short stature, heart defects, presence of an extra (duplicated) thumb, and abnormalities of the kidneys and urinary system (http://ghr.nlm.nih.gov/condition/baraitser-winter-syndrome).

BJORNSTAD SYNDROME

Pili Torti

This is characterized by dry, brittle, flat, twisted hair (pili torti) of scalp, eyebrows, and eyelashes accompanied by moderate to severe bilateral severe sensorineural hearing loss. Pili torti is a rare hair shaft abnormality in which the hair is flattened and intervals twisted at irregular through 180 degrees about its axis. Pili torti may occur as a congenital defect or as an acquired disorder (secondary to patchy alopecia from a variety of causes). When it is congenital, it may be isolated and determined by an autosomal dominant gene or associated with various rare syndromes, including ectodermal dysplasias, neurological defects, and metabolic disturbances. The association of sensorineural hearing loss and pili torti has been recognized as Bjornstad's syndrome since 1965. Fewer than 25 cases of Bjornstad syndrome have been reported (Petit, Dontenwille, Bardon, & Civatte, 1993; Singh & Bresman, 1973; http://www.webmd.com/a-to-z-guides/bjornstad-syndrome).

BRANCHIO-OTO-RENAL SYNDROME (BOR)

Branchio-oto-renal (BOR) syndrome is an autosomal dominant form of inherited hearing impairment that typically disrupts the development of tissues in the neck and causes malformations of the ears and kidneys. The syndrome is characterized by hearing loss due to conductive, sensorineural, or mixed etiologies; preauricular pits or tags; auricular malformations of the outer ear and anatomical defects of the middle and inner ear which may include the Mondini malformation and stapes fixation; branchial fistulae or cysts; and renal anomalies ranging from mild hypoplasia to a lethal condition of bilateral renal agenesis. Like Treacher Collins syndrome, BOR results from abnormal development of the first and second branchial arches. Genetic mutations causing this disorder have been identified in three genes, *EYA1, SIX1,* and *SIX5* (Coppage & Smith, 1995; Kemperman et al., 2002; Kochar et al., 2007; Melnick, Bixler, Nance, Silk, & Yune, 1976; Nance, 2007; http://ghr.nlm.nih.gov/condition/branchiootorenal-syndrome).

CAMURATI-ENGELMANN DISEASE

Craniodiaphyseal Dysplasia; Progressive Diaphyseal Dysplasia

This is a condition that mainly affects the long bones of the body, arms, and legs. Individuals have increased bone density and thickened bones that may include the skull and hips. The increased density of the skull results in increased pressure on the brain and can cause a variety of neurological problems including hearing loss, dizziness, and tinnitus. The disorder is categorized as skeletal with dominant or recessive transmission. Diagnosis is confirmed radiologically. The skull base may be sclerotic. Observed are abnormally long limbs in proportion to height, a decrease in muscle mass and body fat, and delayed puberty. Deafness may appear as progressive sensorineural, mixed, or conductive, possibly accompanied by vestibular disturbance. The apparent cause is a gene mutation of *TGFB1* (Janssens et al., 2006; Nelson & Scott, 1969; Sparkes & Graham, 1972; Wallace, Lachman, Mekikian, Bui, & Wilcox, 2004; Yoshioka et al., 1980; http://ghr.nlm.nih.gov/condition/camurati-engelmann-disease).

CARDIOAUDITORY SYNDROME

(See Jervell and Lange-Nielsen Syndrome)

CEREBRAL PALSY

Cerebral palsy (CP) is a disorder that affects muscle tone, movement, and motor skills (the ability to move in a coordinated and purposeful way). Patients demonstrate some permanent degree of paralysis or lack of coordination due to a defect or lesion of the developing brain, sometimes characterized by uncontrollable motor spasms. Cerebral palsy can also lead to other health issues, including vision, hearing, and speech problems, and learning disabilities. Cerebral palsy involves a wide range of severity of paralysis, weakness, lack of muscle coordination, or other abnormality of motor function due to pathology of the motor control centers of the brain. The prevalence of cerebral palsy is approximately 1.5 to 2 cases per 1,000 live births. The incidence of cerebral palsy has not changed in more than four decades, despite significant advances in the medical care of neonates. There are three types of CP including: (a) spastic, with stiffness and movement difficulties (70% to 80%); (b) athetoid or dyskinesia or involuntary and uncontrolled movements (10% to 15%); and (c) ataxic cerebral palsy that causes a disturbed sense of balance and depth perception (5%).

Damage to the brain may occur during embryonic, fetal, or early infantile life. Essentially nonprogressive, clinical symptoms of the disorder include spasticity (40%), athetosis (40%), ataxia (10%), or combinations of these basic motor dysfunctions. Mental deficiency and convulsive disorders are common. Feeding problems, delayed growth, eye difficulties such as strabismus and nystagmus, developmental delay, orthopedic problems, communication disorders, and educational problems are often evidenced in varying degrees. Different pathogenetic mechanisms of cerebral palsy have been associated with preterm and term births. There is a high risk of cerebral palsy in preterm infants. Nevertheless, most cerebral palsy occurs among term births. Damage to the brain may occur during embryonic, fetal, or early infantile life and may result from an antecedent disorder such as trauma, metabolic disorder of infection, destructive intercranial cerebral processes, or developmental defects of the brain. Children have cerebral palsy as the result of brain damage in the first few months or years of life from infections such as bacterial meningitis or viral encephalitis, or head injury from a motor vehicle accident, a fall, or child abuse. Location of the lesion(s) may be in the cerebral cortex, basal ganglia, or cerebella or other sites in the pyramidal or extrapyramidal systems. The most common are a lack of muscle coordination when performing voluntary movements (ataxia); stiff or tight muscles and exaggerated reflexes (spasticity); walking with one foot or leg dragging; walking on the toes, a crouched gait, or a "scissor" gait; and muscle tone that is either too stiff or too floppy. Management is a multidisciplinary process; although cerebral palsy cannot be cured, appropriate treatment will often improve a child's capabilities. Many children go on to enjoy near-normal adult lives if their disabilities are properly managed. In general, the earlier treatment begins, the better chance children have of overcoming developmental disabilities or learning new ways to accomplish the tasks that challenge them. Treatment may include physical and occupational therapy; speech therapy; drugs to control seizures, relax muscle spasms, and alleviate pain; surgery to correct anatomical abnormalities or release tight muscles; braces and other orthotic devices; wheelchairs and rolling walkers; and communication aids such as computers with attached voice synthesizers. Patients with hearing loss are likely to have mild to moderate sensorineural hearing loss, typically more severe in high frequencies (Goulden & Hodge, 1998; Stanley & Blair, 1994; http://www.ninds.nih.gov/disorders/cerebral_palsy/cerebral_palsy.htm; http://emedicine.medscape.com/article/310740-overview).

CERVICO-OCULO-ACOUSTIC DYSPLASIA

Wildervanck Syndrome, Duane Syndrome, Klippel-Feil Syndrome

Patients typically present with severe deformation of the craniofacial area. Associated eye disorder is seen as an anomaly in Wildervanck syndrome. Intelligence is normal in most, but not all, patients. Congenital paralysis of the sixth cranial nerve (abducens palsy) with retracted globe and severe congenital sensorineural or conductive deafness are shown in 15% of cases. Patients have growth deficiency with striking appearance as head seems to sit directly on shoulders due to fusion of the vertebrae in the neck. Abducens paralysis (known as the Duane anomaly) prevents external rotation of eyes and may be unilateral or bilateral; occasional presentation with cleft palate. Various ear anomalies have been described, including preauricular tags and pits, malformation, atresia or absence of external ear canal, and abnormal middle ear ossicles. Malformed vestibular labyrinth has been reported. It is a recessive disorder with cause unknown (Cross & Pfaffenbach, 1972; Kirkham, 1969; Singh, Rock, & Shulman, 1969; http://www.ncbi.nlm.nih.gov).

CHARGE ASSOCIATION

Initially described by B. Hall (1979), the diagnosis of CHARGE syndrome is based on a combination of major and minor characteristics. The various abnormalities that make up CHARGE association are: (C) coloboma, or hole in one of the structures of the eye, (H) heart defects, (A) atresia of choanae, (R) retarded growth and development, (G) genital hypoplasia, and (E) ear anomalies or deafness. Although the most consistent features are included by the mnemonic, CHARGE, additional abnormalities have been reported including facial palsy, renal abnormalities, orofacial clefts, and tracheoesophageal fistulas. Infants often have multiple life-threatening medical conditions. The etiology is unknown, with most cases being sporadic. Approximately 30% to 35% of patients die within the first 3 months of life. Individuals with CHARGE syndrome often have distinctive facial features, including a square-shaped face and difference in the appearance between the right and left sides of the face (facial asymmetry). Individuals have a wide range of cognitive function, from normal intelligence to major learning disabilities with absent speech and poor communication. Hearing loss may be progressive and present in 85% of reported cases, mild to profound in degree, and conductive, sensorineural, or of mixed etiology. Abnormalities of the pinnae, with or without hearing loss, are a cardinal feature (90%). CHARGE syndrome occurs in approximately 1 in 8,500 to 10,000 individuals. Mutations in the *CHD7* gene cause more than half of all cases of CHARGE syndrome, while one third of individuals with CHARGE syndrome do not have an identified mutation in the *CHD7* gene (Blake, et al., 1998; Blake & Prasad, 2006; Davenport, Hefner, & Thelin, 1986; Dobrowski, Grundfast, Rosenbaum, & Zajtchuk, 1985; Hall, 1979; Lin, Siebert, & Graham, 1990; Thelin, Mitchell, Hefner, & Davenport, 1986; Toriello, 1995; Sanlaville & Verloes, 2007; http://ghr.nlm.nih.gov/condition/charge-syndrome).

CLEFT PALATE AND CLEFT LIP

These are relatively common birth defects resulting from multifactorial inheritance; cleft lip occurs in about 1 in 1,000 births, and cleft palate occurs in about 1 to 2 per 1,000 births making it one of the most common major birth defects. Cleft lip almost always occurs as fissure in the upper lip and may be unilateral or bilateral. Cleft palate may involve only the uvula or both the hard and soft palate. A cleft palate may vary in size, from a defect of the soft palate only to a complete cleft that extends through the hard palate. Because the lips and the palate develop separately, it is possible for a child to be born with a cleft lip only, cleft palate only, or both. Both cleft lip and cleft palate are surgically correctable. Most chil-

dren born with these defects, have surgery to repair these conditions within the first 12 to 18 months of life. Cleft lip with or without cleft palate is generally more common among boys; however, cleft palate occurring alone is more common in girls than boys. Clefts occur more often in children of Asian, Latino, or Native American descent. Cleft lip or palate is a common anomaly associated with many syndromes. The anatomic and physiologic derangement of a cleft palate predisposes patients to a high-risk incidence of middle ear effusion episodes. Otorrhea is a frequent complication during the first year of life. Middle ear disease generally stabilizes or improves by the end of the first decade. Tympanic membrane (TM) perforations and cholesteatoma usually present after preschool age. Approximately 35% to 50% of babies with cleft palate have associated anomalies (Figure A–4). See Chapter 4 for additional information (Arosarena, 2007; Friedman, Wang, & Milczuk, 2005; Kliegman, Behrman, Jenson, & Stanton, 2007; Paradise & Bluestone, 1974; Paradise, 1976b; http://kidshealth.org/parent/medical/ears/cleft_lip_palate.html; http://www.ncbi.nlm.nih.gov/pubmedhealth/PMH0002046).

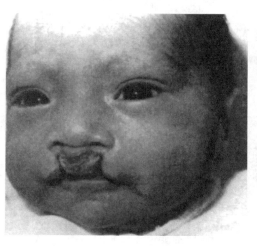

Figure A–4. Bilateral cleft palate and lip.

CLEIDOCRANIAL DYSOSTOSIS

Cleidocranial Dysplasia; Osteodental Dysplasia

Affected individuals present with a cluster of obvious features including defects or absence of the clavicle, late ossification of cranial sutures causing softness of the skull, irregular ossification of bones, and delayed eruption of teeth (Figure A–5). In addition, shortness of stature, narrow drooping shoulders, widely spaced eyes, irregular or absent

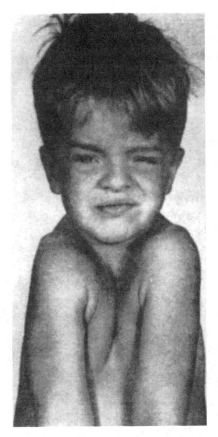

Figure A–5. Cleidocranial dysostosis. Reproduced with permission from "Congenital Shoulder-Neck-Auditory Anomalies," by I. S. Jaffee, 1968, *Laryngoscope*, *58*, pp. 2119–2139.

teeth, and high arched palate or submucous cleft palate have been noted. Concentric narrowing of external auditory canals is present. Some young children with this condition are mildly delayed in the development of motor skills such as crawling and walking, but intelligence is unaffected. Chromosome analyses show normal karyotypes. Inheritance is autosomal dominant with high percentage penetration of defects and wide variability in expression. About one third of the cases appear to be sporadic. Patients may have progressive sensorineural hearing loss and be prone to sinus and ear infections. Progressive deafness is occasionally reported and may be conductive or sensorineural due to retarded bone ossification (Cooper, 2001; Hawkins, Shapiro, & Petrillo, 1975; Jensen, 1990; Mundlos, 1999; Segal, 2007; http://ghr.nlm.nih.gov/condition/cleidocranial-dysplasia).

COCKAYNE'S SYNDROME

Cerebro-Oculo-Facio-Skeletal (Cofs) Syndrome

This is a rare syndrome of progressive growth failure and neurologic deterioration with an incidence of two per one million births. Individuals show dwarfism, mental deficiency, retinal atrophy, and motor disturbances. Growth and development are normal through the first year. During the second year, growth falls below normal range and mental-motor development becomes abnormal. Minimal diagnostic characteristics include dwarfism, retinal degeneration, microcephaly, cataracts, neurologic impairment including progressive mental retardation, sun-sensitive skin, thickening of the skull bones, disproportionately long extremities with large hands and feet, eye disorder, and progressive sensorineural hearing loss of late onset, usually of moderate to severe degree. Prognosis is poor with severe blindness and deafness. Hearing aids are possible; however, mental insufficiency precludes much success. Cockayne syndrome can be divided into subtypes that are distinguished by the severity and age of onset of symptoms. Classical, or type I, Cockayne syndrome is characterized by an onset of symptoms in early childhood (usually after age 1 year). Type II Cockayne syndrome has much more severe symptoms that are apparent at birth (congenital), and death usually occurs by age 6 or 7 years. Type II Cockayne syndrome is sometimes called cerebro-oculo-facio-skeletal (COFS) syndrome or Pena-Shokeir syndrome type II. Type III Cockayne syndrome has the mildest symptoms of the three types and appears later in childhood. It has autosomal recessive inheritance with normal appearance at birth. Cockayne syndrome can result from mutations in either the *ERCC6* gene or the *ERCC8* gene (Nance & Berry, 1992; Pasquier et al., 2006; Riggs & Seibert, 1972; Shemen, Mitchell, & Farkashidy, 1984; Weidenheim, Dickso, & Rapin, 2009; http://ghr.nlm.nih.gov/condition/cockayne-syndrome).

CORNELIA DE LANGE SYNDROME

This multifactorial syndrome is characterized by severe-to-profound intellectual disability and slow growth before and after birth. Although this syndrome affects many parts of the body, the features vary widely among individuals with mild to severe penetrance. Individual features may include microcephaly, hirsutism, and confluent eyebrows often accompanied by anomalies of the external ear, including low-set auricles, and small external auditory canals. Infants generally delivered at full-term although they may be small at birth. The upper limbs are severely malformed; there may be missing toes or fingers and possible webbing between toes. Seizures, eye problems, and cardiac defects are common; possible cleft palate may be accompanied by neonatal feeding and respiratory difficulties. Speech and language problems are severe, and hearing losses attributed to conductive, sensorineural, and mixed etiologies have been reported. Prognosis is poor with diminished life expectancy. There is polygenic inheritance due to mutations in the *NIPBL*, *SMC1A*, and *SMC3* genes (Borck et al., 2007; Fraser & Cambell, 1978; Hall, Prentice, Smiley, & Werkhaven, 1995; Jackson, Kline, Barr, & Koch, 1993; Silver, 1964; http://ghr.nlm.nih.gov/condition/cornelia-de-lange-syndrome).

CROUZON'S SYNDROME

Craniofacial Dysostosis

This condition is usually identified by craniofacial development. The shape of the skull depends on which sutures are involved (Figure A–6). Intelligence may be low when associated with brain damage secondary to increased intracranial pressure. Bifid uvula and cleft palate may be present. Approximately one fourth of reported cases arise as fresh mutations. The disorder is usually detectable at birth or during the first year of life. Ears may be low set. Approximately 50% of patients have nonprogressive conductive hearing impairment; patients may have mixed-type deafness. Middle ear manifestations include deformed stapes with bony fusion of promontory, ankylosis of malleus

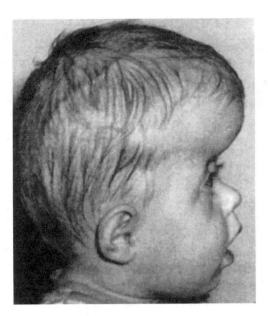

Figure A–6. Crouzon's syndrome.

to outer wall of the epitympanum, distortion and narrowing of middle ear space, absence of the tympanic membrane, and perhaps bilateral atresia. Stenosis or atresia of external canal is common. Early surgical intervention is usually recommended to prevent damage to the brain and eyes. Incidence is approximately 16 per million newborns. This is an autosomal dominant syndrome with variable expression due to mutations in the *FGFR2* gene (Baldwin, 1968; Carinci et al., 2005; Dodge, Wood, & Kennedy, 1959; Vulliamy & Normandale, 1966; http://ghr.nlm.nih.gov/condition/crouzon-syndrome).

CRYPTOPHTHALMOS

Fraser Syndrome

Primarily an eye disorder, cryptophthalmos is a rare congenital anomaly in which the skin is continuous over the eyeball with absence of eyelids. The anomaly is classified into three types: complete, incomplete, and abortive. Failure of eyelid separation can be associated with maldevelopment of the underlying cornea and microphthalmia. Cryptophthalmos usually occurs on both sides and occurs in association with other multiple malformations collectively referred to as Fraser syndrome. In its most severe form, a unilateral or (more often) bilateral extension of skin of the forehead completely covers eye or eyes to the cheeks. In the less severe form, the upper or lower eyelid may simply be absent. Syndactyly of fingers, toes, or both may be present. Laryngeal atresia has been reported. Cleft lip and palate are not uncommon. Hearing loss is mostly conductive; also seen are malformed middle ear ossicles, small and poorly formed pinnae, with stenosis of external auditory canals (Fraser, 1962; Gattuso, Patton, & Baraitser, 1987; Ide & Wollschlaeger, 1969; http://www.ncbi.nlm.nih.gov/pubmed/3099574; http://www.ncbi.nlm.nih.gov/pubmed/19643480).

CUSHING'S SYMPHALANGISM

Cushing's symphalangism, also called proximal symphalangism, is a rare genetic condition characterized by the fusion of the proximal joints in the hands and feet. These individuals usually have straight fingers and are unable to make a fist. Other joints may also be affected, leading to stiff joints in the elbows, ankles, and wrists. Hearing loss due to the fusion of the auditory ossicles is also a characteristic feature. This condition is inherited in an autosomal dominant pattern and is caused by a mutation in the *NOG* gene or *GDF5* gene (Plett et al., 2008; Spoendlin, 1974; http://rarediseases.info.nih.gov/gard/8182/cushings-symphalangism/resources).

CYTOMEGALOVIRUS (CMV)

Disease CMV is one of the most frequently transmitted intrauterine infections in the United States and results in sensorineural hearing loss as its most common sequela. CMV is the leading environmental cause of childhood hearing loss, accounting for approximately 15% to 21% of all hearing loss at birth in the United States. Congenital CMV accounts for more than 6,000 cases of sensorineural hearing loss per year. Typically the mother is asymptomatic but may transmit the CMV to her fetus during pregnancy. An important consideration about CMV-related hearing losses is that they may be progressive or appear as late onset, requiring more frequent audiological monitoring of infants and young children diagnosed with the disease. About 1 in 150 live births is born with congenital CMV infection, and of these infants one of every five will develop significant health problems. Infants and children infected with CMV later after birth rarely have symptoms or problems. As for newborns infected with CMV, 97% of them show no signs of disease during the neonatal period. Most CMV infections are not diagnosed because it usually causes few, if any, symptoms. Congenital CMV is diagnosed when the virus is detected in the newborn's urine, saliva, or blood within 2 to 3 weeks after birth. Transmission of the CMV virus (e.g., in milk or saliva) is common in the perinatal period and early childhood. Infection acquired during birth is usually noticed 3 to 12 weeks after delivery. Infection acquired during infancy may be shed for 5 to 6 years; thus, these patients need to be isolated from other children, even in clinic waiting areas. Approximately 10% of infected children will eventually demonstrate adverse sequelae such as coordination disturbances, hearing loss or deafness, microcephaly, mental deficiency, and moderate enlargement of the spleen and liver with jaundice (yellowing of the skin). There is no vaccination against the disorder, and prevention of CMV infection consists of avoidance of exposure during pregnancy. See Chapter 2 (Adler, Finney, Manganello, & Best, 2004; Barbi et al., 2003; Dahl et al., 2000; Fowler & Boppana, 2006; McCollister et al., 1996; Ross & Fowler, 2008; Strasnick & Jacobson, 1995; http://www.ndmch.com/publications/ DiseaseFactSheets/Cytomegalovirus.pdf; http://www.cdc.gov/cmv/overview.html; http://www.asha.org/Publications/leader/ 2008/080506/f080506b).

DIASTROPHIC DYSPLASIA

Diastrophic Nanism Syndrome

Diastrophic dysplasia is a rare disorder of cartilage and bone development that affects individuals by short stature with very short arms and legs. Most also have early onset joint pain (osteoarthritis) and joint deformities that restrict movement. These joint problems often make it difficult to walk and tend to worsen with age. Additional features of diastrophic dysplasia include an inward- and upward-turning foot (clubfoot), progressive abnormal curvature of the spine, and unusually positioned thumbs (hitchhiker thumbs). About half of infants with diastrophic dysplasia are born with an opening in the roof of the mouth (cleft palate). The auricles show cystic swellings in infancy that later develop into cauliflowerlike deformities that may calcify. The trait is recessive with reported congenital sensorineural hearing loss or external ear canal stenosis, as well as fusion or lack of middle ear ossicles creating conductive hearing loss. This is a rare disorder affecting about 1 in 100,000 newborns. Diastrophic dysplasia is one of several skeletal disorders caused by mutations in the *SLC26A2* gene (Canto, Buixeda, & Ojeda, 2007; Langer, 1965; http://ghr.nlm.nih.gov/condition/diastrophic-dysplasia).

DOWN SYNDROME

Trisomy 21 Syndrome

Down syndrome (Figure A–7) is a chromosomal condition with 47 chromosomes rather than the normal 46 chromosomes. Down syndrome is associated with one of the most common forms of intellectual disability. Down syndrome is the result of a chromosomal abnormality—notably a 21 trisomy, translocation trisomy, or mosaicism. Individuals with Down syndrome exhibit a characteristic facial appearance and generally poor muscle control. A high incidence of occurrence exists (1 in 700 live births) with approximately 5,000 new births with Down syndrome each year in the United States. Clinical findings include

a list of 50 features with varying penetrance. Intellectual disability is almost universal and may vary from mild to severe. These individuals exhibit a characteristic personality that is warm, friendly, and affectionate (Figure A–8). Common diagnostic features include flattened facial features, oblique palpebral fissures, flat occiput, short limbs, short broad hands, short fingers (especially

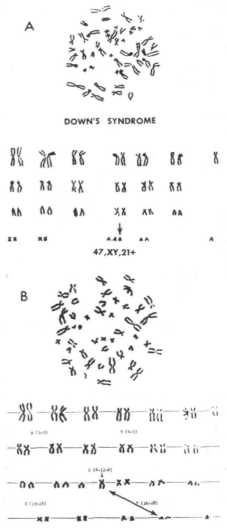

Figure A–8. Karyotypes of Down syndrome. **A.** Extra 21st chromosome. **B.** Translocation. Courtesy of A. Robinson, MD, Cytogenetics Laboratory, University of Colorado Medical Center, Denver, CO.

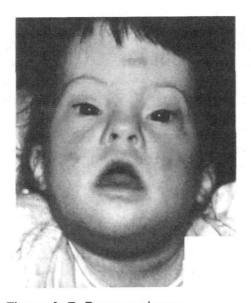

Figure A–7. Down syndrome.

the fifth finger), depressed nasal bridge, congenital hearing defects, absent Moro reflex in infancy, mouth breathing, and dental abnormalities. Ear symptoms include small pinnae, narrow external ear canals, abnormal ear configuration, and a strong tendency for recurrent otitis media. Incidence of hearing loss is very high with implications of sensorineural, conductive, and mixed hearing problems. Anomalies of middle ear ossicles have been reported. Risk of occurrence increases with the age of the mother: 1 in 1,200 at age 25 increasing to 1 in 100 at age 40. Tests such as nuchal translucency ultrasound, amniocentesis, or chorionic villus sampling can be done on a fetus during the first few months during pregnancy to check for Down syndrome. While half of all babies born with Down syndrome have congenital heart defects, new surgical techniques have made repair relatively routine, extending their average lifetime from age 25 in 1983 to 60 in 2012. See Chapter 4 for additional information (Balkany, Mischke, Downs, & Jafek, 1979; Diefendorf et al., 1995; Roizen et al., 1993; Shapiro, 2003; Sherman, Allen, Bean, & Freeman, 2007; http://ghr.nlm.nih .gov/condition/down-syndrome; http:// www.ndss.org; http://www.ncbi.nlm.nih .gov/pubmedhealth).

normally absorbed into the bloodstream by the kidneys are released into the urine instead. It can be caused by faulty genes, or it may result later in life due to kidney damage. Fanconi syndrome has many causes, some of which are inherited and some are yet unknown. Common causes in children are genetic defects that affect the body's ability to break down certain compounds. Exposure to heavy metals such as lead, mercury, or cadmium may directly precede acquired cases. Symptoms include anemia, bone marrow failure, and a variety of birth defects including bone and skeletal problems, eye and ear defects, skin discoloration, and congenital heart defects. Developmental problems may also be associated such as low birth weight, poor appetite, delayed growth, below average height, small head size, learning disabilities, and mental deficiency. In the infantile form, high-frequency sensorineural deafness is noted in infancy; in the adolescent form, slowly progressive sensorineural deafness is noted during the teen years (McDonough, 1970; Walker, 1971; http://www.nhlbi.nih.gov/ health/dci/Diseases/fanconi/fanconi_signs andsymptoms.html; http://www.ncbi.nlm .nih.gov/pubmedhealth/PMH0001374).

DYSCHONDROSTEOSIS

(See Madelung Deformity)

FANCONI'S ANEMIA SYNDROME

Infantile or Adolescent Renal Tubular Acidosis

Fanconi syndrome is a disorder of the kidney tubes in which certain substances

FETAL ALCOHOL SYNDROME (FAS)

Fetal alcohol syndrome refers to growth, mental, and physical problems that may occur in a baby when a mother abuses alcohol during pregnancy. When a pregnant woman drinks alcohol, it easily passes across the placenta to the fetus. Because of this, drinking alcohol during pregnancy can harm the baby's development. Infants with FAS may have the following symptoms: poor growth while the baby is in the womb and after birth; decreased muscle tone and poor coordination; delayed development and significant functional problems in intellect, speech, movement, or social skills; heart defects such as ventricular septal defect or atrial septal defect; significant structural problems with the face; and failure to thrive. Occurrence is estimated at 0.5 to 2 per 1,000 births. Full or partial expression of congenital malformations is associated with prenatal and postnatal growth deficiencies, central nervous system dysfunctions, and anomalies of the skeletal system and internal organs. The syndrome is characterized by a variety of craniofacial disorders such as micrognathia, cleft palate, abnormal pinnae, and hearing loss. It also frequently includes congenital abnormalities of the heart and eyes. Church and Gerkin (1987) noted hearing disorders in 13 of 14 children affected by FAS. Of the 14 study children, 13 had significant recurrent otitis media histories, including four with sensorineural hearing loss. Sparks (1984) described FAS with related speech and language disorders (Church, Edlis, Blakley, & Bawle, 1997; http://www.ncbi.nlm.nih.gov/ pubmedhealth/PMH0001909).

FRAGILE X SYNDROME

Fragile X syndrome is a genetic condition involving changes in part of the X chromosome. Although hearing loss has seldom been associated with fragile X syndrome, it is the most common form of inherited mental retardation in males and a significant cause of mental retardation in females. Fragile X syndrome is caused by a change in the *FMR1* gene. A small section of the gene code *(CGG)* is repeated on a fragile area of the X chromosome. The more repeats, the more likely there is to be a problem. Normally, the *FMR1* gene makes a protein needed for your brain to grow properly. A defect in this gene makes your body produce too little of the protein, or none at all. Boys and girls can both be affected, but because boys have only one X chromosome, a single, fragile X is likely to affect them more severely. Fragile X syndrome can be a cause of autism or related disorders, although not all children with fragile X syndrome have these conditions. Fragile X syndrome is an inherited abnormality of the X chromosome that causes disabilities ranging from severe language delay, behavior problems, autism or autistic-like behaviors (including poor eye contact and hand-flapping), macroorchidism, large, prominent ears, hyperactivity, delayed motor development, and poor sensory skills. Fragile X syndrome affects approximately 1 per 1,000 persons. Most children affected with fragile X syndrome will have some form of speech or language delay. Because they do not speak in short phrases until 2.5 years of age, these children should have routine auditory evaluations to identify otitis media and possible hearing loss. The speech of fragile X children has been described as compulsive, narrative, perseverative, cluttered, and mumbled with poor topic maintenance; syntax is usually appropriate for mental age; a high receptive vocabulary score is usually seen, although auditory memory and processing skills are weak (Hagerman et al., 2009; Hall, Burns, Lightbody, & Reiss, 2008; Paul, Cohen, Breg, Watson, & Herman, 1984; Wolf-Schein et al. 1987; http://www.ncbi.nlm.nih .gov/pubmedhealth/PMH0002633; http:// www.ncbi.nlm.nih.gov/pubmedhealth/ PMH0002633/).

FRIEDREICH ATAXIA

Friedreich's ataxia is an inherited disease that causes progressive damage to the nervous system, resulting in symptoms ranging from gait disturbance to speech problems; it can also lead to heart disease and diabetes. The ataxia results from the degeneration of nerve tissue in the spinal cord, in particular the sensory neurons essential (through connections with the cerebellum) for directing muscle movement of the arms and legs. The spinal cord becomes thinner and nerve cells lose some of their myelin sheath (the insulating covering on some nerve cells that helps conduct nerve impulses). This is an autosomal recessive disorder of the nervous system. Symptoms typically begin between the ages of 5 to 15 years and may include nystagmus, optic atrophy, oculomotor paralysis, retinitis pigmentosa, cataracts, cardiac complications, and organic psychological problems. There is progressive sensorineural deafness of early childhood with better hearing in the middle frequencies (Marmolino, 2011; Pandolfo, 2009; Shanon, Himelfarb, & Gold, 1981; Sylvester, 1958, 1972; http://en.wikipedia.org/wiki/Friedreich's_ataxia; http://www.ninds.nih.gov/disorders/friedreichs_ataxia/detail_friedreichs_ataxia.htm).

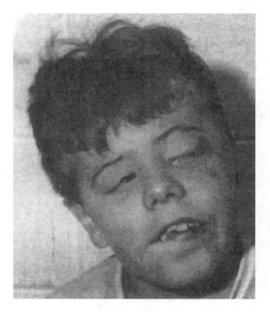

Figure A–9. Goldenhar syndrome.

GOLDENHAR SYNDROME

Oculo-Auriculo-Vertebral Dysplasia

Goldenhar syndrome is a congenital birth defect that involves deformities of the face. It usually affects one side of the face only, reflected as unilateral malformations of craniofacial structures including eye, oral, and musculoskeletal anomalies (Figure A–9). Characteristics include a partially formed or totally absent ear, the chin may be closer to the affected ear, one corner of the mouth may be higher than the other, benign growths of the eye, or a missing eye. Eye abnormalities include cleft or upper lid, epibulbar dermoids, extraocular muscle defects. Auricular abnormalities include auricular appendices, unilateral posteriorly placed ear, unilateral microtia, atresia of external auditory meatus (40%), and blind-ended fistulas. Oral abnormalities include unilateral facial hypoplasia of ramus and condyle, high arched palate, and open bite. Musculoskeletal abnormalities such as hemi-vertebrae and clubfoot are seen. Congenital heart disease may be present. The etiology is unknown but may not be hereditary. Most cases are sporadic with a wide spectrum of anomalies. This may possibly be secondary to vascular abnormality during embryologic development of first and second arches. Conductive hearing loss is present in 40% to 50% of reported cases as a result of atresia of external auditory canals (Bassila & Goldberg, 1989; Feingold & Baum, 1978; Shokeir, 1977; http://www.faces-cranio.org/Disord/Golden.htm; http://www.goldenharsyndrome.org; http://children.webmd.com/goldenhar-syndrome-oculo-auriculo-vertebral-spectrum; http://www.deafblind.com/goldenha.html).

HALLGREN SYNDROME

This syndrome is autosomal recessive, similar to Usher's syndrome. It may include progressive congenital sensorineural hearing loss leading to profound deafness. Symptoms include retinitis pigmentosa, atrophy of the optic nerve, nystagmus, and congenital hearing damage combined with neurological and psychiatric symptoms (Hallgren, 1959; http://www.ncbi.nlm.nih .gov/pubmed/11059142).

HAND-HEARING SYNDROME

This rare syndrome with autosomal dominant inheritance is characterized by hand and finger muscle wasting and sensorineural deafness. Patients manifest familial congenital bilateral or unilateral sensorineural hearing loss of varying degrees. A congenital hand abnormality is seen in both normal-hearing and deaf patients (Figure A–10). Congenital contractures of the digits and wasting of finger muscles are seen. No pain and no other deficits are present (Stewart & Bergstrom, 1971).

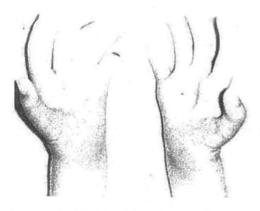

Figure A–10. Hand-hearing syndrome.

HARBOYAN SYNDROME

Corneal Dystrophy

This is an autosomal recessive eye disorder. The ocular manifestations in Harboyan syndrome include diffuse bilateral corneal edema occurring with severe corneal clouding, blurred vision, visual loss, and nystagmus. These symptoms are apparent at birth or within the neonatal period. The age of detectability and onset of slow, progressive hearing loss is usually between 10 and 25 years. There are no reported cases with prelingual deafness; however, a significant hearing loss in children as young as 4 years old has been detected by audiometry, suggesting that hearing may be affected earlier, even at birth. Harboyan syndrome is caused by mutations in the *SLC4A11* gene located at the *CHED2* locus on chromosome 20p13-p12, causing congenital corneal dystrophy with slow progression leading to blindness around age 40 and progressive sensorineural deafness of delayed onset (Harboyan, Mamo, der Kalonstian, & Karam, 1971; Maumenee, 1960; http://www.ncbi .nlm.nih.gov/pmc/articles/PMC1735049; http://www.ncbi.nlm.nih.gov/pmc/articles/ PMC2576053).

HEMIFACIAL MICROSOMIA

Hemifacial microsomia is a condition in which the lower half of one side of the face is underdeveloped and does not grow normally. It is sometimes also referred to as first and second brachial arch syndrome, oralmandibular-auricular syndrome, lateral facial dysplasia, or otomandibular dysostosis. The syndrome varies in severity but always includes maldevelopment of the ear and the mandible. It is a craniofacial disorder with unknown etiology. Abnormalities are unilateral and include ear aplasia and hypoplasia with various pinna malformations. Preauricular tags are present in nearly all cases. External ear canals may be absent or present with the opening covered with skin. Other characteristics include eye abnormalities, such as lower palpebral fissure in the affected side, microphthalmia, cysts, iris, choroid colobomas and strabismus, hypoplastic facial muscles, malocclusion (90%), and hypoplasia of the maxilla and mandible (95%). Unilateral conductive hearing loss may be present (http://www.faces-cranio.org/Disord/Hemi.htm).

HERRMANN SYNDROME

Photomyoclonus, Diabetes Mellitus, Nephropathy, and Sensorineural Deafness

This syndrome is a multisystem disorder beginning in late childhood or early adolescence, with photomyoclonus and hearing loss followed by diabetes mellitus, progressive dementia, pyelonephritis, and glomerulonephritis; progressive sensorineural hearing loss is of later onset. Inheritance is probably autosomal dominant with incomplete penetrance; nervous system disorder, dominant inheritance. Later course of the syndrome includes personality changes leading to severe dementia, slurring of speech, progressive hemiparesis, mild ataxia, renal disease, and diabetes. Age of detectability is third or fourth decade. Progressive sensorineural hearing loss is of late origin (Herrmann, Aguilar, & Sacks, 1964; http://rarediseases.info.nih.gov/GARD/Condition/9267/Herrmann_syndrome.aspx).

HURLER'S SYNDROME/ HUNTER'S SYNDROME

Mucopolysaccharidosis

Hurler syndrome, also known as mucopolysaccharidosis type I (MPS I), also known as gargoylism, is a genetic disorder that results in the buildup of glycosaminoglycans (formerly known as mucopolysaccharides) due to a deficiency of α-L-iduronidase, an enzyme responsible for the degradation of mucopolysaccharides in lysosomes. Lysosomal α-L-iduronidase helps break down long chains of sugar molecules called glycosaminoglycans (formerly called mucopolysaccharides). These molecules are found throughout the body, often in mucus and in fluid around the joints. Without this enzyme, a buildup of heparan sulfate and dermatan sulfate occurs in the body. Symptoms appear during childhood, and early death can occur due to organ damage. MPS I is divided into three subtypes based on severity of symptoms. All three types result from an absence of, or insufficient levels of, the enzyme α-L-iduronidase. MPS I Hurler syndrome is the most severe of the MPS I subtypes. The other two types are MPS I S or Scheie syndrome and MPS I H-S or Hurler-Scheie syndrome.

Hurler is clinically related to Hunter syndrome (Figures A–11 and A–12). Hunter is X-linked while Hurler is autosomal recessive. Although the Hurler and Hunter disorders appear clinically identical, Hunter is generally less severe and affects only males. Hurler's can affect both sexes. Patients with Hunter syndrome usually do not show gross evidence of corneal clouding, a diagnostic symptom of Hurler syndrome. Patients have a normal appearance at birth, but during the early months of life due to an apparent inborn error of metabolism, there is onset of progressive abnormal traits. Diagnostic features include growth failure, marked mental retardation, progressive coarsening of facial features, chronic nasal discharge, joint stiffness, and biochemical evidence of intracellular storage and acid mucopolysaccharides. Death usually occurs at 10 to 14 years of age. Most patients with Hurler's syndrome have some degree of progres-

sive deafness. Hunter's syndrome has been accompanied by deafness in about half the cases, although the loss is usually not severe and most likely mixed sensorineural and conductive. Otolaryngologic manifestations of all affected individuals include upper and lower respiratory infections, narrow nasal passages, hypertrophied adenoids, mucopurulent rhinorrhea, and noisy breathing. Affected individuals are prone to eustachian tube dysfunction and middle ear effusions (Hayes, Babin, & Platz, 1980; Keleman, 1966; Leroy & Crocker, 1966; Peck, 1984; http://www.nlm.nih.gov/medlineplus/ency/article/001204.htm).

HYDROCEPHALUS

Hydrocephalus describes a condition characterized by abnormal accumulation of fluid in and around the brain (Figure A–13). Hydrocephalus is due to a problem with the flow of cerebrospinal fluid, the liquid that surrounds the brain and spinal cord. This problem may be congenital or acquired. It

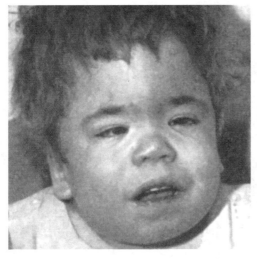

Figure A–11. Hurler's syndrome.

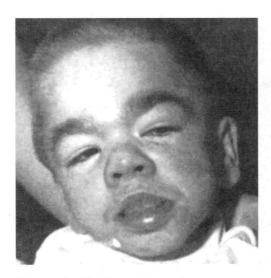

Figure A–12. Hunter's syndrome.

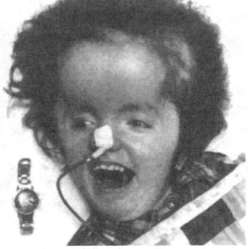

Figure A–13. Hydrocephalus.

is typically detected at birth or within first 3 months of life. Mental deficiency occurs if the condition is not treated. Risk of occurrence is approximately 1 per 2,000 births. The obvious symptoms are enlargement of the head, prominence of the brain, mental deterioration, and convulsions. With successful shunt treatment, 80% of children reach 5 years of age, and 80% of survivors are normal or educable. No reliable or consistent data are available regarding hearing impairment, although Walker, Cervette, Newberg, Moss, and Storrs (1987) discuss auditory evoked brainstem response measurement in neonatal hydrocephalus (http://www.ninds.nih.gov/disorders/hydrocephalus/detail_hydrocephalus.htm; http://www.ncbi.nlm.nih.gov/pubmedhealth/PMH0002538).

JERVELL AND LANGE-NIELSEN SYNDROME (JLNS)

Cardioauditory Syndrome

JLNS is a fairly rare cardiovascular disorder associated with profound sensorineural hearing loss said to affect 0.3% (or 1:1,000 of profoundly deaf children) of congenitally deaf persons. Specifically, the diagnostic marker is the prolongation of the QT interval on the electrocardiogram. This cardiac incident can lead to recurrent attacks of syncope, ventricular arrhythmia, and sudden death. An autosomal recessive arrhythmia trait with consanguinity is identified as one cause. Profound congenital bilateral sensorineural deafness may be accompanied by electrocardiographic abnormalities, fainting attacks, and occasionally sudden death in childhood. Death usually occurs between 3 and 14 years of age in more than 70% of patients. Hearing loss

is usually symmetric. It is often erroneously diagnosed as a seizure disorder and thus is improperly treated. The syndrome is caused by mutations in the *KCNE1* and *KCNQ1* genes (Cusimano, Martines, & Rizzo, 1991; Jervell & Lange-Nielsen, 1957; Nance, 2007; http://ghr.nlm.nih.gov/condition/jervell-and-lange-nielsen-syndrome; http://www.ncbi.nlm.nih.gov/books/NBK1405).

KLIPPEL-FEIL SEQUENCE

Klippel-Feil sequence is a rare craniofacial disorder (Figure A–14) that involves fusion of some or all cervical vertebrae. The sequence is characterized by a short neck with limited mobility, which gives the impression that the head sits on the shoulders. Diagnostic criteria include involvement of ear, eye, and neck anomalies. Other malformations may occur such as clubfoot and cleft palate, and various neurologic

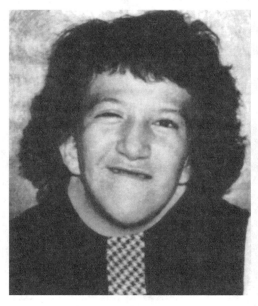

Figure A–14. Klippel-Feil syndrome with right facial paralysis.

disturbances. If familial, there is autosomal dominance with poor penetrance and variable expression. The sequence may be due to faulty segmentation of mesodermal somites in utero, early neural tube development, defects in maternal intestinal tract, or environmental factors. Summary of syndrome characteristics includes multifactorial inheritance, fusion of cervical vertebrae, webbed neck, abducens nerve palsy, occasional cleft palate, torticollis, and severe sensorineural or conductive hearing loss. The hearing loss may range from mild conductive to profound sensorineural. Ear deformities occur in one-third of cases; temporal bone and roentgenogram findings include narrow to absent external auditory meatus or middle ear space, deformed ossicles, narrow oval window niche, underdevelopment of cochlea and vestibular structures, absence of semicircular canals, and absence of eighth cranial nerve. Central nervous system involvement is also frequently described and may contribute to audiologic findings. The frequency is approximately 1:42,000 births with 65% occurring in females (McLay & Maran, 1969; Miyamoto, Yune, & Rosevear, 1983; Nagib, Maxwell, & Chou, 1985; Stewart & O'Reilly, 1989; Windle-Taylor, Emery, & Phelps, 1981; http://www.ninds.nih.gov/disorders/klippel_feil/htm; http://www.klippel-feil.org).

LAURENCE-MOON-BIEDL-BARDET SYNDROME

In general terms, these two syndromes are eye disorders with progressive sensorineural hearing loss of recessive inheritance. Laurence-Moon syndrome is usually considered a separate entity from Biedl-Bardet syndrome. Patients with Laurence-Moon syndrome have retinitis pigmentosa, mental retardation, hypogenitalism, and spastic paraplegia. Biedl-Bardet syndrome is a ciliopathic human genetic disorder that produces many effects and affects many body systems. It is characterized principally by obesity, retinitis pigmentosa, polydactyly, mental retardation, hypogonadism, and renal failure. There have been at least 14 genetic forms of this syndrome identified so far (Konigsmark & Gorlin, 1976; Weinstein, Kliman, & Scully, 1969).

LEOPARD SYNDROME

Multiple Lentigines Syndrome

Multiple lentigines syndrome is an integumentary-pigmentary disorder inherited as an autosomal dominant trait. People with this condition have large numbers of lentigines, which are skin markings somewhat darker than true freckles. They are present from birth and located mostly on the trunk and neck. Affected people also have wide-set eyes (hypertelorism), prominent ears, sensorineural deafness, and cafe-au-lait spots (light brown birthmarks). Additional symptoms include mild pulmonic stenosis and changes in the ECG (electrocardiogram). People with this condition may have abnormal genitalia (cryptorchidism), hypogonadism, or delayed puberty. LEOPARD is an acronym derived from: (L) lentigines, (E) electrocardiographic defects, (O) ocular hypertelorism, (P) pulmonary stenosis, (A) abnormalities of genitalia, (R) retardation of growth, and sensorineural (D) deafness. Hearing loss occurs in approximately 25% of cases and is of marked variation and expressivity, usually detected in childhood (Digilio et al., 2006; Gorlin, Anderson, & Blaw, 1969; Voron, Hatfield, & Kalkhoff, 1976).

LERI-WEILL DISEASE

(See Madelung Deformity)

LONG ARM 18 DELETION SYNDROME

Distal 18q-

Approximately 1 in every 40,000 babies is born with the distal long arm of chromosome 18 deletion. Distal 18q- has been called several different names. This condition may also be called *monosomy 18q, 18q deletion syndrome, partial 18q deletion,* or *de Grouchy syndrome.* Associated symptoms and findings may vary greatly in range and severity from case to case. Abnormalities include mental disabilities, microcephaly, short stature, hearing impairment with malformations of auricles and external auditory canals, retinal changes, facial peculiarities, and a high count of whorls on the fingers. Cleft palate and lip as well as congenital heart disease, horseshoe kidney, cryptorchidism, spinal defects, and foot abnormalities have also been described. It is due to a genetic imbalance involving partial deletion of the long arm of the 18th chromosome (Figure A–15). If translocation is responsible for deletion, transmission to children is possible. Conductive hearing loss is associated with cleft lip and palate or congenital external and middle ear anomalies. Temporal bone study has shown collapsed Reissner's membrane in all turns of the cochlea,

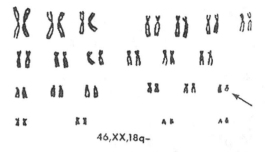

PARTIAL DELETION OF 18 LONG ARM

46,XX,18q-

Figure A–15. Karyotype of partial deletion of the long arm 18 deletion syndrome. Reproduced with permission from *Birth defects compendium,* 2nd ed., by B. Bergsma, 1979, New York, NY: The National Foundation-March of Dimes and Alan R. Liss.

rolled and retracted tectorial membrane, and hypoplastic cochlear aqueduct (Bergstrom, Stewart, & Kenyon, 1974; Cody et al., 2005; Hale et al., 2003; Kos, Schuknecht, & Singer, 1966; Smith, 1962; http://www.chromosome18.org/TheConditions/Distal18q/tabid/127/Default.aspx; http://www.cigna.com/healthinfo/nord967.html).

MADELUNG DEFORMITY

Dyschondrosteosis; Leri-Weill Disease

Madelung's deformity is characterized by malformed wrists and wrist bones and short stature and is often associated with Léri-Weill dyschondrosteosis. Madelung's deformity is a congenital abnormality of the wrist caused by a growth disturbance that retards development of the ulnar and volar portions of the distal radial physis. Associated hearing loss is not common, but congenital bilateral conductive loss with abnormal ossicles and narrow external auditory canals has been reported (Dawe, Wynne-Davies, & Fulford, 1982; Nassif & Harboyan, 1970; http://boneandspine.com/pediatric-disorders/madelung-deformity).

MARSHALL SYNDROME

Stickler Syndrome

Marshall syndrome is a genetic disorder of the connective collagen tissue. The three most common areas to be affected are the eyes, joints, and mouth and facial structures. Marshall syndrome and Stickler syndrome closely resemble each other. Myopia is the most common eye problem in Marshall syndrome. Cataracts also occur more frequently and detached retina less frequently than in Stickler syndrome. The joint changes include hyperextensibility (double-jointedness) and arthritis. Babies and young children with Stickler syndrome usually have very hyperextensible joints. The facial features of Marshall syndrome include a flat midface, the appearance of large eyes, short upturned saddle-like nose, and a round face. The facial features of Stickler syndrome are less prominent but include a rather long flat face, and depressed nasal bridge. The hearing loss associated with Stickler syndrome can be progressive and usually involves the high frequencies. Sensorineural hearing loss has been reported in 20% to 100% of affected individuals. A conductive loss due to otitis media can overlay an existing sensorineural loss and is a frequent problem for children with both Stickler and Marshall syndromes. Occasionally there is dysfunction of central and peripheral vestibular systems. It is a dominant transmission disorder (Admiraal, Szymko, Griffith, Brunner, & Huygen, 2002; Parke, 2002; Ruppert, Buerk, & Pfordresher, 1970; Zellweger, Smith, & Grutzner, 1974; http://www.healthline.com/galecontent/marshall-syndrome).

MEASLES

Measles is a highly contagious viral infection involving the respiratory tract. The infection is spread by contact with droplets from the nose, mouth, or throat of an infected person. Sneezing and coughing can put contaminated droplets into the air. The skin becomes covered with red papules that appear behind the ears and on the face before spreading rapidly down the trunk and onto the arms and legs. Measles may be complicated by bacterial pneumonia, otitis media, and demyelinating encephalitis. Measles may cause hearing loss as a result of invasion of the inner ear via the bloodstream or central nervous system or through purulent labyrinthitis secondary to suppurative otitis media. Hearing loss from measles is now rare due to the use of the measles, mumps, and rubella (MMR) vaccine. Those who have had an active measles infection or who have been vaccinated against the measles have immunity to the disease. See Rubella below and Chapter 2 (http://www.ncbi.nlm.nih.gov/pubmedhealth/PMH0002536).

MENINGITIS

Bacterial meningitis was the leading cause of acquired childhood sensorineural hearing loss until the introduction of the HIB vaccine in 1985. The disease is due to an infection of the meningeal membrane surrounding the brain and spinal cord. The most common causes of meningitis are viral infections that usually get better without treatment. Viral meningitis is milder and occurs more often than bacterial meningitis. It usually develops in the late summer and early fall, and often affects children and adults under age 30. Most infections occur in children under age 5. However, bacterial meningitis infections are also common, extremely serious, and may result in death or brain damage, even if treated. Common bacterial infections include *Haemophilus influenzae*, meningococcal and pneumococcal, staphylococcal, and tuberculosis. The etiology of meningitis is variable, and the disorder may also be caused by chemical irritation, drug allergies, and tumors. Symptoms of meningitis include stiff neck, headache, high fever, nausea, vomiting, and sometimes coma. Approximately 40% of children with deafness due to meningitis have at least one other major handicapping condition. It remains a common cause of sudden, severe to profound sensorineural deafness in developing countries without widespread vaccine programs. Meningitis may be the result of a complication of untreated otitis media. Deafness is usually bilateral but may be unilateral. See Chapter 4 (Finitzo-Hieber, 1981; Liptak, McConnochie, & Roghmann, 1997; Stein & Boyer, 1994; http://www.ncbi.nlm.nih.gov/pubmedhealth/PMH0001700).

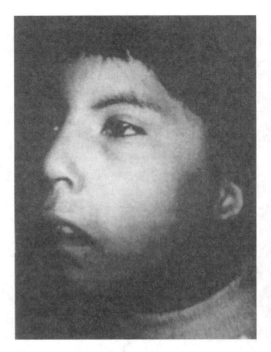

Figure A–16. Moebius syndrome.

MOEBIUS SYNDROME

Moebius syndrome is a rare birth defect caused by the absence or underdevelopment of the sixth and seventh cranial nerves, which control eye movements and facial expression (Figure A–16). Many of the other cranial nerves may also be affected, including the 3rd, 5th, 8th, 9th, 11th, and 12th. The first symptom, present at birth, is an inability to suck. Other symptoms can include feeding, swallowing, and choking problems; excessive drooling; crossed eyes; lack of facial expression; inability to smile; eye sensitivity; motor delays; high or cleft palate; hearing problems; and speech difficulties. Children with Moebius syndrome may have delayed speech because of paralysis of muscles that move the lips, soft palate, and tongue root. Children with Moebius syndrome are unable to move their eyes back and forth. Decreased numbers of muscle fibers have been reported. Deformities of the tongue, jaw, and limbs, such as clubfoot and missing or webbed fingers, may also occur. As children get older, lack of facial expression and inability to smile become the dominant visible symptoms. Approximately 30% to 40% of children with Moebius syndrome have some degree of autism. It is an autosomal dominant syndrome of facial dysplasia with concurrent congenital sensorineural or conductive hearing loss (Bogart & Matsumoto, 2010; Goulden & Hodge, 1998; Kahane, 1979; Meyerson & Foushee, 1978; http://www.ninds.nih.gov/disorders/mobius/moebius.htm; http://www.faces-cranio.org/Disord/Moebius.htm).

MUCKLE-WELLS SYNDROME

Amyloidosis, Nephritis, and Urticaria

Muckle-Wells syndrome is a disorder characterized by periodic episodes of skin rash, fever, and joint pain. Progressive hearing loss and kidney damage also occur in this disorder. People with Muckle-Wells syndrome have recurrent "flare-ups" that begin during infancy or early childhood. These episodes may appear to arise spontaneously or be triggered by cold, heat, fatigue, or other stresses. Affected individuals typically develop a nonitchy rash, mild to moderate fever, painful and swollen joints, and in some cases redness in the whites of the eyes (conjunctivitis). Hearing loss caused by progressive nerve damage (sensorineural deafness) typically becomes apparent during the teenage years. Abnormal deposits of a protein called amyloid (amyloidosis) cause progressive kidney damage in about one third of people with Muckle-Wells syndrome; these deposits may also damage other organs. In addition, pigmented skin lesions may occur in affected individuals. Mutations in the *NLRP3* gene cause Muckle-Wells syndrome. (Haas, Küster, Zuberbier, & Henz, 1978; http://ghr.nlm.nih.gov/condition/muckle-wells-syndrome).

MUCOPOLYSACCHARIDOSIS

(See Hurler's Syndrome/Hunter's Syndrome.)

MUMPS

Mumps is a contagious viral disease occurring mainly in children characterized by swelling of the salivary and parotid glands. It is acquired by aspiration. The incubation period is 18 to 22 days, with fever and painful inflammation of the involved glands. Symptoms are most pronounced during the first 2 days and subside slowly over the next 4 or 5 days. Classic symptoms involve fever, headache, anorexia, malaise, earache, and enlargement of parotids. Prior to availability of the MMR vaccine, mumps was a common cause of sudden, total unilateral sensorineural hearing loss. Bilateral total deafness has been reported, but only in rare instances, usually due to bilateral mumps. Approximately one third of infections are subclinical and nearly asymptomatic. Mumps is now a rare cause of deafness in the United States due to the introduction of the measles, mumps, and rubella (MMR) vaccine. See Chapter 4 (Litman & Baum, 2009; Mason et al., 2007; Roizen, 1999; http://www.ncbi.nlm.nih.gov/pubmedhealth/PMH0002524).

MUSCULAR DYSTROPHY (MD)

Muscular dystrophy is a group of recessive e- or X-linked inherited disorders that involve muscle weakness and loss of muscle tissue, which get worse over time. Muscular dystrophies (MDs), are a group of inherited conditions, which means they are passed down through families. They may occur in childhood or adulthood. There are many different types of muscular dystrophy. Muscle wasting of various types is classified by transmission mode, age of onset, damaged muscle set, rate of disease development, and associated problems. Pseudohypertrophic muscular dystrophy usually begins before age 5 and affects most body muscles including cardiac and pulmonary systems. The facioscapulohumeral type affects face, shoulder, and upper arm muscles; it is slowly progressive with age of onset at 13 to 14 years. *Limb-girdle* type initially affects the muscles of hips and shoulders. Myotonic muscular dystrophy is associated with diabetes mellitus and cataracts, usually of late onset at age 30 to 40 or older. Although generally not associated with hearing loss, severe infantile muscular dystrophy is noted to be accompanied by sloping, mild to moderate sensorineural hearing loss. Risk of occurrence is 1 per 100,000; the childhood form is usually noted during the initial 3 years of life. Genetic counseling is advised when there is a family history of muscular dystrophy. This is extremely rare in women; women may have no symptoms but still carry the gene for the disorder (Black et al. 1971a; Kleigman et al., 2007; http://www .ncbi.nlm.nih.gov/pubmedhealth/PMH 0002172).

NEUROFIBROMATOSIS TYPES 1 AND 2 (NF-1 AND NF-2)

The neurofibromatoses are genetic disorders that cause tumors to grow in the nervous system and produce other abnormalities such as skin changes and bone deformities. The tumors are slow growing and begin in the supporting cells of the nerves and the myelin sheath. Cellular elements from these cell types proliferate excessively throughout the body, forming tumors; melanocytes also function abnormally in this disease, resulting in disordered skin pigmentation and cafe-au-lait spots. The tumors may cause bumps under the skin, colored spots, skeletal problems, pressure on spinal nerve roots, and other neurological problems. Neurofibromatosis also increases the risk of leukemia particularly in children. Children with NF-1 have 200 to 500 times the normal risk of developing leukemia compared to the general population.

The disorders have been classified into categories: neurofibromatosis type 1 (NF-1), neurofibromatosis type 2 (NF-2), and schwannoma. NF-1 is the more common type (1:4,000) accounting for up to 90% of all cases. NF-2 2 has a frequency of 1 in 45,000 people. Symptoms of NF-1, which may be evident at birth and nearly always by the time the child is 10 years old, may include light brown spots on the skin (cafe-au-lait spots), two or more growths on the iris of the eye, a tumor on the optic nerve, a larger than normal head circumference, and abnormal development of the spine, a skull bone, or the tibia. NF-2 is less common (1 per 40,000) and is characterized by slow-growing tumors on the eighth cranial nerves. The tumors create pressure and damage to neighboring nerves causing other symptoms such as headache, facial weakness, sensory or visual changes, and unsteadiness. NF-1 is a multisystem, progressive disorder that can frequently involve portions of the auditory system in diverse and subtle ways for which no characteristic audiologic findings are related. Diagnostic criteria for NF-2 include bilateral eighth nerve tumors and a first-degree relative who also has NF-2 symptoms. The diagnostic criteria for NF-2 are eighth nerve tumors, cataracts at an early age, or changes in the retina that may affect vision, and other nervous system tumors. Surgery is often recommended to remove the tumors. Some NF-1 tumors may become cancerous, and treatment may include surgery, radiation, or chemotherapy. In most cases, symptoms of NF-1 are mild, and individuals live normal and productive lives. In other patients, however, NF-1 can be severely debilitating and may cause cosmetic and psychological issues. The course of NF-2 varies greatly among individuals. In some cases of NF-2, the damage to nearby vital structures, such as other cranial nerves and the brainstem, can be life threatening. It may cause palsies of the 5th, 6th, 7th, 9th, and 10th cranial nerves; cerebellar ataxia may develop. Between 30% and 50% of new cases arise spontaneously through gene mutation. Once this change has taken place, the mutant gene can be passed on to succeeding generations (Korf & Rubenstein, 2005; NIH Consensus Conference, 1988; Pastores, Michels, & Jack, 1991; Pikus, 1995; http:// www.ninds.nih.gov/disorders/neurofibro matosis/neurofibromatosis.htm; http:// www.nfinc.org; http://www.anausa.org).

NORRIE'S DISEASE

Norrie's disease is a rare inherited eye disorder that leads to blindness in male infants at birth or soon after birth. It causes abnormal development of the retina, with masses of immature retinal cells accumulating at the back of the eye. As a result, the pupils appear white when light is shone on them (leukocoria). The irises (colored portions of the eyes) or the entire eyeballs may shrink and deteriorate during the first months of life, and cataracts (cloudiness in the lens of the eye) may eventually develop. About one third of individuals with Norrie disease develop progressive sensorineural hearing loss, and more than half experience developmental delays in motor skills such as sitting up and walking. Other problems may include mild to moderate intellectual disability, often with psychosis, and abnormalities that can affect circulation, breathing, digestion, excretion, or reproduction. Mutations in the *NDP* gene cause Norrie disease (Holmes, 1971; Rehm et al., 2002; Royer et al. 2003; http://ghr.nlm.nih.gov/condition/ norrie-disease).

OPTIC ATROPHY AND POLYNEUROPATHY

Symptoms include progressive visual loss with bilateral and symmetric optic atrophy beginning in the second decade and leading to rapid deterioration of vision. Polyneuropathy continues from childhood. Severe progressive sensorineural deafness in childhood tends to affect high frequencies. Likely a recessive or X-linked transmission occurs. It is sometimes classified as a unique form of Charcot-Marie-Tooth disease. The risk of occurrence is 1 per 100,000 (Iwashita, Inoue, Araki, & Kuroiwa, 1970; http://www .checkorphan.org/disease/optic-atrophy- polyneuropathy-deafness; http://www.ncbi. nlm.nih.gov/pubmed/1292972).

OPTICO-COCHLEO-DENTATE DEGENERATION

This is a rare autosomal recessive eye and nervous system disorder. This syndrome is characterized by progressive visual and sensorineural hearing loss and progressive spastic quadriplegia. The main clinical symptoms consisted of muscle hypotonia (floppy infant), generalized epileptic fits, hypacusis, rotatory nystagmus, insufficient pupillary reactions, and mental deficiency. Vision is normal until about 1 year of age, with total blindness occurring at about age 3 years. Microcephaly, mental deterioration, and speech problems may be evident, with death likely in later childhood (Konigsmark & Gorlin, 1976; Schroder et al., 2004; http://www.springerlink.com/content/vw1193c0d0pgt6j0).

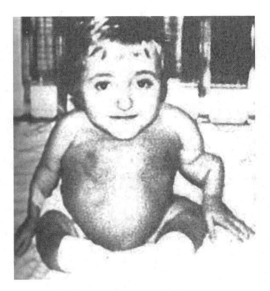

Figure A–17. Osteogenesis imperfecta.

OSTEOGENESIS IMPERFECTA

Also known as "brittle bone" disease, osteogenesis imperfecta (OI) is a congenital disease frequently caused by a defect in the gene that produces type 1 collagen. It is also known as Van Der Hoeve's syndrome. Osteogenesis imperfecta is a heterogeneous group of eight types of disorders of connective tissue characterized by bone fragility with a high percentage of infant death. Multiple fractures may be present at birth. Weak joints, blue sclera, spinal cord and brainstem problems, thin and translucent skin, yellowish-brown and easily broken teeth, and deafness are common symptoms (Figure A–17). Hydrocephalus, nerve root compression, cardiovascular defects, respiratory problems, and pneumonia may also occur. Etiology is hereditary autosomal dominant, present at birth. The majority of severe cases are sporadic, and because of clinical variability, detection may range from birth through adulthood. Eight types of OI exist dependent upon the severity of symptoms and genetic etiology. Of reported cases, 60%

have conductive hearing loss reportedly due to otosclerotic changes and fixation of the stapes. Otologic surgery is usually successful. Temporal bone findings show diminished or immature bone formation in otic capsule and ossicles. Sensorineural hearing loss has also been demonstrated in high frequencies. Genetic counseling, magnesium therapy, and orthopedic correction are recommended. Rate of occurrence is 2 to 5 per 100,000 births. Estimates of hearing loss range between 26% and 60% of cases (Bretlau, Jorgensen, & Johansen, 1970; Cole, 1991; Hall & Rohrt, 1968; Marini, 2007; Quisling, Moore, Jahrsdoerfer, & Cantrell, 1979; Riedner, 1980; http://www.oif.org; http://www.niams.nih.gov/Health_Info/Bone/Osteogenesis_Imperfecta/).

OSTEOPETROSIS

Osteopetroses constitutes a collection of disorders characterized by increased bone density and skeletal modeling abnormalities. Osteopetroses can be categorized based on whether sclerosis or defective skeletal modeling predominates. Some types are comparatively benign; others are progressive and fatal. Bony overgrowth sometimes severely distorts the face. Malocclusion of the teeth may require specialized orthodontic measures. Surgical decompression may be required to relieve elevated intracranial pressure or to release a trapped facial or auditory nerve. The category of osteopetrosis includes Pyle's disease, Albers-Schonberg disease, chalk bone disease, ivory bone disease, and marble bone disease (http://ghr.nlm.nih.gov/condition/osteopetrosis; http://www.osteopetrosis.org).

OTOPALATODIGITAL SYNDROME (OPD I AND II)

This is a sex-linked recessive craniofacial-skeletal disorder with distinctive facial appearance. Otopalatodigital syndrome types I and II are rare X-linked genetic disorders in which complete expression of the disease occurs only in males. Females may be mildly affected with some of the symptoms. OPD type I is the milder form of the disease and is characterized by cleft palate, hearing loss, and skeletal abnormalities in the skull and limbs. OPD type II includes these abnormalities as well as growth deficiency and abnormalities of the brain and is frequently not compatible with life. Infants may have difficulty breathing and require long-term respiratory care. Orthopedic and surgical procedures may be used to correct skeletal deformities. Treatment of hearing loss may be limited due to the severity of deformities within the ear. Individuals with otopalatodigital syndrome type I typically have short stature, an incomplete closure of the roof of the mouth (cleft palate), a downward slant of the opening between the upper and lower eyelids, hearing loss due to a defect of the middle ear (conductive hearing loss), and abnormal shortness of the fingers and toes. Symptoms that are sometimes seen in OPD type I are short, broad thumbs and large toes; wide spaces between the toes; one or more fingers bent to the side; two or more digits united (syndactyly); short fingernails; dislocation of the head of the radius (one of the bones of the forearm); a broad bridge of the nose; underdeveloped bones of the face; or slow speech development. Females with the disorder may have an overhanging brow, a depressed nasal bridge, a wide space between the eyes, and a flat midface. The symptoms expressed in females vary and are fewer. Females do not have the full expression of this disorder. Individuals with otopalatodigital syndrome type II are typically more severely affected, often resulting in stillbirth or early infant death (Buran & Duvall, 1967; Hall et al., 1995; Pazzaglia & Giampiero, 1986; Robertson et al., 2001; Savarirayan et al., 2002, 2003; Rimoin & Edgerton, 1967; Schaefer, Kolodziej, & Olney, 1998; Zaytoun, Harboyan & Kabalan, 2002; http://icmmt.alere.com/kbase/nord/nord878.htm).

PENDRED SYNDROME

Pendred syndrome or Pendred disease is an autosomal recessive genetic disorder with bilateral sensorineural hearing loss and goiter with occasional hypothyroidism (decreased thyroid gland function). There is no specific treatment, other than supportive measures for the hearing loss and thyroid hormone. Pendred's syndrome may account for as many as 7% of all cases of congenital deafness. The goiter may be noted at birth but is usually apparent by age 8 years and is noted in 75% of all cases. If a goiter is present, thyroid function tests are performed to identify mild cases of thyroid dysfunction even if they are not yet causing symptoms. Auditory manifestations are variable but usually demonstrate a moderate-to-profound sensorineural hearing loss. The hearing loss of Pendred's syndrome is often, although not always, present from birth and is typically progressive. MRI scanning of the inner ear usually shows widened or large vestibular aqueducts with enlarged endolymphatic sacs and may show Mondini dysplasia of the cochleae. Genetic testing to identify the Pendrin gene usually establishes the diagnosis. Risk of occurrence is about 1 in 14,500 making it a fairly common disorder related to profound deafness (Batsakis & Nishiyama, 1962; Fraser, 1965; Ilium, Kaier, Hvidberg-Hansen, & Sondergaard, 1972; Johnson et al., 1987; Kabakkaya et al., 1993; Pearce, 2007).

PIERRE ROBIN SEQUENCE

Pierre Robin sequence or complex (pronounced "Roban") is the name given to a birth condition that involves the lower jaw being either small in size (micrognathia) or set back from the upper jaw. As a result, the tongue tends to be displaced back toward the throat, where it can fall back and obstruct the airway. Most infants, but not all, will also have a cleft palate, but none will have a cleft lip. It is a dominant, craniofacial-skeletal disorder. External ears may be low set. Associated congenital amputations, hip dislocation, sternal anomalies, spina bifida, hydrocephaly, and microcephaly have been

reported along with a variety of cardiac and middle ear anomalies. The "sequencing" of events begins with failure of the lower jaw to develop normally before birth. At about 7 to 10 weeks into a pregnancy, the lower jaw grows rapidly, allowing the tongue to descend from between the two halves of the palate. If, for some reason, the lower jaw does not grow properly, the tongue can prevent the palate from closing, resulting in a cleft palate. The small or displaced lower jaw also causes the tongue to be positioned at the back of the mouth, possibly causing breathing difficulty at birth. The presence of cleft palate contributes continually through early childhood development to conductive hearing loss. The placement of ventilation tubes in the eardrums may be recommended to reduce fluid buildup. Because ear infections can cause temporary hearing loss that can affect speech and language development, the patient's hearing should also be monitored routinely. Gould (1989) reported a 50% incidence of conductive hearing loss in a sample of 20 patients with Pierre Robin sequence. Risk of occurrence is varied but estimated by some as 1 in 30,000 (Cohen, 1999; Pashayan & Lewis, 1984; Williams et al., 1981).

PREAURICULAR ANOMALIES

Preauricular Pit, Tag, Cyst, or Sinus

A preauricular pit, sinus, cyst, or tag is a common congenital malformation characterized by a nodule, dent, or dimple located anywhere adjacent to the external ear. These abnormalities are inherited features and include preauricular pits, tags, and fistulas that may be multiple or bilateral in 25% to 50% of cases. Preauricular sinuses and cysts result from developmental defects of the first and second branchial arches. Occasionally a preauricular sinus or a cyst can become infected. This is a dominant craniofacial disorder that may be accompanied by conductive hearing loss or sensorineural hearing loss. Microtia anomaly of the external ear, ear canal atresia, facial paralysis, or mandibular anomalies may also be present. Preauricular tags or pits usually require no treatment except for cosmetic surgery or excision if draining. In rare cases they may be associated with branchio-oto-renal syndrome (Figure A–18; Cremers, Thijssen, & Fischer, 1981; Hayes, 1994; Tan, Constantinides, & Mitchell, 2005; http://www.nlm.nih.gov/medlineplus/ency/article/003304.htm).

PYLE'S DISEASE

Metaphyseal Dysplasia

This is a rare, recessive disorder of the osteopetroses group. Affected people are clinically normal, although scoliosis and bone fragility occasionally occur. The diagnosis is usually made when x-rays are done for an unrelated reason. X-ray changes are striking. Long bones are undermodeled, and bony cortices are generally thin with tubular leg bones. Pelvic bones and thoracic cage are expanded. However, the skull is essentially spared. Nystagmus is common. Progressive sensorineural or conductive hearing loss may be present (Gladney & Monteleone, 1970; Miller, Lehman, & Geretti, 1969; Schaefer et al., 1986).

REFSUM'S DISEASE

Individuals with Refsum disease present with neurologic damage, cerebellar degeneration, and peripheral neuropathy. Onset is most common in childhood/adolescence with a progressive course, although periods of stagnation or remission occur. Symptoms also include ataxia, scaly skin (ichthyosis), difficulty hearing, and eye problems including cataracts and night blindness. Major clinical symptoms include triad of retinitis pigmentosa, peripheral neuropathy, cardiac arrhythmias, loss of the sense of smell (anosmia), problems with balance, and ataxia. Also present is progressive sensorineural hearing loss (Fryer, Winckleman, & Ways, 1971; Nance, 1973; http://www.ninds.nih.gov/disorders/refsum/refsum.htm).

RENAL TUBULAR ACIDOSIS

(See Fanconi's Anemia Syndrome.)

RICHARDS-RUNDLE SYNDROME

Ataxia-Hypogonadism Syndrome

This is a rare nervous system disorder of autosomal recessive inheritance. It begins in early childhood with muscle wasting; nystagmus; congenital, severe to profound,

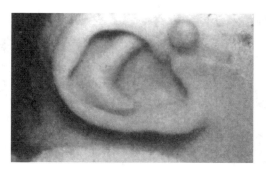

Figure A–18. Preauricular abnormalities.

progressive sensorineural hearing loss; ataxia absent deep tendon reflexes; mental retardation; and failure to develop secondary sexual characteristics (Richards & Rundle, 1959).

RUBELLA

Congenital Rubella Syndrome (CRS)

This disorder presents as a classic triad of symptoms including sensorineural hearing loss, congenital heart disease, and vision problems. Infants with congenital rubella virus infections have a variety of defects of varying severity depending on the embryonic stage during which the infection occurred. Congenital rubella syndrome (CRS) can occur in a developing fetus of a pregnant woman who has contracted the rubella virus. If infection occurs 0 to 28 days before conception, there is a 43% chance the infant will be affected. If the infection occurs 0 to 12 weeks after conception, there is a 51% chance the infant will be affected. If the infection occurs 13 to 26 weeks after conception, there is a 23% chance the infant will be affected by the disease. Infants are not generally affected if rubella is contracted during the third trimester, or 26 to 40 weeks after conception. Problems rarely occur when rubella is contracted by the mother after 20 weeks of gestation, however, she may continue to disseminate the virus after birth. Hearing impairment can result from fetal rubella not only during the first trimester of pregnancy but also in the second and even third trimester. Rubella vaccine is available worldwide and provides lifetime protection to women. However, congenital rubella is still a major prenatal acquired cause of profound childhood deafness in developing countries, In the United States universal application of MMR vaccine to young girls has eliminated CRS.

CRS diagnostic features include transient neonatal manifestations of low birth weight, corneal clouding, and jaundice. Anemia, pneumonia, meningitis, and encephalitis may develop. Associated problems include hearing loss (58%), heart disease (50%), cataract or glaucoma (43%), psychomotor difficulties (45%), cerebral palsy (45%), and mental deficiency (40%). A major feature of rubella embryopathy is a characteristic "salt and pepper" retinal pigmentation that does not interfere with visual acuity. Dental abnormalities, microcephaly, and behavioral problems are common in children with congenital rubella. Rubella deafness is commonly sensorineural and often severe to profound. Children who have been exposed to rubella in the womb should also be watched closely as they age for any indication of developmental delay, autism spectrum disorders, growth retardation, and learning disabilities. Variation in audiometric configuration is common. The pathology of rubella deafness includes a variety of inner ear abnormalities and middle ear and external ear anomalies. Vaccination of females of childbearing age against rubella can prevent congenital rubella syndrome. Termination of pregnancy is often recommended if exposure occurs or CRS is suspected (Roizen, 1999; Roizen et al., 1996; Strasnick & Jacobson, 1995; Stuckless, 1980; http://en.wikipedia.org/wiki/Congenital_rubella_syndrome; http://www.hknc.org/Rubella.htm; http://www.cdc.gov/mmwr/preview/mmwrhtml/rr6204a1.htm; http://www.deafblind.com/crs.html).

SCHWANN SYNDROME

This is a familial dominant syndrome characterized by knuckle pads noted as callous-like thickening over dorsal aspects of interphalangeal joints of fingers and toes and leukonychia or progressive whitening of finger and toenails. Knuckle pads and leukonychia may initially be observed in infancy and early childhood. It is primarily an integumentary-pigmentary disorder that may be associated with congenital sensorineural or conductive-type hearing loss identified in infancy or early childhood. The hearing loss may be mixed mild to moderate in degree (Bart & Pumphrey, 1967; Ramer, Vasily, & Ladda, 1994).

SENSORY RADICULAR NEUROPATHY

Sensory radicular neuropathy is one of a group of hereditary sensory and autonomic neuropathies all characterized by progressive loss of function that predominantly affects the peripheral sensory nerves. Their incidence has been estimated to be about 1 in 25,000. Type 1 is the most common of the hereditary sensory and autonomic neuropathies (HSANs). Charcot-Marie-Tooth syndrome is also within this disorder category. Type 1 is transmitted as an autosomal dominant trait and is characterized by a sensory deficit in the distal portion of the lower extremities, chronic perforating ulcerations of the feet, and progressive destruction of underlying bones. Sweating abnormalities occur along with lightning pains that involve the distal extremities with painless ulcerations of feet. Symptoms appear in late childhood or early adolescence with trophic ulcers as pain sensation is affected more. Many patients have accompanying progressive moderate-to-severe sensorineural deafness and atrophy of the peroneal muscles. Histopathologic examination reveals a marked reduction in the number of unmyelinated fibers. Motor nerve conduction velocities are normal, but the sensory nerve action potentials are absent. Onset may be in late teens or early adult years (Houlden et al., 2006; Mandell & Smith, 1960; Stanley, Puritz, Birggaman, & Wheeler, 1975).

SYPHILIS, CONGENITAL

Syphilis rates of infection have increased since the year 2000, especially in developing countries and often in combination with human immunodeficiency virus (HIV). The number of cases of congenital syphilis has also been increasing in the United States since 1986. This is an infectious disease contracted by the fetus from the infected mother. Syphilis is a sexually transmitted infection caused by the spirochete bacterium *Treponema pallidum* subspecies *pallidum*. The primary route of transmission is through sexual contact; it may also be transmitted from mother to fetus during pregnancy or at birth, resulting in congenital syphilis. Congenital syphilis in the newborn can be prevented by screening mothers during early pregnancy and treating those who are infected. One-third to two-thirds of newborns are typically asymptomatic. Sensorineural hearing impairment of a slow, progressive nature usually begins after 2 years of age. The pattern of deafness shows variation dependent on time of onset and rapidity of progression. The youngster may initially show normal hearing. Hearing loss usually becomes significant in the teens or later, beginning in the high frequencies and progressing to lower frequencies. Congenital syphilis is typically associated with other sensory defects (Chau, Atashband, Chang, Westerberg, & Kozal, 2009; Ikeda & Jensen,

1990; Kerr, Smyth, & Cinnamond, 1973; Roizen, 1999; Strasnick & Jacobson, 1995; http://www.ncbi.nlm.nih.gov/pmc/articles/PMC2819963).

TREACHER COLLINS SYNDROME (TCS)

Mandibular Dysostosis; First Arch Syndrome

The presentation of symptoms in Treacher Collins syndrome (TCS) varies. Some individuals may be so mildly affected that they remain undiagnosed; others can have severe facial bone abnormalities and life-threatening airway compromise. Most of the facial features of TCS are bilateral and recognizable at birth. The most life-threatening problem of individuals with TCS is a constricted airway, because this can give problems with breathing. The external ear anomalies consist of small, rotated, or even absent ears. Also symmetric, bilateral stenosis or atresia of the external auditory canals is common. In most cases, the ossicles and the middle ear cavity are dysmorphic. Even in cases with normal auricles and open external auditory canals, the ossicular chain is often malformed. Inner ear malformations are rarely described. As a result of these abnormalities, a majority of the individuals with TCS are dealing with pure conductive hearing loss. Most TCS patients experience eye problems, varying from colobomata of the lower eyelids and aplasia of lid lashes to short, down-slanting palpebral fissures and missing eyelashes. Vision loss can occur and is associated with strabismus and refractive issues. Cleft palate is often present; dental anomalies are seen in 60% of TCS patients. In some cases dental anomalies in combination with mandible hypoplasia result in a malocclusion, this can lead to problems with food intake and the ability to close the mouth (Figure A–19). General treatment includes genetic counseling, surgical repair of ear anomalies (although severe middle ear malformations make reconstructive surgery difficult), hearing aids, orthodontic treatment, and speech therapy if indicated. Hearing loss in Treacher Collins syndrome is caused by deformed structures in the outer and middle ear. The hearing loss is generally bilateral with a conductive loss of about 50 to 70 dB. Attempts to surgically reconstruct the external auditory canal and improve hearing in children with Treacher Collins syndrome have not yielded positive results. Auditory rehabilitation with Baha or a conventional bone conduction aid has proven preferable to surgical reconstruction. The incidence of TCS is 1:50,000 (Dixon, Trainer, & Dixon, 2007; Dixon et al., 2004; Jahrsdoerfer & Jacobson, 1995; Marres et al., 2002; Sando, Hemenway, & Morgan, 1968; Trainor, Dixon, & Dixon, 2009; Verhagen, Hol, Coppens-Schellenkens, Snik, & Cremers, 2008).

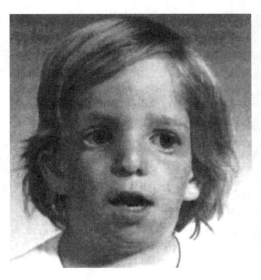

Figure A–19. Treacher Collins syndrome.

TRISOMY 13-15 SYNDROME

Patau Syndrome

Major diagnostic features of Trisomy 13-15, or Patau syndrome, include chromosomal aberration resulting in minimal characteristics of microphthalmia, cleft lip and palate, and polydactyly. A host of other abnormalities may be present, including mental retardation, deafness, broad-nose hypotelorism, microcephaly, heart or skin defects, retroflexed thumbs, "rocker-bottom" feet, seizures, and renal, abdominal, and genitalia abnormalities. Those affected frequently suffer feeding problems, failure to thrive, jitteriness, apneic spells, hypotonia, and jaundice. Trisomy 13-15, or Patau syndrome, is caused by a chromosomal abnormality in which some or all of the cells of the body contain extra genetic material from chromosome 13. This can occur either because each cell contains a full extra copy of chromosome 13 or because each cell contains an extra partial copy of the chromosome. The extra genetic material from chromosome 13 disrupts the normal course of development, causing multiple and complex organ defects (Figure A–20). Low-set external ears or malformed ears and cleft lip and palate are common. Middle ear findings have included deformed stapes, distorted incudostapedial joint, and absence of stapedial muscle and tendon. Inner ear abnormalities have included distorted and shortened cochlea, shortened endolymphatic valve, and degeneration of organ of Corti. Genetic counseling is recommended as indicated. Prognosis is poor as 95% of patients die by 3 years of age. Many infants have difficulty surviving the first few days or weeks due to severe neurological problems or complex heart defects. Surgery may be necessary to repair heart defects or cleft lip and cleft palate. Physical, occupational, and speech therapy will help

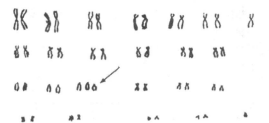

Figure A–20. Trisomy 13-15 (D,) karyotype. Courtesy of A. Robinson, MD, Cytogenetics Laboratory, University of Colorado Medical Center, Denver, CO.

individuals with Patau syndrome reach their full developmental potential. The few surviving children are described as happy, and parents report that they enrich their lives (Black et al., 1971a; Cohen, 1966; Janvier & Farlow, 2012; Maniglia, Wolff, & Herques, 1970; Scherz, Graga, & Reichelderfer, 1972).

TRISOMY 18 SYNDROME

Edwards Syndrome

Trisomy 18 is a genetic disorder caused by the presence of all or part of an extra 18th chromosome (Figure A–21). This genetic condition almost always results from nondisjunction during meiosis. Trisomy 18 syndrome occurs in around one in 6,000 live births, and around 80% of those affected are female. The majority of fetuses with the syndrome die before birth. The syndrome has a very low rate of survival, resulting from heart abnormalities, kidney malformations, and other internal organ disorders. Due to chromosomal aberration, features present at birth include being underweight with an undernourished appearance and microcephaly with triangular shape due to occipital prominence and receding chin. Flexion of hand with overlapping of index finger is characteristic, kidney malformations, struc-

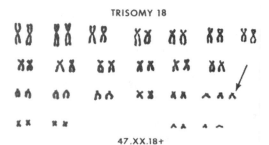

TRISOMY 18

47.XX.18+

Figure A–21. Trisomy 18 karyotype. Courtesy of A. Robinson, MD, Cytogenetics Laboratory, University of Colorado Medical Center, Denver, CO.

tural heart defects at birth (i.e., ventricular septal defect, atrial septal defect, patent ductus arteriosus), intestines protruding outside the body, esophageal atresia, mental retardation, developmental delays, growth deficiency, feeding difficulties, and breathing difficulties are also characteristic of the syndrome. Other malformations associated with Trisomy 18-Edwards syndrome include small head (microcephaly), low-set, malformed ears; abnormally small jaw; cleft lip/cleft palate; upturned nose; narrow eyelid folds (palpebral fissures); widely spaced eyes; drooping of the upper eyelids (ptosis); a short breast bone; clenched hands; choroid plexus cysts; underdeveloped thumbs and or nails, absent radius, webbing of the second and third toes; clubfoot or rocker bottom feet; and in males, undescended testicles. Audiometric testing shows failure to respond to sound. Numerous significant middle ear anomalies as well as cochlea and vestibular anomalies have been noted. Genetic counseling or other treatments are recommended as indicated. Advanced maternal age is common. Half of infants with this condition do not survive beyond the first week of life. The median life span is 5 to 15 days. About 8% of infants survive longer than 1 year; 1% of children live to age 10, typically in less severe cases (Chrysostomidou, Caslaris, Alexiou, & Bartsocas,

1971; Keleman, Hooft, & Kluyskens, 1968; Kos et al., 1966; Smith, 1962; http://www.trisomy18.org).

TRISOMY 21 SYNDROME

(See Down Syndrome.)

TURNER SYNDROME

Gonadal Dysgenesis

Turner syndrome or gonadal dysgenesis encompasses several conditions in females, of which monosomy X (absence of an entire sex chromosome) is most common. It is a chromosomal abnormality in which all or part of one of the sex chromosomes is absent. Unaffected humans have 46 chromosomes, of which two are sex chromosomes. Unaffected females have two X chromosomes, but in Turner syndrome, one of those sex chromosomes is missing or has other abnormalities. In some cases, the chromosome is missing in some cells but not others, a condition referred to as *Turner mosaicism*. As a chromosome defect, Turner syndrome is not inherited. Physical characteristics may include low hairline, webbing of neck, widely spaced or pinpoint nipples, shield-like chest, and webbing of digits, swelling of dorsa of hands and feet, deep creases on thickened palms and soles, hypertelorism, epicanthic folds, ptosis of upper lids, elongated and narrow "gothic" ears, high-arched palate, micrognathia, and enlarged clitoris. Later manifestations include shortness of stature, ocular manifestations, hearing impairment, impairment of taste, congenital cardiovascular disease, anomalies of kidneys, and sexual infantilism. Turner syndrome does not typically cause mental retardation or impair cognition. However, learning difficulties are common among women with Turner syndrome. Conductive hearing loss has been attributed to frequent middle ear infections in infancy and early childhood, but congenital sensorineural hearing loss has also been observed. Occurrence is estimated at 1 in 2,000 (Anderson, Lindsten, & Wedenberg, 1971; Sculerati, Ledesna-Medina, Finegold, & Stool, 1990; Sperling, 2008; Stratton, 1965; Watkin, 1989; http://www.turnersyndrome.org; http://turners.nichd.nih.gov; http://www.ncbi.nlm.nih.gov/pubmedhealth/PMH0001417).

USHER SYNDROME

Usher syndrome is a genetic autosomal recessive trait of congenital deafness and progressive loss of vision leading to eventual blindness. Other names for Usher syndrome include Hallgren syndrome, Usher-Hallgren syndrome, or retinitis pigmentosa-dysacusis syndrome. The hearing loss is bilateral, moderate to profound, and sensorineural. Prevalence among profoundly deaf children has been estimated to be between 3% and 10%. Approximately 3% to 6% of all children who are deaf and another 3% to 6% of children who are hard-of-hearing have Usher syndrome. The hearing loss and vestibular issues are associated with inner ear defects, whereas the vision loss is associated with retinitis pigmentosa caused by degeneration of retinal cells. Usually, the rod cells of the retina are affected first, leading to early night blindness and the gradual loss of peripheral vision. In other cases, there is early degeneration of the cone cells in the macula, leading to a loss of central acuity.

Usher syndrome has three clinical subtypes, denoted as 1, 2, and 3 in order of decreasing severity of deafness. Usher 1 and 2 are the more common forms; together, they account for approximately 90% to 95% of all cases of children who have Usher syndrome. Babies with Usher I are born profoundly deaf, begin to lose their vision in the first decade of life, and often have difficulties maintaining their balance. Usher 1 infants are usually slow to develop motor skills such as walking due to vestibular difficulties. Individuals with Usher 2 are not born deaf but do have hearing loss. They do not seem to have noticeable problems with balance; they begin to lose their vision later during the second decade of life and may preserve some vision even into middle age. Individuals with Usher 2 are generally hard-of-hearing rather than deaf, and their hearing loss does not progress over time; moreover, they generally have a normal vestibular system. Usher syndrome 2 occurs at least as frequently as type I. Usher syndrome 3 is rare, and these individuals are not born deaf but experience a gradual progressive loss of their hearing and vision; they may or may not have balance difficulties.

Usher syndrome is a highly variable condition; the degree of severity is not tightly linked to whether it is Usher 1, 2, or 3. For example, someone with type 3 may be unaffected in childhood but go on to develop a profound hearing loss and a significant loss of sight by early to mid-adulthood. Similarly, someone with type 1, who is therefore profoundly deaf from birth, may keep good central vision until the sixth decade of life, or even beyond. People with type 3, who have useful hearing with a hearing aid, can experience a wide range of severity of their retinitis pigmentosa. Some may maintain good reading vision into their sixties, while others cannot see to read while still in their forties. There is no treatment for retinitis pigmentosa. It occurs in roughly 1 person in 23,000. Usher's syndrome has been the subject of intense gene mapping and found to be associated with a mutation in any one of at least 10 different genes. Early diagnosis of Usher syndrome is important for provision of appropriate educational endeavors, genetic counseling, and screening of relatives (Hallgren, 1959; Kimberling & Moller, 1995; Kloepfer, Laguaite, & McLaurin, 1966; Mets, Young, Pass, & Lasky, 2000; Ouyang et al., 2005; Smith et al., 1994; http://www.nidcd.nih.gov/health/hearing/Pages/usher.aspx; http://www.usher-syndrome.org).

VAN BUCHEM SYNDROME

Hyperostosis Corticalis Generalisata

First described in 1955, Van Buchem syndrome is a rare genetic autosomal recessive disorder of craniofacial and skeletal bone overgrowth. It features a lion-like facial expression with square jaw, also included may by unilateral or bilateral facial paralysis and optic atrophy. Excessive and increased thickening of bone formation is most prominent in the skull, mandible, clavicle, ribs, and diaphyses of long bones, and bone formation occurs throughout life. Skeletal dysplasia is characterized by enlargement of the lower jaw and thickening of the long bones and the top of the skull. The thickening of the bones may compress some nerves resulting in vision and hearing impairment. Paralysis of cranial nerve VII and sensorineural or mixed-type hearing impairments are frequently noted. A large noncoding DNA segment on human chromosome 17 has been identified as being responsible for Van Buchem disease (Fosmoe, Holm, & Hildreth, 1968; Van Hul et al., 1998; http://www.ncbi.nlm.nih.gov/pmc/articles/PMC1376897).

VAN DER HOEVE SYNDROME

(See Osteogenesis Imperfecta.)

VOHWINKEL SYNDROME

Keratoderma Hereditaria Mutilans

Vohwinkel syndrome is a diffuse autosomal dominant keratoderma integumentary disorder with onset in early infancy characterized by a honeycombed keratoderma involving the palmoplantar surfaces including palms, soles, knees, and elbows. Ring-like furrows develop on fingers and toes at about 2 years of age. Mild-to-severe congenital sensorineural hearing loss that may be progressive has been reported. It has been associated with *GJB2*. It may be associated with renal disease (Bitici, 1975; Gedicke, Traupe, Fischer, Tinschert, & Hennies, 2006; http://ghr.nlm.nih.gov/condition/vohwinkel-syndrome; http://ghr.nlm.nih.gov/condition/vohwinkel-syndrome).

WAARDENBURG SYNDROME

Waardenburg syndrome is a group of four genetic conditions distinguished by their physical characteristics, and sometimes by their genetic cause, that can cause hearing loss and changes in coloring (pigmentation) of the hair, skin, and eyes. The features of Waardenburg syndrome have variable penetrance even among members of the same family. Babies born with Waardenburg syndrome may have the characteristic hair and skin changes and hearing loss. However, if the symptoms are mild, Waardenburg syndrome may go undiagnosed until a family member is diagnosed and all family members are examined. Most cases of Waardenburg syndrome have normal hearing, but congenital moderate-to-profound unilateral or bilateral, sometimes progressive, sensorineural hearing loss appears in about 50% of patients. Otologic histopathologic findings include absence of organ of Corti and atrophy of spiral ganglion. Individuals with this condition may have pale blue eyes, different colored eyes, or segments of two different colors in the same eye. Major diagnostic features include white forelock (20%), lateral displacement of medial canthi (95% to 99%); iris bicolor or heterochromia (45%); prominence of root of nose; and hyperplasia of medial portion of eyebrows (50%). Other findings include thin nose with flaring alae nasi, "cupid bow" configuration of lips, prominent mandible, and occasional cleft palate (5%). Waardenburg types I and II have similar features, although type I almost always have eyes that appear widely spaced, and type II do not. In addition, hearing loss occurs less often in type I than in type II. Type III (sometimes called Klein-Waardenburg syndrome) includes abnormalities of the upper limbs in addition to hearing loss and changes in pigmentation. Type IV (also known as Waardenburg-Shah syndrome) has signs and symptoms of both Waardenburg syndrome and Hirschsprung disease, an intestinal disorder that causes severe constipation or blockage of the intestine. Waardenburg syndrome affects an estimated 1 in 40,000 people. It accounts for 2% to 5% of all cases of congenital hearing loss. Types I and II are the most common forms of Waardenburg syndrome, and types III and IV are rare. Mutations in the *EDN3*, *EDNRB*, *MITF*, *PAX3*, *SNAI2*, and *SOX10* genes can cause Waardenburg syndrome. These genes are involved in the formation and development of several types of cells, including pigment-producing cells called

melanocytes. Melanocytes make a pigment called *melanin*, which contributes to skin, hair, and eye color and plays an essential role in the normal function of the inner ear. Mutations in any of these genes disrupt the normal development of melanocytes, leading to abnormal pigmentation of the skin, hair, and eyes and problems with hearing (Figure A–22; Ambani, 1983; Morelli et al., 2007; Nakashima, Sando, Takahashi, & Hashida, 1992; Pantke & Cohen, 1971; http://ghr.nlm.nih.gov/condition/waardenburg-syndrome; http://www.ncbi.nlm.nih.gov/pmc/articles).

WILDERVANCK SYNDROME

Oto-Facio-Cervical Dysmorphia; Cervico-Oculo-Acoustic Dysplasia

Wildervanck syndrome is a rare multifactorial inheritance, genetic disorder that

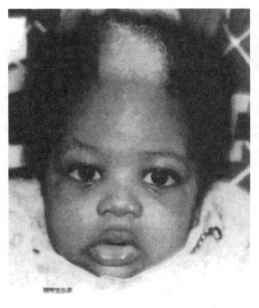

Figure A–22. Waardenburg's syndrome.

primarily affects females. The disorder is characterized by a skeletal condition known as Klippel-Feil syndrome (KFS); abnormalities of certain eye (ocular) movements (i.e., Duane syndrome); and congenital hearing impairment. In some affected individuals, additional physical abnormalities may be present. The occurrence of Wildervanck syndrome appears to be sporadic and random. Depressed nasal root, protruding narrow nose, narrow elongated face, flattened maxilla and zygoma, prominent ears, atresia of external ear canals, preauricular fistulas, and poorly developed neck muscles are seen. Facial asymmetry combines the Klippel-Feil characteristics with retraction of the eyeball (Duane disorder), sixth nerve paralysis, and congenial profound unilateral or bilateral deafness of sensorineural or mixed-type hearing loss in at least 30% of cases (Cremers, Hoogland, & Kuypers, 1984; Gorlin, Cohen, & Hennekam, 2001; Hughes, Davies, Roche, Matthews, & Lane, 1991; Schild, Mafee, & Miller, 1984).

GENERAL REFERENCE AND RESOURCES

Gorlin, R., Cohen, M., & Hennekam, R. (2001). *Syndromes of the head and neck.* New York, NY: Oxford University Press.

Gorlin, R. J., Toriello, H. V., & Cohen, M. M. (Eds.). (1995). *Hereditary hearing loss and its syndromes.* New York, NY: Oxford University Press.

Hennekam, R., Krantz, I., & Allanson, J. (2010). *Gorlin's syndromes of the head and neck. Oxford monographs on medical genetics.* New York, NY: Oxford University Press.

Jones, K. L. (2006). *Smith's recognizable patterns of human malformation* (6th ed.). Philadelphia, PA: Elsevier Saunders.

Konigsmark, B. W., & Gorlin, R. J. (1976). *Genetic and metabolic deafness.* Philadelphia, PA: W. B. Saunders.

Martini, A., Read, A., & Stephens, D. (1996). *Genetics and hearing impairment.* San Diego, CA: Singular.

Morton, C., & Nance, W. (2006). Newborn hearing screening—A silent revolution. *New England Journal of Medicine, 354*(20), 2151–2164.

APPENDIX B

Guidelines for Identification and Management of Infants and Young Children with Auditory Neuropathy Spectrum Disorder*

In June 2008, a panel of experts met in Como, Italy, at the NHS 2008 Conference to develop Guidelines for the Identification and Management of Infants and Young Children With Auditory Neuropathy. Panel members included Deborah Hayes, PhD; Yvonne Sininger, PhD; Arnold Starr, MD; Christine Petit, MD, PhD; Gary Rance, PhD; Barbara Cone, PhD; Kai Uus, MD, PhD; Patricia Roush, AuD; Jon Shallop, PhD; and Charles Berlin, PhD. Following the conference, Hayes and Sininger (2008) summarized the conference and published a set of valuable guidelines based on input from the panel. The Como ANSD guidelines are specific to infants and young children and form an important contribution for the diagnosis and management of this puzzling disorder. We are appreciative to Drs. Hayes and Sininger for their permission to reprint the complete guidelines below.

INTRODUCTION

"Auditory neuropathy" is a relatively recent clinical diagnosis used to describe individuals with auditory disorders due to dysfunction of the synapse of the inner hair cells and auditory nerve and/or the auditory nerve itself. Unlike patients with sensory hearing loss who show clinical evidence of impaired outer hair cell function, patients with "auditory neuropathy" show clinical evidence of normally functioning outer hair cells. Individuals with "auditory neuropathy" typically demonstrate impaired speech understanding and show normal to severely impaired speech detection and pure tone threshold. It has been shown that "auditory neuropathy" affects an individual's ability to process rapidly changing acoustic signals, known as auditory temporal processing.

The range of functional hearing abilities in individuals with "auditory neuropathy" is vast. Some individuals experience little or no difficulty hearing and understanding despite abnormal auditory test results. Others complain of "hearing but not understanding, especially in background noise." Some individuals demonstrate fluctuant hearing abilities, reporting "good hearing days" and "bad hearing days." Finally, some children and adults with "auditory neuropathy" are functionally deaf. For infants and young

*Hayes, Deborah and Sininger, Yvonne S. *Guidelines for identification and management of infants and young children with auditory neuropathy spectrum disorder.* Proceedings from Guidelines Development Conference at NHS 2008, Como, Italy. Monograph published by Bill Daniels Center for Children's Hearing, The Children's Hospital, Denver, CO. 2008. Also available at http://www.childrenscolorado.org/File%20 Library/Conditions-Programs/ASL/ANSD-Monograph-Bill-Daniels-Center-for-Childrens-Hearing.pdf children, the deleterious effect of "auditory neuropathy" on language development and academic achievement can be significant.

Audiological management and speech and language intervention for infants and young children with this disorder is challenging. Because the range of functional hearing ability in "auditory neuropathy" is so great, each child with this diagnosis is unique. Furthermore, because the developmental consequences of "auditory neuropathy" cannot be predicted on the basis of auditory test results obtained in infants, guidelines that exist for identification and management of infants and young children with "typical" sensorineural hearing loss (SNHL) do not entirely fit the special needs of infants with "auditory neuropathy."

To meet the need of the audiologists and other clinicians for guidance in identification and management of infants and young children with "auditory neuropathy," these guidelines were formulated by an expert panel of audiologists, hearing scientists, and physicians to reflect contemporary practice. This document is not intended to duplicate or replace current guidelines for identification and management of children with "typical" SNHL, but rather seeks to supplement these existing documents with recommendations specific to infants and young children with "auditory neuropathy." As new information emerges, new techniques and strategies will undoubtedly evolve. In the interim, these guidelines for identification and management of children with "auditory neuropathy" offer practical guidance to audiologists and other clinicians, and families.

TERMINOLOGY

The term, auditory neuropathy, was originally proposed by Starr and colleagues (Starr et al., 1996), to describe the specific auditory disorder in a series of 10 patients, eight of whom demonstrated evidence of generalized peripheral neuropathy. The auditory disorder was characterized by evidence of normal cochlear outer hair cell function (preservation of otoacoustic emissions and cochlear microphonics) and abnormal auditory pathway function beginning with the VIII nerve (absent or severely abnormal auditory brainstem potentials).

Some investigators (Berlin et al., 2001, 2003; Rapin & Gravel, 2006) have expressed dissatisfaction with the term *auditory neuropathy* because the constellation of test results defining this disorder does not provide direct evidence of auditory nerve dysfunction or "neuropathy." Indeed, only a subset of individuals with this disorder will be found to have abnormal auditory nerve function. Other lesions, for example, mutation of the otoferlin (OTOF) gene, which results in synaptic dysfunction at the junction of the inner hair cell/auditory nerve, will produce the same constellation of auditory test results in affected individuals (Yasunaga et al., 1999; Yasunaga et al., 2000). To address this, and other concerns, Berlin and colleagues (2001a, 2001b) proposed the term "auditory dys-synchronly."

To address the potential confusion that arises from multiple designations for this disorder, the panel sought to identify simplified terminology that would unify the concept of an auditory disorder with a range of presentations secondary to a variety of etiologies. The panel considered multiple suggestions proposed by both panel and audience participants, and concurred that the most appropriate designation was "auditory neuropathy spectrum disorder" (ANSD). Three principle factors drove this consensus. First, despite potentially inexact usage, the term "auditory neuropathy" has gained wide-spread acceptance and usage, both in the professional literature and among parent/consumer organizations. Renaming the disorder could lead to confusion for patients and other professionals whereas retaining current terminology would provide continuity for the scientific community. Second, the expression of this disorder in everyday listening and communication behaviors encompasses a spectrum ranging from limited or mild effects (complaints of difficulty "hearing" in noisy listening conditions) to profound effects (inability to "hear" in any listening condition, functionally "deaf"). Finally, the term "spectrum" was felt to expand the concept of this disorder to include sites of lesion other than the auditory nerve.

Starr et al. (2004) suggested segmenting the term auditory neuropathy into types, for example, Type I (Pre-synaptic), Type II (Post-synaptic). In 2008, Starr et al. proposed refining the terminology by site of disorder. For example, if the auditory nerve was involved but the inner hair cells and synapses were spared, the disorder would be classified as "auditory nerve disorder." Similarly, if the inner hair cells and/or their synapses were disordered but the auditory nerve was normal, then the term "auditory synaptic disorder" would be appropriate. Currently, there are no clinical measures to distinguish site of disorder with this degree of precision. The panel concurred that subtypes or site-specific classification would be helpful to further define the disorder more specifically, and that future research efforts should be directed to develop such a classification scheme.

DIAGNOSTIC CRITERIA

ANSD is characterized by evidence of normal or near normal cochlear hair cell (sensory)

function and absent or abnormal auditory nerve function. Therefore, the (minimum) test battery needed to diagnose ANSD requires tests of cochlear hair cell (sensory) function and auditory nerve function.

Minimum Test Battery Required to Diagnose Individuals with ANSD

Tests Required to Diagnose Individuals with ANSD:

1. Tests of cochlear hair cell (sensory) function:
   a. Otoacoustic emissions (OAEs): Standard screening or diagnostic protocol using Transient-Evoked OAEs (TEOAEs) or Distortion Product OAEs (DPOAEs), and/or
   b. Cochlear microphonics (CM): Click-evoked auditory brainstem response (ABR) to high-level click stimuli (80–90 dB nHL), tested with positive and negative polarity clicks in separate trials, through insert earphones (Berlin et al., 1998; Starr et al., 2001). A trial run with sound-delivery tube clamped should be used to differentiate between the CM and stimulus artifact (Rance et al., 1999).
2. Test of auditory nerve function:
   a. Auditory brainstem response (ABR) to high level click-evoked auditory brainstem response (ABR) to high-level stimuli (80–90 dB nHL). To avoid misinterpreting cochlear microphonics as components of the ABR, responses to positive and negative polarity clicks must be obtained in separate trials as described above. CMs will show a characteristic reversal in polarity

with reversal in polarity of the stimulating click; ABR will show a constant polarity regardless of polarity of the click (Berlin et al., 1998)

Additional Tests Useful for Diagnosing Individuals with ANSD

Middle ear muscle reflexes (acoustic reflexes) are absent in individuals with ANSD (Berlin et al., 2005). Because normative data on acoustic reflex thresholds in very young infants using high probe-tone frequencies (1000 Hz) have not been established, this procedure is not required to diagnose ANSD. Nevertheless, a complete test battery for ANSD should include middle ear muscle reflex testing whenever possible.

Suppression of otoacoustic emissions by contralateral noise is abnormal in individuals with ANSD (Hood et al., 2003). Although this test has not gained widespread clinical usage, it is a potential candidate for further diagnostic studies in individuals with reliably recorded OAES.

Special Considerations in Diagnosing Infants with ANSD

Conventionally-recorded distortion product and transient OAEs are usually normal or near normal in individuals with ANSD. In newborns and very young infants measurement of OAEs may be compromised by presence of residual fluid in the ear canal/middle ear (Doyle et al., 2000) or otitis media with effusion (OME). OAEs may present initially and disappear over time in individuals with ANSD (Starr et al., 1996). Loss of OAEs, however, does not reflect change in auditory function or signal conversion of ANSD to sensorineural hearing loss (SNHL).

Cochlear microphonics also provide a valid measure of hair cell function. CMs remain present in individuals with ANSD despite loss of OAEs (Starr et al., 1996). CMs are easily recorded from standard ABR recording protocols when insert earphones are used (Berlin et al., 2003; Starr et al., 2001). Stimulus artifact precludes effective recording of CMs when electromagnetic circumaural earphones are used (Berlin et al., 2003; Stone et al., 1986).

The auditory brainstem response (ABR) is markedly abnormal in individuals with ANSD. Recordings might appear as (1) a "flat" ABR with no evidence of any peaks or (2) presence of early peaks (waves up to III) with absence of later waves or (3) some poorly synchronized but evident late peaks (wave V) that appear only to stimuli at elevated stimulus levels.

When using these test procedures in newborns and very young infants, recording conditions must be optimum to obtain valid, artifact-free, unambiguous test results. Infants should be quietly sleeping in either natural or sedated sleep to avoid movement artifact or "noisy" recordings. Caution should be used in interpretation of results when these tests are used in infants below 36 weeks gestational age. Repeated measures, over several weeks or months, are recommended to determine the reliability of test results. Because "transient" ANSD has been reported in some infants (Attias & Raveh, 2007; Madden et al., 2002; Psarommatis et al., 2006), particularly those with hyperbilirubinemia, hypoxia, ischemia, and central nervous system immaturity (Attais & Raveh, 2007) frequent monitoring by the ANSD test battery is recommended to establish the stability of test results, especially in the first two years of life.

Once the diagnosis of ANSD has been established, the infant should be referred for comprehensive medical, developmental, and communication assessments.

RECOMMENDED COMPREHENSIVE ASSESSMENT

Many of the assessments recommended for infants with ANSD are similar to assessments recommended for infants with SNHL (JCIH, 2007). The recommended assessments for infants with ANSD include:

1. Pediatric and developmental evaluation and history,
2. Otologic evaluation with imaging of the cochlea and auditory nerve (computed tomography (CT) and magnetic resonance imaging (MRI)),
3. Medical genetics evaluation,
4. Ophthalmologic assessment,
5. Neurological evaluation to assess peripheral and central nerve function, and
6. Communication developmental assessment.

Although not routinely recommended for infants and young children, vestibular assessment should be considered if developmental or otologic evaluation identifies potential vestibular disorder (e.g., nystagmus, delay in walking).

There are three principle reasons for infants with auditory disorders, including infants with ANSD, to receive comprehensive medical, developmental, and communication assessment. First, defining etiology of ANSD is important for predicting if the condition may be transient or is permanent (Attais & Raveh, 2007; Madden et al., 2002; Psarommatis et al., 2006), determining if medical or surgical treatment is needed, and answering parent's questions about cause of their infant's hearing disorder. Second, because infants with ANSD, especially those who received care in the NICU, are at-risk for additional disabilities, early identifica-

tion of developmental delays is important for optimum child development. Third, infants with ANSD may develop additional cranial or peripheral neuropathies secondary to a specific diagnosis (Starr et al., 1996).

ANSD may be unilateral or bilateral. The possibility of cochlear nerve deficiency (absent or small cochlear nerves) should be considered for all children with ANSD, and especially in well-babies with no significant history related to ANSD (Buchman et al., 2006) or infants with unilateral craniofacial anomalies (Carvalho et al., 1999). Contemporary imaging procedures (MRI and/or CT) are useful in these patients to assess integrity of the eighth nerve and internal auditory meatus.

Families of young infants benefit from early referral for communication assessment. Speech-language pathologists and deaf educators with expertise in early communication development can counsel families about the developmental sequence of pre-language, communicative behaviors, and support families in developing language-rich environments. Speech-language pathologists, deaf educators, and early intervention specialists can also help families monitor their infant's language development and assist families in evaluating the effectiveness of their chosen language development strategy.

RECOMMENDED AUDIOLOGIC TEST BATTERY

The audiological test battery recommended for assessing functional hearing and monitoring auditory development in infants and toddlers with SHNL (JCIH, 2007) is appropriate for infants and toddlers with ANSD. This test battery consists of measures of middle ear function, behavioral response to pure-tones, and speech reception and speech recognition. These measures include:

1. Otoscopic examination and acoustic immittance measures of middle ear function. As with any infant, infants with ANSD may develop middle ear dysfunction and otitis media with effusion resulting in mild conductive hearing loss. Because middle ear muscle (acoustic) reflexes are absent or elevated in individuals with ANSD, otoscopy and tympanometry will be most useful for identify infants with middle ear dysfunction.

2. Behavioral assessment of pure-tone thresholds using developmentally-appropriate, conditioned test procedures (visual reinforcement audiometry (VRA), or conditioned orientation reflex (COR) audiometry). For very young or developmentally-delayed infants, behavioral observation audiometry (BOA) may be used to observe the infant's reflexive response to sound, however, results should not be interpreted as representing behavioral threshold or minimal response levels.

3. Speech reception and speech recognition measures. For very young infants, response threshold to repetitive consonant-vowel combinations (e.g., ba-ba, ga-ga) is appropriate; for toddlers, pointing to body parts may yield acceptable speech threshold results. As children's vocabulary develops, speech recognition measures using standardized picture-pointing (e.g., Word Intelligibility by Picture Identification, WIPI {Ross and Lerman, 1970}; Early Speech Perception Test {Moog and Greers, 1990}) or open-set tests should be employed. Standardized taped materials are preferable to live-voice presentation to obtain consistency of stimuli across test sessions and should be employed once children are old enough to repeat recorded materials. Because ANSD can significantly affect speech understanding in background noise, tests of speech recognition in noise or competing messages should be conducted as developmentally appropriate.

4. Otoacoustic emissions utilizing either TEOAEs and/or DPOAEs. Although initially present, OAEs may disappear in individuals with ANSD (Starr et al., 2001; Deltenre et al., 1999).

Obligatory cortical auditory evoked potentials to speech or speech-like signals are not yet a standard clinical measure for infants or toddlers. These measures show promise, however, as objective clinical tools for predicting speech-recognition performance in young children with ANSD (Cone-Wesson et al., 2003; Pearce et al., 2007).

Infants and young children with ANSD should receive frequent audiological evaluation to assess their behavioral response to sound and auditory development. Some youngsters with ANSD will experience fluctuations in detection thresholds for pure-tones (Rance et al., 1999; Rance et al., 2002; Starr et al., 1996). For children who demonstrate consistently elevated pure-tone thresholds, amplification should be considered to improve audibility of speech.

RECOMMENDED AMPLIFICATION STRATEGIES

For infants with typical SNHL, hearing aid fitting can proceed in the earliest months of life based on electrophysiological estimates (e.g., click ABR, ABR to tone bursts, and/or auditory steady state response) of hearing sensitivity. For infants with ANSD, however, electrophysiological methods do not predict auditory detection thresholds. Clinicians and parents must rely upon the infant's or young child's behavioral response to sound to guide the hearing aid fitting decision. If an infant or young child with ANSD demonstrates elevated pure-tone and speech detection thresholds with consistent test-retest reliability, hearing aid fitting should be considered and a trial use of hearing aids should be offered to families.

1. Infants and young children with ANSD should be fitted with amplification as soon as ear-specific elevated pure-tone and speech detection thresholds are demonstrated by conditioned test procedures (VRA or COR, see above). "Thresholds" or minimum response levels obtained by these techniques should be used to set amplification targets.

2. Significant improvement in auditory function, including "recovery" from ANSD has been reported in some infants with this diagnosis (Attias, 2006; Madden et al., 2002; Psarommatis et al., 2006). Careful monitoring of infant's auditory function by ABR and behavioral response by conditioned test procedures is required to adjust and modify amplification as needed. Although some risk factors for "transient" ANAD have been identified (Attias & Raveh, 2007; Madden et al., 2002; Psarommatis et al., 2006), at the present time, all infants and young children with ANSD, regardless of presumed etiology, should be carefully monitored for changes in auditory function and behavioral response to sound.

3. For infants with developmental delay where conditioned test procedures are unsuccessful, amplification fitting may proceed using behavioral observation of auditory behaviors and/or cortical evoked potentials when (a) indications of auditory sensitivity are clearly outside developmental norms until more reliable measures can be obtained, and (b) generally not before 6 months of age.

Temporal processing, or encoding the temporal characteristics of speech, is affected in subjects with ANSD (Zeng et al., 2005; Rance et al., 2004) resulting in a disproportionate loss in speech understanding ability relative to the individual's pure-tone thresholds (Rance et al., 1999; Rance et al., 2002; Starr et al., 1996). Although conventional hearing aids improve sound audibility, they do not resolve temporal processing deficits. Therefore children with ANSD may not experience the same benefits from hearing aids expected from children with typical SNHL in whom temporal processing is relatively unaffected. Parental observation by formal questionnaire or survey) e.g., Infant-Toddler Meaningful Auditory Integration Scale, IT-MAIS [Zimmerman-Phillips et al., 2001]) may be helpful for assessing amplification benefit. In addition, speech recognition testing, including speech-in-nose or competing messages, should be incorporated into the hearing aid monitoring protocol as soon as developmentally appropriate for the child.

Strategies to improve the signal-to-noise ratio for children with ANSD should, theoretically, improve speech recognition and language learning (Hood et al., 2003). Trial use of an FM system, especially in structured and spontaneous language-learning activities, should also be considered for children with ANSD.

SPECIAL CONSIDERATIONS FOR COCHLEAR IMPLANTATION

Despite an adequate trial with appropriately-fitted amplification, some children with

ANSD may demonstrate poor progress in speech understanding ability and aural/auditory language development. For these children, cochlear implantation should be considered, regardless of behavioral audiometric thresholds.

In addition to standard cochlear implantation criteria for children, special considerations for cochlear implantation in children with ANSD include:

1. As noted above, significant improvement in auditory function, including "recovery" from ANSD has been reported in a subset of infants with this diagnosis. Families should be informed that spontaneous improvement in auditory function has been reported up to two years of age. Cochlear implantation, therefore, should not be considered until auditory test results (ABR and estimates of behavioral sensitivity) are stable and demonstrate unequivocal evidence of permanent ANSD (no change or recovery of ABR). Deferring the decision for cochlear implantation until age two years may be appropriate. All infants with ANSD, including those being monitored for possible recovery, should be enrolled in early intervention and language stimulation programs to prevent delay in language acquisition.

2. Evidence of auditory nerve sufficiency should be obtained prior to surgery using appropriate imaging technology (Buchman et al., 2006).

3. Children with ANSD who do not demonstrate good progress with amplification should be considered candidates for cochlear implantation *regardless of audiometric thresholds*. Children in this category with elevated pure-tone and speech detection thresholds should receive a trial of amplification fitted by pediatric amplification guidelines prior to consideration for implantation.

4. Pre-implantation electrical stimulation testing may be useful in determining CI candidacy in some cases but should not be a requirement for implantation.

Emerging data suggest that pre-implantation electrical stimulation testing may be useful in determining CI candidacy in some cases (Gibson et al., 2007). At the present time, pre-implantation electrical stimulation is not a requirement for implantation.

Cochlear implants offer the possibility of improving auditory temporal processing by stimulating synchronous discharge of the auditory nerve. For example, ABR, which requires neural synchrony, can be electrically-evoked in many individuals with cochlear implants (Peterson et al., 2003; Shallop et al., 2003). Furthermore, speech recognition ability measured in cochlear implant users with ANSD to speech recognition ability, which is strongly dependent on temporal processing ability, is similar in many cochlear implant users to speech recognition ability measured in cochlear implant users with typical SNHL (Madden et al., 2002; Mason et al., 2003; Rance & Barker, 2008). For families who wish to consider cochlear implantation for their child with ANSD, referral to a center with experience with managing children with this diagnosis is strongly encouraged.

RECOMMENDED HABILITATION FOR COMMUNICATION DEVELOPMENT

Families of infants with ANSD should be informed that their baby's auditory capacity or speech, language and communication development cannot be predicted on the basis of the initial evaluation. Ongoing monitoring of their infant's auditory, speech, language, communication, and general development monitoring is essential. As with all infants and children with hearing loss (JCIH, 2007), families should be made aware of all communication options presented in an unbiased manner. Informed family choice and desired outcome guide the decision-making process. For most children with ANSD, use of any combination of communication systems that incorporates visual support is appropriate (e.g., auditory/aural with lipreading and natural gesture, cued speech, total communication, sign language). Decisions regarding mode of communication must be ultimately made by the family and respected by all professionals involved.

SCREENING NEWBORNS FOR AUDITORY NEUROPATHY SPECTRUM DISORDER

The panel concurred with the Joint Committee on Infant Hearing 2007 Position Statement in which the definition of targeted hearing loss was expanded to include "neural hearing loss" in infants admitted to the NICU. Because screening by OAEs will fail to detect infants with "neural hearing loss" or ANSD, the panel further concurred with the JCIH recommendation that infants who receive care in the NICU for 5 days or more receive hearing screening by ABR.

Screening well-babies for ANSD is more problematic. In many well-baby nurseries, the hearing screening protocol is screening by OAEs. Although this technology will detect infants with sensory hearing loss, it will "pass" infants with ANSD. Even if the nursery uses a "two-stage" protocol, for example, OAEs followed by automated ABR for those infants who "fail" OAE screening, infants with ANSD will not receive the

second, automated ABR screening because they "passed" OAE screening. In those well-baby nurseries where automated ABR is the first screening technology, infants who fail this test should not be rescreened by OAEs and "passed" because these infants may have ANSD.

Because the probable cause of ANSD in well-babies is genetic, infants with a family history of childhood hearing loss or sensory motor neuropathy should receive hearing screening by ABR.

As more information becomes available on the prevalence of ANSD in the well-baby population, stronger recommendations for screening all infants for ANSD, regardless of nursery care level, may emerge.

For infants who "pass" newborn hearing screening, subsequent parent or caregiver concern about the child's auditory, speech, or language development should trigger a referral for audiological assessment including behavioral pure-tone and speech threshold measures, speech recognition testing (as developmentally appropriate), and tympanometry and middle ear muscle reflexes. Re-screening these infant's or young children's hearing with OAEs is not sufficient because such re-screening will "pass" infants and young children with ANSD.

MONITORING INFANTS WITH "TRANSIENT" ANSD

Some infants with an initial diagnosis of ANSD may demonstrate improved auditory function and even "recovery" on ABR testing (Attias & Raveh, 2007; Madden et al., 2002; Psarommatis et al., 2006). For those infants who "recover" from ANSD, the panel recommends regular surveillance of developmental milestones, auditory skills, parental concerns, and middle ear status consistent with the Joint Committee on Infant Hearing 2007 Position Statement (JCIH, 2007). Because the residual effects of transient ANSD are unknown, ongoing monitoring of the infant's auditory, speech, and language development as well as global (e.g., motor, cognitive, and social) development is critical. Those infants and young children whose speech and language development is not commensurate with their general development should be referred for speech and language evaluation and audiological assessment.

The Joint Committee on Infant Hearing recognizes sensory motor neuropathies such as Friedreich ataxia and Charcot-Marie-Tooth syndrome as risk factors for delayed onset hearing loss (JCIH, 2007). Per the Joint Committee's recommendation, infants with a risk indicator should be referred for an audiological assessment at least once by 24 to 30 months of age. Given the possibility of late onset ANSD in infants with family history of sensory motor neuropathies, audiological assessment including ABR, OAEs, tympanometry and middle ear muscle reflexes is warranted.

COUNSELING FAMILIES OF INFANTS WITH ANSD

Counseling families of infants and young children with ANSD is one of the greatest challenges associated with this disorder. Because the developmental effects of ANSD cannot be predicted from test results obtained in the earliest months or even years of life, families struggle with the uncertainty of what the diagnosis means relative to their infant's growth and development. Many infants with ANSD have had difficult perinatal or neonatal courses with complications including prematurity, birth asphyxia, infections, or other conditions requiring neonatal intensive care. The significance of the ANSD diagnosis may be difficult for families to appreciate as they struggle to understand their infant's complex medical and developmental needs. Strong support systems, including parents of children with similar diagnoses and professionals with expertise in clinical social work and family counseling, should be available to meet the on-going and changing needs of families.

Clinicians working with infants and young children ANSD and their families must remain flexible in approaching habilitative options. All members of the team, including the family, should be encouraged to question specific methodologies and strategies if the child's language and communication development is not commensurate with his or her developmental potential.

Children with ANSD can develop into healthy and dynamic citizens with happy personal lives, successful academic experiences, and satisfying careers. Clinicians should help families realize this goal by identifying and supporting the unique strengths and abilities of the child and family.

Table B–1. Auditory Neuropathy Spectrum Disorder (ANSD): Team Management Protocol for Children Who Demonstrate Age-Appropriate Auditory Responses

Age	Audiological diagnostics	Audiological intervention	Speech-language recommendations	Family consultant or social worker	Additional recommendations
0–2 months	Otoscopy ABR with CM recording protocol OAEs 1 kHz immittance, acoustic reflexes	Parent counseling Parent education	Parent counseling Visual language enhancement techniques Observation of communication	Parent counseling Resources Emotional support Home intervention services	Pediatric/ developmental Otologic Medical genetics Ophthalmologic Neurologic
3–6 months	Otoscopy ABR with CM recording protocol OAEs 1 kHz immittance, acoustic reflexes BOA; startle response Parent auditory questionnaire	Same as above	Counseling to provide language-rich environment Monitor communication success	Connect family to additional community-based resources • Parent organizations	Other as needed
6–9 months	Otoscopy Behavioral assessment (BOA, VRA) attempt ear-specific, frequency-specific warbled tones; speech awareness Immittance, acoustic reflexes OAEs Parent auditory questionnaire	Same as above	Formal communication evaluation including assessment of receptive, expressive, and pragmatic language; play; speech sound production Recommendations based on results	Websites specific to AN Ensure family is receiving visual communication support in the home	Other as needed

continues

Table B–1. *continued*

Age	Audiological diagnostics	Audiological intervention	Speech-language recommendations	Family consultant or social worker	Additional recommendations
9–12 months	Otoscopy Behavioral assessment (BOA, VRA); attempt ear-specific, frequency-specific warbled tones; speech awareness Immittance, acoustic reflexes OAEs Parent auditory questionnaire	Same as above Monitor 6 months	Same as above	Same as above	Optional ABR evaluation under sedation or general anesthesia if child's auditory responses change or per parent request
18 months	Otoscopy Behavioral assessment (BOA, VRA, CPA); attempt ear-specific, frequency-specific warbled tones; speech awareness and speech recognition in quiet and noise Immittance, acoustic reflexes OAEs Parent auditory questionnaire	Parent counseling Monitor 6 months	Formal communication evaluation including assessment of receptive, expressive, and pragmatic language; play; speech sound production Recommendations based on results	Begin support for transition to preschool services	Other as needed
24 months	Same as above	Same as above	Informal reevaluation Monitor vocabulary development	Same as above and Encourage exposure to toddler groups, story time, activities outside the home	Other as needed

Table B–1. *continued*

Age	Audiological diagnostics	Audiological intervention	Speech-language recommendations	Family consultant or social worker	Additional recommendations
3–6 years	Same as above	Same as above Collaboration with educational team	Yearly evaluation including assessment of language and speech sound production	Assist families in obtaining full language access in classroom	Educational consultation services
School age	Same as above	Same as above Collaboration with educational team	Same as above Collaboration with educational speech-language pathologist	Self-advocacy Support with obtaining and using assistive technology as needed	Other as needed

Source: From *Guidelines for Identification and Management of Infants and Young Children With Neuropathy Spectrum Disorder,* by Bill Daniels Center for Children's Hearing, Colorado Children's Hospital, Copyright © 2008.

Table B–2. Auditory Neuropathy Spectrum Disorder: Team Management Protocol for Children Who Demonstrate Variable Auditory Responses/Difficult to Test

Age	Audiological diagnostics	Audiological intervention	Speech-language recommendations	Family consultant or social worker	Additional recommendations
0–2 months	Otoscopy ABR with CM recording protocol OAEs 1 kHz immittance, acoustic reflexes	Parent counseling Parent education	Parent counseling Visual language enhancement techniques Observation of communication	Parent counseling Resources Emotional support Home intervention services	Pediatric/developmental Otologic Medical genetics Ophthalmologic Neurologic
3–6 months	Otoscopy ABR with CM recording protocol; OAEs 1 kHz immittance, acoustic reflexes BOA; startle response Parent auditory questionnaire	Same as above	Counseling to provide language-rich environment including auditory and visual communication systems	Connect family to additional community-based resources • Parent organizations	Other as needed
6–9 months	Otoscopy Behavioral assessment (BOA, VRA); attempt ear-specific, frequency-specific warbled tones; speech awareness Immittance, acoustic reflexes OAEs Parent auditory questionnaire	Same as above	Formal communication evaluation including assessment of receptive, expressive, and pragmatic language; play; speech sound production Recommendations based on results	Websites specific to AN Ensure family is receiving visual communication support in the home	Other as needed

Age	Audiological diagnostics	Audiological intervention	Speech-language recommendations	Family consultant or social worker	Additional recommendations
9–12 months	Otoscopy Behavioral assessment (BOA, VRA); attempt ear-specific, frequency-specific warbled tones; speech awareness Immittance, acoustic reflexes OAEs Parent auditory questionnaire	Same as above or If conditioned behavioral measures demonstrate reliable elevated thresholds, fit with amplification per clinic protocol (see special considerations).	Same as above	Same as above	Optional ABR evaluation under sedation or anesthesia if unable to obtain behavioral auditory responses; child's auditory responses change; per parent request
18 months	Otoscopy Behavioral assessment (BOA, VRA, CPA); attempt ear-specific, frequency-specific warbled tones; speech awareness and speech recognition in quiet and noise Immittance, acoustic reflexes OAEs Parent auditory questionnaire	Monitor 6 months or If conditioned behavioral measures demonstrate reliable elevated thresholds, fit with amplification per clinic protocol (see special considerations)	Formal communication evaluation including assessment of receptive, expressive, and pragmatic language; play; speech sound production Recommendations based on results	Begin support for transition to preschool services	Other as needed
24 months	Same as above	Same as above	Informal reevaluation Monitor vocabulary development	Same as above and Encourage exposure to toddler groups, story time, activities outside the home	Other as needed

continues

Table B–2. *continued*

Age	Audiological diagnostics	Audiological intervention	Speech-language recommendations	Family consultant or social worker	Additional recommendations
3–6 years	Same as above	Same as above	Yearly evaluation including assessment of language; speech sound production	Individual Education Plan (IEP), as appropriate Transition to preschool	Other as needed
School age	Same as above	Same as above	Collaboration with educational speech-language pathologist	Self-advocacy strategies for the parents and child IEP as appropriate	Other as needed

Note: Special considerations: Once frequency-specific/ear-specific audiometric "thresholds" at elevated levels are obtained by conditioned behavioral measures, and remain stable, fit with hearing aids using pediatric fitting strategies and fit to "audiogram." If hearing levels are variable and/or fluctuate, consider multiple HA programs. Monitor and adjust hearing aid fitting based upon hearing thresholds, RECD measurements, parental report, and demonstration of benefit. Add FM as indicated; Parent documentation and input critical for management. If child does not demonstrate benefit from amplification and speech-language skill development is not commensurate with his or her potential, or if child is not making expected progress, then cochlear implantation may be considered *regardless* of audiometric thresholds. CI workup should include surgeon consultation, imaging of cochlear nerve, CT scan, device counseling, team evaluation per CI Center protocol.

Source: From *Guidelines for Identification and Management of Infants and Young Children With Neuropathy Spectrum Disorder,* by Bill Daniels Center for Children's Hearing, Colorado Children's Hospital, Copyright ©2008.

Table B–3. Auditory Neuropathy Spectrum Disorder: Team Management Protocol for Children Who Demonstrate No Response to Auditory Stimulation

Age	Audiological diagnostics	Audiological intervention	Speech-language intervention	Family consultant or social worker	Additional recommendations
0–2 mos	Otoscopy ABR with CM recording protocol; OAEs 1 kHz immittance, acoustic reflexes	Parent counseling Parent education	Parent counseling Visual language enhancement techniques Observation of communication	Parent counseling Resources Emotional support Home intervention services	Pediatric/developmental Otologic Medical genetics Ophthalmologic Neurologic
3–6 mos	Otoscopy ABR with CM recording protocol; OAEs 1 kHz immittance, acoustic reflexes BOA; startle response Parent auditory questionnaire	Same as above	Counseling to provide language-rich environment including auditory and visual communication systems	Connect family to additional community-based resources • Parent organizations	Other as needed
6–9 mos	Otoscopy Behavioral assessment (BOA, VRA); attempt ear-specific, frequency-specific warbled tones; speech awareness Immittance, acoustic reflexes OAEs Parent auditory questionnaire	Same as above and If no auditory response, initiate trial HA fit (begin conservative, then increase gain) Begin conversation re: cochlear implant (CI)	Formal communication evaluation including assessment of receptive, expressive, and pragmatic language; play; speech sound production Recommendations based on results	Websites specific to AN Ensure family is receiving visual communication support in the home	Other as needed

continues

Table B–3. *continued*

Age	Audiological diagnostics	Audiological intervention	Speech-language intervention	Family consultant or social worker	Additional recommendations
9–12 mos	Same as above	If no benefit from amplification, and If parent is interested, proceed with CI evaluation	Same as above	If parent is interested in CI, connect to parent-to-parent support with CI families, CI adult role models	CI workup including surgeon consultation, imaging of cochlear nerve, CT scan, device counseling, team evaluation per CI Center protocol

Note: Ongoing management of children who demonstrate no response to sound should proceed per clinic/team protocol for children who are deaf. Options may include cochlear implant, visual language system, and other supports as selected by the parents.

Source: From *Guidelines for Identification and Management of Infants and Young Children With Neuropathy Spectrum Disorder,* by Bill Daniels Center for Children's Hearing, Colorado Children's Hospital, Copyright © 2008.

REFERENCES

Attias, J., Muller, N., Rubel, Y., & Raveh, E. (2006). Multiple auditory steady-state responses in children and adults with normal hearing, sensorineural hearing loss, or auditory neuropathy. *Annals of Otology, Rhinology, and Larngology, 115*(4), 268–276.

Berlin, C. I., Bordelon, J., & St. John, P. (1998). Reversing click polarity may uncover auditory neuropathy in infants. *Ear and Hearing, 19,* 37–47.

Berlin, C. I., Hood, L. J., Morlet, T., Wilensky, D., St. John, P., Montgomery, E., & Thibodaux, M. (2005). Absent or elecated middle ear muscle reflexes in the presence of normal otoacoustic emissions: A universal finding in cases of auditory neuropathy/dys-synchrony. *Journal of the American Academy of Audiology, 16*(8), 546–553.

Berlin, C. I., Hood, L. J., & Rose, K. (2001). On renaming auditory neuropathy as auditory dys-synchrony. *Audiology Today, 17,* 13–15.

Berlin, C. I., Morlet, T., & Hood, L. J. (2003). Auditory neuropathy/dys-synchrony: Its diagnosis and management. *Pediatric Clinics of North America, 50*(2), 331–340.

Buchman, C. A., Roush, P. A., Teagle, H. F. B., Brown, C. J., Zdanski, C. I., & Grose, J. H. (2006). Auditory neuropathy characteristics in children with cochlear nerve deficiency. *Ear and Hearing, 27*(4), 399–408.

Carvalho, G. J., Song, C. S., Vargervik, K., & Lalwani, A. K. (1999). Auditory and facial nerve dysfunction in patients with hemifacial microsomia. *Archives of Otolaryngology-Head & Neck Surgery, 125*(2), 209–212.

Cone-Wesson, B., Rance, G., & Wunderlich, J. L. (2003). Mismatch negativity in children with auditory neuropathy and sensorineural hearing loss. *Association for Research in Otolaryngology Abstract, 26,* 191.

Deltenre, P., Mansbach, A. L., Bozet, C., Christiaens, F., Barthelemy, P., Paulissen, D., & Renglet, T. (1999). Auditory neuropathy with preserved cochlear microphonics and secondary loss of otoacoustic emissions. *Audiology, 38*(4), 187–195.

Doyle, K. J., Rodgers, P., Fujukawa, S., & Newman, E. (2000). External and middle ear effects on infant hearing screening test results. *Archives of Otolaryngology-Head & Neck Surgery, 122*(4), 477–481.

Gibson, P. R., & Graham, J. M. (2008). Editorial: Auditory neuropathy and cochlear implantation: myths and facts. *Cochlear Implants International.* Retrieved from http://www.interscience.wiley.com

Gibson, W. P., & Sanli, H. (2007). Auditory neuropathy: An update. *Ear and Hearing, 28*(2), 102S–106S.

Hood, L. J., Berlin, C. I., Bordelon, J., & Rose, K. (2003). Patients with auditory neuropathy/dys-synchrony lack efferent suppression of transient evoked otoacoustic emissions. *Journal of the American Academy of Audiology, 14*(6), 302–313.

Joint Committee on Infant Hearing. (2000). Year 2000 Position satement: Principles and guidelines for early hearing detection and intervention program. *Audiology Today,* Special Issue 6, pp. 6–9.

Joint Committee on Infant Hearing. (2007). Year 2007 Position statement: Principles and guidelines for early hearing detection and intervention programs. *Pediatrics, 120,* 898–921.

Madden, C., Rutter, M., Hilbert, L., Greinwald, J., & Choo, D. (2002). Clinical and audiological features in auditory neuropathy. *Archives of Otolaryngology-Head & Neck Surgery, 128,* 1026–1030.

Pearce, W., Golding, M., & Dillon, H. (2007). Cortical auditory evoked potentials in the assessment of auditory neuropathy: Two case studies. *Journal of the American Academy of Audiology, 18,* 380–390.

Pediatric Working Group. (1996). Amplification for infants and children with hearing loss. *American Journal of Audiology, 5,* 53–58.

Peterson, A., Shallop, J., Driscoll, C., Breneman, A., Babb, J., Stoeckel, R., & Fabry, L. (2003). Outcomes of cochlear implantation in children with auditory neuropathy. *Journal of the American Academy of Audiology, 14*(4), 188–201.

Psarommatis, I., Riga, M., Douros, K., Koltsidopoulos, P., Douniadakis, D., Kapetanakis,

I., & Apostolopoulos, N. (2006). Transient infantile auditory neuropathy and its clinical implications. *International Journal of Pediatric Otrorhinolaryngology, 70*(9), 1629–1637.

Rance, G., & Barker, E. J. (2008). Speech perception in children with auditory neuropathy/dys-synchrony managed with either hearing aids or cochlear implants. *Otology & Neurotology, 29*(2), 179–182.

Rance, G., Barker, E., Mok, M., Dowell, R., Rincon, A., & Garratt, R. (2007). Speech perception in noise for children with auditory neuropathy/dys-synchrony type hearing loss. *Ear and Hearing, 28*(3), 351–360.

Rance, G., Beer, D. E., Cone-Wesson, B., Shepherd, R. K., Dowell, R. C., King, A. M., . . . Clark, G. M. (1999). Clinical findings for a group of infants and young children with auditory neuropathy. *Ear and Hearing, 20*, 238–252.

Rance, G., Cone-Wesson, B., Wunderlich, J., & Dowell, R. (2000). Speech perception and cortical event related potentials in children with auditory neuropathy. *Ear and Hearing, 23*, 239–253.

Rance, G., McKay, C., & Graden, D. (2004). Perceptual characterization of children with auditory neuropathy. *Ear and Hearing, 25*, 34–46.

Rance, G., Roper, R., Symons, L., Moody, L. J., Poulis, C., Dourlay, M., & Kelly, T. (2005). Hearing threshold estimation in infants using auditory steady-state responses. *Journal of the American Academy of Audiology, 16*(5), 291–300.

Rapin, I., & Gravel, J. S. (2006). Auditory neuropathy: a biologically inappropriate label unless acoustic nerve is documented. *Journal of the American Academy of Audiology, 17*, 147–150.

Rodríguez-Ballesteros, M., del Castillo, F. J., Martín, Y., Moreno-Pelayo, M. A., Morera, C., Prieto, F., . . . del Castillo, I. (2003). Auditory neuropathy in patients carrying mutations in the otoferlin gene (OTOF). *Human Mutation, 22*, 451–456.

Shallop, J. K., Jin, S. H., & Driscoll, C. L., & Tibesar, R. J. (2003). Characteristics of electrically evoked potentials in patients with auditory neuropathy/auditory dys-synchrony. *International Journal of Audiology, 43*(1), S22–S27.

Starr, A., Isaacson, B., Michalewski, H. J., Zeng, F. G., Kong, Y. Y., Beale, P., . . . Lesperance, M. M. (2004). A dominantly inherited progressive deafness affecting distal auditory nerve and hair cells. *Journal of the Association for Research in Otolaryngology, 5*, 411–426.

Starr, A., Picton, T. W., Sininger, Y. S., Hood, L. J., & Berlin, C. I. (1996). Auditory neuropathy. *Brain, 119*, 741–753.

Starr, A., Sininger, Y. S., Nguyen, T., Michalewski, H. J., Oba, S., & Abdala, C. (2001). Cochlear receptor (microphonic and summating potentials, otoacoustic emissions) and auditory pathway (auditory brainstem potentials) activity in auditory neuropathy. *Ear and Hearing, 22*(2), 91–99.

Starr, A., Zeng, F. G., Michalewski, H. J., & Moser, T. (2008). Perspectives on auditory neuropathy: Disorders of inner hair cells, auditory nerves, and their synapse. In A. I. Basbaum, A. Kaneko, G. M. Shepherd, & G. Westheimer (Eds.), *The senses: A comprehensive reference, Volume 3, Audition* (pp. 397–412). San Diego, CA: Academic Press.

Stone, J. L., Hughes, J. R., Kumar, A., Meyer, D., Subramanian, K. S., Zalkind, M. S., & Fino, J. (1986). Electrocochleograhy recorded noninvasively from the external ear. *Electroencephalography and Clinical Neurophysiology, 63*, 494–496.

Varga, R., Kelley, P. M., Keats, B. J., Starr, A., Leal, S. M., Cohn, E., Kimberling, W. J. (2003). Non-syndromic recessive auditory neuropathy is the result of mutations in the otoferlin (OTOF) gene. *Journal of Medical Genetics, 40*(1), 45–50.

Yasunaga, S., Grati, M., Chardenoux, S., Smith, T. N., Friedman, T. B., Lalwani, A. K., . . . Petit, C. (2000). OTOF encodes multiple long and short isoforms: Genetic evidence that the long ones underlie recessive deafness DFNB9. *American Journal of Human Genetics, 21*, 363–369.

Yasunaga, S., Grati, M., Cohen-Salmon, M., El-Amraoui, A., Mustapha, M., Salem, N., . . . Petit, C. (1999). A mutation of OTOF, encoding otoferlin, a FER-1 like protein, causes

DFNB9, a nonsyndromic form of deafness. *Nature Genetics, 21*, 363–369.

Yellin, M. W., Jerger, J., & Fifer, R. C. (1989). Norms for disproportionate loss in speech intelligibility. *Ear and Hearing, 10*(4), 231–234.

Zeng, F. G., Kong, Y. Y., Michalewski, H. J., & Starr, A. (2005). Perceptual consequences of disrupted auditory nerve activity. *Journal of Neurophysiology, 93*(6), 3050–3063.

Zimmerman-Phillips, S., Robins, A. M., & Osberger, M. J. (2001). *Infant-Toddler Meaningful Auditory Integration Scale.* Sylmar, CA: AdvancedBionicsCorporation.

References

Aarts, N., & Caffee, C. (2005). Manufacturer predicted and measured REAR values in adult hearing aid fitting: Accuracy and clinical usefulness. *International Journal of Audiology*, *44*, 293.

Adler, S. P., Finney, J. W., Manganello, A. M., & Best, A. M. (2004). Prevention of child-to-mother transmission of cytomegalovirus among pregnant women. *Journal of Pediatrics*, *145*(4), 485–491.

Admiraal, R. J., Szymko, Y. M., Griffith, A. J., Brunner, H. G., & Huygen, P. L. (2002). Hearing impairment in Stickler syndrome. *Advances in Otorhinolaryngology*, *61*, 216–223.

Akhtar, N., Jipson, J., & Callanan, M. A. (2001). Learning words through overhearing. *Child Development*, *72*, 416–430.

Alberti, P. W. R. M., & Kristensen, R. (1970). The clinical application of impedance audiometry. *Laryngoscope*, 80, 735–746.

Allen, G. C. (2004). Adhesive otitis media. In C. Cuneyt, C. D. Bluestone, C. Alper, M. Casselbrant, & J. Dohar (Eds.), *Advanced therapy of otitis media*. Hamilton, Ontario, Canada: BC Decker.

Allen, R. L., Stuart, A., Everett, D., & Elangovan, S. (2004). Preschool hearing screening: Pass/ refer rates for children enrolled in a Head Start program in eastern North Carolina. *American Journal of Audiology*, *13*, 29–38.

Ambani, L. M. (1983). Waardenburg and Hirschsprung syndromes. *Journal of Pediatrics*, *102*, 802–806.

American Academy of Audiology. (1992, 1997, Reviewed 2008). *Position statement on guidelines for the diagnosis and treatment of otitis media in children* [Position statement]. Retrieved from http://www.audiology.org

American Academy of Audiology. (1995). Position statement on cochlear implants in children. *Audiology Today*, *7*(3), 14–15.

American Academy of Audiology. (1997). Identification of hearing loss and middle-ear dysfunction in preschool and school-aged children. *Audiology Today*, *9*(3), 18–23.

American Academy of Audiology. (2003). *Pediatric amplification protocol*. Reston, VA.

American Academy of Audiology. (2008). *Clinical practice guidelines: Remote microphone hearing assistance techologies for children and youth*. Reston, VA.

American Academy of Audiology. (2009a). *Position statement and clinical practice guidelines: Ototoxicity monitoring*. Reston, VA.

American Academy of Audiology. (2009b). *Cochlear implants in children* [Position statement]. Retrieved from http://www.audiology.org/resources/documentlibrary/Pages/CochlearChildren.aspx#sthash.DBi1fQQV.dpuf

American Academy of Audiology. (2010). *Practice guidelines for the diagnosis, treatment, and management of children and adults with central auditory processing disorder (CAPD)*. Reston, VA.

American Academy of Audiology. (2011a). *Childhood hearing screening guidelines*. Reston, VA.

American Academy of Audiology. (2011b). *Position statement on classroom acoustics*. Reston, VA.

American Academy of Audiology. (2012). *Audiologic guidelines for the assessment of hearing in infants and young children*. Retrieved from http://www.audiology.org/resources/documentlibrary/Pages/PediatricDiagnostics.aspx#sthash.QnZWku1P.dpuf

American Academy of Audiology. (2013). *Clinical practice guidelines: Pediatric amplification protocol*. Reston, VA.

American Academy of Otolaryngology-Head & Neck Surgery. (2011). Clinical practice guideline: Tonsillectomy in children. *Otolaryngology-Head Neck Surgery, 144*(1), S1–S30. Retrieved from http://oto.sagepub.com/content/144/1_suppl/S1

American Academy of Pediatrics. (1986). Use and abuse of the Apgar score. *Pediatrics, 78*(6), 1148–1149.

American Academy of Pediatrics. (1995). Committee on Genetics and Health: Supervision for children with achondroplasia. *Pediatrics, 95*, 443.

American Academy of Pediatrics. (1999). Newborn and infant hearing loss: Detection and intervention task force on newborn and infant hearing. *Pediatrics, 103*(2), 527–530.

American Academy of Pediatrics. (2013). Supplement to the JCIH 2007 Position statement: Principles and guidelines for early intervention after confirmation that a child is deaf or hard-of-hearing. *Pediatrics, 131*, 4.

American Academy of Pediatrics, Joint Committee on Infant Hearing. (1982). Position statement 1982. *Pediatrics, 70*, 496–497.

American National Standards Institute. (1969). *Specifications for audiometers* (ANSI S3.6-1969). New York, NY.

American National Standards Institute. (2002). *Acoustical performance criteria, design requirements, and guidelines for schools* (S12.60-2002). New York, NY.

American Speech-Language-Hearing Association (ASHA). (1982). Joint Committee on Infant Hearing Position statement. *ASHA, 24*, 1017.

American Speech-Language-Hearing Association (ASHA). (1987). *The short latency auditory evoked potentials*. Rockville, MD.

American Speech-Language-Hearing Association (ASHA). (1990). Guidelines for screening for hearing impairments and middle ear disorders. *ASHA, 32*(Suppl. 2), 17–24.

American Speech-Language-Hearing Association (ASHA). (1992, March). Sedation and topical anesthetics in audiology and speech-language pathology. *ASHA, 34*(Suppl. 7), 41.

American Speech-Language-Hearing Association (ASHA). (1993). Guidelines for audiology services in the schools. *ASHA, 35*(Suppl. 10), 24–32.

American Speech-Language-Hearing Association (ASHA). (1994a). *Guidelines for the audiologic assessment of children from birth to 5 years of age*. Retrieved from http://www.asha.org/policy/GL2004-00002.htm

American Speech-Language-Hearing Association (ASHA). (1994b). Guidelines for the audiologic management of individuals receiving cochleotoxic drug therapy. *ASHA, 36*(Suppl. 12), 11–19.

American Speech-Language-Hearing Association (ASHA). (1995). Report on audiological screening. *American Journal of Audiology, 4*(2), 24–40.

American Speech-Language-Hearing Association (ASHA). (1996). Central auditory processing: current status or research and implications for clinical practice. *American Journal of Audiology, 5*(2), 41–54.

American Speech-Language-Hearing Association (ASHA). (1997). *Guidelines for audiologic screening: Panel on audiologic assessment*. Rockville, MD.

American Speech-Language-Hearing Association (ASHA). (2002). *Guidelines for fitting and evaluation of FM systems*. Rockville, MD.

American Speech-Language-Hearing Association (ASHA). (2005a). *Acoustics in educational settings: Position statement*. Rockville, MD.

American Speech-Language-Hearing Association (ASHA). (2005b). *(Central). Auditory processing disorders* [Technical report]. Rockville, MD.

American Speech-Language-Hearing Association (ASHA). (2005c). *Guidelines for addressing acoustics in educational settings*. Rockville, MD.

American Speech-Language-Hearing Association (ASHA). (2011). *Effects of hearing loss on development*. Audiology Information Series, 796-Y1. Rockville, MD.

Anderson, H., Lindsten, J., & Wedenberg, E. (1971). Hearing defects in males with sex chromosome anomalies. *Acta Oto-Laryngologica (Stockholm), 72*, 55–58.

Anderson, K. L. (1989). Screening Instrument for Targeting Educational Risk (SIFTER). Tampa, FL: Educational Audiology Association.

Anderson, K. L. (2002). *Early Listening Function (ELF)*. Tampa, FL: Educational Audiology Association.

Anderson, K. (2004). The problem of classroom acoustics: The typical classroom soundscape is a barrier to learning. *Seminars in Hearing, 25*(2), 117–129.

Anderson, K. L., & Matkin, N. (1996). Screening Instrument for Targeting Educational Risk in preschool children (age 3 to kindergarten) (preschool SIFTER). Tampa FL: Educational Audiology Association.

Anderson, K. L., & Smaldino, J. (1998). Listening Inventory for Education (LIFE), an efficacy tool. Tampa, FL: Educational Audiology Association.

Anderson, K. L., & Smaldino, J. J. (2000). Children's Home Inventory for Listening Difficulties (CHILD). *Educational Audiology Review, 17*(3).

Aniansson, G., Aim, B., & Andersson, B. (1994). A prospective cohort study on breast-feeding and otitis media in Swedish infants. *Pediatric Infectious Disease Journal, 13*, 183–188.

Anson, B. J. (1963). *An atlas of human anatomy* (2nd ed.). Philadelphia, PA: W. B. Saunders.

Anson, B. J., & Donaldson, J. A. (1967). *The surgical anatomy of the temporal bone and ear.* Philadelphia, PA: W. B. Saunders.

Apgar, V. (1953). A proposal for a new method of evaluation of the newborn infant. *Anesthesiology and Analgesia, 32*, 260.

Apgar, V., & James, L. (1962). Further observations on the newborn scoring system. *American Journal of Diseases of Children, 104*, 419.

Aplin, Y. D., & Rowson, V. J. (1986). Personality and functional hearing loss in children. *British Journal of Clinical Psychology, 25*, 313–314.

Aplin, Y. D., & Rowson, V. J. (1990). Psychological characteristics of children with functional hearing loss. *British Journal of Audiology, 24*(2), 77–87.

Apuzzo, M. L., & Yoshinaga-Itano, C. (1995). Early identification of infants with significant hearing loss and the Minnesota Child Development Inventory. *Seminars in Hearing, 16*, 124–137.

Aragon, M., & Yoshinaga-Itano, C. (2012). Using Language Environment Analysis to improve outcomes for children who are deaf or hard-of-hearing. *Seminars in Speech and Language, 33*(4), 340–353.

Arditi, M., Mason, E., Bradley, J., Tan, T., Barson, W., Schultze, G., & Kaplan, S. (1998). Three-year multicenter surveillance of pneumococcal meningitis in children: Clinical characteristics and outcome related to penicillin susceptibility and dexamethasone use. *Pediatrics, 102*, 1087–1097.

Arehart, K. H., Yoshinaga-Itano, C., Thomson, V., Gabbard, S. A., & Stredler Brown, A. (1980). State of the states: The status of universal newborn screening, assessment, and intervention systems in 16 states. *American Journal of Audiology, 7*, 101–114.

Armitage, S. E., Baldwin, B. A., & Vince, M. A. (1980). The fetal sound environment of sheep. *Science, 208*, 1173–1174.

Arosarena, O. A. (2007). Cleft lip and palate. *Otolaryngologic Clinics of North America, 40*(1), 27–60.

Atkinson, W., Hamborsky, J., McIntyre, L., & Wolfe, S. (Eds.). (2007). Rubella. In *Epidemiology and prevention of vaccine-preventable diseases* (10th ed.). Atlanta, GA: Centers for Disease Control and Prevention (CDC).

Attias, J., Muller, N., Rubel, Y., & Raveh, E. (2006). Multiple auditory steady-state responses in children and adults with normal hearing, sensorineural hearing loss, or auditory neuropathy. *Annals of Otolaryngology, Rhinology, and Laryngology, 115*(4), 268–276.

Avraham, K. B. (2011). The contribution of genetics to hearing impairment. *Audiology Today, 22*, 20–24.

Babson, S. G. (1980). *Diagnosis and management of the fetus and neonate at risk* (4th ed.). St. Louis, MO: Mosby.

Bagatto, M. (2013). The essentials of fitting hearing aids to babies. *Seminars in Hearing, 34*(1), 19–26.

Bagatto, M., Moodie, S., Scollie, S. D., Seewald, R., Moodie, S., Pumford, J., & Liu, K. P. R. (2005).

Clincal protocols for hearing instrument fitting in the desired sensation level method. *Trends in Amplification, 9*(4), 199–225.

Bagatto, M., & Scollie, S. (2011). Current approaches to the fitting of amplification to infants and young children. In R. Seewald & A. M. Tharpe (Eds.), *Comprehensive handbook of pediatric audiology* (pp. 527–552). San Diego, CA: Plural.

Bagatto, M., Scollie, S. D., Hyde, M., & Seewald, R. (2010). Protocol for the provision of amplification within the Ontario infant hearing program. *International Journal of Audiology, 49*(1), S70–S79.

Bagatto, M., Scollie, S., Seewald, R., Moodie, R., & Hoover, B. (2002). Real-ear-to-coupler difference predictions as a function of age for two coupling procedures. *Journal of the American Academy of Audiology, 13*, 407–415.

Baily, D. (1994). Foreword. In J. Rouch & N. Matkin (Eds.), *Infants and toddlers with hearing loss*. Baltimore, MD: York Press.

Bailey, D. (1994). Working with families of children with special needs. In M. Wolery & J. Wilbers (Eds.), *Including children with special needs in early childhood intervention programs* (pp. 23–44). Washington, DC: National Association for the Education of Young Children.

Baker, D. B. (1979). Severely handicapped: Toward an inclusive definition. *AAESPH Review, 4*, 52–65.

Baker, R. B. (1992). Is ear pulling associated with ear infection? *Pediatrics, 90*(6), 1006–1007.

Baker, S., & Baker, K. (1997). Educating children who are deaf or hard-of-hearing: Bilingual-bicultural education. ERIC Digest #E553. *Education Resources Information Center*, ERIC Clearinghouse on Handicapped and Gifted Children.

Baldwin, J. I. (1968). Dysostosis craniofacialis of Crouzon. *Laryngoscope, 78*, 1660–1675.

Baldwin, M., & Watkin, P. (2013). Predicting the degree of hearing loss using click auditory brainstem response in babies referred from newborn hearing screening. *Ear and Hearing, 34*, 361–369.

Baldwin, S. M., Gajewski, B. J., & Widen, J. E. (2011). An evaluation of the cross-check principle using visual reinforecement audi-ometry, otoacoustic emissions, and tympa-nometry. *Journal of the American Academy of Audiology, 21*, 3.

Balkany, T. J. (1980). Otologic aspects of Down's syndrome. *Seminars in Speech, Language, and Hearing, 1*, 39.

Balkany, T. J., Berman, S. A., Simmons, M. A., & Jafek, B. (1978). Middle ear effusion in neonates. *Laryngoscope, 88*, 398–405.

Balkany, T. J., Mischke, R. E., Downs, M. P., & Jafek, B. (1979). Ossicular abnormalities in Down's syndrome. *Otolaryngology-Head and Neck Surgery, 87*, 372.

Balkany, T. J., & Pashley, N. R. T. (Eds.). (1986). *Clinical pediatric otolaryngology*. St. Louis, MO: Mosby.

Bamiou, D., Musiek, F., & Luxon, L. (2001). Aetiology and clinical presentations of auditory processing disorders—A review. *Archives of Diseases in Childhood, 85*(5), 361–365.

Banai, K., Nicol, T., Zecker, S. G., & Kraus, N. (2005). Brainstem timing: Implications for cortical processing and literacy. *Journal of Neuroscience, 25*(43), 9850–9857.

Barbi, M., Binda, S., Caroppa, S., Amborestti, U., Corbetta, C., & Sergi, P. (2003). A wider role for congenital cytomegalovirus infection in sensorineural hearing loss. *Pediatric Infectious Disease Journal, 22*(1), 39–42.

Bart, R. S., & Pumphrey, R. E. (1967). Knuckle pads, leukonychia and deafness; a dominantly inherited syndrome. *New England Journal of Medicine, 276*, 202–207.

Barthes, Roland. (1985). *In the responsibility of forms*. New York, NY: Hill and Wang.

Bartoshuk, A. (1962). Human neonatal cardiac acceleration to sound: Habituation and dishabituation. *Perceptual Motor Skills, 15*, 15–27.

Bartoshuk, A. (1964). Human neonatal cardiac responses to sound: A powerful function. *Psychological Science, 1*, 151–152.

Basser, L. S. (1964). Benign paroxysmal vertigo of childhood: A variety of vestibular neuronitis. *Brain, 87*, 141–152.

Bassila, M. K., & Goldberg, R. (1989). The association of facial palsy and/or sensorineural hearing loss in patients with hemifacial microsomia. *American Journal of Medical Genetics, 26*, 289–291.

Batsakis, J. G., & Nishiyama, R. H. (1962). Deafness with sporadic goiter: Pendred's syndrome. *Archives of Otolaryngology, 76,* 401–406.

Beagley, H. A., & Fisch, L. (1981). Bio-electric potentials available for electric response audiometry: Indications and contraindications. In H. A. Beagley (Ed.), *Audiology and audiological medicine.* Oxford, United Kingdom: Oxford University Press.

Beck, D., & Flexer, C. (2011). Listening is where hearing meets brain . . . in children and adults. *Hearing Review: International Edition,* 24–27.

Beck, D., Moodie, S., & Speidel, D. (2007). Pediatric hearing aid fittings and DSL v5.0. *The Hearing Journal, 60*(6), 54–58.

Beck, D., & Olsen, J. (2008). Extended bandwidths in hearing aids. *Hearing Review, 15*(9).

Beck, D. L., Speidel, D. P., & Petrak, M. (2007). Auditory steady-state response (ASSR): A beginner's guide. *The Hearing Review, 14*(12), 34–37.

Behl, D. D., Houston, T., & Stredler-Brown, A. (2012). The value of a learning community to support telepractice for infants and toddlers with hearing loss. *The Volta Review, 112*(3), 313–328.

Behrens, S., & Blumstein, S. E. (1988). On the role of the amplitude of the fricative noise in the perception of place of articulation in voiceless fricatives. *Journal of the Acoustical Society of America, 84*(3), 861–867.

Bellis, T. J. (2002a). *Assessment and management of central auditory processing disorders in the educational setting* (2nd ed.). Stamford, CT: Thomson Learning.

Bellis, T. J. (2002b). *When the brain can't hear: Unraveling the mystery of auditory processing disorder.* New York, NY: Simon and Schuster.

Bench, J., Collyer, D., Mentz, L., et al. (1977). Studies in behavioral audiometry. III. Six-month-old infants. *Audiology, 15,* 384–394.

Bench, R. J. (1968). Sound transmission to the human foetus through the maternal abdominal wall. *Journal of Genetic Psychology, 113,* 85–87.

Bench, R. J. (1971). Infant audiometry. *Sound, 4,* 72–74.

Benham-Dunster, R. A., & Dunster, J. R. (1985). Hearing loss in the developmentally handicapped: A comparison of three audiometric procedures. *Journal of Auditory Research, 25,* 175–190.

Bennett, M. J. (1980). Trials with the auditory response cradle: Head turns and startles as auditory responses in the neonate. *British Journal of Audiology, 14,* 122.

Bennett, M. J. (1984). Impedance concepts relating to the acoustic reflex. In S. Silman (Ed.), *The acoustic reflex: Basic principles and clinical applications* (pp. 35–61). New York, NY: Academic Press.

Bennett, M. J., & Weatherby, L. (1979). Multiple probe frequency acoustic reflex measurements. *Scandinavian Audiology, 8,* 233–239.

Bennett, M. J., & Weatherby, L. (1982). Newborn acoustic reflexes to noise and pure-tone signals. *Journal of Speech and Hearing Research, 25,* 383–387.

Bentler, R. A. (1989). External ear resonance characteristics in children. *Journal of Speech and Hearing Disorders, 54,* 264–268.

Berg, A. L., Prieve, B. A., Serpanos, Y. C., & Wheaton, M. A. (2011). Hearing screening in a well-infant nursery: Profile of automated ABR-fail/OAE-pass. *Pediatrics, 127*(2), 269–275.

Bergholtz, L. M., Arlinger, S., Kyler, P., & Jerlvall, L. B. (1977). Electrocochleography as a clinical hearing test for difficult-to-test children. *Acta Otolaryngologica, 84,* 385–392.

Bergland, B., Lindvall, T., & Schwela, D. H. (Eds.). (1999). *Guidelines for community noise.* Washington, DC: World Health Organization.

Bergstrom, L. (1984). Congenital hearing loss. In J. L. Northern (Ed.), *Hearing disorders* (2nd ed., pp. 153–160). Boston, MA: Little, Brown.

Bergstrom, L., Neblett, L. M., & Hemenway, W. G. (1972). Otologic manifestations of acrocephalosyndactyly. *Archives of Otolaryngology, 96,* 117–123.

Bergstrom, L., Stewart, J., & Kenyon, B. (1974). External auditory atresia and the deletion chromosome. *Laryngoscope, 84,* 1905–1917.

Berko, J., & Brown, R. (1969). Psycholinguists research methods. In P. H. Mussen (Ed.), *Handbook of research methods in child development.* New York, NY: Wiley.

Berlin, C., & Catlin, F. I. (1965). *Manual of standard pure tone threshold procedure, programmed instruction: Tactics for obtaining valid pure tone clinical thresholds.* Baltimore, MD: Johns Hopkins Medical Institutions.

Berman, S. A., Balkany, T. J., & Simmons, M. A. (1978). Otitis media in the neonatal intensive care unit. *Pediatrics, 62,* 198–202.

Bernstein, R. S., & Gravel, J. (1990). A method for determining hearing sensitivity in infants: The interweaving staircase procedure (ISP). *Journal American Academy of Audiology, 1,* 138–145.

Bess, F. H. (1980). Impedance screening for children: A need for more research. *Annals of Otology, Rhinology, and Laryngology, 89*(Suppl. 68), 228.

Bess, F., Dodd-Murphy, J., & Parker, R. (1998). Children with minimal sensorineural hearing loss: Prevalence, educational performance, and functional status. *Ear and Hearing, 19*(5), 339–354.

Bess, F. H., Klee, T., & Culbertson, J. L. (1986). Identification, assessment and management of children with unilateral sensorineural hearing loss. *Ear and Hearing, 7,* 43–51.

Bess, F. H., & McConnell, F. (1981). *Audiology, education and the hearing-impaired child.* St. Louis, MO: Mosby.

Bess, F. H., & Paradise, J. L. (1994). Universal screening for infant hearing: Not simple, not risk-free, not necessarily beneficial, and not presently justified. *Pediatrics, 98*(2), 330–334.

Bess, F. H., Peek, B., & Chapman, J. (1979). Further observations on noise levels in infant incubators. *Pediatrics, 63,* 100.

Bess, F. H., & Tharpe, A. M. (1984). Unilateral hearing impairment in children. *Pediatrics, 74,* 206–216.

Bhattacharya, J., Bennett, M., & Tucker, S. (1984). Long term follow-up of newborns tested with the auditory response cradle. *Archives of Diseases in Children, 59,* 504.

Bidadi, S., Nejadkazem, M., & Naderpour, M. (2008). The relationship between chronic otitis media-induced hearing loss and the acquisition of social skills. *Otolaryngology-Head and Neck Surgery, 139*(5), 665–670.

Birch, J. W. (1976). Mainstream education for hearing-impaired pupils: Issues and interviews. *American Annals of the Deaf, 121,* 69–71.

Birnholz, J. C., & Benacerraf, B. R. (1983). The development of human fetal hearing. *Science, 22,* 516–518.

Birth Defects Prevention Month and NICHD Research Advances. (2012). *NICHD.* Retrieved from http://www.nichd.nih.gov/news/resources/spotlight/Pages/012913-birth-defects-prevention.aspx

Bitici, O. C. (1975). Familial hereditary progressive sensorineural hearing loss with keratosis and plantaris. *Journal of Laryngology and Otology, 89,* 1143–1146.

Black, F. O., Bergstrom, L., Downs, M. P., & Hemenway, G. (1971a). *Congenital deafness: A new approach to early detection through a high risk register.* Boulder, CO: Colorado Associated University Press.

Black, F. O., Sando, I., Wagner, J. A., et al. (1971b). Middle and inner ear abnormalities, 13-15 (D 1) trisomy. *Archives of Otolaryngology, 93,* 615–619.

Blake, D. T., Strata, F., Churchland, A. K., & Merzenich, M. M. (2002). Neural correlates of instrumental learning in primary auditory cortex. *Proceedings of the National Academy of Sciences, 99*(15), 10114–10119.

Blake, K., Davenport, S. L., Hall, B. D., Hefner, M. A., Pagon, R. A., Williams, M. S., . . . Graham, J. M. (1998). CHARGE association: An update and review for the primary pediatrician. *Clinical Pediatrics, 37,* 159.

Blake, K. D., & Prasad, C. CHARGE syndrome. (2006). *Orphanet Journal of Rare Diseases, 7*(1), 34.

Blanchfield, B., Feldman, J. J., Dunbar, J. L., & Gardner, E. N. (2001). The severely to profoundly hearing-impaired population in the United States: Prevalence estimates and demographics. *Journal of the American Academy of Audiology, 12,* 183–189.

Blennow, F., Svenningsen, N., & Almquist, B. (1974). Noise levels in infant incubators (adverse effects?). *Pediatrics, 53,* 29.

Bluestone, C. D. (1998). Otitis media: A spectrum of diseases. In A. Lalwani & K. Grundfast

(Eds.), *Pediatric otology and neurotology* (pp. 233–240). Philadelphia, PA: Lippincott-Raven.

Bluestone, C. D., Beery, Q. C., & Paradise, J. (1973). Audiometry and tympanometry in relation to middle ear effusions in children. *Laryngoscope, 83*, 594–604.

Boatman, D., Freeman, J., Vining E., Pulister, M., Miglioretti, D., Minaham, R., & McKhann, G. (1999). Language recovery after left hemispherectomy in children with late-onset seizures. *Annals of Neurology, 46*, 579–586.

Bodner-Johnson, B., & Sass-Lehrer, M. (Eds.). (2003). *The young deaf or hard-of-hearing child: A family-centered approach to early education.* Baltimore, MD: Brookes.

Bogart, K. R., & Matsumoto, D. (2010). Living with Moebius syndrome: adjustment, social competence, and satisfaction with life. *Cleft Palate Craniofacial Journal, 47*(2), 134–142.

Bollerslev, J., Grodum, E., & Grontved, A. (1987). Autosomal dominant osteopetrosis. *Journal of Laryngology and Otology, 101*, 1088–1091.

Boney, S. (2007). Adult amplification. In R. S. Ackley, T. N. Decker, & C. J. Limb (Eds.), *An essential guide to hearing and balance disorders.* Mahwah, NJ: Lawrence Erlbaum.

Bonfils, P., Vziel, A., & Pujol, R. (1988). Screening for auditory dysfunction in infants by evoked oto-acoustic emissions. *Otolaryngology-Head and Neck Surgery, 114*, 887–890.

Boothroyd, A. (1991). Speech perception measures and their role in the evaluation of hearing aid performance in a pediatric population. In J. A. Feigin & P. G. Stelmachowicz (Eds.), *Pediatric amplification: Proceedings of the 1991 national conference* (pp. 77–91). Omaha, NE: Boys Town National Research Hospital.

Boothroyd, A. (1993). Profound deafness. In R. Tyler (Ed.), *Cochlear implants: Audiological foundations* (pp. 1–34). San Diego, CA: Singular.

Boothroyd, A. (2004). Measuring auditory speech perception capacity in very young children. In R. T. Miyamoto (Ed.), *Cochlear implants.* International Congress Series 1273 (pp. 292–295). Amsterdam, the Netherlands: Elsevier.

Borck, G., Zarhrate, M., Bonnefont, J. P., Munnich, A., Cormier-Daire, V., & Colleaux, L.

(2007). Incidence and clinical features of X-linked Cornelia de Lange syndrome due to SMC1L1 mutations. *Human Mutations, 28*(2), 205–206.

Bornstein, H. (1973). A description of some current sign systems designed to represent English. *American Annals of the Deaf, 188*, 454–463.

Bornstein, H. (1978). Sign language in the education of the deaf. In I. Schlesinger & L. Namir (Eds.), *Sign language of the deaf: Psychological linguistics and social perspectives* (pp. 333–359). New York, NY: Academic Press.

Bornstein, H. (1979). Systems of sign. In L. Bradford & W. Hardy (Eds.), *Hearing and hearing impairment* (pp. 331–361). New York, NY: Academic Press.

Bosman, A., Snik, A., Emmanuel, A., Mylanus, C., & Cremers, W. (2009). Fitting range of the Baha Intenso. *International Journal of Audiology, 48*(6), 346–352.

Bowd, A. D. (2005). Otitis media: Health and social consequences for Aboriginal youth in Canada's north. *International Journal of Circumpolar Health, 64*, 1.

Bower, T. (1975). Competent newborns. In R. Levin (Ed.), *Child alive.* Garden City, NY: Anchor Press/Doubleday.

Boymans, M., Goverts, S. T., Kramer, S. E., Festen, J. M., & Dreschler, W. A. (2008). Understanding the benefits of bilateral hearing aids. *Ear and Hearing, 29*(6), 930–941.

Brackett, D., & Maxon, A. B. (1986). Service delivery alternatives for the mainstreamed hearing-impaired child. *Language, Speech, and Hearing Services in Schools, 17*, 115–125.

Bradford, L. (1975). Respiration audiometry. In L. Bradford, (Ed.), *Physiological measures of the audiovestibular system.* New York, NY: Academic Press.

Bretlau, P., Jorgensen, M. B., & Johansen, H. (1970). Osteogenesis imperfecta: Light and electron microscopic studies of the stapes. *Acta Oto-Laryngologica (Stockholm), 69*, 172–184.

Bright, K. E. (1997). Spontaneous otoacoustic emissions. In M. Robinette & T. Glattke (Eds.), *Otoacoustic emissions: Clinical applications* (pp. 46–62). New York, NY: Thieme.

British Society of Audiology. (2011). *Auditory processing disorder (APD).* British Society of Audiology APD Special Interest Group. MRC Institute of Hearing.

Brody, J. A. (1964). Notes on the epidemiology of draining ears and hearing loss in Alaska with comments on future studies and control measures. *Alaska Medicine, 6,* 1.

Brody, J. A., Overfield, T., & McAlister, R. (1965). Draining ears and deafness among Eskimos. *Archives of Otolaryngology, 81,* 29–33.

Brooks, D. (1968). An objective method of detecting fluid in the middle ear. *International Audiology, 7,* 280–286.

Brooks, D. (1971). Electroacoustic impedance bridge studies on normal ears of children. *Journal of Speech and Hearing Research, 14,* 247–253.

Brown, J. B., Fryer, M. P., & Morgan, L. R. (1969). Problems in reconstruction of the auricle. *Plastic and Reconstructive Surgery, 43,* 597–604.

Brownell, W. E. (1983). Observations on a motile response in isolated outer hair cells. In W. R. Webster & L. M. Aitken (Eds.), *Mechanisms of hearing* (pp. 5–10). Clayton, Australia: Monash University Press.

Brownell, W. E., Bader, C. R., Bertrend, D., & de Ribaupierre,Y. (1985). Evoked mechanical responses of isolated cochlear hair cells. *Science, 227,* 194–196.

Buck, M. L. (2005). The use of chloral hydrate in infants and children. *Pediatric Pharmacology, 11*(9).

Buckman, R. (1992). *How to break bad news: A guide for health care professionals.* Baltimore, MD: Johns Hopkins University Press.

Buran, D. J., & Duvall, A. J. (1967). The oto-palato-digital (OPD) syndrome. *Archives of Otolaryngology, 85,* 394–399.

Busby, P. A., Dettman, J., Altidis, P. M., Blarney, P. J., & Roberts, S. A. (1990). Assessment of communication skills in implanted deaf children. In G. M. Clark, Y. C. Tong, & J. F. Patrick (Eds.), *Cochlear prostheses.* Edinburgh: Churchill Livingstone.

Calderon, R. (2000). Parental involvement in deaf children's education programs as a predictor of child's language, early reading, and social-emotional development. *Journal of Deaf Studies and Deaf Education, 5*(2), 140–155.

Calderon, R., & Low, S. (1998). Early social-emotional, language, and academic development in children with hearing loss: Families with and without fathers. *American Annals of the Deaf, 143*(3), 225–234.

Caleffe-Schenck, N., & Baker, D. (2011). *Speech sounds: A guide for parents and professionals.* Centennial, CO: Cochlear Americas.

Callison, D. M., & Horn, K. L. (1998). Large vestibular aqueduct syndrome: An overlooked etiology for progressive childhood hearing loss. *Journal of the American Academy of Audiology, 9,* 285–291.

Cameron, S., & Dillon, H. (2007). Development of the Listening in Spatialized Noise–Sentences Test (LISN-S). *Ear and Hearing, 28*(2), 196–211.

Campbell, K. C. M. (2011). Detection of ototoxicity. *Seminars in Hearing, 32,* 2, 196–202.

Canto, M. J., Buixeda, M., J., & Ojeda, F. (2007). Early ultrasonographic diagnosis of diastrophic dysplasia at 12 weeks of gestation in a fetus without previous family history. *Prenatal Diagnosis, 27*(10), 976–978.

Capute, A. J., Palmer, F. B., Shapiro, B. K., Watchtel, R., Schmidt, S., & Ross, A. (1986). The Clinical Linguistic and Auditory Milestone Scale of Infancy (CLAMS): Prediction of cognition in infancy. *Developmental Medicine and Child Neurology, 28,* 762–771.

Carhart, R., & Jerger, J. (1959). Preferred method for clinical determination of pure tone thresholds. *Journal of Speech and Hearing Disorders, 24,* 330–345.

Carinci, F., Pezzetti, F., Locci, P., Becchetti, E., Carls, F., Avantaggiato, A., . . . Bodo, M. (2005). Apert and Crouzon syndromes: Clinical findings, genes and extracellular matrix. *Journal of Craniofacial Surgery, 16*(3), 361–368.

Carnegie Corporation. (1994). *Starting points: Meeting the needs of our youngest children. Report of the Carnegie Task Force.* New York, NY.

Carney, A. (1996). Audition and the development of oral communication competency. In

F. Bess, J. Gravel, & A. Tharpe (Eds.), *Amplification for children with auditory deficits* (pp. 29–54). Nashville, TN: Bill Wilkerson Center Press.

Carney, A. (1999). Auditory system development and dysfunction: What do we really know about childhood hearing loss? *Trends in Amplification, 4*(2), 32–38.

Carney, A., & Moeller, M. P. (1998). Treatment efficiency: Hearing loss in children. *Journal of Speech, Language, and Hearing Research, 41*, 61–84.

Carter, L., Golding, M., Dillon, H., & Seymour, J. (2010). The detection of infant cortical auditory evoked potentials (CAEPs) using statistical and visual detection techniques. *Journal of the American Academy of Audiology, 21*, 347–356.

CASTLE Staff, University of North Carolina. (2011). *Speech sounds: Vowels—A guide for parents and professionals.* Centennial, CO: Cochlear Americas.

Centers for Disease Control and Prevention. (1988). Universal precautions for the prevention of transmission of HIV, HBV, and other blood-borne pathogens in health care settings. *Morbidity and Mortality Weekly Report (MMWR), 37*(24), 377–388.

Centers for Disease Control and Prevention. (2005). Elimination of rubella and congenital rubella syndrome—United States, 1969–2004. *Morbidity and Mortality Weekly Report (MMWR), 54*(11), 279–282.

Champion, R. H. J. (1989). Muckle-Wells syndrome (urticaria, amyloidosis and deafness). *British Journal of Dermatology, 121*(34), 75.

Charles, J., & Key, L. (1998). Developmental spectrum of children with osteopetrosis. *Journal of Pediatrics, 132*, 371.

Chau, J., Atashband, S., Chang, E., Westerberg, B., & Kozal, F. (2009). A systematic review of pediatric sensorineural hearing loss in congenital syphilis. *International Journal of Pediatric Otorhinolaryngology, 73*(6), 787–792.

Chen, S. J., Yang, E. Y., Kwan, M. L., Chang, P., Shiao, A., & Lien, C. F. (1996). Infant hearing screening with an automated auditory brainstem response screener and the audi-

tory brainstem response. *Acta Paediatrica, 85*, 14–28.

Chermak, G., & Musiek, F. (Eds). (2007). *Handbook of (central) auditory processing disorders: Comprehensive intervention* (Vol. 2). San Diego, CA: Plural.

Chermak, G. D., Pederson, C. M., & Bendel, R. B. (1984). Equivalent forms and split-half reliability of the NU-CHIPS administered in noise. *Journal of Speech and Hearing Disorders, 49*, 196–201.

Chial, M. (1998). Yet another audiogram. *ASHA Hearing and Hearing Disorders: Research and Diagnostics Newsletter, 2*(1), 2–3.

Chianese, J., Hoberman, A., Paradise, J. L., Colborn, D. K., Kearney, D., Rockett, H., & Kurs-Losky, M. (2007). Spectral gradient acoustic reflectometry compared with tympanometry in diagnosing middle ear effusion in children aged 6 to 24 months. *Archives of Pediatric Adolescent Medicine, 161*(9), 884–888.

Ching, T., Dillon, H., Seewald, R., Britton, L., Joyce, J., & Scollie, S. (2006). *Hearing aid prescription for children: NAL-NL1 and DSL[i/o].* Paper presented at the Fourth Widex Congress of Paediatric Audiology, Ottawa, Ontario, Canada.

Chomsky, N. (1966). *Aspects of the theory of syntax.* Cambridge, MA: MIT Press.

Chomsky, N. (1995, June 6). Chimp talk debate: Is it really language? *The New York Times.*

Chrysostomidou, D. M., Caslaris, E., Alexiou, D., & Bartsocas, C. (1971). Trisomy 18 in Greece. *Acta Paediatrica Scandinavica, 69*, 591–593.

Chugani, H. (1993). Positron emission tomography scanning in newborns. *Clinics in Perinatology, 20*(2), 398.

Chugani, H. (1997). How to build a baby's brain. *Newsweek, Special Edition*, pp. 29–30.

Chugani, H., Phelps, M., & Mazziotta, J. (1987). Positron emission tomography study of human brain functional development. *Annals of Neurology, 22*(4), 495.

Church, M., Edlis, F., Blakley, B. W., & Bawle, E. V. (1997). Hearing, language, speech, vestibular and dentofacial disorders in fetal alcohol syndrome. *Alcoholism, Clinical and Experimental Research, 21*(3), 495–512.

Church, M. W., & Gerkin, K. P. (1987). Hearing disorders in children with fetal alcohol syndrome: Findings from case reports. *Pediatrics, 82,* 147–154.

Church, M., & Kaltenbach, J. A. (1997). Hearing, speech, language, and vestibular disorders in the fetal alcohol syndrome: Literature review. *Alcoholism, Clinical and Experimental Research, 21*(3), 495–512.

Churchland, P. (1997). *The engine of reason, the seat of the soul: Philosophical journey into the brain.* Boston, MA: MIT Press.

Clark, G. M., Cowan, R., & Dowell, R. C. (Eds.). (1997). *Cochlear implantation for infants and children.* San Diego, CA: Singular.

Clark, J. G. (2002). If it's not hearing loss, then what? Confronting nonorganic hearing loss in children. *AudiologyOnline.* Retrieved from http://www.audiologyonline.com/articles/if-it-s-not-hearing-1153

Clark, M. (2007). *A practical guide to quality interaction with children who have a hearing loss.* San Diego, CA: Plural.

Clifton, R. K. (1998). The development of spatial hearing in human infants. In L. A. Werner & E. W. Rubel (Eds.), *Developmental psychoacoustics* (pp. 135–148). Washington, DC: American Psychological Association.

Clopton, B. M., & Silverman, M. S. (1977). Plasticity of binaural interactions, II: Critical periods and changes in midline response. *Journal of Neurophysiology, 40,* 1275–1280.

Cody, J. D., Semrud-Clikeman, M., Hardies, L. J., Lancaster, J., Ghidoni, P. D., Schaub, R. L., . . . Hale, D. E. (2005). Growth hormone benefits children with 18q deletions. *American Journal of Medical Genetics, 137*(1), 9–15.

Cohen, D., & Sade, J. (1972). Hearing in secretory otitis media. *Canadian Journal of Otology, 1,* 27.

Cohen, M. E. (1967). Neurological abnormalities in achondroplastic children. *Journal of Pediatrics, 71,* 367.

Cohen, M. M., Jr. (1999). Robin sequence and complexes. *American Journal of Medical Genetics 84,* 311–315.

Cohen, M. M., & Kreiborg, S. (1993). The growth pattern in the Apert syndrome. *American Journal of Medical Genetics, 47,* 617–623.

Cohen, N., & Waltzman, S. (1996). Cochlear implants in infants and young children. *Seminars in Hearing, 17*(2), 215–222.

Cohen, R. E. (1966). The "D" syndrome. *American Journal of Diseases in Children, 111,* 235.

Cohn, E. S., & Kelley, P. M. (1999). Clinical phenotype and mutations in connexin 26 (DFNB1/GJB2), the most common cause of childhood hearing loss. *American Journal of Medical Genetics, 89*(3), 130–136.

Cole, D. E., & Cohen, M. M. (1991). Osteogenesis imperfecta: An update. *Journal of Pediatrics, 119,* 73–74.

Cole, E., & Flexer, C. (2008). *Children with hearing loss: Developing listening and talking (birth to six).* San Diego, CA: Plural.

Collet, L., Gartner, M., Moulin, A., Kauffman, I., Disant, F., & Morgon, A. (1989). Evoked otoacoustic emissions and sensorineural hearing loss. *Otolaryngology-Head and Neck Surgery, 115,* 1060–1062.

Condon, W. S., & Sander, L. W. (1974). Neonate movement is synchronized with adult speech: Interactional participation and language structure. *Science, 183,* 99–101.

Cone-Wesson, B., Dowell, R. C., Tomlin, D., Rance, G., & Ming, W. J. (2002). The auditory steady-state response: Comparisons with the auditory brainstem response. *Journal of the American Academy of Audiology, 13,* 173–187.

Cone-Wesson, B., Vohr, B. R., Sininger, Y. S., Widen, J. E., Folsom, R. C., Gorga, M. P., & Norton, S. J. (2000). Identification of neonatal hearing impairment: Infants with hearing impairment. *Ear and Hearing, 21*(5), 488–507.

Cooper, J., Langley, L., Meyerhoff, W., & Gates, G. (1977). The significance of negative middle ear pressure. *Laryngoscope, 87,* 92–97.

Cooper, J. C., Gates, G. A., Owen, J. H., & Dickson, H. G. (1975). An abbreviated impedance bridge technique for school screening. *Journal of Speech and Hearing Disorders, 40,* 260–269.

Cooper, L. F., & Jabs, E. W. (1987). Aural atresia associated with multiple congenital anomalies and mental retardation: A new syndrome. *Journal of Pediatrics, 110*(5), 747–750.

Cooper, S., Flaitz, C., Johnston, D., Lee, B., & Hecht, J. (2001). A natural history of cleidocranial dysplasia. *American Journal of Medical Genetics, 104,* 1.

Coplan, J., Gleason, J. R., Ryan, R., Burke, M. G., & Williams, M. L. (1982). Validation of an early language milestone scale in a high-risk population. *Pediatrics, 70*(5), 677–683.

Coppage, K. B., & Smith, R. J. (1995). Branchio-oto-renal syndrome. *Journal of the American Academy ofAudiology, 6*(1), 103–110.

Cornett, R. O. (1985). Diagnostic factors bearing on the use of cued speech with hearing-impaired children. *Ear and Hearing, 6*(1), 33–35.

Corriveau, K. H., Goswami, U., & Thomson, J. M. (2010). Auditory processing and early literacy skills in a preschool and kindergarten population. *Journal of Learning Disabilities, 43*(4), 369–382.

Crandell, C. C. (1991). Classroom acoustics for normal-hearing children: Implications for rehabilitation. *Educational Audiology Monographs, 2,* 18–38.

Crandell, C., & Smaldino, J. (1996). An update of classroom acoustics for children with hearing impairment. *Volta Review, 1,* 4–12.

Crandell, C., Smaldino, J., & Flexer, C. (1995). *Sound-field FM amplification: Theory and practical applications.* San Diego, CA: Singular.

Crandell, C., Smaldino, J., & Flexer, C. (2005). Sound field amplification: Applications to speech perception and classroom acoustics (2nd ed.). Clifton Park, NY: Thomson Delmar Learning.

Cremers, C. W., Wijdeveld, P. G., & Pinckers, A. J. (1977). Juvenile diabetes mellitus, optic atrophy, hearing loss, diabetes insipidus, atonia of the urinary tract and bladder and other abnormalities (Wolfran syndrome). *Acta Paediatrica, 264,* 1–16.

Cremers, C. W. R. J., Thijssen, H. O. M., & Fischer, A. J. E. M. (1981). Otological aspects of the earpit-deafness syndrome. *Journal of Otolaryngology, 43,* 223–239.

Cremers, W. R. J., Hoogland, G. A., & Kuypers, W. (1984). Hearing loss in the cervico-oculo-acoustic (Wildervanck) syndrome. *Archives of Otolaryngology, 110,* 54–57.

Cross, H. E., & Pfaffenbach, D. D. (1972). Duane's retraction syndrome and associated congenital malformations. *American Journal of Ophthalmology, 73,* 442–449.

Cullen, K. A., Hall, M. J., & Golosinskiy, A. (2009). Ambulatory surgery in the United States: 2006. *National Health Statistics Report.* Washington, DC.

Culpepper, B., & Thompson, G. (1994). Effects of reinforcer duration on the response behavior of pre-term 2-year-olds in visual reinforcement andrometry. *Ear and Hearing, 15,* 161–167.

Cunningham, G. C. (1970). Biochemical screening programs and problems. In E. M. Gold (Ed.), *Earlier recognition of handicapping conditions in childhood: Proceedings of a biregional institute* (pp. 37–41). Berkeley, CA: University of California School of Public Health.

Cunningham, M., & Cox, E. O. (2003). Hearing assessment in infants and children: Recommendations beyond neonatal screening. *Pediatrics, 111*(2): 436–440.

Cusimano, F., Martines, E., & Rizzo, C. (1991). The Jervell and Lange-Nielsen syndrome. *International Journal of Pediatric Otolaryngology, 22,* 49–55.

Cyr, D. G. (1980). Vestibular testing in children. *Annals of Otology, Rhinology, Laryngology, 89*(5, Pt. 2), 63–69.

Cyr, D. G. (1983). The vestibular system: Pediatric considerations. *Seminars in Hearing, 4*(1), 33–46.

Cyr, D. G., Brookhouser, P. E., Valente, M., & Grossman, A. (1985). Vestibular evaluation of infants and preschool children. *Otolaryngology-Head and Neck Surgery, 93*(4), 463–468.

Dahl, H. A. (1979). Progressive hearing impairment in children with congenital CMV. *Journal of Speech and Hearing Disorders, 44,* 220.

Dahle, A., Fowler, K. B., Wright, J., Boppana, S., Britt, W., & Pass, R. (2000). Longitudinal investigation of hearing disorders in children with congenital cytomegalovirus. *Journal of the American Academy of Audiology, 11,* 283–290.

Dahle, A. J., & McCollister, F. P. (1983). Considerations for evaluating hearing in multiply handicapped children. *The multiply handicapped child (Proceedings of a symposium in Edmonton, Alberta)*. New York, NY: Grune & Stratton.

Dallos, P. (1973). *The auditory periphery: Biophysics and physiology.* New York, NY: Academic Press.

Dallos, P. (2008). Cochlear amplification, outer hair cells and prestin. *Current Opinion in Neurobiology. 18*(4), 370–376.

Dalzell, L., Orlando, M., MacDonald, M., Berg, A., Bradley, M., Cacace, A., . . . Prieve, B. (2000). The New York State Universal Newborn Hearing Screening Demonstration Project: Ages of hearing loss identification, hearing aid fitting, and enrollment in early intervention. *Ear and Hearing, 21*(2), 118–130.

Danenberg, M. A., Loos-Cosgrove, M., & LoVerde, M. (1987). Temporary hearing loss and rock music. *Language, Speech, and Hearing Services in Schools, 18*, 267–274.

Davenport, S. L., Hefner, M. A., & Thelin, J. W. (1986). CHARGE syndrome: Part I: External ear anomalies. *International Journal of Pediatric Otorhinolaryngology, 12*, 137–143.

Davidson, L. S., Geers, A. E., Blarney, P. J., Tobey, E. A., & Brenner, C. A. (2011). Factors contributing to speech perception scores in long-term pediatric cochlear implant users. *Ear and Hearing, 32*(Suppl. 1), 19S–26S.

Davis, A., & Wood, S. (1992). The epidemiology of childhood hearing impairment: Factors relevant to planning of services. *British Journal of Audiology, 26*, 77–90.

Davis, H. (1976). Brainstem and other responses in electric response audiometry. *Annals of Otology, 85*, 3–13.

Davis, J. M., Elfenbein, J., Schum, R., & Bentler, R. (1986). Effects of mild and moderate hearing impairments on language, educational, and psychosocial behavior of children. *Journal of Speech and Hearing Disorders, 51*, 53–62.

Davis, J. M., Shepard, N. T., Stelmachowicz, P. G., & Gorga, M. P. (1981). Characteristics of hearing-impaired children in the public schools. Part II: Psychoeducational data. *Journal of Speech and Hearing Disorders, 46*, 130–137.

Davis, P. A. (1939). Effects of acoustic stimuli on the waking human brain. *Journal of Neurophysiology, 2*, 444–499.

Davis, R., & Stiegler, L. N. (2005). Toward more effective audiological assessment of children with autism spectrum disorder. *Seminars in Hearing, 26*(4), 241–252.

Dawe, C., Wynne-Davies, R., & Fulford, G. E. (1982). Clinical variation in dyschondrosteosis: A report on 13 individuals in 8 families. *Journal of Bone and Joint Surgery, 64B*, 377–381.

Day, J., Bamford, J., Parry, G., Shepherd, M., & Quigley, A. (2000). Evidence on the efficacy of insert earphone and sound field VRA with young infants. *British Journal of Audiology, 34*, 329–334.

DeCasper, A. J., & Fifer, W. P. (1980). Of human bonding: Newborns prefer their mothers' voices. *Science, 208*, 1174–1176.

DeCasper, A. J., & Spence, M. J. (1986). Prenatal maternal speech influences newborns' perception of speech sounds. *Infant Behavior and Development, 9*, 133–150.

Delgado, J. L., Johnson, C. L., Roy, I., & Trevino, P. M. (1990). Hispanic health and nutrition examination survey: Methodological considerations. *American Journal of Public Health, 80*(Suppl.), 6–10.

Demany, I., McKenzie, B., & Vurpillot, E. (1977). Rhythm perception in early infancy. *Nature, 266*, 718–719.

Denton, D. M., Brill, R. B., Kent, M. S., et al. (1974). Schools for deaf children. In P. J. Fine (Ed.), *Deafness in infancy and early childhood.* New York, NY: Medicom Press.

Derbyshire, A. J., & Davis, H. (1935). The action potential of the auditory nerve. *American Journal of Physiology, 113*, 476–504.

Dhar, S., & Hall, J. W., III. (2012). *Otoacoustic emissions: Principles, procedures and protocols.* San Diego, CA: Plural.

Diefendorf, A. (2003). Behavioral hearing assessment: Considerations for the young child with developmental disabilities. *Seminars in Hearing, 24*(3), 189–200.

Diefendorf, A. (2011). Behavioral audiometry with children. In R. Seewald & A. M. Tharpe (Eds.), *Comprehensive handbook of pediat-*

ric audiology (pp. 497–509). San Diego, CA: Plural.

Diefendorf, A., Allen, R. K., Burch, M. L., Corbin, K. R., Griffiths, C. E., Rehal, B. K., & Weinzierl, A. A. (2011). Audiologic considerations for children with multiple modality involvement. In R. Seewald & A. M. Tharpe (Eds.), *Comprehensive handbook of pediatric audiology* (pp. 713–730). San Diego, CA: Plural.

Diefendorf, A. O., Bull, M. J., Casey-Harvey, D., Miyamoto, R. T., Pope, M. L., Renshaw, J. J., . . . Wagner-Escobar, M. (1995). Down syndrome: A multidisciplinary perspective. *Journal of the American Academy of Audiology*, *6*(1), 39–46.

Digilio, M. C., Sarkozy, A., de Zorzi, A., Pacileo, G., Limongelli, G., Mingarell, R., . . . Dallapiccola, B. (2006). "LEOPARD" syndrome: Clinical diagnosis in the first year of life. *American Journal of Medical Genetics*, *140*(7), 740–746.

Dillon, H. (2005). So, baby, how does it sound? Cortical assessment of infants with hearing aids. *Hearing Journal*, *58*(10), 10–17.

Dillon, H. (2012). *Hearing aids* (2nd ed.). Sydney, Australia: Boomerang Press.

Dillon, H., Ching, T., & Golding, M. (2008). Hearing aids for infants and children. In J. Madell & C. Flexer (Eds.), *Pediatric audiology: Diagnosis, technology, and management*. New York, NY: Thieme.

Dillon, H., & Storey, L. (1998). National acoustic laboratories' procedures for selecting the saturation sound pressure level of hearing aids: Theoretical derivation. *Ear and Hearing*, *19*(4), 255–266.

Dixon, J., Trainer, P., & Dixon, M. J. (2007). Treacher Collins syndrome. *Orthodondics and Craniofacial Research*, *10*, 88.

Dobie, R. A., & Berlin, C. I. (1979). Influence of otitis media on hearing and development. *Annals of Otology, Rhinology, and Laryngology*, *88*(60), 48–53.

Dobrowski, J. M., Grundfast, K. M., Rosenbaum, K. N., & Zajtchuk, J. T. (1985). Otorhinolaryngic manifestations of CHARGE association. *Otolaryngology-Head and Neck Surgery*, *93*, 798–803.

Dockrell, J., & Shield, B. (2012). The impact of sound-field systems on learning and attention in elementary school classrooms. *Journal of Speech, Language, and Hearing Research*, *55*, 1163–1177.

Dodge, H. W., Jr., Wood, M. W., & Kennedy, R. J. (1959). Craniofacial dysostosis: Crouzon's disease. *Pediatrics*, *23*, 98.

Dodge, P. R., Davis, H., Feigin, R. D., Holmes, S. J., Kaplan, Sj. L., Jubellier, D., . . . Hirsh, S. K. (1984). Prospective evaluation of hearing impairment as a sequela of acute bacterial meningitis. *New England Journal of Medicine*, *311*(14), 869–874.

Dolnick, E. (1993). Deafness as a culture. *Atlantic Monthly*, *272*(3), 37–53.

Douek, E., Dodson, H., Banister, L., Ashcroft, P., & Humphries, K. N. (1976). Effects of incubator noise on the cochlea of the newborn. *Lancet*, *2*, 1110–1113.

Doupe, A. J., & Kuhl, P. K. (1999). Birdsong and human speech: Common themes and mechanisms. *Annual Review of Neuroscience*, *22*, 567–631.

Downs, D., Schmidt, B., & Stephens, T. J. (2005). Auditory behaviors of children and adolescents with pervasive developmental disorders. *Seminars in Hearing*, *26*(4), 226–240.

Downs, M. P. (1970). The identification of congenital deafness. *Transactions of the American Academy of Ophthalmology and Otolaryngology*, *741*, 208–214.

Downs, M. P. (Ed.). (1980). Communication disorders in Down's syndrome. *Seminars in Speech, Language, and Hearing*, *1*, 1.

Downs, M. P. (1986). The rationale for neonatal hearing screening. In E. T. Swigard (Ed.), *Neonatal hearing screening* (pp. 3–16). San Diego, CA: College-Hill Press.

Downs, M. P., & Hemenway, W. G. (1969). Report on the hearing screening of 17,000 neonates. *International Audiology*, *8*, 72–76.

Downs, M. P., & Silver, H. K. (1972). The A.B.C.D.'s to H.E.A.R.: Early identificatiction in nursery, office and clinic of the infant who is deaf. *Clinical Pediatrics*, *11*, 563–566.

Downs, M. P., & Sterritt, G. M. (1964). Identification audiometry for neonates: A preliminary report. *Journal of Auditory Research*, *4*, 69–80.

Doyle, K. J., Fuikawa, S., Rogers, P., & Newman, E. (1998). Comparison of newborn hearing screening by transient otoacoustic emissions and auditory brainstem response using ALGO-2. *International Journal of Pediatric Otorhinolaryngology, 43,* 207–211.

Dreschler, W. A., & Boymans, M. (1994). Clinical evaluation on the advantage of binaural hearing aid fittings. *Audiologische Akustik, 5,* 12–23.

Drubach, D. (2000). *The brain explained.* Upper Saddle River, NJ: Prentice-Hall.

Duncan, B., Ey, J., Holberg, C., Wright, A., Martinez, F., & Taussig, L. (1993). Exclusive breastfeeding for at least four months protects against otitis media. *Pediatrics, 91,* 867–872.

Dunn, J., & Shatz, M. (1989). Becoming a conversationalist despite (or because of) having an older sibling. *Childhood Development, 60,* 399–410.

Dunst, C., Trivette, C., Starnes, A., Hamby, D., & Gordon, N. (1993). *Building and evaluating family support initiatives: A national study of programs for persons with developmental disabilities.* Baltimore, MD: Paul H. Brookes.

Dupertius, S. M., & Musgrave, R. H. (1959). Experiences with the reconstruction of the congenitally deformed ear. *Plastic and Reconstructive Surgery, 23,* 361–373.

Durieux-Smith, A., Picton, T., Edwards, C., Goodman, J., & MacMurray, B. (1985). The crib-o-gram in the NICU: An evaluation based on brainstem electric response audiometry. *Ear and Hearing, 6,* 20.

Eagles, E. L., Wishik, S. M., & Doerfler, L. G. (1967). Hearing sensitivity and ear disease in children: A prospective study. *Monographs in Laryngoscope* (Suppl.), 1–274.

Edwards, C. (1991). Assessment and management of listening skills in school-aged children. *Seminars in Hearing, 12,* 389–401.

Edwards, C. (1996). Auditory intervention for children with mild auditory deficits. In F. Bess, J. Gravel, & A. Tharpe (Eds.), *Amplification for children with auditory deficits* (pp. 383–398). Nashville, TN: Bill Wilkerson Center Press.

Edwards, E. P. (1968). Kindergarten is too late. *Saturday Review,* pp. 60–79.

Egelhoff, K., Whitelaw, G., & Rabidouxs, P. (2005). What audiologists need to know about autism spectrum disorder. *Seminars in Hearing, 24*(4), 202–209.

Eggermont, J. J., Ponton, C. W., Don, M., Waring, M. D., & Kwong, B. (1997). Maturational delays in cortical evoked potentials in cochlear implant users. *Acta Otolaryngologica, 117*(2), 161–163.

Eichwald, J., & Gabbard, S. A. (Eds.). (2008). Mild and unilateral hearing loss in children. *Seminars in Hearing, 29,* 2.

Eilers, R., & Oiler, K. (1994). Infant vocalizations and the early diagnosis of severe hearing impairment. *Journal of Pediatrics, 124*(2), 199–203.

Eilers, R., Widen, J., Urbano, R., Hudson, T., & Gonzales, L. (1991). Optimization of automated hearing test algorithms: A comparison of data from simulations and young children. *Ear and Hearing, 12*(3), 199–203.

Eilers, R. E., Wilson, W. R., & Moore, J. M. (1977). Developmental changes in speech discrimination in infants. *Journal of Speech and Hearing Research, 20*(4), 766–779.

Eimas, P. D., Siqueland, E. R., Juscyzk, P., & Vigorito, J. (1972). Speech perception in infants. *Science, 171,* 303.

Eimas, P. D., & Tartter, V. C. (1979). On the development of speech perception: Mechanisms and analogies. *Advances in Child Development and Behavior, 13,* 155–193.

Eisele, W., Berry, R., & Shriner, T. (1975). Infant sucking response patterns as a conjugate function of change in the sound pressure level of auditory stimuli. *Journal of Speech and Hearing Research, 18,* 296–307.

Eisenberg, R. B. (1970). The development of hearing in man: An assessment of current status. *Asha, 12,* 119–123.

Eisenberg, R. B. (1976). *Auditory competence in early life.* Baltimore, MD: University Park Press.

Eisenberg, L. S. (2009). *Clinical management of children with cochlear implants.* San Diego, CA: Plural.

Eisenberg, L. S., Johnson, K. C., & Martinez, M. A. (2005). Clinical assessment of speech perception for infants and toddlers. *Audiology-*

Online. Retrieved September 12, from http://www.audiologyonline.com/articles/clinical-assessment-speech-perception-for-1016

Eiserman, W., Hartel, D., Shisler, L., Buhrmann, J., White, K., & Foust, T. (2008). Using otoacoustic emissions to screen for hearing loss in early childhood care settings. *International Journal of Pediatric Otorhinolaryngology, 72,* 475–482.

El-Darouti, M. A., Marzouk, S. A., & Abdel-Halim, M. R. (2006). Muckle-Wells syndrome: Report of six cases with hyperpigmented sclerodermoid skin lesions. *International Journal of Dermatology, 45*(3), 239–244.

Eliachar, I., Sando, I., & Northern, J. L. (1974). Simultaneous manometric and tympanometric measurements of middle-ear pressures in guinea pigs. *Archives of Otolaryngology, 99*(3), 172–176.

Elliot, G. B., & Elliot, K. A. (1964). Some pathological, radiological and clinical implications of the precocious development of the human ear. *Laryngoscope, 74,* 1160–1171.

Elliott, L. (1982). Effects of noise on perception of speech of children and certain handicapped individuals. *Sound Vibration, 16,* 12.

Elliott, L. L., & Katz, D. R. (1980). Children's pure-tone detection. *Journal of the Acoustical Society of America, 67,* 343–344.

Elssman, S., Matkin, N., & Sabo, M. (1987). Early identification of congenital sensorineural hearing impairment. *Hearing Journal, 40*(9), 13–17.

Elverland, H. H., & Torbergsen, T. (1991). Audiologic findings in a family with mitochondrial disorder. *American Journal of Otology, 12,* 459–465.

English, G. M., Northern, J. L., & Fria, T. J. (1973). Chronic otitis media as a cause of sensorineural hearing loss. *Archives of Otolaryngology, 98,* 17–22.

Erber, N. (1982). *Auditory training.* Washington, DC: Alexander Graham Bell Association for the Deaf.

Erber, N. P. (1980). Use of the auditory numbers test to evaluate speech perception abilities of hearing-impaired children. *Journal of Speech and Hearing Disorders, 45,* 527.

Erber, N. P., & Alencewicz, C. M. (1972). Audiologic evaluation of deaf children. *Journal of Speech and Hearing Disorders, 41,* 256–267.

Erdman, S. A., & Sedge, R. K. (1981). Subjective comparisons of binaural versus monaural amplification. *Ear and Hearing, 2,* 225–229.

Estabrooks, W., & Marlow, J. (2000). *The baby is listening* (pp. 22–25). Washington, DC: Alexander Graham Bell Association.

Estabrooks, W. I. (2000). Auditory-verbal practice. In S. B. Waltzman & N. L. Cohen (Eds.), *Cochlear implants.* New York, NY: Thieme Medical.

Evans, G. W., Gonnella, C., Marcynyszyn, L. A., Gentile, L., & Salpekar, N. (2005). The role of chaos in poverty and children's socioemotional adjustment. *Psychological Science, 16*(7).

Ewing, I. R., & Ewing, A. W. G. (1944). The ascertainment of deafness in infancy and early childhood. *Journal of Laryngology and Otology, 59,* 309–338.

Falk, S., & Farmer, J. (1973). Incubator noise and possible deafness. *Archives of Otolaryngology, 97,* 385.

Falk, S. A., & Woods, N. F. (1973). Hospital noise-levels and potential health hazards. *New England Journal of Medicine, 289,* 774.

Fausti, S., Henry, J., & Frey, R. (1996). In J. Northern (Ed.), *Hearing disorders* (pp. 149–164). Needham Heights, MA: Allyn & Bacon.

Feingold, M., & Baum, J. (1978). Goldenhar's syndrome. *American Journal of Diseases in Children, 132,* 136–138.

Fernald, A. (1985). Four-month-old infants prefer to listen to "motherese." *Infant Behavior and Development, 8,* 181–195.

Fernald, A., & Kuhl, P. (1987). Acoustic determinants of infant preference for "motherese" speech. *Infant Behavior and Development, 10,* 279–293.

Ferrari, D. (2012). Patient therapeutic education via tele-audiometry: The Brazilian experience. *Hearing Review, 19*(10), 40–43.

Ferraro, J. A. (1986). Electrocochleography. *Seminars in Hearing, 7*(3), 239–337.

Ferraro, J. A. (2010). Electrocochleography: A review of recording approaches, clinical applications, and new findings in adults and children. *Journal of the American Academy of Audiology, 21*(3), 145–152.

Ferraro, J. A., Beck, D. L., & Speidel, D. P. (2011). Developments in electrocochleography. *Hearing Review, 18*(7), 38–42.

Field, T. M., Woodson, R., Greenberg, R., & Cohen, D. (1982). Discrimination and imitation of facial expressions by neonates. *Science, 218,* 179–181.

Finitzo, T., Albright, K., & O'Neal, J. (1998). The newborn with hearing loss: Detection in the nursery. *Pediatrics, 102,* 1452–1460.

Finitzio, T., & Crumley, W. (1999). The role of the pediatrician in hearing loss. From detection to connection. *Pediatric Clinics of North America, 46*(1), 15–34.

Finitzo-Hieber, T. (1982). Auditory brainstem response: Its place in infant audiological evaluations. *Seminars in Speech, Language, and Hearing, 3,* 76–87.

Finitzo-Hieber, T. (1988). Classroom acoustics. In R. Roeser (Ed.), *Auditory disorders in school children* (2nd ed., pp. 221–233). New York, NY: Thieme-Stratton.

Finitzo-Hieber, T., Gerling, I. J., Matkin, N. D., & Cherow-Skalka, E. (1980). A sound effects recognition test for the pediatric audiologic evaluation. *Ear and Hearing, 1,* 271.

Finitzio-Hieber, T., McCracken, G., & Brown, K. (1985). Prospective controlled evaluation of auditory function in neonates given netilmicin or amikacin. *Pediatrics, 106,* 129–135.

Finitzo-Hieber, T., McCracken, G., Roeser, R., Allen, D. A., Chrarne, D. F., & Morrow, J. (1979). Ototoxicity in neonates treated with gentamicin and kanamycin: Results of a four-year controlled follow-up study. *Pediatrics, 63,* 443.

Finitzo-Hieber, T., Simhadri, R., & Hieber, J. P. (1981). Auditory brainstem response assessment of postmeningitic infants and children. *International Journal of Pediatric Otorhinolaryngology, 3,* 275.

First, L. R., & Palfrey, J. S. (1994). The infant or young child with developmental delay. *New England Journal of Medicine, 330*(7), 478–483.

Firszt, J., & Reeder, R. (1996). Cochlear implants and children: Device programming and considerations for young children. *Seminars in Hearing, 17*(4), 337–351.

Fischler, R. S., Todd, W. N., & Feldman, C. M. (1985). Otitis media and language performance in a cohort of Apache Indian children. *American Journal of Diseases in Children, 139,* 355–360.

Fish, A., & Morford, J. (2012). *The benefits of bilingualism: Impacts on language and cognitive development.* NSF Science of Learing Center on Visual Language and Visual Learning, Research Brief No. 7. Washington, DC: Gallaudet University.

Fitzpatrick, E., Durieux-Smith, A., Eriks-Brophy, A., Olds, J., & Gaines, R. (2007). The impact of newborn hearing screening on communication development. *Journal of Medical Screening, 14,* 123–131.

Fitzpatrick, E. M., Durieux-Smith, A., & Whittingham, J. (2010). Clinical practice for children with mild bilateral and unilateral hearing loss. *Ear and Hearing, 31,* 392–400.

Fletcher, H. (1953). *Speech and hearing in communication.* New York, NY: Van Nostrand.

Flexer, C. (1990). Audiological rehabilitation in the schools. *ASHA, 32*(4), 44–45.

Flexer, C. (2004). The impact of classroom acoustics: Listening, learning, and literacy. *Seminars in Hearing, 25*(2), 131–140.

Flexer, C. (2012). *Auditory brain development: The key to developing listening, language and literacy.* Retrieved from http://hearinghealth matters.org/hearingandkids/2012/auditory-brain-development

Flexer, C., & Gans, D. P. (1982). Evaluating behavioural observation audiometry with handicapped children. *Exceptional Children, 29,* 217–224.

Flexer, C., & Gans, D. P. (1985). Comparative evaluation of the auditory responsiveness of normal infants and profoundly multihandicapped children. *Journal of Speech and Hearing Research, 28,* 163–168.

Flexer, C., & Gans, D. P. (1986). Distribution of auditory response behaviors in normal infants and profoundly multihandicapped children. *Journal of Speech and Hearing Research*, 29, 425–429.

Fligor, B. J., & Cox, L. C. (2004). Output levels of commercially available portable compact disc players and the potential risk to hearing. *Ear and Hearing*, 25, 513–527.

Foerst, A., Beutner, D., Lang-Roth, R., Huttenbrink, K. B., von Wedel, H., & Walger, M. (2006). Prevalence of auditory neuropathy/synaptopathy in a population of children with profound hearing loss. *International Journal of Pediatric Otorhinolaryngology*, 70(8), 1415–1422.

Forget-Dubois, N., Dionne, G., Lemelin, J. P., Perusse, D., Tremblay, R. E., & Boivin, M. (2009). Early child language mediates the relation between home environment and school readiness. *Child Development*, 80(3).

Fosmoe, R. J., Holm, R. S., & Hildreth, R. C. (1968). Van Buchem's disease (hyperostosis corticalis generalisata familiaris). *Radiology*, 90, 771–774.

Fowler, K. B., & Boppana, S. B. (2006). Congenital cytomegalovirus (CMV): Infection and hearing deficit. *Journal of Clinical Virology*, 35(2), 226–231.

Fowler, K. B., McCollister, F. P., Dahle, A. J., Boppana, S., Britt, W. J., & Pass, R. F. (1997). Progressive and fluctuating sensorineural hearing loss in children with asymptomatic congenital cytomegalovirus infection. *Journal of Pediatrics*, 130, 624–630.

Fowler, K. B., Stagno, S., Pass, R. F., Brittm, W. J., Boll, T. J., & Alford, C. A. (1992). The outcome of congenital cytomegalovirus infection in relation to maternal antibody status. *New England Journal of Medicine*, 326, 663–667.

Frankenburg, W. K., & Camp, B. W. (1975). *Pediatric screening tests*. Springfield, IL: Charles C Thomas.

Fraser, G. R. (1962). Our genetical load. *Annals of Human Genetics*, 25, 387–415.

Fraser, G. R. (1965). Association of congenital deafness with goiter (Pendred's syndrome). A study of 207 families. *Annals of Human Genetics*, 28, 201–249.

Fraser, W. I., & Cambell, B. M. (1978). A study of six cases of de Lange Amsterdam syndrome, with special attention to voice, speech, and language characteristics. *Developmental Medicine and Child Neurology*, 20, 189–198.

Freitas, V. S., Alvarenga, K., Bevilacqua, M. C., Martinez, M. A., & Costa, O. A. (2009). Critical analysis of three newborn hearing screening protocols. *Pro Fono*, 21(3), 201–206.

French, N. R., & Steinberg, J. C. (1979). Factors governing the intelligibility of speech sounds. *Journal of Acoustical Society of America*, 19, 90–119.

Fria, T. (1980). The auditory brainstem response: Background and clinical applications. *Monographs in Contemporary Audiology*, 2(2), 37.

Fria, T., LeBlanc, J., Kristensen, R., & Alberti, P. (1975). Ipsilateral acoustic reflex stimulation in normal and sensorineural impaired ears: A preliminary report. *Canadian Journal of Otology*, 4, 695–703.

Fria, T. J., Cantekin, E. I., & Eichler, J. A. (1985). Hearing acuity of children with otitis media with effusion. *Otolaryngology-Head and Neck Surgery*, 111, 10–16.

Friederichs, E., & Friederichs, P. (2005). Electrophysiologic and psycho-acoustic findings following one-year application of a personal ear-level device in children with attention deficit and suspected central auditory processing disorder. *Journal of Educational Audiology*, 12, 31–36.

Friedman, A., Schulman, R., & Weiss, S. (1975). Hearing and diabetic neuropathy. *Archives of Internal Medicine*, 135, 573–576.

Friedman, O., Wang, T. D., & Milczuk, H. A. (2005). Cleft lip and palate. In C. W. Cummings, P. W. Flint, B. H. Haughey, et al. (Eds.), *Otolaryngology: Head and neck surgery* (4th ed.). Philadelphia, PA: Mosby Elsevier.

Froding, C. (1960). Acoustic investigation of newborn infants. *Acta Oto-Laryngologica*, 52, 31–41.

Froeschels, E., & Beebe, H. (1946). Testing hearing of newborn infants. *Archives of Otolaryngology*, 44, 710–714.

Fromkin, V., Krashen, S., Curtiss, S., Rigler, D., & Rigler, M. (1974). The development of language in Genie: A case of language acquisition beyond the "critical period." *Brain and Language*, 1, 81–107.

Fryauf-Bertschy, H., Tyler, R., Kelsay, M. R., Gantz, B. J., & Woodworth, G. G. (1997). Cochlear implant use by prelingually deafened children: The influences of age at implant and length of device use. *Journal of Speech, Language, and Hearing Research, 40*, 183–199.

Fryer, D. A., Winckleman, A. C., & Ways, P. O. (1971). Refsum's disease. *Neurology, 21*, 162–167.

Fujikawa, S., Yang, L., Waffarn, F., & Lerner, M. (1997). Persistent pulmonary hypertension of the newborn (PPHN) treated with inhaled nitric oxide: Preliminary hearing outcomes. *Journal of the American Academy of Audiology, 8*, 263–268.

Fuller, D., Pimente, J., & Peregoy, B. (2011). *Applied anatomy and physiology for speech-language pathology and audiology.* Baltimore, MD: Lippencott Williams & Wilkins.

Fulton, R. T., Gorzycki, P. A., & Hull, W. L. (1975). Hearing assessment with young children. *Journal of Speech and Hearing Disorders, 40*, 397–404.

Gabbard, S. A., Northern, J. L., & Yoshinaga-Itano, C. (1999). Hearing screening in newborns under 24 hours of age. *Seminars in Hearing, 20*(3), 291–305.

Gaffney, M., Eichwald, J., Grosse, S. D., & Mason, C. A. (2010). Identifying infants with hearing loss—United States, 1999 to 2007. *Morbidity and Mortality CDC Weekly Report, 59*(8), 220–223.

Galambos, R., Hicks, G., & Wilson, M. (1982). Hearing loss in graduates of a tertiary intensive care nursery. *Ear and Hearing, 3*(1), 87–90.

Galambos, R., Hicks, G., & Wilson, M. (1984). The auditory brainstem response reliably predicts hearing loss in graduates of a tertiary intensive care nursery. *Ear and Hearing, 5*(4), 254–260.

Gallaudet Research Institute. (2003). *Regional and national summary report of data from the 2001–2002 annual survey of deaf and hard-of-hearing children and youth.* Washington, DC: GRI, Gallaudet University. Retrieved from http://research.gallaudet.edu/Demographics/2002_National_Summary.pdf

Gallaudet Research Institute. (2008). *Regional and national summary report of data from the 2001–2002 annual survey of deaf and hard-of-hearing children and youth.* Washington, DC: Gallaudet University.

Gallaudet University Center for Assessment and Demographic Study. (1998). Thirty years of the annual survey of deaf and hard-of-hearing children and youth: A glance over the decades. *American Annals of the Deaf, 142*(2), 72–76.

Galster, J. A., & Abrams, H. (2012). Are you ready for remote hearing aid programming? *Hearing Review, 19*(10), 26–29.

Galster, J. A., Valentine, S., Dundas, J. A., & Fitz, K. (2011). *Spectral iQ: Audibly improving access to high-frequency sounds* [White paper from Starkey Labs, Eden Prairie, MN]. Retrieved from http://www.spectraliq.com/pdfs/spectral-iq-wht-paper.pdf

Gans, D. P. (1987). Improving behavioral observation audiometry testing and scoring problems. *Ear and Hearing, 8*, 92–99.

Gans, D. P., & Flexer, C. (1982). Observer bias in the hearing testing of profoundly involved multiply handicapped children. *Ear and Hearing, 3*, 309–313.

Gans, D. P., & Flexer, C. (1983). Auditory response behavior of severely and profoundly multiply handicapped children. *Journal of Auditory Research, 23*, 137–146.

Gans, R. (2014). Evaluation and management of vestibular function in infants and children with hearing loss. In J. Madell & C. Flexer (Eds.), *Pediatric audiology: Diagnosis, technology, and management* (2nd ed.). New York, NY: Thieme.

Gans, R. E. (2012). *Online Global Education and Training Hearing Review, 19*(10), 34–38.

Gates, G. A. (1988). Adenoidectomy in the management of otitis media in children. In A. Lalwani & K. Grundfast (Eds.), *Pediatric otology and neurotology* (pp. 241–250). Philadelphia, PA: Lippincott-Raven Publishers.

Gattuso, J., Patton, M. A., & Baraitser, M. (1987). The clinical spectrum of the Fraser syndrome: Report of three new cases and review. *Journal of Medical Genetics, 24*(9), 549–555.

Gedicke, M. M., Traupe, H., Fischer, B., Tinschert, S., & Hennies, H. C. (2006). Towards characterization of palmoplantar keratoderma caused by gain-of-function mutation in loricrin: Analysis of a family and review of the literature. *British Journal of Dermatology, 154*(1), 167–171.

Geers, A. E. (2003). Predictors of reading skill development in children with early cochlear implantation. *Ear and Hearing, 24*(1), 59S–68S.

Geers, A. E. (2006). Factors influencing spoken language outcomes in children following early cochlear implantation. *Advances in Oto-Rhino-Laryngology, 64,* 50–65.

Geers. A., & Brenner, C. (2003). Background and educational characteristics of prelingually deaf children implanted by five years of age. *Ear and Hearing,* 24(1), 2S–14S.

Geers, A., & Moog, J. (1990). *Early speech perception test.* St. Louis, MO: Central Institute for the Deaf.

Geers, A. E., & Moog, J. (1994). Effectiveness of cochlear implant and tactile aids for deaf children: the sensory aids study at the Central Institute for the Deaf. *Volta Review, 96,* 5.

Geers, A. E., Moog, J., & Schick, B. (1984). Acquisition of spoken and signed English by profoundly deaf children. *Journal of Speech and Hearing Disorders, 49,* 378–388.

Geers, A. E., & Schick, B. (1988). Acquisition of spoken and signed English by hearing-impaired children of hearing-impaired or hearing parents. *Journal of Speech and Hearing Disorders, 53,* 136–143.

Geers, A. E., Tobey, E. A., & Moog, J. S. (2011). Editorial: Long-term outcomes of cochlear implantation in early childhood. *Ear and Hearing, 32*(1).

Geffner, D., & Ross-Swain, D. (2006). *The listening inventory manual.* Novato, CA: Academic Therapy.

Geffner, D., & Ross-Swain, D. (2013). *Auditory processing disorders: Assessment, management and treatment* (2nd ed.). San Diego, CA: Plural.

Gelfand, S. A., Silman, S., & Ross, L. (1987). Long-term effects of monaural, binaural and no amplification in subjects with bilateral hearing loss. *Scandinavian Audiology, 16,* 201–207.

Gifford, R. H. (2011). Who is a cochlear implant candidate? *The Hearing Journal, 64*(6), 14–18.

Gifford, R. H. (2012). FDA indications for pediatric cochlear implantation fail to reflect current research. *The Hearing Journal, 63*(10), 12–14.

Gifford, R. H. (2013). *Cochlear implant patient assessment: Evaluation of candidacy, performance, and outcomes.* San Diego, CA: Plural.

Gilley, P., Sharma, A., Mitchell, T., & Dorman, M. (2010). The influence of a sensitive period for auditory-visual integration in children with cochlear implants, *Restorative Neurology and Neuroscience, 28*(2), 207–218.

Gladney, J. H., & Monteleone, P. I. (1970). Metaphysical dysplasia. Genetic and otolaryngologic aspects. *Archives of Otolaryngology, 92,* 147–153.

Glass, L., Shapiro, I., Hodge, S. E., Bergstrom, L., & Rimoin, D. L. (1981). Audiologic findings of patients with achondroplasia. *International Journal of Pediatric Otorhinolaryngology, 3,* 129–135.

Glattke, T., & Fujikawa, S. (1991). Otoacoustic emissions. *American Journal of Audiology, 1,* 29–49.

Glista, D., Scollie, S., Bagatto, M., Seewald, R., Parsa, V., & Johnson, A. (2009). Evaluation of nonlinear frequency compression: Clinical outcomes. *International Journal of Audiology, 48*(9), 632–644.

Goehring, J. L., Hughes, M. L., & Baudhuin, J. L. (2012). Evaluating the feasibility of using remote technology for cochlear implants. *The Volta Review, 112*(3), 255–266.

Goldstein, R., & Rodman, L. B. (1967). Early components of averaged evoked responses to rapidly repeated auditory stimuli. *Journal of Speech and Hearing Research, 10,* 697–705.

Gopnik, A., Meltzoff, A., & Kuhl, P. (1999). *The scientist in the crib: What early learning tells us about the mind.* New York, NY: HarperCollins.

Gorga, M. P., Kaminski, J. R., & Beauchaine, K. A. (1988). Auditory brainstem responses from graduates of an intensive care nursery using an insert earphone. *Ear and Hearing, 9*(3), 144–147.

Gorga, M. P., Kaminski, J. R., Beauchaine, K. L., Jesteadt, W., & Neely, S. T. (1989). Auditory brainstem responses from children three months to three years of age: Normal patterns of response II. *Journal of Speech and Hearing Research, 32*, 281–288.

Gorga, M. P., Reiland, J. K., Beauchaine, K. A., Worthington, D. W., & Jesteadt, W. (1987). Auditory brainstem responses from graduates of an intensive care nursery: Normal patterns of response. *Journal of Speech and Hearing Research, 30*, 311–318.

Gorga, M. P., Worthington, D. W., Reiland, J., Beauchaine, K. A., & Goldgar, D. E. (1985). Some comparisons between auditory brainstem response thresholds, latencies and the pure tone audiogram. *Ear and Hearing, 6*(2), 105–112.

Gorlin, R., Cohen Jr., M., & Hennekam, R. (2001). *Syndromes of the head and neck.* Oxford, United Kingdom: Oxford University Press.

Gorlin, R. J., Anderson, R. C., & Blaw, M. (1969). Multiple lentigines syndrome. *American Journal of Diseases in Children, 117*, 652–662.

Gould, H. J. (1989). Audiologic findings in Pierre Robin. *Ear and Hearing, 10*, 211–213.

Gould, J. H., & Caldarelli, D. D. (1982). Hearing and otopathology in Apert syndrome. *Archives of Otolaryngology, 108*, 347–349.

Goulden, K., & Hodge, M. (1998). Neurogenic communicative disorders of childhood. In A. F. Johnson & B. H. Jacobson (Eds.), *Medical speech-pathology: A practitioner's guide* (pp. 409–422). New York, NY: Thieme Medical.

Gravel, J. (1989). Behavioral assessment of auditory function. *Seminars in Hearing, 10*, 217–228.

Gravel, J., Berg, A., Bradley, M., Cacace, A., Campbell, D., Dalzell, L., . . . Prieve, B. (2000). The New York State universal newborn hearing screening demonstration project: Effects of screening protocol on inpatient outcome measures. *Ear and Hearing, 21*(2), 131–140.

Gravel, J., & Ellis, M. (1995). The auditory consequences of otitis media with effusion: The audiogram and beyond. *Seminars in Hearing, 16*(1), 44–59.

Gravel, J., Fischer, R. M., & Chase, P. (2009). Bess and hearing screening; portending the challenges in children. *Seminars in Hearing, 30*(2), 71–79.

Gravel, J., & Traquina, D. (1992). Experience with the audiological assessment of infants and toddlers. *International Journal of Pediatric Otorhinology, 23*(1), 59–72.

Gravel, J., & Wallace, I. (1992). Listening and language at 4 years of age. *Journal of Speech and Hearing Research, 35*, 588–595.

Gravel, J., & Wallace, I. (1995). Early otitis media, auditory abilities and educational risk. *American Journal of Speech-Language Pathology, 4*(3), 9–94.

Gravel, J., & Wallace, I. (1998). Audiologic management of otitis media. In F. Bess (Ed.), *Children with hearing impairments: Contemporary trends* (pp. 215–227). Nashville, TN: Vanderbilt Bill Wilkerson Center Press.

Gravel, J., & Wallace, I. (2000). Effects of otitis media with effusion on hearing in the first 3 years of life. *Journal of Speech and Hearing Research, 43*, 631–644.

Greenberg, M. T. (1975). Hearing families with deaf children: Stress and functioning as related to communication method. *American Annals of the Deaf, 125*, 1063.

Greenberg, M. T., Calderon, R., & Kusche, C. (1984). Early intervention using simultaneous communication with deaf infants: The effect on communication development. *Child Development, 55*, 607–616.

Grieser, D. L., & Kuhl, P. K. (1988). Maternal speech to infants in a tonal language: Support for universal prosodic features in motherese. *Developmental Psychology, 24*, 14–20.

Grosse, S. D. (2007). Education cost savings from early detection of hearing loss: New findings. *Volta Voices, 14*(6), 38–40.

Guly, A. J. (2007). *Anatomy of the temporal bone with surgical implications* (3rd ed.). New York, NY: Informa Healthcare USA.

Haapaniemi, J. J. (1996). The hearing threshold levels of children at school age. *Ear and Hearing, 17*(6), 469–477.

Haas, N., Küster, W., Zuberbier, T., & Henz, B. M. (1978). Muckle-Wells syndrome: Clinical and histological skin findings compatible with cold air urticaria in a large kindred. *British Journal of Dermatology, 151*(1), 99–104.

Hagerman, R. J., Berry-Kravis, E., Kaufmann, W. E., Ono, M. Y., Tartaglia, N., Lachiewicz, A., . . . Tranfaglia, M. (2009). Advances in the treatment of fragile X syndrome. *Pediatrics, 123*(1), 378–390.

Hakansson, B., Carlsson, P., Tjellstrom, A., & Liden, G. (1994). The bone-anchored hearing aid: Principal design and audiometric results. *Ear Nose and Throat Journal, 73*(9), 670–675.

Hale, D. E., Cody, J. D., Baillargeon, J., Schaub, R., Danney, M. M., & Leach, R. J. (2003). The spectrum of growth abnormalities in children with 18q deletions. *Journal of Clinical Endocrinology and Metabolism, 85*(12), 4450–4454.

Hall, B. (1979). Choanal atresia and associated multiple anomalies. *Journal of Pediatrics, 95*, 395.

Hall, J. G., & Rohrt, T. (1968). The stapes in osteogenesis imperfecta. *Acta Oto-Laryngologica (Stockholm), 65*, 345–348.

Hall, J. W, III. (1978). Predicting hearing loss from the acoustic reflex: A comparison of three methods. *Archives of Otolaryngology, 104*, 601–605.

Hall, J. W., III. (2000). *Handbook of otoacoustic emissions*. San Diego, CA: Singular.

Hall, J. W., III. (2007). *New handbook of auditory evoked potentials*. Boston, MA: Allyn & Bacon.

Hall, J. W., III., Bantwal, A., Ramkumar, V., & Chhabria, N. (2011). Electrophysiologic assessment of hearing with auditory middle latency and auditory late responses. In R. Seewald & A.M. Tharpe (Eds.), *Comprehensive handbook of pediatric audiology* (pp. 449–482). San Diego, CA: Plural.

Hall, J. W., III, & Johnston, K. (2007). Electroacoustic and electrophysiologic auditory measures on the assessment of (central) auditory processing disorder. In F. Musiek & G. Chermak (Eds.), *Handbook of (central) auditory processing disorder: Vol I: Auditory neuroscience and diagnosis* (pp. 287–315). San Diego, CA: Plural.

Hall, J. W., III, Johnston, K. N., John, A. B., Kreisman, N. V., & Crandell, C. C. (2010). *Multiple benefits of Phonak Edulink use by children with auditory processing disorder (APD)*. Naperville, IL: Phonak.

Hall, J. W., III, Prentice, C. H., Smiley, G., & Werkhaven, J. (1995). Auditory dysfunction in selected syndromes and patterns of malformations. *Journal of the American Academy of Audiology, 6*(1), 80–92.

Hall, J. W., III, & Swanepoel, D. W. (2010). *Objective assessment of hearing*. San Diego, CA: Plural.

Hall, S., Burns, D., Lightbody, A., & Reiss, A. (2008). Longitudinal changes in intellectual development in children with fragile X syndrome. *Journal of Abnormal Child Psychology, 36*(6), 927–939.

Hallgren, V. (1959). Retinitis pigmentosa combined with congenital deafness; with vestibulo-cerebellar ataxia and mental abnormality in a portion of cases. *Acta Psychiatrica Scandinavica Supplementum, 138*, 1–101.

Harboyan, G., Mamo, J., der Kalonstian, V., & Karam, F. (1971). Congenital corneal dystrophy. Progressive sensorineural deafness in a family. *Archives of Ophthalmology, 75*, 27–32.

Harris, S., Ahlfors, K., Ivarsson, S., Lemmark, B., & Svanberg, L. (1984). Congenital cytomegalo-virus infection and sensorineural hearing loss. *Ear and Hearing, 5*, 352–355.

Harrison, J., & Hutsell, G. (2009). What is auditory-oral education? In L. Seaver (Ed.), *Book of choice: Support for parenting a child who is deaf or hard-of-hearing* (2nd ed.). Boulder, CO: Hands and Voices.

Hart, B., & Risley, T. (1995). *Meaningful differences in the everyday experience of young American children*. Baltimore, MD: Paul H. Brookes.

Harvey, A. S. (1991). CHARGE association: Clinical manifestations and developmental outcome. *American Journal of Medical Genetics, 39*, 48–55.

Haskins, H. (1949). *A phonetically balanced test of speech discrimination for children*. (Unpublished master's thesis). Northwestern University, Evanston, IL.

Hawkins, D., & Cook, J. (2003). Hearing aid software predictive gain values: How accurate are they? *Hearing Journal, 56*(7).

Hawkins, D., & Yacuillo, W. W. (1984). Signal-to-noise ratio advantage of binaural hearing aids and directional microphones under different levels of reverberation. *Journal of Speech and Hearing Disorders, 49*, 278–286.

Hawkins, D. B. (1984). Comparisons of speech recognition in noise by mildly-to-moderately hearing-impaired children using hearing aids and FM systems. *Journal of Speech and Hearing Disorders, 49*, 409–418.

Hawkins, D. B., Prosek, R., Walden, B., & Montgomery, A. (1987). Binaural loudness summation in the hearing-impaired. *Journal of Speech and Hearing Research, 30*, 37–43.

Hawkins, H. B., Shapiro, R., & Petrillo, C. J. (1975). The association of cleidocranial dysotosis with hearing loss. *American Journal of Roentgenology, 125*, 944–947.

Hayes, D. (1994). Hearing loss in infants with craniofacial anomalies. *Archives of Otolaryngology-Head and Neck Surgery, 110*(1), 39–46.

Hayes, D. (1999). State programs for universal newborn hearing screening. *Pediatric Clinics of North America, 46*(1), 89–93.

Hayes, D. (2000). The New York State Project: A leap to the future. *Ear and Hearing, 21*(2), 83.

Hayes, D. (2012). Infant diagnostic evaluations using tele-audiology. *Hearing Review, 19*(10), 30–31.

Hayes, D., Eclavea, E., Dreith, S., & Habte, B. (2012). From Colorado to Guam: Infant diagnostic audiological evaluations by telepractice. *Volta Review, 112*(3), 243–254.

Hayes, D., & Jerger, J. (1978). Response detection in respiration audiometry. *Archives of Otolaryngology, 104*, 183–185.

Hayes, D., & Northern, J. L. (1996). *Infants and hearing.* San Diego, CA: Singular.

Hayes, D., & Sininger, Y. (Eds.). (2008). *Guidelines to identification and management of infants and young children with auditory neuropathy spectrum disorder.* Denver, CO: Bill Daniels Center for Children's Hearing, The Children's Hospital.

Hayes, E., Babin, R., & Platz, C. (1980). The otologic manifestations of mucopolysaccharidoses. *American Journal of Otology, 2*, 65.

Healey, B. (1996). The Council for Exceptional Children. *CEC Today, 3*(5).

Hecox, K., & Jacobson, J. (1984). Auditory evoked potentials. In J. L. Northern (Ed.), *Hearing disorders.* Boston, MA: Little, Brown & Co.

Hecox, K., Squires, N., & Galambos, R. (1976). Brainstem auditory evoked responses in man. Effect of stimulus rise-fall time and duration. *Journal of the Acoustical Society of America, 60*, 1187–1192.

Hegyi, T., Carbone, T., Anwar, M., Ostfeld, B., Hiatt, M., Koons, A., . . . Paneth, N. (1998). The Apgar score and its components in the preterm infant. *Pediatrics, 101*(1), 77–81.

Helenius, K. K., Laine, M. K., Tähtinen, P. A., Laht, E., & Ruohola, A. (2012). Tympanometry in discrimination of otoscopic diagnoses in young ambulatory children. *Pediatric Infectious Disease Journal, 31*(10), 1003–1006.

Hendricks-Munoz, K. D., & Walton, J. P. (1988). Hearing loss in infants with persistent fetal circulation. *Pediatrics, 81*(5), 650–656.

Hepper, P., & Shahidullah, B. (1994). Development of fetal hearing. *Archives of Diseases in Children and Fetal Neonatal Education, 71*(2), F81–F87.

Herrmann, C., Jr., Aguilar, M. J., & Sacks, O. W. (1964). Hereditary photomyoclonus associated with diabetes mellitus, deafness, nephropathy and cerebral dysfunction. *Neurology, 14*, 212–221.

Herrmann, B. S., Thornton, A. R., & Joseph, J. M. (1995). Automated infant hearing screening using the ABR: Development and validation. *American Journal of Audiology, 4*, 6–14.

Hicks, T., Fowler, K., Richardson, M., Dahl, A., Adams, L., & Pass, R. (1993). Congenital cytomegalovirus infection and neonatal auditory screening. *Journal of Pediatrics, 123*, 779–782.

Hoberman, A., Paradise, J. L., Rockette, H. E., Shaikh, N., Wald, E. R., Kearney, D. H., . . . Barbadora, K. A. (2011). Treatment of acute otitis media in children under two years of age. *New England Journal of Medicine, 364*(2), 105–115.

Hodges, A., & Ruth, R. (1987). Subject related factors influencing the acoustic reflex. *Seminars in Hearing, 8,* 339–357.

Hoff, E. (2012). Interpreting the early language trajectories of children from low-SES and language minority homes: Implications for closing achievement gaps. *Developmental Psychology, 49*(1), 4–14.

Holmes, E. M. (1949). The microtia ear. *Archives of Otolaryngology, 49,* 243–265.

Holmes, L. B. (1971). Nome's disease; An X-linked syndrome of retinal malformation, mental retardation, and deafness. *Journal of Pediatrics, 70,* 89–92.

Hood, D. C. (1975). Evoked cortical response audiometry. In L. Bradford (Ed.), *Physiological measures of the audio-vestibular system.* New York, NY: Academic Press.

Hood, L. (2011). Variation in auditory neuropathy spectrum disorder: Implications for evaluation and management. *Seminars in Hearing, 32*(2), 117–122.

Hood, L. J. (1998). *Clinical applications of the auditory brainstem response.* San Diego, CA: Singular.

Hood, L. J., & Berlin, C. I. (1996). Central auditory function and disorders. In J. L. Northern (Ed.), *Hearing disorders* (3rd ed., pp. 227–244). Needham Heights, MA: Allyn & Bacon.

Hornickel, J., Zecker, S., Bradlow, A., & Kraus, N. (2012). Assistive listening devices drive neuroplasticity in children with dyslexia. *Proceedings of the National Academy of Sciences. 109*(41), 16731–16736.

Horton, K. B. (1975). Early intervention through parent training. *Otolaryngology Clinics of North America, 8,* 143–157.

Hosford-Dunn, H., Johnson, S., Simmons, F. B., Malachowski, N., & Low, K. (1987). Infant hearing screening: Program implementation and validation. *Ear and Hearing, 8*(1), 12–20.

Houlden, H., King, R., Blake J., Groves, M., Love, S., Woodward, C., . . . Reilly, M. (2006). Clinical, pathological and genetic characterization of hereditary sensory and autonomic neuropathy type 1 (HSANI). *Brain, 129*(2), 411–425.

Houston, K. T., Stredler-Brown, A., & Alverson, D. C. (2012). More than 150 years in the making: The evolution of telepractice for hearing. *Volta Review, 112*(10), 195–206.

Houston, T., & Stredler-Brown, A. (2012). A model of early intervention for children with hearing loss provided through teleprac-tice. *Volta Review, 112*(3), 283.

Howie, V. M., Ploussard, J. H., & Sloyer, J. (1975). The "otitis-prone" condition. *American Journal of Diseases in Children, 129,* 676–678.

Hughes, P. J., Davies, P. T., Roche, S. W., Matthews, T. D., & Lane, R. J. (1991). Wilder-vanck or cervico-oculo-acoustic syndrome and MRI findings. *Journal of Neurology, Neurosurgery and Psychiatry, 54,* 503–504.

Hull, F. M., Mielke, P. W., Timmons, R. J., & Williford, J. (1971). The national speech and hearing survey: Preliminary results. *Asha, 13,* 501–509.

Hunter, L. L., Davey, C. S., Kohtz, A., & Daly, K. A. (2007). Hearing screening and middle ear measures in American Indian infants and toddlers. *International Journal of Pediatric Otorhinolaryngology, 71*(9), 1429–1438.

Hunter, L. L., & Margolis, R. H. (1992). Multifrequency tympanometry: Current clinical application. *American Journal of Audiology, 1,* 33–43.

Hunter, L. L., & Margolis, R. H. (2011). Middle ear measurement. In R. Seewald & A. M. Tharpe (Eds.), *Comprehensive handbook of pediatric audiology.* San Diego, CA: Plural.

Huttenlocher, J., Waterfall, H., Vasilyeva, M., Vevea, J., & Hedges, L. V. (2010). Sources of variability in children's language growth. *Cognitive Psychology, 61*(4), 343–365.

Ide, C. H., & Wollschlaeger, P. P. (1969). Multiple congenital abnormalities associated with cryptophthalmia. *Archives of Ophthalmology, 81,* 640–644.

IHAFF. (1994). *Independent hearing aid fitting forum manual.* Yorba Linda, CA: Dennis Van Vliet.

Ikeda, M. K., & Jenson, H. B. (1990). Evaluation and treatment of congenital syphilis. *Journal of Pediatrics, 117,* 843.

Ilium, P., Kaier, H. W., Hvidberg-Hansen, J., & Sondergaard, G. (1972). Fifteen cases of Pendred's syndrome. *Archives of Otolaryngology, 96*, 297–304.

Individuals with Disabilities Education Act (IDEA). (2004). Retrieved from http://idea .ed.gov/

Ireton, H., & Thwing, E. (1972). *The Minnesota Child Development Inventory.* Minneapolis, MN: University of Minnesota.

Irwin, O. C. (1947). Infant speech: Consonantal sounds according to manner of articulation. *Journal of Speech and Hearing Disorders, 12*, 402–404.

Isaacs, J. B. (2012). *Starting school at a disadvantage: The school readiness of poor children.* Retrieved from http://www.brookings.edu/ research/papers/2012/03/19-school-disad vantage-isaacs

Iwashita, H., Inoue, N., Araki, S., & Kuroiwa, Y. (1970). Optic atrophy, neural deafness and distal neurogenic amyotrophy. *Archives of Neurology, 22*, 357–364.

Jackson, L., Kline, A. D., Barr, M. A., & Koch, S. (1993). Cornelia de Lange syndrome: A clinical review of 310 individuals. *American Journal of Medical Genetics, 47*(7), 940–946.

Jacobson, J. T. (1996). Short-latency auditory evoked potentials. In J. Northern (Ed.), *Hearing disorders* (3rd ed., pp. 73–97). Needham Heights, MA: Allyn & Bacon.

Jacobson, J. T., & Jacobson, C. A. (1987). Application of test performance characteristics in newborn auditory screening. *Seminars in Hearing, 8*(2), 133–141.

Jahrsdoerfer, R. A., & Hall, J. W., III. (1986). Congenital malformations of the ear. *American Journal of Otology, 7*, 267–269.

Jahrsdoerfer, R. A., & Jacobson, J. T. (1995). Treacher Collins syndrome: Otologic and auditory management. *Journal of the American Academy of Audiology, 6*(1), 93–102.

Janssens, K., Vanhoenacker, F., Bonduelle, M., Verbruggen, L., Van Maldergem, L., Ralston, S., . . . Van Hul, W. (2006). Camurati-Engelmann disease: Review of the clinical, radiological, and molecular data of 24 families and implications for diagnosis and treatment. *Journal of Medical Genetics, 43*(1), 1–11.

Janvier, A., & Farlow, W. (2012). The experience of families with children with trisomy 13 and 18 in social networks. *Pediatrics, 130*(2), 293–298.

Jensen, B. L. (1990). Somatic development in cleidocranial dysplasia. *American Journal of Medical Genetics, 35*, 69–74.

Jerger, J. (1970). Clinical experience with impedance audiometry. *Archives of Otolaryngology, 92*, 311–324.

Jerger, J., Anthony, L., Jerger, S., & Mauldin, L. (1974a). Studies in impedance audiometry: III. Middle ear disorders. *Archives of Otolaryngology, 99*, 165–171.

Jerger, J., Burney, P., Mauldin, L., & Crump, B. (1974b). Predicting hearing loss from the acoustic reflex. *Journal of Speech and Hearing Disorders, 39*, 11–22.

Jerger, J., Chmiel, R., Frost, J., & Coker, N. (1986). Effect of sleep on the auditory steady state evoked potential. *Ear and Hearing, 7*(4), 240–245.

Jerger, J., & Hayes, D. (1976). The cross-check principle in pediatric audiometry. *Archives of Otolaryngology, 102*, 614–620.

Jerger, J., & Hayes, D. (1980). Diagnostic applications of impedance audiometry: Middle ear disorder: Sensorineural disorder. In J. Jerger & J. L. Northern (Eds.), *Clinical impedance audiometry* (2nd ed., pp. 109–127). Acton, MA: American Electromedics.

Jerger, J., Hayes, D., Anthony, L., & Mauldin, L. (1978). Factors influencing prediction of hearing level from the acoustic reflex. *Contemporary Monographs in Audiology, 1*, 1.

Jerger, J., Hayes, D., & Jordon, C. (1980). Clinical experience with auditory brainstem response audiometry in pediatric assessment. *Ear and Hearing, 1*, 19–25.

Jerger, J., & Jerger, S. (1970). Temporary threshold shift in rock-and-roll musicians. *Journal of Speech and Hearing Research, 13*, 218–224.

Jerger, J., Jerger, S., & Mauldin, L. (1972). Studies in impedance audiometry: I. Normal and sensorineural ears. *Archives of Otolaryngology, 96*, 513–523.

Jerger, J., & Musiek, F. (2000). Report of the consensus conference on the diagnosis of auditory processing disorders in school-aged children.

Journal of the American Academy of Audiology, 11(9), 467–474.

Jerger, J., Oliver, T., & Chmiel, R. (1988). The auditory middle latency response. *Seminars in Hearing, 9*(1), 75–86.

Jerger, S. (1983). Decision matrix and information theory analyses in the evaluation of neuroaudiologic tests. *Seminars in Hearing, 4*(2), 121–132.

Jerger, S., & Jerger, J. (1983). Pediatric speech intelligibility test: Performance-intensity characteristics. *Ear and Hearing, 4*, 138–145.

Jerger, S., Jerger, J., Alford, B., & Abrams, S. (1983). Development of speech intelligibility in children with recurrent otitis media. *Ear and Hearing, 4*, 138–145.

Jerger, S., Jerger, J., & Lewis, S. (1981). Pediatric speech intelligibility test: II. Effect of receptive language age and chronological age. *International Journal of Pediatric Otorhinolaryngology, 3*, 101–118.

Jerger, S., Jerger, J., Mauldin, L., & Segal, P. (1974). Studies in impedance audiometry: II. Children less than 6 years old. *Archives of Otolaryngology, 99*, 1–9.

Jerger, S., Lewis, S., Hawkins, J., & Segal, M. (1980). Pediatric Speech Intelligibility Test: I. Generation of test materials. *International Journal of Pediatric Otorhinolaryngology, 2*, 217–230.

Jervell, A., & Lange-Nielsen, F. (1957). Congenital deaf-mutism, functional heart disease with prolongation of the QT interval, and sudden death. *American Heart Journal, 54*, 59–68.

Jewett, D., & Williston, J. S. (1971). Auditory evoked far fields averaged from the scalp of humans. *Brain, 94*, 681–696.

Johansson, B., Wedenberg, E., & Westin, B. (1964). Measurement of tone response by the human fetus. *Acta Oto-Laryngologica (Stockholm), 57*, 188–192.

Johnsen, T., Larsen, C., Friis, J., & Hougaard-Jensen, F. (1987). Pendred's syndrome: Acoustic, vestibular and radiological findings in 17 unrelated patients. *Journal of Laryngology and Otology, 101*, 1187–1192.

Johnson, C. D., Benson, P. V., & Seaton, J. B. (1997). *Educational audiology handbook*. San Diego, CA: Singular.

Johnson, C. D., & Von Almen, P. (1997). Functional listening evaluation. In C. D. Johnson, P. V. Benson, & J. B. Seaton, *Educational audiology handbook* (pp. 336–339). San Diego, CA: Singular.

Johnson, G. (1995, June 6). Chimp talk debate: Is it really language? *The New York Times*.

Johnson, J. L., White, K. R., Widen, J. E., Gravel, J. S., James, M., Kennalley, J. M., . . . Holstrum, J. (2005). A multicenter evaluation of how many infants with permanent hearing loss pass a two-stage otoacoustic emissions/automated auditory brainstem response newborn hearing screening protocol. *Pediatrics, 116*(3), 663–670.

Johnson, J. S., & Watrous, B. S. (1978). An acoustic impedance screening program with an American Indian population. In E. R. Harford, F. H. Bess, C. D. Bluestone, & J. O. Klein (Eds.), *Impedance screening for middle ear disease in children*. New York, NY: Grune & Stratton.

Johnson, L. G., & Arenberg, K. (1981). Cochlear abnormalities in Alport's syndrome. *Otolaryngology-Head and Neck Surgery, 107*, 340–349.

Johnson, R. L. (1967). Chronic otitis media in school-age Navajo Indians. *Laryngoscope, 77*, 1990–1995.

Johnston, C. C., Lawy, N.. Lord, T., Vellios, F., Nerritt, A. D., & Deiss, W. P. (1968). Osteopetrosis: A clinical, genetic, metabolic, and morphologic study of the dominantly inherited benign form. *Medicine, 47*, 149–167.

Johnston, K. N., John, A. B., Kreisman, N., Hall, J., & Crandell, C. C. (2009). Multiple benefits of personal FM system use by children with auditory processing disorder (APD). *International Journal of Audiology, 48*, 371–383.

Joint Committee on Infant Hearing. (1971). Retrieved from http://www.jcih.org/JCIH 1971.pdf

Joint Committee on Infant Hearing. (1973). Retrieved from http://www.jcih.org/JCIH 1973.pdf

Joint Committee on Infant Hearing. (1982). Retrieved from http://www.jcih.org/JCIH 1982.pdf.

Joint Committee on Infant Hearing. (1994). Retrieved from http://www.jcih.org/JCIH 1994.pdf

Joint Committee on Infant Hearing. (1995). Retrieved from http://www.jcih.org/JCIH 1995.pdf.

Joint Committee on Infant Hearing. (2000). Retrieved from http://www.jcih.org/JCIH 2000.pdf.

Joint Committee on Infant Hearing. (2007). Retrieved from http://www.jcih.org/JCIH 2007.pdf.

Jones, F. R., & Simmons, F. B. (1977). Early identification of significant hearing loss: The Crib-o-gram. *Hearing Instruments, 28,* 8–10.

Jones, S. M. (2011). *Genetics, embryology and development of auditory and vestibular systems.* San Diego, CA: Plural.

Jordan, O. (1972). Mental retardation and hearing defects. *Scandinavian Audiology, 1,* 29–32.

Jordan, R. E., & Eagles E. L. (1961). *Annals of Otology, Rhinology, and Laryngology, 102,* 285–288.

Kabakkaya, Y., Bakan, E., Yiğitoglu, M. R., Gökçe, G., & Doğan, M. (1993). Pendred's syndrome. *Annals of Oto-Rhino-Laryngology, 102,* 285–288.

Kahane, J. C. (1979). Pathophysiologic effects of Mòbius syndrome on speech and hearing. *Archives of Otolaryngology-Head and Neck Surgery, 105,* 29–34.

Kamhi, A. G. (1982). Developmental vs. difference theories of mental retardation: A new look. *American Journal of Mental Deficiencies, 86,* 1–7.

Kankkunen, B., & Thuringer, R. (1987). Hearing impairment in connection with preauricular tags. *Acta Paediatrica Scandinavica, 76,* 143–146.

Kaplan, S. L., Catlin, F., Weaver, T., & Feigin, R. D. (1984). Onset of hearing loss in children with bacterial meningitis. *Pediatrics, 73,* 575–579.

Karver, S. (1998). Otitis media. *Primary Care: Clinics in Office Practice, 25,* 691–692.

Katz, J., & Elliott, L. L. (1978). *Development of a new children's speech discrimination test.* Paper presented at the American Speech and Hearing Association Convention, Chicago, IL.

Kavanagh, K. T., Gould, H., McCormick, G., & Franks, R. (1989). Comparison of the iden-tifiability of the low intensity ABR and MLR in the mentally handicapped patient. *Ear and Hearing, 10*(2), 124–130.

Kearsley, R., Snider, M., Richie, R., Crawford, J. D., & Talbot, N. B. (1962). Study of relations between psychologic environment and child behavior. *American Journal of Diseases in Children, 104,* 12–20.

Keats, B. J. B. (1996). Genes and hearing impairment. *Audiology Today, 8*(5), 11–13.

Keefe, D. H., & Levi, E. (1996). Maturation of the middle and external ears: acoustic power-based responses and reflectance tympanometry. *Ear and Hearing, 17,* 361.

Keidser, G., Brew, C., & Peck, A. (2003). How proprietary fitting algorithms compare to each other and to some generic algorithms. *Hearing Journal, 56*(3), 28.

Keith, R. (1973). Impedance audiometry with neonates. *Archives of Otolaryngology, 97,* 465–467.

Keith, R. W. (1975). Middle ear functions in neonates. *Archives of Otolaryngology, 101,* 376–379.

Keith, R. W. (1978). Commentary. Letter to the Editor. *Audiology Hearing Education, 4,* 28.

Keith, R. W. (1986). *SCAN: A screening test for auditory processing disorders.* San Antonio, TX: Psychological Corporation/Harcourt Brace Jovanovich.

Keith, R. W. (1999). Diagnosing central auditory processing disorders in children. In R. Roeser, M. Hosford-Dunn, & M. Valente (Eds.), *Audiology: Diagnosis, treatment strategies and practice management.* New York, NY: Thieme Medical.

Keith, R. W. (2000a). *SCAN-C: Test of auditory processing disorders in children* (Revised). San Antonio, TX: Psychological Corporation.

Keith, R. W. (2000b). Development and standardization of SCAN-C test for auditory processing disorders in children. *Journal of the American Academy of Audiology, 11*(8), 438–445.

Keith, R. W. (2009). *SCAN–3:C tests for auditory processing disorders for children (SCAN-3:C).* San Antonio, TX: Pearson.

Keith, W. J., & Smith, R. P. (1987). Automated pediatric hearing assessment using interactive video images. *Hearing Instruments, 38*(9), 27–28.

Keleman, G. (1966). Hurler's syndrome and the hearing organ. *Journal of Laryngology, 80,* 791–803.

Keleman, G., Hooft, C., & Kluyskens, P. (1968). The inner ear in autosomal trisomy. *Practices in Otorhinolaryngology (Basel), 30,* 251–258.

Kelly, A. American Sign Language. (2010). In L. Seaver (Ed.), *The book of choice: Support for parenting a child who is deaf or hard-of-hearing* (2nd ed.). Boulder, CO: Hands and Voices.

Kelley, M., Wu, D., Popper, A., & Fay, R. (Eds.). (2005). *Development of the inner ear (Springer handbook of auditory science).* New York, NY: Springer Science.

Kemp, D., & Ryan, S. (1993). The use of transient evoked otoacoustic emissions in neonatal hearing screening programs. *Seminars in Hearing, 14,* 30–45.

Kemp, D. T. (1978). Stimulated acoustic emissions from the human auditory system. *Journal of the Acoustical Society of America, 64,* 1386–1391.

Kemp, D. T. (1980). Towards a model for the origin of cochlear echos. *Hearing Research, 2,* 533–548.

Kemperman, M. H., Hoefsloot, L. H., & Cremers, C. W. (2002). Hearing loss and connexin 26. *Royal Journal of Social Medicine, 95*(4), 171–177.

Kemperman, M. H., Koch, S. M., Joosten, F. B., Kumar, S., Huygen, P. L., & Cremers, C. W. (2002). Inner ear anomalies are frequent but nonobligatory features of the branchio-otorenal syndrome. *Archives of Otolaryngology-Head Neck Surgery, 128*(9), 1033–1038.

Kenna, M. A., Feldman, H. A., Neault, M. W., Frangulov, B. S., We, B. L., Fligor, B., & Rehn, H. L. (2010). Audiologic phenotype and progression in *GJB2* (connexin 26) hearing loss. *Archives of Otolaryngology-Head Neck Surgery, 136*(1), 81–87.

Kennedy, C. R., McCann, D. C., Campbell, M. J., Law, C. M., Mullee, M., Petrou, S., . . . Stevenson, J. (2006). Language ability after early detection of permanent childhood hearing impairment. *New England Journal of Medicine, 354,* 2131–2141.

Kent, R. D. (1976). Anatomical and neuromuscular maturation of the speech mechanism: Evidence from acoustical studies. *Journal of Speech and Hearing Research, 19*(3), 421–427.

Kent, R. D., Osberger, M. J., Netsell, R., & Hustedde, C. G. (1987). Phonetic development in identical twins differing in auditory function. *Journal of Speech and Hearing Disorders, 52,* 64–75.

Kerr, G., Smyth, G. D., & Cinnamond, M. (1973). Congenital syphilitic deafness. *Journal of Laryngology and Otology, 87,* 1–12.

Kessels, R. P. C. (2003). Patient's memory for medical information. *Journal of the Royal Society of Medicine, 96*(5), 219–222.

Killion, M., & Mueller, G. (2010). Twenty years later: A new count-the-dots method. *Hearing Journal, 63,* 1, 10–17.

Kimberling, W. J., & Moller, C. (1995). Clinical and molecular genetics of Usher syndrome. *Journal of the American Academy of Audiology, 6*(1), 63–72.

Kimberling, W. J., & Pieke-Dahl, S. (1998). Decoding Usher syndrome. *Hearing Health,* 52–54.

Kirk, K. I., Miyamoto, R. T., Lento, C. I., Yang, E., O'Neill, T., & Fears, B. (2002). Effects of age at implantation in young children. *Annals of Otology, Rhinology, and Laryngology, 189,* 69–73.

Kirk, K. I., Pisoni, D. B., & Osberger, M. J. (1995). Lexical effects on spoken word recognition by pediatric cochlear implant users. *Ear and Hearing, 16,* 470–481.

Kirkham, T. H. (1969). Duane's syndrome and familial perceptive deafness. *British Journal of Ophthalmology, 53,* 335–339.

Kirkim, G., Serbetcioglu, B., Erdag, T. K., & Ceryan, K. (2008). The frequency of auditory neuropathy detected by universal newborn hearing screening program. *Inernational Journal of Pediatric Otolaryngology, 72*(10), 1461–1469.

Klatte, M., Hellbruck, J., Seidel, J., & Leistner, P. (2010). Effects of classroom acoustics on performance and well-being in elementary school children: A field study. *Environment and Behavior, 42*(5), 659–692.

Klein, J. O. (2011a). Children under 2 years of age with acute otitis media benefit from antibiotic treatment. *Journal of Pediatrics, 159*(3), 514–515.

Klein, J. O. (2011b). Is acute otitis media a treatable disease? (2011). *New England Journal of Medicine, 364*(2), 168–169.

Kliegman, R. M., Behrman, R. E., Jenson, H. B., & Stanton, B. F. (Eds.). (2007). *Nelson textbook of pediatrics* (18th ed.). Philadelphia, PA: Saunders Elsevier.

Klinke, R., Kral, A., Heid S., Tilleinj, J., & Hartmann, R. (1999). Recruitment of the auditory cortex in congenitally deaf cats by long-term cochlear electrostimulation. *Science, 285*, 1729–1733.

Kloepfer, H. W., Laguaite, J. K., & McLaurin, J. W. (1966). The hereditary syndrome of deafness in retinitis pigmentosa. *Laryngoscope, 76*, 850–862.

Knight, K. R. G., Kraemer, D. F., & Neuwelt, E. A. (2005). Ototoxicity in children receiving platinum chemotherapy: Underestimating a commonly occurring toxicity that may influence academic and social development. *Journal of Clinical Oncology, 23*(34), 8588–8596.

Knight, K. R. G., Kraemer, D. F., Winter, C., & Neuwelt, E. A. (2007). Early changes in auditory function as a result of platinum chemotherapy: Use of extended high-frequency audiometry and evoked distortion-product otoacoustic emissions. *Journal of Clinical Oncology, 25*(10), 1190–1195.

Kobler, S., & Rosenhall, U. (2002). Horizontal localization and speech intelligibility with bilateral and unilateral hearing aid amplification. *International Journal of Audiology, 45*, 63–71.

Koch, M. (2009). Total communication. In L. Seaver (Ed.), *The book of choice: Support for parenting a child who is deaf or hard-of-hearing* (2nd ed.). Boulder, CO: Hands and Voices.

Kochhar, A., Fischer, S. M., Kimberling, W. J., & Smith, R. J. (2007). Branchio-oto-renal syndrome. *American Journal of Medical Genetics, 143*(14), 1671–1678.

Kochkin, S. (2005). MarkeTrak VII: Hearing loss population tops 31 million people. *Hearing Review, 12*(7), 16–29.

Kochkin, S., Beck, D. L., Christensen, L. A., Compton-Conley, C., Kricos, P. B., Fligor, B. J., . . . Turner, R. G. (2010). MarkeTrak VIII: The impact of the hearing healthcare professional on hearing aid user success. *Hearing Review, 17*(4), 12–34.

Kochkin, S., Luxford, W., Northern, J., Mason, P., & Tharpe, A. M. (2007). Are 1 million dependents with hearing loss in America being left behind? *Hearing Review, 14*(10), 10–37.

Kolb, B. (1989). Brain development, plasticity, and behavior. *American Psychologist, 44*(9), 1203–1212.

Konigsmark, B. W., & Gorlin, R. J. (1976). *Genetic and metabolic deafness.* Philadelphia, PA: W. B. Saunders.

Konigsmark, B. W., Hollander, M. B., & Berlin, C. I. (1968). Familial neural hearing loss and atopic dermatitis. *Journal of the American Medical Association, 204*, 953–957.

Konigsmark, B. W., Mengel, M. C., & Haskins, H. (1970). Familial congenital moderate neural hearing loss. *Journal of Laryngology, 84*, 495–506.

Koop, C. E. (1989). *Importance of early identification of children with hearing problems.* Washington, DC: U. S. Public Health Service, Department of Health and Human Resources Statement.

Koop, C. E. (2010). Pursuing excellence in early hearing detection and intervention programs. *Pediatrics, 126*(Suppl. 1), S1–S2.

Korczak, P., Smart, J., Delgado, R., Strobel, T. M., & Bradford, C. (2012). Auditory steady state responses: A tutorial. *Journal of the American Academy of Audiology, 23*(3), 146–170.

Korf, B., & Rubenstein, A. (Eds.). (2005). *Neurofibromatosis: A handbook for patients, families and healthcare professionals.* New York, NY: Thieme.

Kos, A. O., Schuknecht, H. F., & Singer, J. D. (1966). Temporal bone studies in 13-15 and 18 trisomy syndrome. *Archives of Otolaryngology, 83*, 439–445.

Kral, A., Hartmann, R., Tillein, J., Heide, S., & Klinke, R. (2000). Congenital auditory deprivation reduces synaptic activity within the auditory cortex in a layer-specific manner. *Cerebral Cortex, 10*(7), 714–726.

Kraus, N., Bradlow, A. R., Cheatham, M. A., Cunningham, J., King, C. D., Koch, D. B., . . . Wright, B. A. (2000). Consequences of neural asynchrony: A case of auditory neuropathy. *Journal of the Association of Research in Otolarygology. 1*, 33–45.

Kraus, N., McGee, T., & Comperatore, C. (1989). MLRs in children are consistently present during wakefulness, stage I, and REM sleep. *Ear and Hearing, 10*(6), 339–345.

Kraus, N., Ozdamar, O., Stein, L., & Reed, N. (1984). Absent auditory brainstem response: Peripheral hearing loss or brainstem dysfunction? *Laryngoscope, 94*, 400–406.

Kruger, B. (1987). An update on the external ear resonance in infants and young children. *Ear and Hearing, 8*(6), 333–336.

Kryter, K. D., & Ades, H. W. (1943). Studies on the function of the higher acoustic nervous centers in the cat. *Americal Journal of Psychology, 56*, 501–536.

Kuczwara, L. A., Birnholz, J. C., & Klodd, D. A. (1984). Auditory responsiveness in the fetus. *National Student Speech, Language, and Hearing Association Journal, 14*, 12–20.

Kuhl, P. (2011). Early language learning and literacy: Neuroscience implications for education. *Mind, Brain and Education. 5*(1), 128–142.

Kuhl, P., Williams, K., Lacerda, F., Stebens, K., & Lindblom, B. (1992). Lingusistic experience alters phonetic perception in infants by 6 months of age. *Science, 255*, 606–608.

Kuhl, P. K. (1988). Auditory perception and the evolution of speech. *Human Evolution, 3*, 19–43.

Kuhl, P. K., Andruski, J. E., Chistovich, I. A., Chistovich, L. A., Kozhevnikova, E. V., Ruskiner, V. L., & LaCerda, F. (1997). Cross-language analysis of phonetic units in language addressed to infants. *Science, 277*, 684–686.

Kuhl, P. K., & Meltzoff, A. N. (1982). The bimodal perception of speech in infancy. *Science, 10*(218), 1138–1141.

Kuhl, P. K., & Meltzoff, A. (1996). Infant vocalizations in response to speech: Vocal imitation and developmental change. *Journal of the Acoustical Society of America, 100*(4, Pt. 1), 2425–2438.

Kuhl, P. K., & Meltzoff, A. (1997). Evolution, nativism, and learning in the development of language and speech. In M. Gopnik (Ed.), *The inheritance and innateness of grammers* (pp. 7–44). New York, NY: Oxford University Press.

Kuk, F. (2011). Hearing aids for children with auditory processing disorders? *Seminars in Hearing, 32*(2), 189–195.

Kuk, F., Jackson, A., Keenan, D., & Lau, C. (2008). Personal amplification for school-age children with auditory processing disorders. *Journal of the American Academy of Audiology, 19*, 465–480.

Kulig, S. G., & Bakler, K. (1973). *Physician's developmental quick screen for speech disorders.* Galveston, TX: University of Texas Medical Branch.

Lane, H. (1977). *The wild boy of Aveyron.* Cambridge, MA: Harvard University Press.

Langer, L. O., Jr. (1965). Diastrophic dwarfism in early infancy. *American Journal of Roentgenology, 93*, 399.

Langer, S. K. (1957). *Philosophy in a new key.* Cambridge, MA: Harvard University Press.

Langford, C., Bench, J., & Wilson, I. (1975). Some effects of prestimulus activity and length of prestimulus observations on judgments of newborns' responses to sounds. *Audiology, 14*, 44–52.

Lantz, J., Petrakk, M., & Prigge, L. (2004). Using the 1000-Hz probe tone for immittance measurements in infants. *The Hearing Journal, 57*(10).

Laugen, N. J. (2013). Providing information to families in newborn hearing screening follow-up: Professional challenges. *Seminars in Hearing, 34*(1), 11–18.

Laughton, J. (1994). Models and current practices in early intervention with hearing-impaired infants. *Seminars in Hearing, 15*(2), 148–158.

League, R., Parker, J., Robertson, M., Valentine, V., & Powell, J. (1972). Acoustical environments in incubators and infant oxygen tents. *Preventive Medicine, 1,* 231.

Lee, D. J., Gomez-Marion, O., & Lee, H. M. (1996). Prevalence of childhood hearing loss. The Hispanic health and nutrition examination survey and the national health and nutritional examination survey II. *American Journal of Epidemiology, 144,* 442–449.

Lee, D. J., Gomez-Marion, O., & Lee, H. M. (1998). Prevalence of unilateral hearing loss in children: The national health and nutrition examination survey II and the Hispanic health and nutrition examination survey. *Ear and Hearing, 19*(4), 329–332.

Lempert, J., Wever, E. G., & Lawrence, M. (1947). The cochleogram and its clinical application. *Archives of Otolaryngology-Head and Neck Surgery, 45,* 61–67.

LENA Foundation. (2011). *Automatic language assessment in three easy steps.* Retrieved from http://www.lenafoundation.org/ProSystem/Overview.aspx

Lenneberg, E. H. (1967). *Biological foundations of language.* New York, NY: Wiley.

Leroy, J. G., & Crocker, A. C. (1966). Clinical definition of Hunter-Hurler phenotypes. A review of 50 patients. *American Journal of Diseases in Children, 112,* 518–530.

Leske, M. C. (1981). Prevalence estimates of communicative disorders in the U.S.: Language, hearing and vestibular disorders. *Asha, 23,* 229–236.

Levitt, H., McGarr, N., & Geffner, D. (1987). Development of language and communication skills in hearing-impaired children. *Asha Monographs* (No. 126). Rockville, MD: American Speech and Hearing Association.

Lewis, D. (1994). Assistive devices for classroom listening: FM systems. *American Journal of Audiology, 3,* 70–83.

Lewis, D. (1999). Selecting and pre-setting amplification for children: Where do we begin? *Trends in Amplification, 4*(2), 72–89.

Libby, E. R. (1982). In search of transparent insertion gain hearing aid responses. In G. Studebaker & F. Bess (Eds.), *Monographs in contemporary audiology* (pp. 112–123). Nashville, TN: Vanderbilt Hearing Aid Report.

Liden, G., & Kankkonen, A. (1969). Visual reinforcement audiometry. *Acta Oto-Laryngologica (Stockholm), 67,* 281–292.

Lieberman, P. (1975). *On the origins of language.* New York, NY: Macmillan.

Lightfoot, G., & Kennedy, V. (2006). Cortical electric response audiometry hearing threshold evaluation: Accuracy, speed, and the effects of stimulus presentation features. *Ear and Hearing, 27*(5), 443–456.

Lin, A. E., Siebert, J. R., & Graham, J. M., Jr. (1990). Central nervous system malformations in the CHARGE association. *American Journal of Medical Genetics, 37,* 304–310.

Lindsay, J. R., Black, F. O., & Donnelly, W. N. (1975). Acrocephalosyndactyly (Apert's syndrome): Temporal bone findings. *Annals of Otology, Rhinology, and Laryngology, 84,* 174–178.

Lindsay, R. L. (2005). Medical perspectives on autism spectrum disorders. *Seminars in Hearing, 26*(4), 191–201.

Ling, D. (1975). Recent developments affecting the education of hearing-impaired children. *Public Health Review, 4,* 117–152.

Ling, D., Ling, A. H., & Doehring, D. G. (1970). Stimulus response and observer variables in the auditory screening of newborn infants. *Journal of Speech and Hearing Research, 13,* 9–18.

Lins, O. G., Picton, T. W., Boucher, B. L., Durieux-Smith, A., Champagne, S. C., Moran, L. M., . . . Savio, G. (1996). Frequency-specific audiometry using steady-state responses. *Ear and Hearing, 17,* 81–96.

Lipscomb, D. (1996). The external and middle ear. In J. Northern (Ed.), *Hearing disorders* (3rd ed., pp. 1–14). Needham Heights, MA: Allyn & Bacon.

Liptak, G. S., McConnochie, K. M., & Roghmann, K. J. (1997). Decline of pediatric admissions with *Haemophilus influenzae* type b in New York State, 1982–1983: Relation to immunizations. *Journal of Pediatrics, 130,* 923.

Litke, R. E. (1971). Elevated high-frequency hearing in school children. *Archives of Otolaryngology, 94,* 255–257.

Litman, N., & Baum, S. G. (2009). Mumps virus. In G. L. Mandell, J. E. Bennett, & R. Dolin

(Eds.), *Principles and practice of infectious diseases* (7th ed.). Philadelphia, PA: Elsevier Churchill Livingstone.

Littman, T., Demmoer, G., Williams, S., Istas, A., & Griesser, C. (1995). Congenital asymptomatic cytomegalovirus infection and hearing loss. *Abstracts for the Association for Research in Otolaryngology, 19*, 40.

Lloyd, L. I., Spradlin, J. E., & Reid, M. J. (1968). An operant audiometric procedure for difficult-to-test patients. *Journal of Speech and Hearing Disorders, 33*, 236–245.

Loeb, G. E. (1985a, February). The functional replacement of the ear. *Scientific American, 252*(2), 104–111.

Loeb, G. E. (1985b). Single and multichannel cochlear prostheses: Rationale, strategies, and potential. In R. Schindler & M. Merzenich (Eds.), *Cochlear implants* (pp. 17–28). New York, NY: Raven Press.

Long, J., Lucey, J., & Philip, A. (1980). Noise and hypoxemia in the intensive care nursery. *Pediatrics, 65*, 143.

Lonsbury-Martin, B., & Martin, G. (1990). The clinical utility of distortion product emissions. *Ear and Hearing, 11*(2), 144–154.

Los Angeles County, Office of the Los Angeles County Superintendent of Schools, Audiology Services, and Southwest School for the Hearing-Impaired. (1980). *Test of auditory comprehension*. North Hollywood, CA: Forworks.

Lotke, M. (1995). She won't look at me. *Annals of Internal Medicine, 123*, 54–57.

Loy, B., & Roland, P. (2009). *Cochlear implants: What parents should know*. San Diego, CA: Plural.

Luterman, D. (1979). *Counseling parents of hearing-impaired children*. Boston, MA: Little, Brown.

Luterman, D. M. (1976). A comparison of language skills of hearing-impaired children trained in a visual/oral method and an auditory/oral method. *American Annals of the Deaf, 121*, 389–393.

Luterman, D. M. (1996). *Counseling persons with communication disorders and their families* (3rd ed.). Austin, TX: Pro-Ed.

Luterman, D. M., Kurtzer-White, E., & Seewald, R. (1999). *The young deaf child*. Baltimore, MD: York Press.

Lutman, M. E., Davis, A. C., Fortnum, H. M., & Wood, S. (1997). Field sensitivity of targeted neonatal hearing screening by transient-evoked otoacoustic emissions. *Ear and Hearing, 18*(4), 265–276.

MacDonald, H. M. (1980). Neonatal asphyxia: I. Relationship of obstetric and neonatal complications to neonatal mortality in consecutive deliveries. *Journal of Pediatrics, 96*, 898–902.

MacDonald, J. T., & Feinstein, S. (1984). Hearing loss following *Haemophilus influenzae* meningitis in infancy. *Archives of Neurology, 41*, 1058–1059.

Macrae, J. H. (1968a). TTS and recovery from TTS after use of powerful hearing aids. *Journal of the Acoustical Society of America, 44*, 1445–1446.

Macrae, J. H. (1968b). Recovery from TTS in children with sensorineural deafness. *Journal of the Acoustical Society of America, 44*, 1451.

Macrae, J. H., & Farrant, R. H. (1965). The effect of hearing aid use on the residual hearing of children with sensorineural deafness. *Annals of Otology, Rhinology, and Laryngology, 74*, 407–419.

Madden, C., Halsted, M., Benton, C., Greinwald, J., & Choo, D. (2003). Enlarged vestibular aqueduct syndrome in the pediatric population. *Otology and Neurotology, 24*, 625–632.

Madden, C., Rutter, M., Hilbert, L., Greinwald, J., & Choo, D. (2002). Clinical and audiological features in auditory neuropathy. *Archives of Otolaryngology-Head and Neck Surgery, 128*, 1026–1030.

Madell, J. (1998). *Behavioral evaluation of hearing in infants and children*. New York, NY: Thieme Medical.

Mahoney, T. M. (1984). High-risk hearing screening of large general newborn populations. *Seminars in Hearing, 5*(1), 25–36.

Maniglia, J. M., Wolff, D., & Herques, A. S. (1970). Congenital deafness in 13-15 syndrome. *Archives of Otolaryngology, 92*, 181–188.

Marchant, C. D., McMillan, P. M., & Shurin, P. A. (1984). Objective diagnosis of otitis media in early infancy by tympanometry and ipsilateral acoustic reflex thresholds. *Journal of Pediatrics, 109,* 590–595.

Margolis, R. M. (1978). Tympanometry in infants: State-of-the-art. In E. R. Harford, F. H. Bess, C. D. Bluestone, & J. Klein. (Eds.), *Impedance screening for middle ear disease in children* (pp. 41–56). New York, NY: Grune & Stratton.

Margolis, R. M. (2004, August 3). Boosting memory with informational counseling. *ASHA Leader.*

Margolis, R. M., Bass-Ringdahl, S., Hanks, W. D., Hotte, L., & Zapala, D. A. (2003). Tympanometry in newborn infants: 1-kHz norms. *Journal of the American Academy of Audiology, 14*(7), 383–392.

Marini, J. C. (2007). Osteogenesis imperfecta. In R. M. Kliegman, R. E. Behrman, H. B. Jenson, & B. F. Stanton (Eds.), *Nelson textbook of pediatrics* (18th ed.). Philadelphia, PA: Saunders Elsevier.

Markides, A. (1986). Speech levels and speech-to-noise ratios. *British Journal of Audiology, 20,* 115–120.

Marmolino, D. (2011). Friedreich's ataxia: Past, present and future. *Brain Research Reviews, 67*(1–2), 311–330.

Marple, B., & Meyerhoff, W. (1998). Perilymphatic fistula. In A. Lalwani & K. Grundfast (Eds.), *Pediatric otology and neurotology* (pp. 635–644). Philadelphia, PA: Lippincott-Raven.

Marres, H. A. (2002). Hearing loss in the Treacher Collins syndrome. *Advances in Otorhinolaryngology, 61,* 209–215.

Marron, J., Crisafi, M., Driscoll, J., Wung, J., Driscoll, Y., Fay, T., & James, L. (1992). Neurodevelopmental outcome in survivors of persistent pulmonary hypertension of the newborn. *Pediatrics, 90,* 392–396.

Marschark, M., Lang, H. G., & Albertini, J. A. (2002). *Educating deaf students.* New York, NY: Oxford University Press.

Martin, G., Probst, R., & Lonsbury-Martin, B. (1990). Otoacoustic emissions in human ears: Normative findings. *Ear and Hearing, 11*(2), 106–120.

Mason, J. A., & Herrmann, K. R. (1998). Universal hearing screening by automated auditory brainstem response measurement. *Pediatrics, 101*(2), 221–229.

Mason, W. H. (2007). Mumps. In R. M. Kliegman, R. E. Behrman, H. B. Jenson, & B. F. Stanton, (Eds.), *Kliegman: Nelson textbook of pediatrics* (18th ed.). Philadelphia, PA: Saunders Elsevier.

Mathers, R. (2009). Mainstreaming. In L. Seaver (Ed.), *The book of choice: Support for parenting a child who is deaf or hard-of-hearing* (2nd ed.). Boulder, CO: Hands and Voices.

Matkin, A., & Matkin, N. (1985). Benefits of total communication as perceived by parents of hearing-impaired children. *Language, Speech, and Hearing Services in Schools, 16,* 64–74.

Matkin, N. D. (1977). Assessment of hearing sensitivity during the preschool years. In F. Bess (Ed.), *Childhood deafness* (pp. 127–134). New York, NY: Grune & Stratton.

Matkin, N. D. (1984). Early recognition and referral of hearing-impaired children. *Pediatrics in Review, 6*(5), 151–155.

Matkin, N. D., & Wilcox, A. (1999). Considerations in the education of children with hearing loss. *Pediatric Clinics of North America, 46*(1), 143–151.

Mauk, G. W., White, K. R., Mortensen, L. B., & Behrens, T. R. (1991). The effectiveness of screening programs based on high-risk characteristics in early identification of hearing impairment. *Ear and Hearing, 12,* 312–319.

Maumenee, A. E. (1960). Congenital hereditary corneal dystrophy. *American Journal of Ophthalmology, 50,* 1114–1123.

Maxon, A. B., White, K. R., Behrens, T. R., & Vohr, B. R. (1995). Referral rates and cost efficiency in a universal newborn hearing screening program using transient evoked otoacoustic emissions. *Journal of the American Academy of Audiology, 6,* 271–277.

McCabe, B. F. (1989). Perilymph fistula: The Iowa experience to date. *American Journal of Otology, 1*(10), 262.

McCandless, G. A., & Allred, P. L. (1978). Tympanometry and emergence of the acoustic reflex in infants. In E. R. Harford, F. H. Bess, C. D. Bluestone, & J. Klein (Eds.), *Impedance* screening for middle ear disease in children (pp. 56–67). New York, NY: Grune & Stratton.

McCandless, G. A., & Best, L. (1964). Evoked responses to auditory stimuli in man using a summing computer. *Journal of Speech and Hearing Research, 7*, 193–202.

McCarthy, M., Duncan, J., & Leigh, G. (2012). Telepractice: The Australian experience in an international context. *Volta Review, 112*(3), 297–312.

McCollister, F. P., Simpson, L. C., Dahle, A. J., & Pass, B. F. (1996). Hearing loss and congenital symptomatic cytomegalovirus infection. *Journal of the American Academy of Audiology, 7*(2), 57–62.

McCreery, R. (2010). Small ears, BIG decisions. *Hearing Journal, 63*(7), 10–17.

McCroskey, J., & Meezan, W. (1998). Family-centered services: Approaches and effectiveness. In *The future of children: Protecting children from abuse and neglect, 8*, 1. Retrieved from http://futureofchildren.org/futureof children/publications/docs/08_01_03.pdf

McDonough, E. R. (1970). Fanconi anemia syndrome. *Archives of Otolaryngology, 92*, 284–285.

McFarlan, D. (1927). The Voice Test of Hearing. *Archives of Otolaryngology, 5*, 1–5.

McFarland, D. H. (2008). *Netter's atlas of anatomy for speech, swallowing and hearing.* St. Louis, MO: Mosby Elsevier.

McGee, T., & Kraus, N. (1996). Auditory development reflected by middle latency response. *Ear and Hearing, 17*(5), 419–429.

McLay, K., & Maran, A. G. D. (1969). Deafness and the Klippel-Feil syndrome. *Journal of Laryngology and Otology, 83*, 175–184.

McMillan, P., Bennett, M., Marchant, C., & Shurin, P. (1985). Ipsilateral and contralateral acoustic reflexes in neonates. *Ear and Hearing, 6*(6), 320–324.

McNellis, E. L., & Klein, A. J. (1997). Pass/fail for repeated click-evoked otoacoustic emission and auditory brainstem response screenings in newborns. *Otolaryngology-Head and Neck Surgery, 116*(4), 431–437.

McPherson, B., Law, M. M., & Wong, M. S. (2010). Hearing screening for school children: Comparison of low-cost, computer-based and conventional audiometry. *Child Care and Health Development, 36*(3), 323–331.

McWilliam, R., Tocci, L., & Harbin, G. (1998). *Family-centered services: Early intervention service providers' constructed meanings.* Retrieved from http://ccu.opac2.marmot .org/Record/.b20173118

Meadow, K. P. (1968). *The effect of early manual communication and family climate* (Doctoral dissertation). University of California-Berkeley.

Meadow, K. P., & Trybus, R. J. (1979). Behavioral and emotional problems of deaf children: An overview. In L. J. Bradford & W. G. Hardy (Eds.), *Hearing and hearing impairment.* New York, NY: Grune & Stratton.

Meadow-Orlans, K. P. (1987). An analysis of the effectiveness of early intervention programs for hearing-impaired children. In M. J. Guralnick & F. C. Bennet (Eds.), *The effectiveness of early intervention for at-risk and handicapped children* (pp. 325–357). New York, NY: Academic Press.

Meadow-Orlans, K. P., Mertens, D. M., Sass-Lehrer, M., & Scott-Olson, K. (1997). Support services for parents and their children who are deaf or hard-of-hearing. *American Annals of the Deaf, 142*, 278–288.

Meadow-Orlans, M., Mertens, D., & Sass-Lehrer, M. (2003). *Parents and their deaf children: The early years.* Washington, DC: Gallaudet University Press.

Mehl, A., & Thomson, V. (1998). Newborn hearing screening: The great omission. *Pediatrics, 101*, 34.

Meinke, D. K., & Dice, N. (2007). Comparison of audiometric screening criteria for the identification of noise-induced hearing loss in adolescents. *American Journal of Audiology, 16*(2), S190–S202.

Melnick, M., Bixler, D., Nance, W. E., Silk, K., & Yune, H. (1976). Familial branchio-oto-renal dysplasia. A new addition to the branchial arch syndrome. *Clinical Genetics, 9*, 25–34.

Mendel, M. (1980). Clinical use of primary cortical responses. *Audiology, 19*, 1–15.

Mendel, M. (1985). Middle and late auditory evoked potentials. In J. Katz (Ed.), *Handbook of clinical audiology* (3rd ed., pp. 565–581). Baltimore, MD: Williams & Wilkins.

Mendel, M., & Goldstein, R. (1969). The effect of test conditions on the early components of the averaged electroencephalic response. *Journal of Speech and Hearing Research, 12,* 344.

Mendel, M., & Goldstein, R. (1971). Stability of the early components of the averaged electroencephalographic response. *Journal of Speech and Hearing Research, 14,* 829–840.

Mendel, M., Hosick, E., Windman, T., Davis, H., Hirsh, S. K., & Dinges, D. F. (1975). Audiometric comparison of the middle and late components of the adult auditory evoked potential awake and sleep. *Electroencephalography and Clinical Neurophysiology, 38,* 27–33.

Menyuk, P. (1972). *The development of speech.* New York, NY: Bobbs-Merrill.

Merchant, S. N., Burgess, B. J., Adams, J. C., Kashtan, C. E., Gregory, M. C., Santi, P. A., . . . Nadol, J. B., Jr. (2004). Temporal bone histopathology in Alport syndrome. *Laryngoscope, 114*(9), 1609–1618.

Mets, M. B., Young, N. M., Pass, A., & Lasky, J. B. (2000). Early diagnosis of Usher syndrome in children. *Transactions of the American Ophthalmological Society, 98,* 237–245.

Mettler, G., & Fraser, F. (2000). Reoccurrence risk for sibs of children with "sporadic" achondroplasia. *American Journal of Medical Genetics, A90,* 250.

Metz, O. (1946). The acoustic impedance measured on normal and pathological ears. *Acta Oto-Laryngologica (Stockholm), 63,* 11–253.

Metz, O. (1952). Threshold of reflex contractions of muscles of middle ear and recruitment of loudness. *Archives of Otolaryngology, 55,* 536–543.

Meyer, S. E., Jardine, C. A., & Deverson, W. (1997). Developmental changes in tympanometry: A case study. *British Journal of Audiology, 31,* 189–195.

Meyer, T., & Pisoni, D. (1999). Some computational analyses of the PBK test: Effects of frequency and lexical density on spoken word recognition. *Ear and Hearing, 20*(4), 363–370.

Meyerson, M. D., & Foushee, D. R. (1978). Speech, language and hearing in Moebius syndrome: A study of 22 patients. *Developmental Medicine and Child Neurology, 20*(3), 357–365.

Miller, A. L., Lehman, R. H., & Geretti, R. (1969). Unusual audiological findings in cranial-metaphysical dysplasia. *Archives of Otolaryngology, 89,* 861–864.

Mills, J. H. (1975). Noise and children: A review of literature. *Journal of the Acoustical Society of America, 58,* 768–779.

Mills, J. H., Gengel, R. W., Watson, C. S., & Miller, J. D. (1970). Temporary changes for the auditory system due to exposure to noise for one or two days. *Journal of the Acoustical Society of America, 48,* 524–530.

Mitchell, O., & Richards, G. (1976). Effects of various anesthetic agents on normal and pathological middle ears. *Ear, Nose, and Throat Journal, 55,* 36.

Mitchell, R. E., & Karchmer, M. A. (2004). When parents are deaf versus hard-of-hearing: Patterns of sign use and school placement of deaf and hard-of-hearing children. *Journal of Deaf Studies and Deaf Education, 9*(2).

Miyamoto, R. T., Kirk, K. I., Robbins, A. M., Todd, S., & Riley, A. (1996). Speech perception and speech production in children with multichannel cochlear implants. *Acta Oto-Laryngologica, 116,* (2), 240–243.

Miyamoto, R. T., Kirk, K. I., Robbins, A. M., Todd, S., Riley, A., & Pisoni, D. B. (1997). Speech perception and speech intelligibility in children with multichannel cochlear implants. *Advances in Oto-Rhino-Laryngology, 52,* 198–203.

Miyamoto, R. T., Yune, H. Y., & Rosevear, W. H. (1983). Klippel-Feil syndrome and associated ear deformities. *American Journal of Otology, 1*(5), 113–119.

Moller, A. (1962). The sensitivity of the contraction of the tympanic muscles in man. *Annals of Otology, Rhinology, and Laryngology, 71,* 86–95.

Moller, A. (2000). *Hearing: Its physiology and pathophysiology.* New York, NY: Academic Press.

Moeller, M. P. (2000). Early intervention and language development in children who are deaf and hard-of-hearing. *Pediatrics, 106*, E43.

Moeller, M. P. (2010). Optimizing early word learning in infants with hearing loss. *Audiology Today, 3*, 19–26.

Moeller, M. P., Hoover, B., Putman, C., & Arbataitis, K. (2007). Vocalizations of infants with hearing loss compared with infants with normal hearing: part II: Transition to words. *Ear and Hearing, 28*, 628–642.

Moncrieff, D., & Wertz, D. (2008). Auditory rehabilitation for interaural asymmetry: Preliminary evidence of improved dichotic listening performance following intensive training. *International Journal of Audiology, 47*, 84–97.

Moncrieff, D. W. (2011). Dichotic listening in children: Age-related changes in direction and magnitude of ear advantage. *Brain and Cognition, 76*(2), 316–322.

Moncur, J. (1968). Judge reliability in infant testing. *Journal of Speech and Hearing Research, 11*, 348–357.

Montgomery, D. E., & Matkin, N. D. (1992). Hearing-impaired children in schools: Integrated or isolated? In F. H. Bess & J. W. Hall, III (Eds.), *Screening children to auditory function*. Nashville, TN: Bill Wilkerson Center Press.

Moodie, K., Seewald, R., & Sinclair, S. (1994). Procedure for predicting real-ear hearing aid performance in young childen. *American Journal of Audiology, 3*, 23–31.

Moog, J. S., & Geers, A. E. (1990). *Early speech perception test for profoundly hearing-impaired children*. St. Louis, MO: Central Institute for the Deaf.

Moog, J. S., & Geers, A. E. (2003). Epilogue: Major findings, conclusions and implications for deaf education. *Ear and Hearing, 24*(1), 121S–125S.

Moon, C., Cooper, R. P., & Fifer, W. P. (1993). Two-day olds prefer their native language. *Infant Behavior and Development, 16*, 495–500.

Moore, D. (2007). Auditory processing disorders: Acquisition and treatment. *Journal of Communication Disorders, 40*, 295–304.

Moore, J. (1999). Comparison of risk of conductive hearing loss among three ethnic groups of Arctic audiology patients. *Journal of Speech, Language, and Hearing Research, 42*, 1069–1079.

Moore, J. M., Thompson, G., & Thompson, M. (1975). Auditory localization of infants as a function of reinforcement conditions. *Journal of Speech and Hearing Disorders, 40*, 29–34.

Moore, J. M., Wilson, W. R., Lillis, K. E., et al. (1976). *Earphone auditory threshold of infants utilizing visual reinforcement auditory reinforcement (VRA)*. Poster session presented at the American Speech and Hearing Association meeting, Houston, TX.

Moore, J. M., Wilson, W. R., & Thompson, G. (1977). Visual reinforcement of head-turn responses in infants under twelve months of age. *Journal of Speech and Hearing Disorders, 42*, 328–334.

Moores, D. F. (2000). *Educating the deaf: Psychology, principles and practices* (5th ed.). Independence, KY: Cengage Learning.

Morelli, J. G. (2007). Hypopigmented lesions. In R. M. Kliegman, R. E. Behrman, H. B. Jenson, & F. Stanton (Eds.), *Nelson textbook of pediatrics* (18th ed.). Philadelphia, PA: Saunders Elsevier.

Morton, C. C., & Nance, M. D. (2006). Newborn hearing screening—A silent revolution. *New England Journal of Medicine, 354*(20), 2151–2164.

M'Rad, R., Sanak, M., Deschenes, G., Zhou, J., Bonaiti-Pellie, C., Holvoet-Vermaut, L., . . . Grunfeld, J. P. (1992). Alport syndrome: A genetic study of 31 families. *Human Genetics, 90*, 420–426.

Muckle, T. J. (1979). The "Muckle-Wells" syndrome. *British Journal of Dermatology, 100*, 87–92.

Mueller, H. G., Bentler, R., & Wu, Y. H. (2008). Prescribing maximum hearing aid output. *The Hearing Journal, 61*(3), 32–36.

Mueller, H. G., & Hall, J. W., III. (1998). *Audiologists' desk reference* (Vol. I and Vol II). San Diego, CA: Singular.

Mueller, H. G., & Hawkins, D. B. (1990). Three important considerations in hearing aid selection. In R. E. Sandlin (Ed.), *Handbook of hearing aid amplification* (Vol. II, pp. 31–60). Boston, MA: Little, Brown.

Mueller, H. G., Hawkins, D. B., & Northern, J. L. (1992). *Probe microphone measurements: Hearing aid selection and assessment.* San Diego, CA: Singular.

Mueller, H. G., & Killion, M. (1990). An easy method for calculating the articulation index. *The Hearing Journal, 43*(9), 14–17.

Mueller, H. G., & Picou, E. M. (2010). Survey examines popularity of real-ear probe-microphone measures. *The Hearing Journal, 63*(3), 27–32.

Mueller, H. G., Ricketts, T. A., & Bentler, R. (2013). *Modern hearing aids: Pre-fitting testing and selection considerations.* San Diego, CA: Plural.

Mundkur, N. (2005). Neuroplasticity in children. *Indian Journal of Pediatrics, 72*, 855–857.

Mundlos, S. (1999). Cleidocranial dysplasia: Clinical and molecular genetics. *Journal of Medical Genetics, 36*, 177.

Murphy, K. P. (1962). Development of hearing in babies. *Child and Family, 1*(1).

Murphy, K. P. (1979, September). A developmental approach to pediatric audiometry. *Hearing Aid Journal,* 6–32.

Musiek, F. R., & Chermak, G. (Eds.). (2007). *Handbook of (central) auditory processing disorder. Volume I: Auditory neuroscience and diagnosis.* San Diego, CA: Plural.

Musiek, F. R., & Schochat, E. (1998). Auditory training and central auditory processing disorders: A case study. *Seminars in Hearing, 19*(4), 357–366.

Musselman, C. R., Lindsay, P. H., & Wilson, A. K. (1988). An evaluation of recent trends in preschool programming for hearing-impaired children. *Journal of Speech and Hearing Disorders, 53*, 71–88.

Myer, C. M., Farrer, S. M., Drake, A. F., & Cotton, R. T. (1989). Perilymphatic fistulas in children: Rationale for therapy. *Ear and Hearing, 10*, 112–116.

Myers, F. N., & Stool, S. (1969). The temporal bone in osteoporosis. *Archives of Otolaryngology, 89*, 44–53.

Nadol, J. B., & McKenna, M. J. (2004). *Surgery of the ear and temporal bone.* Baltimore, MD: Lippincott Williams & Wilkins.

Nagib, M. G., Maxwell, R. E., & Chou, S. N. (1985). Klippel-Feil syndrome in children: Clinical features and management. *Child's Nervous System, 1*, 255–263.

Nahmias, A. J. (1974). The TORCH complex. *Hospital Practice, 9*, 65–72.

Nahmias, A. J., & Norrild, B. (1979). Herpes simplex virus 1 and 2: Basic and clinical aspects. *Disease Monographs, 25*(10), 1–49.

Nakashima, S., Sando, I., Takahashi, H., & Hashida, Y. (1992). Temporal bone histopathologic findings of Waardenburg's syndrome. *Laryngoscope, 102*, 563–567.

Nance, M. A., & Berry, S. A. (1992). Cockayne syndrome: A review of 140 cases. *American Journal of Medical Genetics, 42*, 68–84.

Nance, W. (2007). The genetics of deafness. In R. Ackley, T. Decker, & C. Limb (Eds.), *An essential guide to hearing and balance disorders.* Mahwah, NJ: Lawrence Erlbaum.

Nance, W., & Kearsey, M. J. (2004). Relevance of connexin deafness (DFNB1) to human evolution. *American Journal of Human Genetics, 74*, 1081–1087.

Nance, W. E. (1973). *Symposium on Usher's syndrome.* Public Service Programs. Gallaudet College, Washington, DC.

Nassif, R., & Harboyan, G. (1970). Madelung's deformity with conductive hearing loss. *Archives of Otolaryngology, 91*, 175–178.

National Assessment of Educational Progress. (2007). http://nces.ed.gov/pubsearch/pubs info.asp?pubid=2007496

National Center for Family Literacy. (2007). *Developing early literacy: Report of the National Early Literacy Panel.* Jessup, MD: National Institute for Literacy.

National Council on Disability. (2000). *Transition and post-school outcomes for youth with disabilities: Closing the gaps to post-secondary ed and employment.* Retrieved from http://www.ncd.gov/publications/2000/

National Institutes of Health Consensus Development Conference statement: Neurofibromatosis. (1988). *Archives of Neurology, 45*(5), 575–578.

Naulty, C. M., Weiss, I. P., & Herer, G. R. (1986). Progressive sensorineural hearing loss in survivors of persistent fetal circulation. *Ear and Hearing, 7,* 74–77.

Neff, W. B. D. (1947). The effects of partial section of the auditory nerve. *Journal of Comprehensive Physiology, 40,* 203–216.

Neighbors, M., & Tannehill-Jones, R. (2010). Childhood diseases and disorders. In *Human diseases* (3rd ed., pp. 457–479). Clifton Park, NY: Cengage Learning.

Nelson, M., & Scott, C. I. (1969). Engelmann's disease (a form of craniodiaphysial dysplasia). *Birth Defects, 5*(4), 301.

Nelson, P. B., & Soli, S. D. (2000). Acoustical barriers to learning: Children at risk in every classroom. *Language, Speech, and Hearing Services in Schools, 31,* 356–361.

Neuman, A. C., Wroblewski, M., Hajicek, J., & Rubinstein, A. (2010). Effects of noise and reverberation on speech recognition peformance of normal-hearing children and adults. *Ear and Hearing, 31*(3), 336–344.

Nicholas, J. G., & Geers, A. E. (2008). Effects of early auditory experiences on the spoken language of deaf children at 3 years of age. *Ear and Hearing, 27,* 286–298.

Nichols, P. T., Ramadan, H. H., Wax, M. K., & Santrock, R. D. (1998). Relationship between tympanic membrane perforations and retained ventilation tubes. *Archives of Otolaryngology-Head and Neck Surgery, 124,* 417–419.

NIDCE, 2010, CDC. 2011. Annual data Early Hearing Detection and Intervention (EHDI) program. Retrieved from http://www.cdc.gov/ncbddd/hearingloss/ehdi-data.html

Niemeyer, W., & Sesterhenn, G. (1972). Calculating the hearing threshold from the stapedius reflex threshold for different sound stimuli. *Journal of Audiological Communication, 11,* 84.

Niskar, A., Kieszak, M., Holmes, A., Esteban, E., Rubin, C., & Brody, D. (1998). Prevalence of hearing loss among children 6 to 19 years of age. *Journal of the American Medical Association, 279,* 1071–1075.

Niskar, A. S., Kieszak, S. M., Holmes, A. E., Esteban, E., Rubin, C., & Brody, D. J. (2001). Estimated prevalence of noise-induced hearing threshold shifts among children 6 to 19 years of age: The Third National Health and Nutri-

tion Examination Survey, 1988–1994, United States. *Pediatrics, 108*(1), 40–43.

Noback, C. R., Strominger, N. L., & Demarest, R. J. (1996). *Human nervous system: Structure and function* (5th ed.). Philadelphia, PA: Williams & Wilkins.

Nobel, W. (2006). Bilateral hearing aids: A review of self-reports of benefit in comparison with unilateral fitting. *International Journal of Audiology, 45,* 63–71.

Nolte, J. (2008). *The human brain: An introduction to its functional anatomy* (3rd ed.). Philadelphia, PA: Mosby Elsevier.

Northern, J. L. (1977). Acoustic impedance in the pediatric population. In F. Bess (Ed.), *Childhood deafness: Causation, assessment, and management.* New York, NY: Grune & Stratton.

Northern, J. L. (1978). Impedance screening in special populations: State of the art. In E. R. Harford, F. H. Bess, C. D. Bluestone, & J. Klein, (Eds.), *Impedance screening for middle ear disease in children* (pp. 229–248). New York: Grune & Stratton.

Northern, J. L. (1980a). Acoustic impedance measures in the Down's population. *Seminars in Speech, Language, and Hearing, 1,* 81.

Northern, J. L. (1980b). Impedance screening: An integral part of hearing screening. *Annals of Otology, Rhinology, and Laryngology, 89*(68), 3.

Northern, J. L. (1986). Selection of children for cochlear implantation. *Seminars in Hearing, 7,* 341–347.

Northern, J. L. (1988). Recent developments in acoustic immittance measurements in children. In F. Bess (Ed.), *Hearing impairment in children* (pp. 176–189). Parkton: York Press.

Northern, J. L. (1992). Special issues concerned with screening for middle ear disease in children. In F. H. Bess & J. W. Hall, III (Eds.), *Screening children for auditory function* (pp. 39–60). Nashville, TN: Bill Wilkerson Center Press.

Northern, J. L. (1996). Acoustic immittance measurements. In J. Northern (Ed.), *Hearing disorders* (3rd ed.). Needham Heights, MA: Allyn & Bacon.

Northern, J. L. (2012). Extending hearing healthcare: Tele-audiology. *Hearing Review, 19*(10), 12–16.

Northern, J. L., & Downs, M. P. (1974). *Hearing in children* (1st ed.). Baltimore, MD: Williams & Wilkins.

Northern, J. L., & Hayes, D. (1994). Universal screening for infant hearing impairment: Necessary, beneficial and justifiable. *Audiology Today, 6*(2), 10–13.

Norton, S. J. (1993). Application of transient evoked otoacoustic emissions to pediatric populations. *Ear and Hearing, 14*, 64–73.

Norton, S. J., Gorga, M. P., Widen, J. E., Folsom, R. C., Sinninger, Y. S., Cone-Wesson, B., . . . Fletcher, K. (2000). Identification of neonatal hearing impairment: A multi-center intervention. *Ear and Hearing, 21*(5), 348–356.

Norton, S. J., & Widen, J. E. (1990). Evoked otoacoustic emissions in normal-hearing infants and children: Emerging data and issues. *Ear and Hearing, 11*, 121–127.

Nozza, R. J. (1995). Critical issues in acoustic immittance screening for middle-ear effusion. *Seminars in Hearing, 16*(1), 86–98.

Nozza, R. J., Bluestone, C. D., Kardatzke, D., & Bachman, R. (1992). Towards the validation of aural acoustic immittance measures for the diagnosis of middle ear effusion in children. *Ear and Hearing, 13*, 442–453.

Nozza, R. J., Bluestone, C. D., Kardatzke, D., & Bachman, R. N. (1994). Identification of middle ear effusion by aural acoustic admittance and otoscopy. *Ear and Hearing, 15*, 310–323.

Nozza, R. J., & Wilson, W. R. (1984). Masked and unmasked pure-tone thresholds of infants and adults: development of auditory frequency selectivity and sensitivity. *Journal of Speech and Hearing Research, 27*, 613–622.

Oller, D. K. (1978). Infant vocalizations and the development of speech. *Allied Health & Behavioral Sciences, I*, 523–549.

Oller, D. K. (1980). The emergence of the sounds of speech in infants. In G. Komshian-Yeni, J. F. Kavanagh, & C. A. Ferguson (Eds.), *Child phonology: Production, 1* (pp. 83–112). New York, NY: Academic Press.

Oller, D. K, & Eilers, R. (1988). The role of audition in infant babbling. *Child Development, 59*, 441–449.

Olsen, S., Fiechtl, B., & Rule, S. (2012). An evaluation of virtual home visits in early intervention: the feasibility of virtual intervention. *The Volta Review, 112*(3), 267–282.

Olsen, W. (2008). Hearing dogs. In *Mayo Clinic on better hearing in balance* (pp. 132–133). Rochester, NY: Mayo Clinic Health Solutions.

Olsen, W. O., & Matkin, N. D. (1979). Speech audiometry. In W. F. Rintelmann (Ed.), *Hearing assessment*. Baltimore, MD: University Park Press.

Orchik, D. J., Dunn, J. W., & McNutt, L. (1978a). Tympanometry as a predictor of middle ear effusion. *Archives of Otolaryngology, 104*, 4–6.

Orchik, D. J., Morff, R., & Dunn, J. W. (1978b). Impedance audiometry in serous otitis media. *Archives of Otolaryngology, 104*, 409–412.

O'Reilly, R. C., Morlet, T., Nicholas, B. D., Josephson, G., Horlbeck, D., Lundy, L., & Mercado, A. (2010). Prevalence of vestibular and balance disorders in children. *Otology & Neurotology, 31*(9), 1441–1444.

Osberger, M. J., & Hesketh, L. J. (1988). Speech and language disorders related to hearing impairment. In N. Lass, McReynolds, L. V., Northern, J. L., & Yoder, D. E. (Eds). *Handbook of speech-language pathology & audiology* (pp. 858–885). Toronto, Canada: BC Decker.

Ouyang, X. M., Yan, D., Du, L. L., Hejtmancik, J. F., Jacobson, S. G., Nance, W. E . . . & Liu, X. Z. (2005). Characterization of Usher syndrome type I gene mutations in an Usher syndrome patient population. *Human Genetics, 116*(4), 292–299.

Owens, E., Kessler, D. K., Raggio, M. W., & Schubert, E. D. (1985). Analysis and revision of the minimal auditory capabilities (MAC) battery. *Ear and Hearing, 6*, 280–290.

Oyler, R. F, Oyler, A. L., & Matkin, N. D. (1987). Warning: A unilateral hearing loss may be detrimental to a child's academic career. *Hearing Journal, 40*(9), 18–22.

Oyler, R. F, Oyler, A. L., & Matkin, N. D. (1988). Unilateral hearing loss: Demographics and educational impact. *Language, Speech, and Hearing Services in Schools, 19,* 201–210.

Ozdamar, O., & Kraus, N. (1983). Auditory middle-latency response in human. *Audiology, 22,* 34–49.

Palmer, C. (2007). An evidence-based approach to applying hearing instrument technology in pediatrics. In *Sound foundations through early amplification* (pp. 121–126). Warrenville, IL: Phonak.

Palmer, C., & Mormer, E. (1999). Goals and expectations of the hearing aid fitting. *Trends in Amplification, 4*(2), 61–71.

Palmer, J., & Yantis, P. A. (1990). *Survey of communication disorders.* Baltimore, MD: Williams & Wilkins.

Pandolfo, M. (2009). Friedreich ataxia: The clinical picture. *Journal of Neurology, 256*(1), 3–8,

Pantke, O. A., & Cohen, M. M., Jr. (1971). The Waardenburg syndrome. *Birth Defects, 7*(7), 147–152.

Paparella, M. M., & Brady, D. R. (1970). Sensorineural hearing loss in chronic otitis media and mastoiditis. *Archives of Otolaryngology, 74,* 108–115.

Pappas, D. G., Sr. (1998). *Diagnosis and treatment of hearing impairment in children* (2nd ed). San Diego, CA: Singular.

Paradise, J. L. (1976a). Pediatrician's view of middle ear effusions: more questions than answers. *Annals of Otology, Rhinology, and Laryngology, 85*(25), 20–24.

Paradise, J. L. (1976b). Management of middle ear effusions in infants with cleft palate. *Annals of Otology, Rhinology, and Laryngology, 85*(25), 285–288.

Paradise, J. L. (1980). Otitis media in infants and children. *Pediatrics, 65,* 917–943.

Paradise, J. L. (1982). Editorial retrospective: tympanometry. *New England Journal of Medicine, 307,* 1074–1076.

Paradise, J. L. (1995). Managing otitis media: A time for change. *Pediatrics, 96*(4), 712–715.

Paradise, J. L., & Bluestone, C. D. (1969). Diagnosis and management of ear disease in cleft palate infants. *Transactions of the American Academy of Ophthalmology and Otolaryngology, 73,* 709–714.

Paradise, J. L., & Bluestone, C. D. (1974). Early treatment of the universal otitis media of infants with cleft palate. *Pediatrics, 53,* 48–54.

Paradise, J. L, Elster, B., & Tan, L. (1994). Evidence in infants with cleft palate that breast milk protects against otitis media. *Pediatrics, 94,* 853–860.

Paradise J. L., Feldman, H. M., Campbell, T. F., Dollaghan, C. A., Rockette, H. E., Pitcairn, D. L . . . Pelham, W. E. (2007). Tympanostomy tubes and developmental outcomes at 9 to 11 years of age. *New England Journal of Medicine, 356,* 248–261.

Paradise, J. L., Smith, C., & Bluestone, C. D. (1976). Tympanometric detection of middle ear effusion in infants and young children. *Pediatrics, 58,* 198–206.

Parke, D. W. (2002). Stickler syndrome: clinical care and molecular genetics. *American Journal of Ophthalmology, 134*(5), 746–748.

Parnes, L. S., & McCabe, B. F. (1987). Perilymph fistula: An important cause of deafness and dizziness in children. *Pediatrics, 80*(4), 524–528.

Parring, A. (1988). Hearing disabled children: Epidemiology and identification. *Scandinavian Audiology, 30,* 21–23.

Parry, G., Hacking, C., Bamford, J., & Day, J. (2003). Minimal response levels for visual reinforcement audiometry in infants. *International Journal of Audiology, 42,* 413–417.

Pascoe, D. (1980). Clinical implications of nonverbal methods of hearing aid selections and fitting. *Seminars in Hearing, 1*(4).

Pashayan, H. M., & Lewis, M. B. (1984). Clinical experience with Robin Sequence. *Cleft Palate Journal, 21,* 270–276.

Pashayan, H. M., Pruzansky, S., & Solomon, L. (1974). The EEC syndrome. *Birth Defects, 10*(7), 105–127.

Pasquier, L., Laugel, V., Lazaro, L., Dollfus, H., Journel, H., Edery, P . . . .Cormier-Daire V. (2006). Wide clinical variability among 13 new Cockayne syndrome cases confirmed by biochemical assays. *Archives of Diseases in Children, 91*(2), 178–182.

Pastores, G. M., Michels, V. V, & Jack, C. R., Jr. (1991). Early childhood diagnosis of acoustic neuromas in presymptomatic individuals at risk for neurofibromatosis. *American Journal of Medical Genetics, 41,* 325–329.

Paul, R., Cohen, D., Breg, W., Watson, M., & Herman, S. (1984). Fragile X syndrome: Its relations to speech and language disorders. *Journal of Speech and Hearing Disorders, 49,* 326–336.

Pazzaglia, V. E., & Giampiero, B. (1986). Oto-palato-digital syndrome in four generations of a large family. *Clinical Genetics, 30,* 338–344.

Pearce, J. M. (2007). Pendred's syndrome. *European Neurology, 58*(3), 189–190.

Peck, J. E. (1984). Hearing loss in Hunter's syndrome: Mucopolysaccharidosis II. *Ear and Hearing, 5*(4), 243–246.

Peckham, C. S., Stark, O., Dudgeon, J. A., Martin, J. A., & Hawkins, G. (1987). Congenital cytomegalovirus infection: A cause of sensorineural hearing loss. *Archives of Diseases in Childhood, 62,* 1233–1237.

Pediatric Working Group of the Conference on Amplification for Children with Auditory Deficits. (1996). Amplification for infants and children with hearing loss. *American Journal of Audiology, 5,* 77–88.

Pehringer, J. (2011). VRA: Blending skill and technology. *Hearing Journal, 64*(1), 43.

Pelton, S., Shurin, P., & Klein, J. (1977). Persistence of middle ear effusion after otitis media. *Pediatric Research, 11,* 504.

Penn, T. O. (1999). School-based hearing screening in the United States. *Audiology Today, 11*(6), 20–21.

Petit, A., Dontenwille, M., Bardon, C., & Civatte, J. (1993). Pili torti with congenital deafness (Bjornstad's syndrome): Report of three cases in one family, suggesting autosomal dominant transmission. *Clinical and Experimental Dermatology, 18*(1), 94–95.

Petitto, L. A., & Marentette, P. F. (1991). Babbling in the manual mode: Evidence for the ontogeny of language. *Science, 251,* 1493–1495.

Petroff, M. A., Simmons, F. B., & Winzelberg, J. (1986). Two emerging perilymph fistula "syndromes" in children. *Laryngoscope, 96,* 498–501.

Picton, R. W., Hillyard, S. A., Krausz, H. I., & Galambos, R. (1974). Human auditory evoked potentials. I. Evaluation of components. *Electroencephalography and Clinical Neurophysiology, 36,* 179–190.

Picton, T. W. (2013). Hearing in time: Evoked potential studies of temporal processing. *Ear and Hearing, 34*(4), 385–401.

Picton, T. W., Vajsra, J., Rodriquez, R., & Campbell, K. B. (1987). Reliability estimates from steady-state evoked potentials. *Electroencephalography and Clinical Neurophysiology, 68,* 119–131.

Pikus, A. T. (1995). Pediatric audiologic profile in type I and type 2 neurofibromatosis. *Journal of the American Academy of Audiology, 6*(1), 54–62.

Pikus, A. T. (2002). Heritable vestibular disorders. *Seminars in Hearing, 23*(2), 129–142.

Pisoni, D. B. (2000). Cognitive factors and cochlear implants: Some thoughts on perception, learning and memory in speech perception. *Ear and Hearing, 21*(1), 70–78.

Pittman, A. (2008). Short-term world-learning rate in children with normal hearing and children with hearing loss in limited and extended high-frequency bandwidths. *Journal of Speech, Language, and Hearing Research, 51,* 785–797.

Plant, G., & Spens, K. E. (Eds.). (1995). *Profound deafness and speech communication.* London, UK: Whurr.

Plett, S. K., Berdon, W. E., Cowles, R. A., Oklu, R., & Campbell, J. B. (2008). Cushing proximal symphalangism and the NOG and GDF5 genes. *Pediatric Radiology, 38*(2), 209–215.

Pollack, D. (1982). Amplification and auditory/verbal training for the limited hearing infant 0 to 30 months. *Seminars in Speech, Language, and Hearing, 3,* 52–67.

Porter, H., & Bess, F. H. (2011). Children with unilateral hearing loss. In R. Seewald & A. M. Tharpe (Eds.). *Comprehensive handbook of pediatric audiology* (pp. 175–191). San Diego, CA: Plural.

Portmann, D., Boudard, P., & Herman, D. (1997). Anatomical results with titanium implants in the mastoid region. *Ear, Nose, and Throat Journal, 76*(4), 231–236.

Potts, P., & Greenwood, J. (1983). Hearing aid monitoring. *Language, Speech, and Hearing Services in Schools, 14,* 163.

Pratt, S. R. (1999). Post-fitting issues: A need for parent counseling and instruction. *Trends in Amplification, 4*(2), 103–107.

Prezant, T. R., Shohat, M., Jaber, L., Pressman, S., & Fischel-Ghodsian, N. (1992). Biochemical characterization of a pedigree with mitochondrially inherited deafness. *American Journal of Medical Genetics, 44,* 465–472.

Prieve, B. A., Dalzell, L., Berg, A., Bradley, M., Cacace, A., Campbell, D., . . . Stevens, F. (2000). The New York State Universal Newborn Hearing Screening Demonstration Project: Outpatient outcome measures. *Ear and Hearing, 21*(2), 131–140.

Prieve, B. A., & Stevens, F. (2000). The New York State Universal Newborn Hearing Screening Demonstration Project: Introduction and overview. *Ear and Hearing, 21*(2), 85–91.

Primus, M. A. (1987). Response and reinforcement in operant audiometry. *Journal of Speech and Hearing Disorders, 52,* 294–299.

Primus, M. A. (1992). The role of localization in visual reinforcement audiometry. *Asha, 35*(3), 1137–1141.

Primus, M. A., & Thompson, G. (1985). Response strength of young children in operant audiometry. *Journal of Speech and Hearing Research, 28,* 539–547.

Pryor, S. P., Madeo, A. C., Reynolds, J. C., Sarlis, N. J., Arnos, K. S., Nance, W. E. . . . Griffith, A. J. (2005). SLC26A4/PDS genotype-phenotype correlation in hearing loss with enlargement of the vestibular aqueduct (EVA): Evidence that Pendred syndrome and non-syndromic EVA are distinct clinical and genetic entities. *Journal of Medical Genetics, 42,* 159–165.

Quar, T. K., Ching, T. Y. C., Newall, P., & Sharma, M. (2013). Evaluation of real-world preferences and performance of hearing aids fitted according to the NAL-NL1 and DSL v5 procedures in children with moderately severe to profound hearing loss. *International Journal of Audiology, 52,* 322–332.

Querleu, Q., Renard, Z., & Crepin, G. (1981). Perception auditive et reactivite foetale aux stimulations sonores. *Journal de Gynecologie, Obstetrique et Biologie de la Reproduction, 10,* 307–314.

Quisling, R. W., Moore, G. R., Jahrsdoerfer, R. A., & Cantrell, R. W. (1979). Osteogenesis imperfecta: A study of 160 family members. *Archives of Otolaryngology, 105,* 207–211.

Raff, M., Barres, B., Burne, J., Coles, H., Ishizaki, Y., & Jacobson, M. (1993). Programmed cell death and control of cell survival: Lessons from the nervous system. *Science, 622,* 695–700.

Ramer, J. C., Vasily, D. B., & Ladda, R. L. (1994). Familial leukonychia, knuckle pads, hearing loss, and palmoplantar hyperkeratosis: An additional family with Bart-Pumphrey syndrome. *Journal of Medical Genetics, 31,* 68–71.

Rance, G. (2008). Auditory capacity in children with auditory neuropathy spectrum disorder. In D. Hayes & Y. S. Sininger (Eds.), *Guidelines to identification and management of infants and young children with auditory neuropathy spectrum disorder* (pp. 17–19). Denver, CO: Bill Daniels Center for Children's Hearing, The Children's Hospital.

Rance, G., & Rickards, F. (2002). Prediction of hearing threshold in infants using auditory steady-state evoked potentials. *Journal of the American Academy of Audiology, 13,* 236–245.

Rance, G., Rickards, F. W., Cohen, L. T., DeVidi, S., & Clark, G. M. (1995). The automated prediction of hearing thresholds in sleeping subjects using auditory steady-state potentials. *Ear and Hearing, 16,* 499–507.

Ranee, G., Beer, D. E., Cone-Wesson, B., Shepherd, R. C., Dowell, R. C., King, A. M. . . . Clark, G. M. (1999). Clinical findings for a group of infants and young children with auditory neuropathy. *Ear and Hearing, 20*(3), 238–252.

Raynor, D. B. (1993). Cytomegalovirus infection in pregnancy. *Seminars in Perinatalogy, 17,* 394–402.

Redding, J., Hargest, T., & Minsky, S. (1977). How noisy is intensive care? *Critical Care Medicine, 5,* 275.

Reed, D., & Dunn, W. (1970). Epidemiological studies of otitis media among Eskimo children. *Public Health Report, 85,* 699–706.

Reed, D., Struve, S., & Maynard, J. E. (1967). Otitis media and hearing deficiency among Eskimo children; a cohort study. *American Journal of Public Health, 57,* 1657–1662.

Reef, S. (2006). Rubella mass campaigns. *Current Topics in Microbiologic Immunology, 304,* 221–229.

Rehm, H. L., Zhang, D. S., Brown, M. C., Burgess, B., Halpin, C., Berger, W., . . . Chen, Z. Y. (2002). Vascular defects and sensorineural deafness in a mouse model of Norrie disease. *Journal of Neuroscience, 1*(22), 4286–4292.

Reilly, J. (1989). Congenital perilymph fistula: A prospective study in infants and children. *Laryngoscope, 99,* 393–397.

Reilly, S., Wake, M., Ukoumunne, O. C., Bavin, E., Prior, M., Cini, E., . . . Bretherton, L. (2010). Predicting language outcomes at 4 years of age: Findings from Early Language in Victoria Study. *Pediatrics, 126*(6), e1530–1537. Retrieved from http://peds.2010-0254[pii] 10.1542/peds.2010-0254

Reisen, A. H. (1947). The development of visual perception in man and chimpanzee. *Science, 106,* 107–108.

Reisen, A. H. (1960). Effects of stimulus deprivation on the development and atrophy of the visual sensory system. *American Journal of Orthopsychiatry, 30,* 23–36.

Renshaw, J., & Diefendorf, A. (1998). Adapting the test battery for the child with special needs. In F. Bess (Ed.), *Children with hearing impairment* (pp. 83–103). Nashville, TN: Bill Wilkerson Center Press.

Richards, B. W., & Rundle, A. T. (1959). A familial hormonal disorder associated with mental deficiency, deaf mutism and ataxia. *Journal of Mental Deficiencies Research, 3,* 33–35.

Richburg, C. M., & Smiley, D. F. (2012). *School-based audiology.* San Diego, CA: Plural.

Richieri-Costa, A., DeMirander, E., Kamiya, T. Y., & Freire-Maia, D. V. (1990). Autosomal dominant tibial hemimelia-poly-syndactyly-tripha-langeal thumbs syndrome: Report of a Brazilian family. *American Journal of Medical Genetics, 36,* 1–6.

Rickards, F. W., & Clark, G. M. (1982). Steady-state evoked potentials in humans to amplitude-modulated tones. *Journal of the Acoustical Society of America, 72*(1), S54.

Rickards, F. W., Tan, L. E., Cohen, L. T., Wilson, O. J., Drew, J. H., & Clark, G. M. (1994). Auditory steady-state evoked potentials in newborns. *British Journal of Audiology, 28,* 327–337.

Rickards, F. W., Wilson, O. J., Tan, L. E., & Cohen, L. T. (1990). Steady-state evoked potentials in normal neonates. *Australian Journal of Audiology, 21*(4).

Ricketts, T., Dittberner, A., & Johnson, E. (2008). High frequency amplification and sound quality in listeners with normal through moderate hearing loss. *Journal of Speech, Language, and Hearing Research, 51,* 160–172.

Ridgeway, J. (1969, August). Dumb children. *Saturday Review,* 19–21.

Riedner, E. D., Levin, S., & Holliday, M. J. (1980). Hearing patterns in dominant osteogenesis imperfecta. *Otolaryngology-Head and Neck Surgery, 106,* 737–740.

Ries, P. (1994). Prevalence and characteristics of persons with hearing trouble: United States, 1990–1991. *Vital Health Statistics, 10*(188), 9–10.

Riggs, W., Jr., & Seibert, J. (1972). Cockayne's syndrome; roentgen findings. *American Journal of Roentgenology, 116,* 623–633.

Rimoin, D. L., & Edgerton, M. T. (1967). Genetic and clinical heterogeneity in the oral-facial-digital syndrome. *Journal of Pediatrics, 71,* 94–102.

Rintelmann, W. F., & Bess, F. H. (1988). High-level amplification and potential hearing loss in children. In F. H. Bess (Ed.), *Hearing impairment in children* (pp. 278–309). Parkton, MD: York Press.

Robbins, A., & Osberger, M. J. (1991). *Meaningful use of speech scale.* Indianapolis, IN: Indiana Univeristy, School of Medicine.

Robbins, A. M., Bollard, P., & Green, J. (1999). Language development in children implanted with the Clarion cochlear implant. *Annals of Otology, Rhinology, and Laryngology, 177*(108), 2113–2118.

Robbins, A. M., Renshaw, J. J., & Berry, S. W. (1991). Evaluating meaningful auditory integration in profoundly hearing-impaired children. *American Journal of Otology, 12,* 144–150.

Robertson, S. P., Walsh, S., Oldridge, M., Gunn, T., Becroft, D., & Wilkie, A. O. (2001). Linkage of otopalatodigital syndrome type 2 (OPD2) to distal Xq28: Evidence for allelism with OPD1. *American Journal of Human Genetics, 69,* 223–227.

Robillard, T., & Gersdorff, M. (1986). Prevention of pre and perinatal acquired hearing defects. *Journal of Auditory Research, 26,* 207–237.

Robinette, M. S., Rhodes, D. P., & Marion, M. W. (1974). Effects of secobarbital on impedance audiometry. *Archives of Otolaryngology, 100,* 351–354.

Robinshaw, H. M. (1995). Early intervention for hearing impairment: Differences in the timing of communicative and linguistic development. *British Journal of Audiology, 29,* 314–334.

Robinson, J. D., Baer, T., & Moore, B. C. (2007). Using transposition to improve consonant discrimination and detection for listeners with severe high-frequency hearing loss. *International Journal of Audiology, 46,* 293–308.

Roeser, R., & Downs, M. (2004). *Auditory disorders in school children* (4th ed.). New York, NY: Thieme-Stratton.

Roeser, R., & Northern, J. (1981). Screening for hearing loss and middle ear disorders. In R. Roeser & M. Downs (Eds.), *Auditory disorders in school children* (pp. 120–150). New York. NY: Thieme-Stratton.

Roeser, R. J., Glorig, A., Gerken, G. M., & Kessinger, R. (1977). A hearing aid malfunction detection unit. *Journal of Speech and Hearing Disorders, 42,* 351–357.

Roizen, N. J. (1999). Etiology of hearing loss in children: Nongenetic causes. In N. J. Roizen & A. O. Diefendorf (Eds.), *Pediatric Clinics of North America, 46*(1), 49–64.

Roizen, N. J., & Johnson, D. (1996). Congenital infections. In A. J. Capute, & P. J. Accardo (Eds.), *Developmental disabilities in infancy and childhood* (2nd ed.). Baltimore, MD: Paul H. Brookes.

Roizen, N. J., Walters, C., Nicol, T., & Blondis, T. (1993). Hearing loss in children with Down syndrome. *Journal of Pediatrics, 123*(1), 9–11.

Rolffe, S. (2009). Cued speech. In L. Seaver (Ed.), *The book of choice: Support for parenting a child who is deaf or hard-of-hearing* (2nd ed.). Boulder, CO: Hands and Voices.

Rosenberg, G. G. (1995). *The improving classroom acoustics project.* Sarasota, FL: Florida Department of Education, Bureau of Student Services and Exceptional Education, 1993–1995.

Rosenfeld, R. (1997). Answers to parent's questions about otitis media. *Audiology Today, 9*(3), 12–13.

Rosenhall, U., Nordin, V., Sandstrom, M., Ahlsen, G., & Gillberg, C. (1999). Autism and hearing loss. *Journal of Autism and Developmental Disorders, 29*(5), 349–357.

Ross, D., & Fowler, K. (2008, May). Cytomegalovirus: A major cause of hearing loss in children. *ASHA Leader,* p. 6.

Ross, D. S., Gaffney, M., Green, D., & Holstrum, W. (2008). Prevalence and effects. *Seminars in Hearing, 29*(2), 141–148.

Ross, M. (1969). Changing concepts in hearing aid candidacy. *Eye, Ear, Nose, and Throat Monographs, 48,* 27–34.

Ross, M., & Lerman, J. (1970). A picture identification test for hearing-impaired children. *Journal of Speech and Hearing Research, 13,* 44–53.

Ross, M., & Seewald, R. C. (1988). Hearing aid selection and evaluation with young children. In F. Bess (Ed.), *Hearing impairment in children* (pp. 190–213). Parkton, MD: York Press.

Roush, J. (2000). What happens after screening? *Hearing Journal, 53,* 56–60.

Roush, J., Bryant, K., Mundy, M., Zeisel, S., & Roberts, J. (1995). Developmental changes in static admittance and tympanometric width in infants and toddlers. *Journal of the American Academy of Audiology, 6*(4), 334–338.

Roush, J., Holcomb, M., Roush, P., & Escolar, M. (2004). When hearing loss occurs with multiple disabilities. *Seminars in Hearing, 25*(4), 333–345.

Roush, J., & Kamo, G. (2008). Counseling and collaboration with parents of children with hearing loss. In J. Madell & C. Flexer (Eds.), *Pediatric audiology: Diagnosis, technology and management* (p. 273). New York, NY: Thieme.

Roush, J., & Matkin, N. (Eds.). (1994). *Infants and toddlers with hearing loss.* Baltimore, MD: York Press.

Roush, J., & McWilliam, R. A. (1994). Family-centered early intervention: Historical, philosophical and legislative issues. In J. Roush & N. Matkin (Eds.), *Infants and toddlers with hearing loss* (pp. 3–94). Baltimore, MD: York Press.

Roush, P. A. (2008). Management of children with auditory neuropathy spectrum disorder: Hearing aids. In D. Hayes & Y. S. Sininger (Eds.), *Guidelines to identification and management of infants and young children with auditory neuropathy spectrum disorder* (pp. 30–32). Denver, CO: Bill Daniels Center for Children's Hearing, The Children's Hospital.

Roush, P. A., & Seewald, R. C. (2009). Acoustic amplification for infants and children: Selection, fitting and management. In L. S. Eisenberg (Ed.), *Clinical management of children with cochlear implants* (pp. 35–57). San Diego, CA: Plural.

Rowe, M. L. (2008). Child-directed speech: Relation to socioeconomic status, knowledge of child development and child vocabulary skill. *Journal of Child Language, 35*(1), 185–205.

Rowe, M. L., & Goldin-Meadow, S. (2009). Differences in early gesture explain SES disparities in child vocabulary size at school entry. *Science, 323,* 5916.

Royer, G., Hanein, S., Raclin, V, Gigarel, N., Rozet, J. M., Munnich, A., . . . Bonnefont, J. P. (2003). NDP gene mutations in 14 French families with Norrie disease. *Human Mutatations, 22*(6), 499.

Ruben, R. J., & Rapin, I. (1980). Plasticity of the developing auditory system. *Annals of Otology, Rhinology, and Laryngology, 89,* 303–311.

Rudnick, C. M., & Hoekzema, G. S. (2002). Neonatal herpes simplex virus infection. *American Family Physician, 65*(6), 1138–1142.

Ruppert, E. S., Buerk, E., & Pfordresher, M. F. (1970). Hereditary hearing loss with saddle nose and myopia. *Archives of Otolaryngology, 92,* 95–98.

Rushmer, N. (1994). Supporting families of hearing-impaired infants and toddlers. *Seminars in Hearing, 15*(2), 160–171.

Rutter, M. (1978). Diagnosis and definition. In M. Rutter & E. Schopler (Eds.), *Autism: A reappraisal of concepts and treatments* (pp. 1–26). New York, NY: Plenum Press.

Ryan, A. F., & Dallos, P. (1996). The physiology of the cochlea. In J. Northern (Ed.), *Hearing disorders* (3rd ed.). Needham Heights, MA: Allyn & Bacon.

Sabo, D. L., Paradise, J. L., Kurs-Lasky, M., & Smith, C. G. (2003). Hearing levels in infants and young children in relation to testing technique, age group, and the presence or absence of middle-ear effusion. *Ear and Hearing, 24,* 38–47.

Salamy, A., Eldredge, L., & Tooley, W. H. (1989). Neonatal status and hearing loss in high-risk infants. *Journal of Pediatrics, 114,* 847–852.

Samples, J. M., & Franklin, B. (1978). Behavioral responses in 7 to 9-month-old infants to speech and non-speech stimuli. *Journal of Auditory Research, 18,* 115–123.

Sando, I., Hemenway, W. G., & Morgan, R. W. (1968). Histopathology of the temporal bone in mandibulofacial dysostosis. *Transactions of the American Academy of Ophthalmology and Otolaryngology, 72,* 913–924.

Sanlaville, D., & Verloes, A. (2007). CHARGE syndrome: An update. *European Journal of Human Genetics, 15*(4), 389–399.

Sarnat, H., & Menkes, J. (2000). Neuroembryology: Genetic programming and malformations of the nervous system. In J. Menkes & H. Sarnat (Eds.), *Child neurology.* Baltimore, MD: Lippincott Williams & Wilkins.

Savage-Rumbaugh, E., Taylor, T., & Shanker, S. (1998). *Apes, language and the human mind.* London, UK: Oxford University Press.

Savarirayan, R. (2003). Oto-palato-digital syndrome. In *The NORD guide to rare disorders* (pp. 239–240). Philadelphia, PA: Lippincott Williams & Wilkins.

Savarirayan, R., Cornmier-Daire, V., Unger, S., Lachman, R. S., Roughley, P. J., Wagner, S. F.,

. . . Wilcox, W. R. (2000). Oto-palato-digital syndrome, type II: Report of three cases with further delineation of the chrondro-osseous morphology. *American Journal of Medical Genetics, 95,* 193–200.

Schaefer, B., Stein, S., Oshman, D., Rennert, O., Thumau, G., Wall, J., . . . Brown, O. (1986). Dominantly inherited craniodiaphysial dysplasia. *Clinical Genetics, 30,* 381–391.

Schafer, E., & Kleineck, M. (2009). Improvements in speech recognition using cochler implants and three types of FM systems: A meta-analytic approach. *Journal of Educational Audiology, 15,* 4–14.

Schaefer, G. B., Kolodziej, P., & Olney, A. (1998). Oto-palatal-digital syndromes. *Ear, Nose, and Throat Journal, 77*(8), 586–587.

Schein, J. D., & Delk, M. T. (1974). *The deaf population of the United States.* Silver Spring, MD: National Association of the Deaf.

Scherz, R. G., Graga, J. R., & Reichelderfer, T. E. (1972). A typical example of 13-15 trisomy in a Negro boy. *Clinical Pediatrics, 11,* 246–248.

Schild, J. A., Mafee, M. G., & Miller, M. F. (1984). Wildervanck syndrome: The external appearance and radiographic findings. *International Journal of Pediatric Otorhinolaryngology, 7,* 305–310.

Schildroth, A. (1988). Recent changes in the educational placement of deaf students. *American Annals of the Deaf, 133*(2), 61–67.

Schildroth, A., & Hotto, S. (1993). Annual survey of hearing-impaired children and youth: 1991–1992 school year. *American Annals of the Deaf, 138*(2), 239–243.

Schlesinger, H. S., & Meadow, K. P. (1972). Emotional support to parents. In D. L. Lillie (Ed.), *Monograph on parent programs in child development centers* (pp. 13–25). Chapel Hill, NC: University of North Carolina Press.

Schröder, J. M., Hackel, V., Wanders, R. J., Göhlich-Ratmann, G., & Voit, T. (2004). Optico-cochleo-dentate degeneration associated with severe peripheral neuropathy and caused by peroxisomal D-bifunctional protein deficiency. *Acta Neuropathologica, 108*(2), 154–167.

Schuknecht, H. F. (1993). *Pathology of the ear* (2nd ed.). Philadelphia, PA: Lea and Febiger.

Schulman-Galambos, C., & Galambos, R. (1979). Brainstem evoked response audiometry in newborn hearing screening. *Archives of Otolaryngology, 105,* 86–90.

Schultz, L. F., Vase, P., & Schmidt, H. (1978). Atopic dermatitis and congenital deafness. *British Journal of Dermatology, 99,* 325–328.

Schwartz, D. M., & Schwartz, R. H. (1978). A comparison of tympanometry and acoustic reflex measurements for detecting middle ear effusion in infants below seven months of age. In E. R. Harford, F. H. Bess, C. D. Bluestone, & J. Klein (Eds.), *Impedance screening for middle ear disease in children* (pp. 91–96). New York, NY: Grune & Stratton.

Schwartz, D. M., & Schwartz, R. H. (1980). Tympanometric findings in young infants with middle ear effusion: Some further observations. *International Journal of Pediatric Otolaryngology, 2,* 67–72.

Schwartz, S. (1987). *Choices in deafness: A parent's guide.* Bethesda, MD: Woodbine House.

Scollie, S. D. (2006). The DSL method: Improving with age. *Hearing Journal, 59*(6), 10–16.

Scollie, S. D., Ching, T. Y. C., Seewald, R. C., Dillon, H., Britton, L. Steinberg, J., & Corcoran, J. (2010). Evaluation of the NAL-NAL1 and DSL v4.1 prescriptions for children: Preferences in real world use. *International Journal of Audiology, 49,* S49–S63.

Scollie, S. D., & Seewald, R. (2002). Hearing aid fitting and verification procedures for children. In J. Katz (Ed.), *Handbook of clinical audiology* (pp. 687–706). New York, NY: Lippincott William & Wilkins.

Scollie, S. D., Seewald, R., Cornelisse, L., Moodie, S., Bogatto, M., Launagaray, D., . . . Dumford, J. (2005). The desired sensation level multistage input/output algorithm. *Trends in Amplification, 9*(4), 159–197.

Sculerati, N., Ledesna-Medina, J., Finegold, D. N., & Stool, S. E. (1990). Otitis media and hearing loss in Turner syndrome. *Archives of Otolaryngology-Head and Neck Surgery, 116*(4), 707.

Seaver, L. (Ed.). (2009). *The book of choice: Support for parenting a child who is deaf or hard-of-hearing.* Boulder, CO: Hands and Voices.

Seewald, R. C. (1991). Hearing aid output limiting considerations for children. In J. Feigin & P. Stelmachowicz, (Eds.), *Pediatric amplification: Proceedings of the 1991 national conference* (pp. 19–35). Omaha, NE: Boys Town National Hospital Press.

Seewald, R. C. (2013). *A retrospective on the development of a science-based approach to pediatric hearing aid fittings: What a difference 40 years makes.* Presented at Marion Downs Lecture in Pediatric Audiology, AudiologyNOW, Anaheim, CA.

Seewald, R. C., Mills, J., Bagatto, M., Scollie, S., & Moodie, S. (2008). A comparison of manufacturer-specific prescriptive procedures for infants. *Hearing Journal, 61*(11), 26–34.

Seewald, R. C., Moodie, S., Scollie, S., & Bagatto, M. (2005). The DSL method of pediatric hearing instrument fitting: Historical perspective and current issues. *Trends in Amplification, 9*(4), 145–157.

Seewald, R. C., Ross, M., & Spiro, M. K. (1985). Selecting amplification characteristics for young hearing-impaired children. *Ear and Hearing, 6*(1), 48–53.

Seewald, R. C., & Scollie, S. (1999). Infants are not average adults: Implications for audiometric testing. *Hearing Journal, 52*, 64–72.

Segal, N., & Puterman, M. (2007). Cleidocranial dysplasia: Review with an emphasis on otological and audiological manifestations. *International Journal of Pediatric Otorhinolaryngology, 71*(4), 523–526.

Sekhar, L., Zalewski, T. R., & Pau, I. M. (2013). Variability of state school-based hearing screening protocols in the United States. *Journal of Community Health, 38*(3), 569–574.

Sell, E. J., Gaines, J. A., Gluckman, C., & Williams, E. (1985). Persistent fetal circulation neurodevleopmental outcome. *American Journal of Diseases in Children, 139*, 25–28.

Serpanos, Y. C., & Jarmel, F. (2007). Quantitative and qualitative follow-up outcomes from a preschool audiologic screening program: Perspectives over a decade. *American Journal of Audiology, 16*(1), 4–12.

Shanon, E., Himelfarb, M., & Gold, S. (1981). Auditory function in Friedreich's ataxia. *Otolaryngology-Head and Neck Surgery, 107*, 254–256.

Shapiro, B. L. (2003). Down syndrome and associated congenital malformations. *Journal of Neural Transmission, 67*(Suppl.), 207–214.

Shapiro, F. (1993). Osteopetrosis: Current clinical considerations. *Clinical Orthopedics, 294*, 34.

Shargorodsky, J., Curhan, S. G., Curhan, G. C., & Eavey, R. (2010). Change in prevalence of hearing loss in U.S. adolescents. *Journal of the American Medical Association, 304*(7), 772–778.

Sharma, A., Cardon, G., Henion, K., & Roland, P. (2011). Cortical maturation and behavioral outcomes in children with auditory neuropathy spectrum disorder. *Internatational Journal of Audiology, 50*, 98–106.

Sharma, A., & Dorman, M. (2005). The clinical use of P[1] latency as a bio-marker for assessment of central auditory development in children with hearing impairment. *Audiology Today, 17*(3), 18–19.

Sharma, A., Dorman, M., & Spahr, A. (2002). A sensitive period for the development of the central auditory system in children with cochlear implants: Implications for age of implantation. *Ear and Hearing, 23*(6), 532–539.

Sharma, A., Martin, K., Roland, P., Bauer, P., Sweeny, M., Gilley, P., & Dorman, M. (2005). P[1] latency as a biomarker for central auditory development in children with hearing impairment. *Journal of the American Academy of Audiology, 16*, 568–577.

Sharma, A., Nash, A., & Dorman, M. (2009). Cortical development, plasticity and re-organization in children with cochlear implants. *Journal of Communication Disorders, 42*, 272–279.

Sharma, A., Purdy, S. C., & Kelly, A. S. (2009). Comorbidity of auditory processing, language, and reading disorders. *Journal of Speech, Language, and Hearing Research, 52*(3), 706.

Sharma, A., Purdy, S., & Kelly, A. (2012). A randomized control trial of interventions in school-aged children with auditory processing disorders. *International Journal of Audiology, 51*(7), 506–518.

Sharma, A., Purdy, S. C., Newall, P., Wheldall, K., Beaman, R., & Dillon, H. (2006). Electrophysiological and behavioral evidence of auditory processing deficits in children with reading disorder. *Clinical Neurophysiology*, *117*, 1130–1144.

Sharma, A., Tobey, E., Dorman, M., Martin, K., Gilley, P., & Kunkel, F. (2004). Central auditory maturation and babbling development in infants with cochlear implants. *Archives of Otolaryngology-Head Neck Surgery*, *130*(5), 511–516.

Shemen, L. J., Mitchell, D. P., & Farkashidy, J. (1984). Cockayne syndrome—An audiologic and temporal bone analysis. *American Journal of Otology*, *5*, 300–307.

Sherman, S. L., Allen, E. G., Bean, L. H., & Freeman, S. B. (2007). Epidemiology of Down syndrome. *Mental Retardation and Development Disabilities Research Review*, *13*(3), 221–227.

Shohat, M., Flaum, E., Cobb, S. R., Lachman, R., Rubin, C., Ash, C., & Rimoin, D. L. (1993). Hearing loss and temporal bone structure in achondroplasia. *American Journal of Medical Genetics*, *45*, 548–551.

Shokeir, M. K. (1977). The Goldenhar syndrome: A natural history. *Birth Defects*, *13*(3C), 67–83.

Shroder, J., Hackel, V., Wanders, R., Gohlich-Ratmann, G., & Voit, T. (2004). Opticocochleo-dentate degeneration associated with severe peripheral neuropathy and caused by peroxisomal D-bifunctional protein deficiency. *Acta Neuropathology*, *108*(2), 154–167.

Shurin, P. A., Pelton, S. I., Donner, A., & Klein, J. (1979). Persistence of middle ear effusion after acute otitis media in children. *New England Journal of Medicine*, *300*, 1121–1123.

Shurin, P. A., Pelton, S. I., & Klein, J. O. (1976). Otitis media in the newborn infant. *Annals of Otolology, Rhinolology, and Laryngology*, *85*, 216–222.

Siegenthaler, B., & Haspiel, G. (1996). *Development of two standardized measures of hearing for speech by children*. Washington, DC: Cooperative Research Program, Project 2372, U. S. Office of Education.

Silman, S., Gelfand, S., & Silverman, C. (1984). Late-onset auditory deprivation: Effects of monaural versus bilateral hearing aids. *Journal of the Acoustical Society of America*, *76*(5), 1357–1362.

Silver, H. K. (1964). The de Lange syndrome. *American Journal of Diseases of Children*, *108*, 523–529.

Silverman, C. A., & Emmer, M. B. (1993). Auditory deprivation and recovery in adults with asymmetric sensorineural hearing impairment. *Journal of the American Academy of Audiology*, *4*, 338–346.

Silverman, C. A., & Silman, S. (1990). Apparent auditory deprivation from monaural amplification and recovery with binaural amplification. *Journal of the American Academy of Audiology*, *1*, 175–180.

Simmons, F. B. (1976). Automated hearing screening test for newborns: The Crib-o-Gram. In G. Mencher (Ed.), *Early identification of hearing loss* (pp. 171–180). Basel, Switzerland: Karger.

Simmons, F. B. (1982). Comment on hearing loss in graduates of a tertiary intensive care nursery. *Ear and Hearing*, *3*, 188.

Simmons, F. B., & Russ, F. (1974). Automated newborn hearing screening: The Crib-o-Gram. *Archives of Otolaryngology*, *100*, 1.

Simmons, J., Beauchaine, K. L., & Eiten, L. R. (2007). Hearing instrument fitting for infants and young children. In R. S. Ackley, T. N. Decker, & C. J. Limb (Eds.), *The essential guide to hearing and balance disorders* (pp. 217–247). Mahwah, NJ: Lawrence Erlbaum.

Singh, S., & Bresman, M. J. (1973). Menkes' "kinky hair syndrome" (trichopolio dystrophy). *American Journal of Diseases in Children*, *125*, 572–578.

Singh, S. P., Rock, E. H., & Shulman, A. (1969). Klippel-Feil syndrome with unexplained conductive hearing loss. *Laryngoscope*, *79*, 113–117.

Sininger, Y. S. (2008). Auditory neuropathy spectrum disorder: Challenges and questions. In D. Hayes & Y. Sininger (Eds.), *Guidelines to identification and management of infants and young children with auditory neuropathy spectrum disorder* (pp. 9–14). Denver, CO: Bill Daniels Center for Children's Hearing, The Children's Hospital.

Sininger, Y. S., Doyle, K. J., & Moore, J. K. (1999). The case for early identification of hearing loss in children. *Pediatric Clinics of North America, 46*(1), 1–13.

Sininger, Y. S., Hood, L. J., Starr, A., Berlin, C. I., & Picton, T. W. (1995). Hearing loss due to auditory neuropathy. *Audiology Today, 7*(2), 10–12.

Sininger, Y. S., Martinez, A., Eisenberg, L. S., Christnsen, E., Grimes, A., & Hu, J. (2009). Newborn hearing screening speeds diagnosis and access to intervention by 20–24 months. *Journal of American Academy of Audiology, 20*, 49–57.

Sininger, Y. S., & Starr, A. (2001). *Auditory neuropathy: A new perspective on hearing disorders.* San Diego, CA: Singular.

Siqueland, E. R., & DeLucia, C. A. (1969). Visual reinforcement of nonnutritive sucking in human infants. *Science, 165*, 1144–1146.

Skinner, M. W. (1978). The hearing of speech during language acquisition. *Otolaryngologic Clinics of North America, 11*, 631–650.

Smaldino, J., & Crandell, C. (2000). Classroom amplification technology: Theory and practice. *Language, Speech, and Hearing Services in Schools, 31*, 371–376.

Smaldino, J., & Crandell, C. C. (2004). Classroom acoustics. *Seminars in Hearing, 25*(2).

Smart, J., Purdy, S., & Kelly, A. (2008). Personal FM systems for children with auditory processing disorder: Successfully fitting this heterogeneous population. *Access 2: Achieving clear communication employing sound solutions–2008: Proceedings of the first international virtual conference on FM* (pp. 38–44).

Smiley, D. F., & Richburg, S. (2012a). Classroom acoustics. In S. Richburg & D. F. Smiley (Eds.), *School-based audiology.* San Diego, CA: Plural.

Smiley, D. F., & Richburg, S. (2012b). Amplification for the classroom. In S. Richburg & D. F. Smiley (Eds.), *School-based audiology.* San Diego, CA: Plural.

Smith, C. G., Paradise, J. L., Sabo, D. L., Rockette, H. E., Kars-Lasky, M., & Bernard, B. S. (2006). Tympanonometric findings and the probability of middle-ear effusion in 3686 infants and young children. *Pediatrics, 118*, 1–13.

Smith, D. W. (1962). The number 18 trisomy syndrome. *Journal of Pediatrics, 60*, 513.

Smith, K., & Hodgson, W. (1970). The effects of systematic reinforcement on the speech discrimination responses of normal and hearing-impaired children. *Journal of Auditory Research, 10*, 110–117.

Smith, R. J., Berlin, C. I., Hejtmancik, J. F., Keats, B. J., Kimberling, W. J., Lewis, R. A., . . . Tranebjaerg, L. (1994). Clinical diagnosis of the Usher syndromes. Usher syndrome consortium. *American Journal of Medical Genetics, 50*(1), 32–38.

Smoski, W. J., Brunt, M. A., & Tannahill, J. C. (1992). Listening characteristics of children with central auditory processing disorders. *Language, Speech, and Hearing Services in Schools, 23*, 145–152.

Sohmer, H., & Feinmesser, M. (1967). Cochlear action potentials recorded from the external ear in man. *Annals of Otolaryngology, 76*, 427–435.

Solomon, M., Pistrang, N., & Barker, C. (2004). The benefits of mutual support groups for parents of children with disabilities. *American Journal of Communication Psychology, 29*(1), 113–132.

Sousa, D. A. (2011). *How the brain learns* (4th ed.). Thousand Oaks, CA: Corwin Press.

Sparkes, R. S., & Graham, C. B. (1972). Camurati-Englemann disease: Genetics and clinical manifestations with a review of the literature. *Journal of Medical Genetics, 9*, 73–85.

Sparks, S. (1984). Speech and language in fetal alcohol syndrome. *Asha, 26*, 27–31.

Sperling, M. (2008). *Pediatric endocrinology* (p. 615). New York, NY: Elsevier Health Sciences.

Spitz, R. A. (1959). *A genetic field theory of ego formation. Its implications for pathology.* New York, NY: International Universities Press.

Spivak, L. (1998). *Universal newborn hearing screening.* New York, NY: Thieme Medical.

Spoendlin, H. (1967). The innervation of the organ of Corti. *Journal of Laryngology and Otology, 81*, 717–738.

Spoendlin, H. (1969). Innervation patterns in the organ of Corti of the cat. *Acta Oto-Laryngologica (Stockholm), 67*, 239–254.

Spoendlin, H. (1974). Congenital stapes ankylosis and fusion of carpal and tarsal bones as a dominant hereditary syndrome. *Acta Oto-Rhino-Laryngologica, 206*, 173–179.

Sprague, B., Wiley, T., & Goldstein, R. (1985). Tympanometric and acoustic reflex studies in neonates. *Journal of Speech and Hearing Research, 28*, 265–272.

Spring, D. R., & Dale, P. A. (1977). Discrimination of linguistic stress in early infancy. *Journal of Speech and Hearing Research, 20*, 224–232.

Stach, B. (1998). Central auditory disorders. In A. Lalwani & K. Grundfast (Eds.), *Pediatric otology and neurotology* (pp. 387–396). Philadelphia, PA: Lippincott-Raven.

Stach, B. (2002). The auditory steady-state response: A primer. *Hearing Journal, 55*(9), 10–18.

Stach B. (2008). *Clinical audiology: An introduction.* San Diego, CA: Plural.

Stach, B. A., & Jerger, J. F. (1990). Immittance measures in auditory disorders. In J. Jacobson & J. Northern (Eds.), *Diagnostic audiology.* Boston, MA: College-Hill Press.

Stagno, S., Pass, R. F., Dworsky, M. E., Henderson, R. E., Moore, E. G., Walton, P., & Alford, C. A. (1982). Congenital cytomegalovirus infection: The relative importance of primary and recurrent maternal infection. *New England Journal of Medicine, 306*, 945–949.

Stanley, F. J., & Blair, E. (1994). Cerebral palsy. In I. B. Pless (Ed.), *The epidemiology of childhood disorders* (pp. 473–497). New York, NY: Oxford University Press.

Stanley, R. J., Puritz, E. M., Birggaman, R. A., & Wheeler, C. E., Jr. (1975). Sensory radicular neuropathy. *Archives of Dermatology, 111*, 760–762.

Stapells, D. R., & Oats, P. (1997). Estimation of the pure-tone audiogram by the auditory brainstem response: A review. *Audiology and Neurotology, 2*, 257–280.

Starr, A. (2008). Auditory neurosciences and the recognition of auditory neuropathy. In D. Hayes, & Y. S. Sininger (Eds.). *Guidelines to identification and management of infants and young children with auditory neuropathy spectrum disorder* (pp. 15–16). Aurora, CO: Bill Daniels Center for Children's Hearing, The Children's Hospital.

Starr, A., Arnlie, R. N., Martin, W. H., & Sanders, S. (1977). Development of auditory function in newborn infants revealed by auditory brainstem potentials. *Pediatrics, 60*, 831–839.

Starr, A., Picton, T. W., Sininger, Y. S., Hood, L. J., & Berlin, C. I. (1996). Auditory neuropathy. *Brain, 119*, 741–753.

Stein, L. (1999). Factors influencing the efficacy of universal newborn hearing screening. *Pediatric Clinics of North America, 46*(1), 95–105.

Stein, L., & Boyer, K. (1994). Progress in the prevention of hearing loss in infants. *Ear and Hearing, 15*, 116–124.

Stein, L., Clark, S., & Kraus, N. (1983). The hearing-impaired infant: Patterns of identification and habilitation. *Ear and Hearing, 4*(5), 232–236.

Stein, L., Ozdamar, O., & Schnabel, M. (1981). Auditory brainstem responses (ABR) with suspected deaf-blind children. *Ear and Hearing, 1*(2), 30–40.

Stein, L., Tremblay, K., Pasternak, J., Banerjee, S., Lindemann, K., & Kraus, N. (1996). Brainstem abnormalities in neonates with normal otoacoustic emissions. *Seminars in Hearing, 17*, 197–213.

Stein, L. K., & Boyer, K. M. (1994). Progress in the prevention of hearing loss in infants. *Ear and Hearing, 15*(2), 116–125.

Stein, L. K., & Jabaley, T. (1981). Early identification and parent counseling. In L. Stein, E. Mendel, & T. Jabaley (Eds.), *Deafness and mental health.* New York, NY: Grune & Stratton.

Stein, L. K., Jabaley, T., Spitz, R., Stoakley, D., & McGee, T. (1990). Hearing-impaired infants: Patterns of identification and habilitation revisited. *Ear and Hearing, 11*(3), 201–205.

Stein, L. K., & Kraus, N. (1988). Auditory evoked potentials with special populations. *Seminars in Hearing, 9*(1), 35–46.

Stein, L. K., Kraus, N., Ozdamar, O., Cartee, C., Jabaley, T., Jeantet, C., & Reed, N. (1987). Hearing loss in an institutionalized mentally retarded population. *Otolaryngology-Head and Neck Surgery, 113,* 32–35.

Stelmachowicz, P., Hoover, B. M., Lewis, D. E., & Kortekaas, R. (2000). The relation between stimulus context, speech audibility, and perception for normal-hearing and hearing-impaired children. *Journal of Speech, Language, and Hearing Research, 43*(4), 902–914.

Stelmachowicz, P., Lewis, D., Choi, S., & Hoover, B. (2007). Effect of stimulus bandwidth on auditory skills in normal hearing and hearing-impaired children. *Ear and Hearing, 28,* 483–494.

Stelmachowicz, P., Pittman, A., Hoover, B., & Lewis, D. (2001). The effect of stimulus bandwidth on the perception of /s/ in normal and hearing impaired children and adults. *Journal of the Acoustical Society of America, 110,* 2183–2190.

Stelmachowicz, P., Pittman, A., Hoover, B., Lewis, D., & Moeller, M. (2004). The importance of high-frequency audibility in the speech and language development of children with hearing loss. *Archives of Otolaryngology-Head & Neck Surgery, 130,* 556–562.

Stelmachowicz, P., Seewald, R., & Gorga, M. (1998). Strategies for fitting amplification in early infancy. In F. Bess (Ed.), *Children with hearing impairment: Contemporary trends.* Nashville, TN: Vanderbilt Bill Wilkerson Center Press.

Stender, T., Appleby, R., & Hallenbeck, S. (2011). V & V and its impact on user satisfaction. *Hearing Review, 12,* 16–18–21.

Stephenson, P., & Zawolkow, E. (2009). Signing Exact English (SEE). In L. Seaver (Ed.), *The book of choice: Support for parenting a child who is deaf or hard-of-hearing.* Boulder, CO: Hands and Voices.

Stewart, E. J., & O'Reilly, B. F. (1989). Klippel-Feil syndrome and conductive deafness. *Journal of Laryngology and Otology, 103,* 947–949.

Stewart, J. M., & Bergstrom, L. (1971). Familial hand abnormality and sensorineural deafness: A new syndrome. *Journal of Pediatrics, 78,* 102–110.

Stockard, J. E., Stockard, J. J., Westmoreland, B., & Corfits, J. L. (1979). Brainstem auditory evoked responses: Normal variation as a function of stimulus and subject characteristics. *Archives of Neurology, 36,* 823–831.

Stockard, J. E., & Westmoreland, B. F. (1981). Technical considerations in the recording and interpretation of the brainstem auditory evoked potential for neonatal neurologic diagnosis. *American Journal of EEG Technology, 21,* 31–54.

Stoel-Gammon, C., & Otomo, K. (1986). Babbling development of hearing-impaired and normally hearing subjects. *Journal of Speech and Hearing Disorders, 51,* 33–41.

Strasnick, B., & Jacobson, J. T. (1995). Teratogenic hearing loss. *Journal of the American Academy of Audiology, 6*(1), 29–38.

Stratton, H. J. M. (1965). Gonadal dysgenesis and the ears. *Journal of Laryngology and Otology, 79,* 343–346.

Stredler-Brown, A. (2008). The importance of early intervention for infants and children with hearing loss. In J. Madell & C. Flexer (Eds.), *Pediatric audiology: Diagnosis, technology, and management* (pp. 239). New York, NY: Thieme.

Stredler-Brown, A., & Johnson, C. D. (2004). *Functional auditory performance indicators: An integrated approach to auditory skill development.* Retrieved from http://www.cde.state.co.uscdesped/download/FAPI_3-1-04g.pdf

Strong, C. J., Clark, T. C., & Walden, B. E. (1994). The relationship of hearing loss severity to demographic, age, treatment and intervention effectiveness variables. *Ear and Hearing, 15*(2), 126–137.

Stuckless, E. R. (Ed.). (1980). Deafness and rubella: Infants in the 60s, adults in the 80s. *American Annals of the Deaf, 125,* 959.

Suzuki, T., & Ogiba, Y. (1961). Conditioned orientation audiometry. *Archives of Otolaryngology, 74,* 192–198.

Swanepoel, D. W. (2012). The need for tele-audiology. *Hearing Review, 19*(10), 18–25.

Sweetow, R. W. (2009). Time-based expectations and the communication needs assessment. *Starkey Audiology Series, 1*(3).

Sybert, V. P., & McCauley, E. (2004). Turner's syndrome, *New England Journal of Medicine, 351*(12), 1227–1238.

Syka, J., & Meerzenich, M. (Eds.). (2011). *Plasticity and signal representation in the auditory system.* New York, NY: Springer Sciences+Business Media.

Sylvester, P. E. (1958). Some unusual findings in a family with Friedreich's ataxia. *Archives of Diseases in Childhood, 33,* 217–221.

Sylvester, P. E. (1972). Spino-cerebellar degeneration, hormonal disorder, hypogonadism, deaf-mutism, and mental deficiency. *Journal of Mental Deficiencies Research, 16,* 203–214.

Tahtinen, P. A., Laine, M. K., Houvinen, P., Jalava, J., Ruuskanen, O., & Ruohola, A. (2011). A placebo-controlled trial of antimicrobial treatment for acute otitis media. *New England Journal of Medicine, 364*(2), 116–126.

Tait, M., Nikolopoulos, T. P., DeRaeve, L., Johnson, S., Datta, G., Karltorp, E., . . . Frijns, J. H. (2010). Bilateral versus unilateral cochlear implantation in young children. *International Journal of Pediatric Otorhinolarngology, 74,* 206–211.

Tan, T., Constantinides, H., & Mitchell, T. (2005). The preauricular sinus: A review of its aetiology, clinical presentation and management. *International Journal of Pediatric Otorhinolaryngology, 69,* 1469–1474.

Taylor, B., & Mueller, H. G. (2011). *Fitting and dispensing hearing aids.* San Diego, CA: Plural.

Teele, D. W. (1994). Long term sequela of otitis media: Fact or fiction? *Pediatric Infectious Disease Journal, 13,* 1069–1073.

Teele, D. W., Klein, J. O., & Rosner, B. A. (1989). Epidemiology of otitis media during the first seven years of life in children in greater Boston: A prospective, cohort study. *Journal of Infectious Disease, 160*(1), 83–94.

Templin, M. (1966). Vocabulary problems of the deaf child. *International Audiology, 5,* 349.

Tervoort, B. (1964). Development of languages and the critical period; the young deaf child: Identification and management. *Acta Oto-Laryngologica Supplement (Stockholm), 206,* 247–251.

Tharpe, A. M., & Ashmead, D. (1993). Computer simulation technique for assessing pediatric auditory test protocols. *Journal of the American Academy of Audiology, 4*(2), 80–90.

Tharpe, A. M., Sladen, D. P., Dodd-Murphy, J., & Boney, S. J. (2009). Minimal hearing loss in children: Miminal but not inconsequential. *Seminars in Hearing, 30*(2), 80–91.

Thelin, J. W., Mitchell, J. A., Hefner, M. A., & Davenport, S. L. (1986). CHARGE syndrome: Part II. Hearing loss. *International Journal of Pediatric Otorhinolaryngology, 12,* 145–163.

The State of America's Children. (2011). Children's Defense Fund. Retrieved from http://www.childrensdefense.org/child-research-data-publications/data/state-of-americas-2011.pdf

Thomas, I. T., Frias, J. L., Felix, V., Sanchez de Leon, L., Hernandez, R. A., & Jones, M. C. (1986). Isolated and syndromic cryptophtalmos. *American Journal of Medical Genetics, 25*(1), 85–98.

Thompson, G. (1983). Structure and function of the central auditory system. *Seminars in Hearing, 4,* 81–95.

Thompson, G., & Folsom, R. C. (1984). A comparison of two conditioning procedures in the use of visual reinforcement audiometry (VRA). *Journal of Speech and Hearing Disorders, 49,* 241–245.

Thompson, G., Wilson, W., & Moore, J. (1979). Application of visual reinforcement audiometry (VRA) to low-functioning children. *Journal of Speech and Hearing Disorders, 44,* 80–90.

Thompson, M., & Thompson, G. (1972). Responses of infants and young children as a function of auditory stimuli and test month. *Journal of Speech and Hearing Research, 15,* 699–707.

Thompson, M., Thompson, G., & Vethivelu, S. (1989). A comparison of audiometric test methods for 2-year-old children. *Journal of Speech and Hearing Disorders, 54,* 174–179.

Thomsen, K. A., Terkildsen, K., & Arnfred, J. (1965). Middle ear pressure during anesthesia. *Archives of Otolaryngology-Head and Neck Surgery, 82*, 609.

Tietz, W. (1963). A syndrome of deaf-mutism associated with albinism showing dominant autosomal inheritance. *American Journal of Human Genetics, 15*, 259–264.

Time. (2012, October 22). *180*(17).

Tjellstrom, A., & Hakansson, B. (1995). The bone-anchored hearing aid: Design principles, indications, and long-term clinical results. *Otolaryngology Clinics of North America, 28*(1), 53–72.

Tobey, E. (2010, February 16). The changing landscape of pediatric cochlear implantation. *ASHA Leader*, p. 1.

Tompkins, S. M., & Hall, J. W., III. (1990). Comparison of two gradient methods in normal ears versus otitis media [Abstract]. *Journal of the American Academy of Audiology, 1*, 49–50.

Toriello, H. (1995). CHARGE association. *Journal of the American Academy of Audiology, 6*(1), 47–53.

Trainor, P. A., Dixon, J., & Dixon, M. J. (2009). Treacher Collins syndrome: Etiology, pathogenesis and prevention. *European Journal of Human Genetics, 4*, 275–283.

Tremblay, K. L. (2003). Central auditory plasticity: Implications for auditory rehabilitation. *The Hearing Journal, 56*(1), 10–13.

Tremblay, K. L., & Kraus, N. (2002). Auditory training induces asymmetrical changes in cortical neural activity. *Journal of Speech, Language, and Hearing Research, 45*(3), 564–572.

Trevarthen, C. (1975). Early attempts at speech. In R. Levin (Ed.), *Child alive*. Garden City, NY: Anchor Press/Doubleday.

Tyler, R. S. (Ed.). (1993). *Cochlear implants: Audiological foundations*. San Diego, CA: Singular.

Umat, C., Mukari, S., Ezan, N., & Din, N. (2011). Changes in auditory memory performance following the use of frequency-modulated system in children with suspected auditory processing disorders. *Saudi Medical Journal, 32*(8), 818–824.

Upfold, L. (1988). Children with hearing aids in the 80s: Etiologies and severity of impairment. *Ear and Hearing, 9*, 75–80.

U.S. Department of Education. (2005). *The condition of education 2005*. Retrieved from http://files.eric.ed.gov/fulltext/ED492631.pdf

U. S. Department of Health and Human Services. (2000, January). *Healthy People 2010*. Retrieved from http://www.health.gov/healthypeople/

Uus, K. (2008). Identification of neonates with auditory neuropathy spectrum disorder. In D. Hayes & Y. S. Sininger (Eds.), *Guidelines to identification and management of infants and young children with auditory neuropathy spectrum disorder* (pp. 28–29). Denver, CO: Bill Daniels Center for Children's Hearing, The Children's Hospital.

Valente, M. (Ed.). (2002a). *Strategies for selecting and verifying hearing aid fittings* (2nd ed.). New York, NY: Thieme Medical.

Valente, M. (Ed.). (2002b). *Hearing aids: Standards, options, and limitations* (2nd ed.). New York, NY: Thieme Medical.

Valente, M. (2007). Maturational effects of the vestibular system: A study of rotary chair, computerized dynamic posturography and vestibular evoked myogenic potentials with children. *Journal of the American Academy of Audiology, 18*(6), 461–481.

Valente, M., & Oeding, K. (2009). Recent fitting options for single-sided deafness. *Starkey Audiology Series, 1*(4).

Van der Pouw, K., Snik, A., & Cremers, C. (1998). Audiometric results of bilateral bone-anchored hearing aid applications in patients with bilateral congenital aural atresia. *Laryngoscope, 108*(4), 548–553.

Van Hul, W., Balemans, E., Van Hul, F. G., Dikkers, H., Obee, R. J., Stokroos, P., . . . Willems, P. J. (1998). Van Buchem disease (hyperostosis corticalis generalisata). Maps to chromosome 17q12-q21. *American Journal of Human Genetics, 62*(2), 391–399.

Van Tasell, D. (1993). Hearing loss, speech, and hearing aids. *Journal of Speech and Hearing Research, 36*, 228–244.

Vander Werff, K. R., Brown, C. J., Gienapp, B. A., & Schmidt- Clay, K. M. (2002). Comparison of auditory steady-state response and auditory brainstem response thresholds in children. *Journal of the American Academy of Audiology, 13*, 227–235.

Verhagen, C. V., Hol, M. K., Coppens-Schellenkens, W., Snik, A. F., & Cremers, C. W. (2008). The Baha softband: A new treatment for young children with bilateral congenital aural atresia. *International Journal of Pediatric Otorhinolaryngology, 72*(10), 1455–1459.

Vickers, D. A., Backus, B. C., Macdonald, N. K., Rostamzadeh, N. K., Mason, N. K., Pandua, R., . . . Mahon, M. H. (2013). Using personal response systems to assess speech perception within the classroom: An approach to determine the efficacy of sound field amplification in primary school classrooms. *Ear and Hearing, 34*, 491–502.

Vohr, B., Carty, L., Moore, P., & Letourneau, K. (1998). The Rhode Island hearing assessment program: Experience with statewide hearing screening. *Journal of Pediatrics, 133*, 353–357.

Vohr, B., & Maxon, A. (1996). Screening infants for hearing impairment. *Journal of Pediatrics, 128*, 710–714.

Vohr, B. R., Widen, J. E., Cone-Wesson, B., Sininger, Y. S., Gorga, M. P., Folsom, R. C., & Norton, S. J. (2000). Identification of neonatal hearing impairment: Characteristics of infants in the neonatal intensive care unit (NICU) and well-baby nursery. *Ear and Hearing, 21*(5), 373–382.

Von Almen, P., Allen, L., Adkins, J., Anderson, K., Blake-Rahter, T., English, K., & DeConde-Johnson, C. (1994). Letter to editor. *Pediatrics, 94*(6), 957.

Von Almen, P., Allen, L., Adkins, T., Anderson, K., Blake-Rahter, T., English, K., & Johnson, C. D. (1994). Universal screening for infant hearing impairment. Executive Board of the Educational Audiology Association. *Pediatrics, 94*(6), 957.

Voron, D. A., Hatfield, H. H., & Kalkhoff, R. K. (1976). Multiple lentigines syndrome. *American Journal of Medicine, 60*, 447–456.

Vulliamy, D. G., & Normandale, P. A. (1966). Craniofacial dysostosis in a Dorset family. *Archives of Diseases in Childhood, 41*, 375.

Wake, M., Poulakis, Z., Hughes, E. K., Carey-Sargeant, C., & Richards, F. W. (2005). Hearing impairment: A population study of age at diagnosis, severity, and language outcomes at 7 to 8 years. *Archives of Diseases in Children, 90*, 238–244.

Waldman, D., & Roush, J. (2010). *Your child's hearing loss.* San Diego, CA: Plural.

Waldman, E. H., & Brewer, C. C. (2007). Medical diseases and disorders of the ear. In R. S. Ackley, T. N. Decker, & C. J. Limb (Eds.), *An essential guide to hearing and balance disorders* (pp. 13–41). Mahweh, NJ: Lawrence Erlbaum.

Walker, D., Downs, M. P., Gugenheim, S., & Northern, J. L. (1989). Early language milestone scale and language screening of young children. *Pediatrics, 83*(2), 284–288.

Walker, M. L., Cervette, M. J., Newberg, N., Moss, S. D., & Storrs, B. B. (1987). Auditory brainstem responses in neonatal hydrocephalus. *Concepts in Pediatric Neurosurgery, 7*, 142–152.

Walker, W. G. (1971). Renal tubular acidosis and deafness. *Birth Defects, 7*(4), 126.

Wallace, I. F., Gravel, J. S., McCarton, C. M., Stapells, D. R., Bernstein, R. S., & Ruben, R. J. (1988). Otitis media, auditory sensitivity, and language outcomes at one year. *Laryngoscope, 98*, 64–70.

Wallace, S. E., Lachman, R. S., Mekikian, P. B., Bui, K. K., & Wilcox, W. R. (2004). Marked phenotypic variability in progressive diaphyseal dysplasia (Camurati-Engelmann disease): Report of a four-generation pedigree, identification of a mutation in TGFB1, and review. *American Journal of Medical Genetics, 129*(3), 235–247.

Watkin, P. (1996). Neonatal acoustic emission screening and the identification of deafness. *Archives of Disease in Childhood, 74*, F16–F25.

Watkin, P. M. (1989). Otologic disease in Turner's syndrome. *Journal of Laryngology and Otology, 103*, 731–738.

Watkins, S. (1987). Long-term effects of home intervention with hearing-impaired children. *American Annals of the Deaf, 132,* 267–271.

Weatherby, L., & Bennett, M. (1980). The neonatal acoustic reflex. *Scandanavian Audiology, 9,* 103–110.

Weber, B. (1969). Validation of observer judgments in behavioral observation audiometry. *Journal of Speech and Hearing Disorders, 34,* 350–355.

Weber, H. J. (1987). Colorado's statewide hearing screening program utilizing visual reinforcement audiometry. *Hearing Instruments, 38*(9), 22–24.

Webster, D. B., & Webster, M. (1977). Neonatal sound deprivation affects brainstem auditory nuclei. *Archives of Otolaryngology, 103,* 392–396.

Webster, D. B., & Webster, M. (1979). Effects of neonatal conductive loss on brainstem auditory nuclei. *Annals of Otology, Rhinology, and Laryngology, 88,* 684–688.

Webster, D. B., & Webster, M. (1980). Mouse brainstem auditory nuclei development. *Annals of Otology, Rhinology, and Laryngology, 89*(68), 254–256.

Wedenberg, E. (1956). Auditory tests on newborn infants. *Acta Otolaryngologica, 46,* 446–461.

Weidenheim, K. M., Dickso, D. W., & Rapin, I. (2009). Neuropathology of Cockayne syndrome: Evidence for impaired development, premature aging, and neurodegeneration. *Mechanisms of Ageing and Development, 130*(9), 619–636.

Weinstein, R. L., Kliman, B., & Scully, R. E. (1969). Familial syndrome of primary testicular insufficiency with normal virilization, blindness, deafness, and metabolic abnormalities. *New England Journal of Medicine, 281,* 969–977.

Weir, R. H. (1966). Some questions on the child's learning of phonology. In F. Smith & G. Miller (Eds.), *The genesis of language* (pp. 153–169). Cambridge, MA: MIT Press.

Weiss, K. L., Goodwin, M. W., & Moores, D. F. (1975). *Characteristics of young deaf children and early intervention programs* (Research Report 91). Washington, DC: Department of HEW, Bureau of Education for the Handicapped.

Wepman, D. (1987). *Helen Keller: Humanitarian.* New York, NY: Chelsea House.

Werner, L. A., Mancl, L. R., & Folsom, R. C. (1996). Preliminary observations on the development of auditory sensitivity in infants with Down syndrome. *Ear and Hearing, 17,* 455–468.

Wester, D. C., Atkin, C. L., & Gregory, M. C. (1995). Alport syndrome: Clinical update. *Journal of the American Academy of Audiology, 6*(1), 73–79.

Wetherby, A. M., Koegal, R., & Mendel, M. (1981). Central auditory nervous system dysfunction in autistic individuals. *Journal of Speech and Hearing Research, 24,* 420–429.

Wetherby, A. M., Prizant, B., & Hutchinson, T. (1998). Communicative, social/affective, and symbolic profiles of young children with autism and pervasive developmental disorders. *American Journal of Speech Language Pathology, 7,* 79–91.

Wever, E. G., & Bray, C. W. (1930). Auditory nerve impulses. *Science, 71,* 215.

Wever, E. G., & Lawrence, M. (1954). *Physiological acoustics* (pp. 187–194). Princeton, NJ: Princeton University Press.

Wever, E. G., & Neff, W. D. (1947). A further study of the effects of partial section of the auditory nerve. *Journal of Comparative Physiology and Psychology, 40,* 217–226.

White, K. R. (1996). Universal newborn hearing screening using transient evoked otoacoustic emissions: Past, present and future. *Seminars in Hearing, 17*(2), 171–183.

White, K. R. (2004). Early hearing detection and intervention programs: Opportunities for genetic services. *American Journal of Medical Genetics, 130,* 29–36.

White, K. R., & Behrens, T. R. (Eds.). (1993). The Rhode Island hearing assessment project: Implications for universal newborn hearing screening. *Seminars in Hearing, 14*(1), 1–122.

White, K. R., Vohr, B., Maxon, B., Behrens, T., McPherson, M., & Mark, G. (1994). Screening all newborns for hearing loss using transient evoked oto-acoustic emissions.

International Journal of Pediatric Otorhino-laryngology, 29(3), 203–217.

Whitton, J., & Polley, D. (2012). Ear infection today, "lazy ear" tomorrow? *Audiology Today, 24*(4), 32–37.

Widen, J. E. (1997). Evoked otoacoustic emissions in evaluating children. In M. Robinette & T. Glattke (Eds.), *Otoacoustic emissions: Clinical applications* (pp. 271–306). New York, NY: Thieme Medical.

Widen, J. E. (2011). *Behavioral audiometry with infants.* In R. Seewald & A. M. Tharpe (Eds.), *Comprehensive handbook of pediatric audiology* (pp. 483–493). San Diego, CA: Plural.

Widen, J. E., Folsom, R. C., Cone-Wesson, B., Carty, L., Dunnell, J. J., Koebsel, K., . . . Norton, S. (2000). Identification of neonatal hearing impairment: Hearing status at 8 to 12 months corrected age using a visual reinforcement audiometry protocol. *Ear and Hearing, 21*, 471–487.

Widen, J. E., Johnson, J. L., White, K. R., Gravel, J. S., Vohr, B. R., James, M., . . . Norton, S. (2005). A multisite study to examine the efficacy of the otoacoustic emission/automated auditory brainstem response newborn hearing screening protocol: Results of visual reinforcement audiometry. *American Journal of Audiology, 14*, 200–216.

Wilber, R. B. (1987). *American sign language: Linguistic and applied dimensions.* Boston, MA: Little, Brown.

Wiley, T., & Fowler, C. (1997). *Acoustic immittance measures in clinical audiology: A primer.* San Diego, CA: Singular.

Williams, A., Williams, M., Walker, C., et al. (1981). The Robin anomaly (Pierre Robin syndrome): Follow-up study. *Archives of Diseases in Childhood, 56*, 663–668.

Williams, C. J., & Jacobs, A. M. (2009). The impact of otitis media on cognitive and educational outcomes. *Medical Journal of Australia, 191*(9), S69–S72.

Williamson, W. D., Demmler, G. J., Percy, A. K., & Catlin, F. I. (1992). Progressive hearing loss in infants with asymptomatic congenital cytomegalovirus infection. *Pediatrics, 90*(6), 862–866.

Wilson, W., Marinac, J., Pitty, K., & Burrows, C. (2011). The use of sound-field amplification devices in different types of classrooms. *Language, Speech, and Hearing Services in Schools, 42*, 395–407.

Wilson, W. R., Folson, R. C., & Widen, J. E. (1982). *Hearing impairment in Down's syndrome children.* Paper presented at the Elks 1982 International Symposium, The Multiply Handicapped Hearing-Impaired Child. Edmonton, Canada.

Wilson, W. R., & Thompson, G. (1984). Behavioral audiometry. In J. Jerger (Ed.), *Pediatric audiology* (pp. 1–44). San Diego, CA: College-Hill Press.

Windle-Taylor, P., Emery, P. J., & Phelps, P. D. (1981). Ear deformities associated with the Klippel-Feil syndrome. *Annals of Otology, 90*, 210–216.

Wing, L. (1993). The definition and prevalence of autism: A review. *European Child & Adolescent Psychiatry, 2*(1), 1–14.

Winter, M. E. (2010). Hearing aid amplificatoin in pediatric patients. In M. J. Derebery & W. M. Luxford (Eds.), *Hearing loss: The otolaryngologist's guide to amplification* (pp. 83–94). San Diego, CA: Plural.

Wolf-Schein, E., Sudhalter, V., Cohen, I., Fisch, G. S., Hanson, D., Pfadt, A. G., . . . Brown, W. T. (1987). Speech-language and the fragile X syndrome: Initial findings. *Asha, 29*, 35–38.

Worthington, D. W., & Peters, J. F. (1980). Quantifiable hearing and no ABR: Paradox or error? *Ear and Hearing, 1*, 281–285.

Wright, L. B., & Rybak, L. P. (1983). Crib-o-gram (COG) and ABR: Effect of variables on test results. *Journal of the Acoustical Society of America, 74*(1), 540–544.

Yilmaz, S., Karasalihoglu, A. R., Tas, A., Yagiz, R., & Tas, M. (2006). Otoacoustic emissions in young adults with a history of otitis media. *Journal of Laryngology and Otology. 120*(2), 103–107.

Yoshinaga-Itano, C. (1994). Language assessment of infants and toddlers with significant hearing loss. *Seminars in Hearing, 15*(2), 128–140.

Yoshinaga-Itano, C. (1995). Efficacy of early identification and intervention. *Seminars in Hearing, 16,* 115–120.

Yoshinaga-Itano, C. (1999). Early identification: An opportunity and challenge for audiology. *Seminars in Hearing, 20*(4), 317–333.

Yoshinaga-Itano, C., & Apuzzo, M. (1995). Early identification of infants with significant hearing loss and the Minnesota child development inventory (MCDI). *Seminars in Hearing, 16*(2), 124–135.

Yoshinaga-Itano, C., Baca, R. L., &. Sedey, A. L. (2010). Describing the trajectory of language development in the presence of severe to profound hearing loss: A closer look at children with cochlear implants versus hearing aids. *Otology and Neurotology, 31*(8), 1268–1274.

Yoshinaga-Itano, C., Sedey, A., Coulter, D., & Mehl, A. (1998). Language of early- and later-identified children with hearing loss. *Pediatrics, 102*(5), 1161–1171.

Yoshioka, H., Mino, M., Kiyosawa, N., Hirasawa, Y., Morikora, Y., Kasubuchi, Y., & Kusunoki, T. (1980). Muscular changes in Engelmann's disease. *Archives of Diseases in Childhood, 55,* 716–719.

Yost, W. A. (2007). *Fundamentals of hearing: An introduction* (5th ed.). San Diego, CA: Academic Press.

Zaytoun, G., Harboyan, G., & Kabalan, W. (2002). The oto-palatal-digital syndrome: Variable clinical expressions. *Archives of Otolaryngology-Head Neck Surgery, 126,* 129.

Zeaman, D., & Wegner, N. (1954). The role of drive reduction in the classical conditioning of an autonomically mediated response. *Journal of Experimental Psychology, 48,* 349–354.

Zeaman, D., & Wegner, N. (1956). Cardiac reflex to tones of threshold intensity. *Journal of Speech and Hearing Disorders, 21,* 71–75.

Zellweger, H., Smith, J. K., & Grutzner, P. (1974). The Marshall syndrome: Report of a new family. *Journal of Pediatrics, 84,* 868–871.

Zigler, E. (1969). Developmental versus different theories in mental retardation and the problem of motivation. *American Journal of Mental Deficiencies, 73,* 536–556.

Zimmerman, S., Osberger, M. J., & Robbins, A. M. (1998). Infant-Toddler: Meaningful Auditory Integration Scale (IT-MAIS). In W. Estabrooks (Ed.), *Cochlear implants for kids.* Washington DC: AG Bell Association for the Deaf.

Zwislocki, J. (1963). An acoustic method for clinical examination of the ear. *Journal of Speech and Hearing Research, 6,* 303–314.

Author Index

A

Ades, H.W., 19
Ahlfors, K., 104
Akhtar, N., 35
Alberti, P.W.R.M., 316
Albright, K., 393
Alencewicz, C.M., 292
Allen, R.L., 408
Allred, P.L., 336
Altidis, P.M., 290
American Academy of Audiology, 157, 158, 163, 193, 274, 411, 412, 416, 424, 447, 449
American Academy of Otolaryngology-Head & Neck Surgery, 182
American Academy of Pediatrics, 391
American Speech-Language-Hearing Association, 157, 161, 193, 327, 365, 417
Anderson, K., 525–526
Anderson, K.L., 154
Anthony, L., 337
Apgar, V., 164
Apuzzo, M., 145
Apuzzo, M.L., 218
Arditi, M., 200
Arlinger, S., 364
Armitage, S.E., 120
Arnlie, R.N., 347, 358
Ashmead, D., 277

B

Bader, C.R., 338
Bagatto, M., 453, 454
Baker, D., 33
Baldwin, M., 444
Balkany, T.J., 188, 205
Bantwal, A., 357
Barthes, R., 149
Bartoshuk, A., 388
Basser, L.S., 367

Baudhuin, J.L., 243
Beagley, H.A., 367
Beauchaine, K.A., 350, 351, 352
Beck, D., 149, 362, 459
Beck, D.L., 365
Beebe, H., 310
Beery, Q.C., 321, 323
Bellis, T.J., 152
Benacerraf, B.R., 119
Bench, R.J., 119, 126
Benham-Dunster, R.A., 297
Bennett, M., 336
Bennett, M.J., 336
Bentler, R., 29
Bergholtz, L.M., 364
Bergstrom, L., 213
Berlin, C., 294
Berlin, C.I., 29, 207, 208, 586, 588
Bernstein, R.S., 277
Berry, R., 270
Bertrend, D., 338
Bess, F., 29
Bess, F.H., 96, 191, 392, 416, 526
Birch, J.W., 521
Birnholz, J.C., 119
Blarney, P.J., 290, 293
Blondis, T., 205
Bluestone, C.D., 203, 321, 323, 332
Bodner-Johnson, B., 232
Boothroyd, A., 38
Bornstein, H., 514
Boyer, K.M., 101, 105
Boymans, M., 457
Brackett, D., 522
Bradford, L., 388–389
Brady, D.R., 185
Bray, C.W., 363
Brenner, C.A., 293
Bright, K.E., 340
British Society of Audiology, 152
Brody, J.A., 189

Brookhouser, P.E., 368
Brooks, D., 315, 323
Brownell, W.E., 338
Bryant, K., 323
Buckman, R., 237
Busby, P.A., 290

C

Caleffe-Schenck, N., 33
Callanan, M.A., 35
Campbell, K.C.M., 193
Cantekin, E.I., 175
Cardon, G., 359
Carnegie Corp., 531
Carney, A., 35, 130, 218
Carter, L., 358
Catlin, E.I., 294
Catlin, F., 200
Cervette, M.J., 513
Chapman, J., 96
Chermak, G., 161
Chhabria, N., 357
Chmiel, R., 355
Chomsky, N., 1
Clark, G.M., 480
Clerc, Laurent, 514
Clifton, R.K., 143
Cogswell, Alice, 513
Cohen, D., 139
Cohen, L.T., 361
Cohen, N., 480
Coker, N., 355
Collet, L., 343
Collyer, D., 126
Comperatore, C., 357
Condon, W.S., 125, 128
Cone-Wesson, B., 397
Cooper, J., 325
Cooper, J.C., 376
Cornett, R.O., 498
Cowan, R., 480
Crawford, J.D., 121
Crandell, C., 526
Crandell, C.C., 209
Crepin, G., 120
Crumley, W., 393
Culbertson, J.L., 191

Culpepper, B., 275
Cunningham, G.C., 374
Curhan, G.C., 27
Curhan, S.G., 27
Cyr, D.G., 368

D

Dahle, A.J., 299
Dale, P.A., 125
Dallos, P., 16, 19
Davidson, L.S., 293
Davis, A.C., 402
Davis, H., 346, 348, 363
Davis, J.M., 29, 522
Davis, P.A., 345
Davis, R., 303–304
de Ribaupierre, Y., 338
DeCasper, A.J., 119
Delgado, J.L., 25
DeLucia, C.A., 270
Demany, I., 125
Denton, D.M., 495
Derbyshire, A.J., 363
Dettman, J., 290
Dhar, S., 340, 341
Dice, N., 414
Dickson, H.G., 376
Diefendorf, A., 249
Dillon, H., 358, 456
Disant, F., 343
Dittberner, A., 459
Dobie, R.A., 29
Dodd-Murphy, J., 29
Dodge, P.R., 200
Dolnick, E., 497
Dorman, M., 476, 478
Doupe, A.J., 121
Dowell, R.C., 480
Downs, D., 303
Downs, M., 411
Downs, M.P., 205, 264, 310, 386, 387, 390, 394
Doyle, K.J., 118
Dreith, S., 243
Dreschler, W.A., 457
Dundas, J.A., 458–459
Dunn, J., 35
Dunn, J.W., 320

Dunster, J.R., 297
Durieux-Smith, A., 29, 389

E

Eagles, E.L., 416
Eavey, R., 27
Eclavea, E., 243
Edwards, C., 29, 389
Edwards, E.P., 146
Eichler, J.A., 175
Eilers, R., 138, 277
Eimas, P.D., 125
Eisele, W., 270
Eisenberg, L.S., 293, 480
Eisenberg, R.B., 125, 127
Elangovan, S., 408
Eldredge, L., 192–193
Elfenbein, J., 29
Elliot, G.B., 119
Elliot, K.A., 119
Elliott, L.L., 289
English, G.M., 185
Erber, N.P., 288, 292
Escolar, M., 213
Estabrooks, W., 148
Everett, D., 408
Ewing, Sir Alexander, 248, 309

F

Fausti, S., 193
Feigin, R.D., 200
Feinmesser, M., 347
Ferraro, J.A., 365
Festen, J.M., 457
Field, T.M., 139
Fifer, W.P., 119
Finitzo, T., 393
Finitzo-Hieber, T., 289, 352, 397
Fisch, L., 356
Fischel-Ghodsian, N., 193
Fitz, K., 458–459
Fitzpatrick, E., 191, 192
Fitzpatrick, E.M., 29
Flexer, C., 149, 263, 265, 270, 297, 506, 525, 526
Folson, R.C., 272, 300
Fortnum, H.M., 402

Fowler, C., 318
Fowler, K.B., 104
Franklin, B., 267
Franks, R., 357
Fria, T.J., 175, 185
Froding, C., 386
Froeschels, E., 310
Frost, J., 355
Fujikawa, S., 99
Fuller, D., 12
Fulton, R.T., 282

G

Gabbard, S.A., 403
Gaines, J.A., 99
Galambos, R., 347, 348
Gallaudet, E.M., 514
Gallaudet, T.H., 513, 514
Galster, J.A., 458–459
Gans, D.P., 244, 263, 265, 297, 367, 368
Gartner, M., 343
Gates, G., 325
Gates, G.A., 183, 376
Geers, A.E., 292, 293, 475–476, 480, 498
Geffner, D., 154, 161, 217
Gelfand, S., 457–458
Gelfand, S.A., 458
Gesell, A.L., 490
Gifford, R.H., 467, 480
Gluckman, C., 99
Goehring, J.L., 243
Gold, T., 338
Goldgar, D.E., 350
Golding, M., 358
Goldstein, R., 336, 356
Goodman, J., 389
Goodwin, M.W., 512
Gorga, M.P., 350, 351, 352, 449, 522
Gorzycki, P.A., 282
Gould, H., 357
Gould, H.J., 573
Goverts, S.T., 457
Gravel, J., 272, 277
Greenberg, M.T., 533
Greenberg, R., 139
Greenwood, J., 464
Gregg, N. McAllister, 101

Grossman, A., 368
Guly, A.J., 12

H

Haapaniemi, J.J., 28
Habte, B., 243
Hall, J., 209
Hall, J.W., III, 158, 169, 323, 325, 337, 340, 341,
    347, 357, 371, 443
Harbin, G., 238
Harris, J.D., 426
Harris, S., 104
Hart, B., 220, 492
Haspiel, G., 288
Hawkins, D.B., 456, 457, 529
Hayes, D., 39, 41, 157, 209, 243, 248, 260, 337,
    355, 388, 391, 392
Hecox, K., 347
Helenius, K.K., 323
Henion, K., 359
Hepper, P., 120
Herer, G.R., 99
Herrmann, B.S., 400
Herrmann, K.R., 393, 405
Hesketh, L.J., 494
Hicks, T., 104
Hillyard, S.A., 348
Hodges, A., 337
Hodgson, W., 288
Holcomb, M., 213
Hood, D.C., 356
Hood, L., 209
Hood, L.J., 207, 208, 347, 586
Hoover, B., 459
Horton, K.B., 532
Houston, T., 244
Howie, V.M., 188
Hughes, M.L., 243
Hull, F.M., 25
Hull, W.L., 282
Huntre, L.L., 317
Hustedde, C.G., 137

I

Irwin, O.C., 130
Ivarsson, S., 104

J

Jabaley, T., 231
Jaber, L., 193
Jacobson, C.A., 377
Jacobson, J.T., 377
Jacobson, R., 113
Jahrsdoerfer, R.A., 169
James, William, 114
Jarmel, F., 408
Jerger, J., 157, 197, 231, 248, 289, 290, 315, 316,
    321, 330, 337, 355, 388, 420
Jerger, J.F., 326
Jerger, S., 24, 197, 288, 289, 290, 326, 330, 348,
    357
Jerlvall, L.B., 364
Jesteadt, W., 352
Jewett, D., 347
Jipson, J., 35
Johansson, B., 119
John, A.B., 209
Johnson, C.D., 411
Johnson, C.L., 25
Johnson, E., 459
Johnson, J.L., 404
Johnston, K., 158
Johnston, K.N., 209
Joint Committee on Infant Hearing, 391, 392,
    395, 396, 397, 398, 399, 427, 443, 592, 593
Jordan, O., 314
Jordan, R.E., 416
Juscyzk, P., 125

K

Kaminski, J.R., 351
Kamo, G., 237
Kankkunen, B., 168, 271
Kaplan, S.L., 200
Katz, D.R., 289
Kauffman, I., 343
Kavanagh, K.T., 357
Kearsley, R., 121
Keith, R.W., 154, 157, 335, 336
Keith, W.J., 277
Keller, H., 2
Kemp, D.T., 338
Kennedy, C.R., 428

Kennedy, V., 359
Kent, R.D., 137, 139
Killion, M., 450, 451
Klatte, M., 526
Klee, T., 191
Klein, J.O., 181, 182
Klodd, D.A., 119
Koch, M., 515
Konigsmark, B.W., 367–368
Koop, C. Everett, 4, 7
Kramer, S.E., 457
Kraus, N., 116, 207, 346, 357
Krausz, H.L., 348
Kreisman, N., 209
Kristensen, R., 316
Kryter, K.D., 19
Kuczwara, L.A., 119
Kuhl, P., 2
Kuhl, P.K., 121, 129
Kurtzer-White, E., 228, 232
Kyler, P., 364

L

Laht, E., 323
Laine, M.K., 323
Langley, L, 325
Laugen, N.J., 238
Lawrence, M., 328, 363
Lemmark, B., 104
Lempert, J., 363
Lenneberg, E.H., 2, 145
L'Epèe, L'Abbè de, 513
Lerman, J., 288
Lerner, M., 99
Leske, M.C., 25
Levitt, H., 217, 220
Lewis, D., 456, 459, 529
Libby, E.R., 446
Liden, G., 271
Lieberman, P., 126, 129
Lightfoot, G., 359
Ling, D., 266, 522
Litke, R.E., 197
Lloyd, L.I., 282–283
Loeb, G.E., 468
Long, J., 96
Loy, B., 480

Lucey, J., 96
Luterman, D.M., 212, 228, 229, 232, 424, 511
Lutman, M.E., 402

M

MacMurray, B., 389
Madell, J., 270
Mancl, L.R., 300
Marchant, C., 336
Margolis, R.H., 317
Margolis, R.M., 334
Marlow, J., 149
Martin, W.H., 347, 358
Mason, J.A., 393, 405
Matkin, A., 517–518
Matkin, N., 154, 517–518
Matkin, N.D., 37, 136, 192, 271, 275, 286, 288, 484, 491
Mauldin, L., 330, 337
Maxon, A.B., 522
McAlister, R., 189
McCandless, G.A., 336
McCollister, F.P., 299
McConnell, F., 526
McCormick, G., 357
McFarlan, D., 12
McGarr, N., 217
McGee, T., 357
McKenzie, B., 125
McMillan, P., 336
McNutt, L., 320
McWilliam, R., 238
McWIlliam, R.A., 228
Meadow, K.P., 234, 235, 533
Mehl, A., 376, 385, 393
Meinke, D.K., 414
Meltzoff, A.N., 129
Mendel, G., 64
Mendel, M., 356
Mentz, L., 126
Menyuk, P., 132, 136
Metz, O., 316, 328
Meyer, T., 288
Meyerhoff, W., 325
Mielke, P.W., 25
Mills, J., 453
Miyamoto, R.T., 290

Moeller, M., 459
Moeller, M.P., 219, 428
Moller, A., 35, 151
Montgomery, A., 456
Montgomery, D.E., 491
Moodie, S., 453
Moog, J., 280, 292, 494
Moore, J.K., 118
Moore, J.M., 271–272, 275
Moores, D.F., 499, 512
Morff, R., 320
Morgon, A., 343
Moss, S.D., 513
Moulin, A., 343
Mueller, H.G., 441, 443, 450, 451, 456, 457
Mundy, M., 323
Murphy, K.P., 264, 300
Musiek, F.R., 24, 161
Musselman, C.R., 509

N

Nadol, J.B., 12
Nance, W., 535
National Assessment of Educational Progress,
    491
National Institutes of Health Consensus
    Development Conference, 391, 392, 399, 474
Naulty, C.M., 99
Neely, S.T., 352
Nelson, P.B., 525
Netsell, R., 137
Newberg, N., 513
Nicol, T., 205
Niemeyer, W., 337
Northern, J.L., 185, 264, 315, 316, 392, 416
Norton, S.J., 275
Nozza, R.J., 323

O

Oats, P., 349
Ogiba, Y., 271
Oliver, T., 355
Oller, K., 138
Olsen, J., 459
Olsen, W.O., 286, 288
Orchik, D.J., 320, 336

Osberger, M.J., 137, 494
Otomo, K., 137, 138, 139
Overfield, T., 189
Owen, J.H., 376
Oyler, A.L., 192
Oyler, R.F., 192, 242
Ozdamar, O., 207, 305, 357

P

Palmer, C., 449
Paparella, M.M., 185
Paradise, J., 321, 323
Paradise, J.L., 203, 323, 325, 335, 392
Parker, R., 29
Pascoe, D., 426
Paul, J., 220
Paul, T., 220
Peek, B., 96
Peters, J.F., 207
Petroff, M.A., 195
Philip, A., 96
Picton, R.W., 348
Picton, T., 389
Picton, T.W., 207, 208
Pikus, A.T., 368
Pisoni, D., 288
Pittman, A., 459
Plant, G., 290
Ploussard, J.H., 188
Pollack, D., 511
Porter, H., 191
Potts, P., 464
Pratt, S.R., 232
Pressman, S., 193
Prezant, T.R., 193
Primus, M.A., 270, 271, 275
Prosek.R., 456

Q

Querleu, Q., 120

R

Ramkumar, V., 357
Rance, G., 208
Rapin, I., 147

Reed, N., 207
Reid, M.J., 282–283
Reiland, J., 350
Reiland, J.K., 352
Reisen, A.H., 146
Renard, Z., 120
Richburg, C.M., 411
Richburg, S., 526
Richie, R., 121
Rickards, F.W., 361
Ricketts, T., 459
Ridgeway, J., 514
Ries, P., 25
Risley, T., 220, 492
Roberts, J., 323
Roberts, S.A., 290
Robinshaw, H.M., 217
Rodman, L.B., 356
Roeser, R., 411
Roizen, N.J., 205
Roland, P., 359, 480
Rose, K., 586
Rosenberg, G.G., 528
Rosenfeld, R., 183
Rosner, B.A., 181
Ross, M., 288, 423, 426, 460
Ross-Swain, D., 154, 161
Roush, J., 213, 228, 237, 323, 326
Roush, P., 213
Roush, P.A., 454, 455
Roy, I., 25
Ruben, R.J., 147
Ruohola, A., 323
Ruth, R., 337
Ryan, A.F., 16, 19
Rybak, L.P., 389

S

Salamy, A., 192–193
Samples, J.M., 267
Sander, L.W., 125, 128
Sanders, S., 347, 358
Sass-Lehrer, M., 232
Schick, B., 494, 498
Schlesinger, H.S., 234, 495
Schmidt, B., 303
Schnabel, M., 305

Schuknecht, H.F., 12
Schum, R., 29
Schwartz, D.M., 336
Schwartz, R.H., 336
Schwartz, S., 498
Scollie, S., 453
Scollie, S.D., 47, 431, 439, 453, 454
Seewald, R., 47, 228, 232, 431, 439, 449
Seewald, R.C., 453, 454, 455, 460
Sekhar, L., 414
Sell, E.J., 99
Serpanos, Y.C., 408
Sesterhenn, G., 337
Seymour, J., 358
Shahidullah, B., 120
Shargorodsky, J., 27
Sharma, A., 359, 476, 477–478
Shatz, M., 35
Shepard, N.T., 522
Shohat, M., 193
Shriner, T., 270
Shurin, P., 336
Siccard, L'Abbè, 513, 514
Siegenthaler, B., 288
Silman, S., 457–458
Silver, H.K., 387
Silverman, C., 457–458
Simmons, F.B., 195, 389
Simmons, J., 454
Sininger, Y., 209
Sininger, Y.S., 118, 143, 146, 207, 208, 209, 428
Siqueland, E.R., 125, 270
Skinner, B.F., 268
Skinner, M.W., 30, 33
Sloyer, J., 188
Smaldino, J., 526
Smiley, D.F., 411, 526
Smith, C., 323
Smith, C.G., 323
Smith, K., 288
Smith, R.P., 277
Snider, M., 121
Sohmer, H., 347
Soli, S.D., 525
Solomon, M., 227
Sparks, S., 558
Speidel, D.P., 365
Spens, K.E., 290

Spiro, M.K., 460
Spoendlin, H., 17
Spradlin, J.E., 282–283
Sprague, B., 336
Spring, D.R., 125
Squires, N., 347
Stach, B., 362
Stach, B.A., 326
Stapells, D.R., 349
Starr, A., 207, 208, 347, 358, 587
Stein, L., 207, 305, 384
Stein, L.K., 101, 105, 231, 346, 420
Stelmachowicz, P., 449, 459
Stelmachowicz, P.G., 522
Stephens, T.J., 303
Sterritt, G.M., 386, 387
Stiegler, L.N., 303–304
Stoel-Gammon, C., 137, 138, 139
Storrs, B.B., 513
Stredler-Brown, A., 244
Stuart, A., 408
Suzuki, T., 271
Svanberg, L., 104
Swanepoel, D.W., 323, 326, 347, 371

T

Tähtinen, P.A., 323
Tait, M., 469
Talbot, N.B., 121
Tan, L.E., 361
Tartter, V.C., 125
Taylor, B., 441
Teele, D.W., 181
Templin, M., 145
Tharpe, A.M., 191, 277
Thompson, G., 265, 267, 269, 270, 271–272, 275
Thompson, M., 267, 271–272, 275
Thomson, V., 376, 385, 393
Thornton, A.R., 400
Thuringer, R., 168
Timmons, R.J., 25
Tobey, E.A., 293
Tocci, R., 238
Tompkins, S.M., 323
Tooley, W.H., 192–193
Traquina, D., 272

Tremblay, K.L., 116
Trevarthen, C., 129
Trevino, P.M., 25
Trybus, R.J., 533
Tyler, R.S., 290

U

U.S. Department of Education, 297

V

Valente, M., 368
Valentine, S., 458–459
Van Tasell, D., 16
Vethivelu, S., 275
Vickers, D.A., 525
Vigorito, J., 125
Vurpillot, E., 125

W

Waffarn, F., 99
Walden, B., 456
Walker, M.L., 513
Wallace, I.F., 239
Walters, C., 205
Waltzman, S., 480
Watkin, P., 444
Watkins, S., 217
Weatherby, L., 336
Weaver, T., 200
Weber, B., 263
Weber, H.J., 406
Wedenberg, E., 386, 387
Wedenberg, F., 119
Wegner, N., 388
Weiss, I.P., 99
Weiss, K.L., 512
Werner, L.A., 300
Westin, B., 119
Wever, E.G., 328, 363
White, K.R., 216
Whittingham, J., 29
Widen, J.E., 272, 300, 339
Wilber, R.B., 514
Wilcox, W., 484

Wiley, T., 318, 336
Williams, E., 99
Williford, J., 25
Williston, J.S., 347
Wilson, O.J., 361
Wilson, W.R., 265, 269, 270, 272, 275, 300
Winzelberg, J., 195
Wohlner, L.W., 37
Wood, S., 402
Woodson, R., 139
Worthington, D.W., 207, 350, 352
Wright, L.B., 389

Y

Yang, L., 99
Yoshinaga-Itano, C., 145, 217, 218, 219, 428
Yost, W.A., 9, 12

Z

Zalewski, T.R., 414
Zeaman, D., 388
Zeisel, S., 323
Zigler, E., 265

Subject Index

Note: Page numbers in **bold** reference non-text material.

A

A-ABR. *See* Automated ABR

A-O communication. *See* Auditory-oral (A-O) communication methods

A-V communication. *See* Auditory-verbal (A-V) communication methods

AAA. *See* American Academy of Audiology

"ABCD's of the High Risk Register for Deafness," 387

Abducens palsy, 550

Abducens paralysis, 550

Abortion, ethical dilemma of, 110

ABR. *See* Auditory brainstem response (ABR) tests

ABR audiometry. *See* Auditory brainstem response (ABR) audiometry

Achondroplasia, **537**, 543–544, **544**

Acoustic coupling, hearing aids, 463

Acoustic cues, 126

Acoustic immittance, 315–316, **413**

Acoustic immittance measures, 315–331, 416, 417, 418

  acoustic reflex thresholds, 327–331, **329, 330**

  clinical applications of, 331–337

  equivalent ear canal volume (Veq), 326–327, **326, 327**

  in infants, 334–337

  screening pitfalls, **413**

  static admittance, 325–326

  tympanometry, **318**, 319–321, **320, 322**, 323, **324**, 325

Acoustic neuromas, 55, 544

Acoustic phonetics, 32

Acoustic reflex sensation level (SL), 330

Acoustic reflex tests, hearing loss prediction with, 337

Acoustic reflex thresholds, 327–331, **329, 330**

Acoustic screening. *See* Auditory screening

Acoustic speech cues, 34, 35

  hearing loss and, 35

Acoustic stapedial reflex (ASR), 328, 331

Acoustic stapedial reflex responses, in infants, 335, 336

Acoustic stapedial reflex tests, 328–331

Acoustics

  classroom acoustics, 159, 522, 524–526

  of speech, 30–35

Acoustics of speech, hearing loss and its effect on speech and language, 35–39, **40**, 41

Action potential (AP), 363

Acute mastoiditis, 186–187

Acute otitis media, 177–178

Adenine, in DNA, 53, **54**

Adenoidectomy, 181

Adenoids, 181

Adhesive otitis media, 179–180, **180**

Adolescent renal tubular acidosis, 557

Advocacy, for hearing-impaired children, 486, 506

AEP. *See* Auditory evoked potential

Afferent auditory pathway, 17–19, **18, 19, 20**

Affricatives, 33

AGC. *See* Automatic gain control

AI. *See* Audibility index

Air-bone gap, 22, 332–333

Albers-Schonberg disease, **537**, 544–545, 572

Albinism, **537**, 545

Alport's syndrome, 46, **537**, 545–546

Alveolar sounds, 33

Ambient noise, hearing loss and, 36

Amblyaudia, 154, 160

American Academy of Audiology (AAA), 239–240

  2008 statement on classroom acoustics, 525

  2012 Pediatric Assessment Guidelines, 274, 447–448

  2013 Pediatric Amplification Guidelines, 424, 461

  Screening Guidelines, 412–413

  Specialty Certification in Pediatrics, 48

American Academy of Pediatrics, 391
American Recovery and reinvestment Act of
2009 (ARRA), 290
American School for the Deaf, 514
American Sign Language (ASL), 498, 513–515,
516, 517
American Speech-Language-Hearing
Association (ASHA), Guidelines for
Audiology Screening, 411
Americans with Disabilities Act, 244
Amikacin, 192, **541**
Amino acids, in protein synthesis, 56–57
Aminoglycosides, 192, 193, 201
Amniocentesis, 63
Amniotic fluid, 63
Amplification
classroom amplification, 525
by ear structures, 14
See also Hearing aids
Anencephaly, 76
ANSD. *See* Auditory neuropathy spectrum
disorder
ANT. *See* Auditory Numbers Test
Antibiotics
for bacterial sepsis, 201
for otitis media, 181, 182
ototoxicity of, 192, 368, 397, **541**
Antiretroviral therapy (ARV), for HIV,
107–108
Aortic arch arteries, 84
AP. *See* Action potential
Apert syndrome, 170, **537**, 546–547, **546**
Apgar evaluation, 164, **165**
Aplasia, 198, **537**
Apoptosis, 116
ARRA. *See* American Recovery and
reinvestment Act of 2009
Ascending auditory pathway, 17–19, **18, 20**
ASD. *See* Autism spectrum disorder
ASHA. *See* American Speech-Language-
Hearing Association
ASL. *See* American Sign Language
Asperger disorder, 302
Asphyxia at birth, **537**
Aspirin, 193
ASR. *See* Acoustic stapedial reflex
Assistive devices, personal FM systems for
children, 160, 209, 526, 527–530

Association, 155, 535
ASSR. *See* Auditory steady-state response
Ataxia-hypogonadism syndrome, 574–575
Atopic dermatitis, 547
Atresia, 168–169, **168, 538**
Attention, 155
Audibility index (AI), 450
Audiograms, examples of, **23**
Audiologists
as advocates, 486
auditory maturation and, 121, **122**, 123–127,
250–252, 264–265
case history, 255, **256–257**, 257–258,
259–260
counseling parents, 47, 229, 231–233, 237,
420, 594
in education setting, 474–487, 506
empathy by, 236
expectations from children, 251–253
fitting pediatric hearing aids, 426–428,
438–439, **439**
informing parents about diagnosis, 212,
227–237, 414–415
knowledge of medical disorders, 163
literacy role of, 491–495
medical exam by, 167, 258, 260, **261**
rapport with children, 249–253, 267–268,
278–279, 294–295, 309
self-understanding by, 233–239
specialty training for, 47–49
tele-educational online teaching programs
for, 244
telepractice, 242–244
as treatment team partners, 45, 398
use of assistant, 260–265, **262**, 271, 310
"virtual home visits" by, 243
Audiology, use of assistant, 260–265, **262**, 271,
310
Audiometric assistant, 260–265, **262**, 271, 310
Audiometry
in infants, 126
periodic reassessment, 46
See also Auditory brainstem response
(ABR) audiometry; Behavioral
observation audiometry; Conditioned
play audiometry; Operant reinforcement
audiometry; Physiologic hearing
tests; Tangible reinforcement operant

conditioning audiometry; Visual
reinforcement audiometry
Auditory brainstem response (ABR)
audiometry, 347–353, **347**, **348**, **350–355**,
355
for ANSD diagnosis, 587–588, 593
on developmentally delayed children,
418–419
disadvantages of, 349, 353
maturation of, 351–353, **351–355**, 355
on newborns, 205, 266, 392, 444, 587–588,
593
Auditory cortex, 19
Auditory discrimination tests, 156
Auditory dys-synchonly, 586
Auditory evoked potential (AEP), 345, **345**
Auditory evoked responses (AERs), 158
Auditory localization, 143, 155, 267
Auditory maturation index, 264–265
Auditory maturation responses, 121, **122**,
123–127, 250–252, 264–265
Auditory middle-latency evoked response
(MLR), 355–357, **356**
Auditory nerve, 17
Auditory neuropathy, 206, 585, 586
Auditory neuropathy spectrum disorder
(ANSD), 206–209, 403–404, 585–594
cochlear implants for, 591–592
communication systems for, 592–593
counseling families dealing with, 594
diagnostic criteria, 587–588
in infants, 588
monitoring infants with "transient" ANSD,
593–594
recommended amplification strategies,
590–591
recommended audiologic test battery,
589–590
recommended comprehensive assessment,
589
screening newborns for, 155, 594
team management protocol, **595–602**
terminology, 586–587
use of term, 585, 586
Auditory Numbers Test (ANT), **287**, 289
Auditory-oral (A-O) communication methods,
508–512
Auditory pathway, 7–8, **8**, **9**, 14–16

Auditory processing, in children, 151–161
Auditory processing disorders (APD), 151,
159–161
See also Central auditory processing
disorder
Auditory Response Cradle, 389
Auditory screening, 248, 373–421
behavioral hearing tests, 247–307
case history, 255, **256–257**, 257–258,
259–260
central auditory processing disorder
(CAPD), 154–159
of children with autism spectrum disorder
(ASD), 302–304
of children with brain injury, 300–302
of children with deafness and blindness,
304–305
of children with intellectual disability,
299–300
of children with multiple handicaps,
296–299, **298**
of children with otitis media, 240–241
of children with pervasive developmental
disorders (PDDs), 302–304
cost of, 376
cross-check principle, 248–249, 276, 297
decision matrix analysis, 377–378, **377**
of developmentally delayed children,
418–419, 591
of difficult-to-test children, 295–305, 309,
314, 315, 316, 365–367
follow-up, 419–421
Head Start Performance Standards, 405, 408,
409
hearing and speech developmental
questionnaire for parents, 132, **133–134**,
135–136, 253, **254**, 256–257
hospital-based hearing screening protocols,
403
of infants, 121, **122**, 123–127, 271–277, **273**,
276
insert earphones, 249, **249**
objective hearing tests, 309, 310
of older child (5 years and older), 294–295,
295
pass-fail criteria, 381–382, **381**, 408
pediatric speech audiometry, 283–286
physiologic hearing tests, 309–371

Auditory screening *(continued)*
  pitfalls of, **413**
  predictive value of, 379–381, **380**
  of preschool children, 409–410, **410**
  prevalence vs. incidence, 378–379
  principles of, 374–382
  of school-age children, 410–415, **412**, **413**
  in schools, 408, 410–411, **415**
  sensitivity of, 378
  specificity of, 378
  statistics for, 4
  of toddlers, 277–283, **280**, 310–315, **312**
  of uncooperative children, 309
  for unilateral sensorineural hearing loss, 191
  vestibular evaluation, 367–368
  volunteers and, 398–399
  See also Language and speech screening;
    Newborn hearing screening
Auditory steady-state response (ASSR),
    359–363, **360**, **361**, 444
Auditory system
  fetal development, 118–119
  plasticity of, 118
Auditory temporal processing and patterning
    tests, 157
Auditory thresholds, 11
Auditory-verbal (A-V) communication
    methods, 508–512
Auditory-verbal practice method, 511
Auditory-Verbal Therapists, 508
Aural approach, 511
Auricle
  anatomy of, 166–167, **167**
  embryology of, 82, **83**, 167–168
  shape of, 168
Auricular hillocks, 75, 82, 84
Auropalpebral reflex, 310, 386
Autism spectrum disorder (ASD), 205–206,
    302–304
Automated ABR (A-ABR), 399–401, **400**,
    404–405
Automated evoked otoacoustic emissions, for
    newborn screening, 399, 401–405, **402**,
    404
Automatic gain control (AGC), 460
Autosomal dominant disorders, 64–65, **66**
Autosomal recessive disorders, 65, **66**
Autosomes, 56

B

Babbling, 130, 132, 135, 137, 138
Background noise, 34
Bacterial meningitis, 455, **537**
Bacterial sepsis, 201
BAHA. *See* Bone anchored hearing aids
Balance translocations, 69
Baraitser-Winter syndrome, 547–548
Base-pair arrangement, 53, **54**
Basilar membrane, 16
Behavioral hearing tests, 247–307
  audiometric assistant in, 260–262, **261**, 271
  bracketing protocol, 274
  case history for, 255, **256–257**, 257–258,
    259–260
  children's response to sound, 121, **122**,
    123–126, 250–252
  conditioned play audiometry, 277–283, **280**
  cross-check protocol, 248–249, 276, 297
  for developmentally delayed children, 419,
    591
  Interweaving Staircase Procedure, 277
  in newborns, 266–268
  observer bias in, 263–264
  Optimized Hearing Test Algorithm, 277
  reinforcement theory, 268–271
  speech sample, 258, 279
  tangible reinforcement operant conditioning
    audiometry (TROCA), 282–283
Behavioral observation audiometry (BOA), 263
Behaviorists, 268–269
Behind-the-ear (BTE) hearing aids, 428, **429**,
    434–435
Biedl-Bardet syndrome, 564
Bilabial sounds, 33
Bilateral acoustic neuromas, 55
Bilateral cochlear implants, 469
Bilateral hearing loss, **23**, 25, 26, 37
Bilateral microtia, 169
Bilateral sensorineural hearing loss, **375**
Bilingual-bicultural education, 520
Bilirubin, 95, 165, 166
Binaural hearing aids, 456–458
Binaural interaction tests, 157
Binaural separation, 155
Binaural squelch, 457
Binaural summation, 456

Binaural synthesis, 155

Biobehavioral function, 1

Birth, perinatal care following, 90–93, **91**

Birth defects, genetics of, 56

Bjornstad syndrome, **537**, 548

Blastocyst, 70, 72

Blending, 155

Blindness, screening children with deafness and blindness, 304–305

Blood circulation. *See* Circulatory system

Bluetooth, 434

BOA. *See* Behavioral observation audiometry

Body-type hearing aids, 423

Boil, of the external ear canal, 172

Bone anchored hearing aids (BAHA), 436–437, **437**

Bone conduction hearing aids, 436

Bone conduction pathway, 8–9, **9**

Bone conduction threshold, 444

Bony exostoses, 171

Bony labyrinth, 85

BOR. *See* Branchio-oto-renal syndrome

Bottom-up treatments, 159

Boxer's ears, 172

BPD. *See* Bronchopulmonary dysplasia

Bracketing protocol, 274

Brain

    brainstem auditory pathway, 17–20, **18–20**

    embryology of, 115

    hydrocephalus, **539**, 562–563, **562**

    of infants, 115, 117

    lesions, hearing and, 19

    meningitis, 199–200, **540**, 566–567

    neuroplasticity of, 114–118, 143–144

    synaptic pruning, 116

Brain lesions, hearing and, 19

Brainstem auditory pathway, 17–20, **18–20**

Branchial arch disorders, 170, 194, **537**, 548

Branchial arches, 74

Branchial grooves, 81, 82

Branchial membranes, 81, 82

Branchial structures, fetal development, 81–82, **81**

Branchio-oto-renal syndrome (BOR), 194, **537**, 548, 574

"Brittle bone" disease, 571

Brodmann's areas, 19

Bronchopulmonary dysplasia (BPD), 98–99

BTE hearing aids. *See* Behind-the-ear (BTE) hearing aids

Bullous myringitis, 178–179

Bush, George W., 490

C

C-levels, 471

CAEP. *See* Cortical auditory evoked potential

Camurati-Engelmann disease, **537**, 548–549

Cancer treatment drugs, ototoxicity of, 193, **537**, **541**

Canonical babble, 137, 138

Canonical stage, 137, 138

CANS. *See* Central auditory nervous system

CAPD. *See* Central auditory processing disorder

Carboplatin, 193

Cardioauditory syndrome. *See* Jervell and Lange-Nielsen syndrome

Cardiovascular system, embryology of, 72, 76

Cardiovascular system disorders, in newborns, 99–100

Carnegie Task Force on Meeting the Needs of Young Children (1994), 531

Caroplatin, 193

Carraro syndrome, **537**, 543

Carriers, 65, **66**

Case history, 255, **256–257**, 257–258, **259–260**

Cauliflower ears, 172

Cell division, 55, **55**, 57–59

    defined, 57

    gametogenesis, 59

    meiosis, 57, 58–59, **59**

    mitosis, 57–58, **58**

Central auditory nervous system (CANS), 152

Central auditory processing disorder (CAPD), 24, 151–161

    causes of, 152

    co-morbidities, 152

    defined, 152

    screening for, 154–159

    symptoms of, 152–154

    treatment of, 159–161

Central nervous system

    disorders, in newborns, 100

    embryology of, 71, 74, 76

Centromeres, 55, **55**, 56

Cerebral palsy (CP), **538**, 549–550
Cerebro-oculo-facio-skeletal (COFS)
    syndrome, 553
Cerumen. *See* Earwax
Cervico-oculo-acoustic dysplasia, 550, 582
CFAs. *See* Craniofacial anomalies
Chalk bone disease, 572
CHAPS. *See* Children's Auditory Performance
    Scale
Charcot-Marie-Tooth disease, 570, 576, 594
CHARGE association, 100
CHARGE syndrome, 194, **538**, 550–551
CHD. *See* Congenital heart disease
CHD7 gene, 551
Chemotherapy drugs, ototoxicity of, 193, **537**,
    541
CHILD. *See* Children's Home Inventory for
    Listening Difficulties
Child development
    auditory developmental milestones, **122**
    auditory maturation index, 264–265
    auditory maturation responses, 121, **122**,
        123–127, 250–252, 264–265
    developmental speech milestones, 130–132,
        131, **259–260**
    hearing and speech developmental
        questionnaire for parents, 132, **133–134**,
        135–136, 253, **254**, 256–257
    hearing loss and, 6–7
Childhood hearing loss
    child development and, 6–7
    childhood infections associated with,
        199–202
    defining, 27–28
    demographics of, 25–27
    Down syndrome associated with, 205
    early detection of, 2–7
    economic burden of, 41–43
    education and training expenses, 42, 43
    educationally significant hearing loss,
        483–484, **484**
    functional hearing loss, 305–307
    grammatical rules and, 36, 38
    incidence statistics, 3–4
    lifetime loss of income and, 42
    medical and audiologic expenses, 41–42
    medical disorder syndrome and condition
        list for, **537–543**, 543–583

minimal hearing loss, 28–30
normal family communications and, 43
otitis media and, 406, 416–418
ototoxicity, 100, 192–193, 368, 397, **541**
perilinguistically deafened children, 472
periodic reassessment, 46
postlinguistically deafened children, 472
prelinguistically deafened children, 472
prevalence of, 26–27
referral guidelines, 136, **136**, 417–418
school problems and, 43–44
special living expenses, 42
statistics, 394
team management of, 45–47, 398
treatment of. *See* Treatment plan
See also Hearing-impaired children
Childhood infections, **539–540**
    bacterial sepsis, 201
    hearing loss and, 199–202
    herpes simplex virus (HSV), 200–201
    meningitis, 199–200
    mumps, 201–202
    viral diseases, 202
Children
    audiologists' rapport with, 249–253,
        267–268, 278–279, 294–295, 309
    auditory processing in, 151–161
    development of oral communication,
        127–132
    difficult-to-test children, 295–305, 309, 314,
        315, 316, 365–367
    High-Risk Register for Deafness, 387–388,
        390
    parents influence in children's development,
        123–132, 531
    referral guidelines for children with speech
        delay, 136, **136**
    responses to sound, 250–252
    risk factors for deafness, 390, 395–398
    See also Child development; Childhood
        hearing loss; Childhood infections;
        Hearing-impaired children; Infants;
        Newborns
Children with autism spectrum disorder
    (ASD), 302–304
Children with brain injury, 300–302
Children with deafness and blindness, 304–305
Children with intellectual disability, 299–300

Children with multiple handicaps, 296–299, **298**

Children with pervasive developmental disorders (PDDs), 302–304

Children's Auditory Performance Scale (CHAPS), 154, 303

Children's Home Inventory for Listening Difficulties (CHILD), 154

Children's Spondee Word List, 274

Chloral hydrate, 366

Cholesteatoma, 180, 181, 185–186, 187, **187**

Chorionic villus sampling (CVS), 63

Chromatids, 55

Chromosomal abnormalities, 67–69, **68**

Chromosomal nondisjunctions, 68

Chromosomal rearrangement, 68, 69

Chromosomes, 55–56, **55**

changes in number, 68–69

changes in structure, 68

chromosomal abnormalities, 67–69, **68**

Denver system, 60

karyotype, 60, 61, 67

meiosis, 57, 58–59, **59**

mitosis, 57–58, **58**

Chronic mastoiditis, 187

Chronic suppurative otitis media (CSOM), 180, 186

CIC hearing aids. *See* Completely in-the-canal (CIC) hearing aids

Circulatory system, fetal, 79–80

Cisplatin, 193

Clarke School for the Deaf, 510

Classical Cockayne syndrome, 553

Classical conditioning, 268

Classroom amplification, 525

Classrooms, as difficult listening environment, 159, 522, 524–526

Cleft lip, 90, 203–204, 551, **551**

Cleft palate, 90, 203–204, **538**, 551, **551**

Cleidocranial dysostosis, **538**, 552, **552**

Clinical Guidelines for Pediatric Amplification (American Academy of Audiology), 424

Cloaca, embryology of, 76

Closed-response testing, 287

Closure, 155

CM. *See* Cochlear microphonic

CMV infection. *See* Cytomegalovirus (CMV) infection

Cochlea
anatomy of, 14
electrocochleography, 363–365, **363**
fetal development of, 86
neural impulses and, 17
otoacoustic emissions (OAEs), 193, 337–338, 412–413, 587, 593
ototoxic pathology in, 193

Cochlear duct, 15, 16

Cochlear hearing loss, 330

Cochlear implants, 464–481
for auditory neuropathy spectrum disorder (ANSD), 591–592
benefits of, 474–476, 496
bilateral implants, 469
bimodal use, 468
components of, 467–468, **467**
"hybrid" cochlear implant, 469
selection of pediatric candidates, 471–474, **474**, 512
sensitive period for implantation in children, 476–478
speech intelligibility and, 478
speech perception testing with, 290, 292–293, **292**
speech production and, 494
success with, 478–481
surgery for, 469–470
training for, 471

Cochlear microphonic (CM), 363, **370**, 587, 588

Cochlear nerve, 16

Cochlear nuclei, 17, 18–19, **18**

Cochlear pouch, 85

Cockayne's syndrome, **538**, 552–553

Codon, 56

COFS syndrome. *See* Cerebro-oculo-facio-skeletal (COFS) syndrome

Cognition, 155

COL4A5 gene, 546

Colorado, universal newborn hearing screening, 393

Combined method, 515

Communication
American Sign Language (ASL), 498, 513–515, **516**, 517
auditory-oral (A-O) and auditory-verbal (A-V) methods, 508–512

Communication *(continued)*
  combined method, 515
  cued speech, 519
  deaf culture, 497–499, 514
  families and, 532
  fingerspelling, 512, 513, 514
  interpreters for the deaf, 515, 521, 522
  lip reading, 513
  Listening and Spoken Language, 511
  manual communication, 508, 512
  manually coded English (MCE), 518–519
  methods of, 507–520
  personal FM systems for children, 160, 209, 526, 527–530
  Rochester method, 515, 517
  signing, 496, 512–513, 518–522
  Signing Exact English (SEE), 519–522
  speechreading, 513
  stages of, 503
  total communication (TC), 508, 517–518
  visual-oral methods, 512–513
  See also Language; Oral communication
Completely in-the-canal (CIC) hearing aids, 436
Compression circuits, in hearing aids, 461
Computerized probe-microphone measurements, 440–441, **441**, 442
Computerized stimulus presentations, 271
Conditioned orientation reflex, 272
Conditioned orientation reflex (COR) audiometry, 272
Conditioned play audiometry (CPA), 277–283, **280**, 444–445
Conductive hearing loss, 21–22, **23**, 173, 330–331
Congenital, use of term, 52
Congenital anomalies of ears, face, and palate, 89–90
  See also Genetic disorders
Congenital cholesteatomas, 186
Congenital deafness, 39, 89
Congenital heart disease (CHD), 99
Congenital infections of newborns, 100–109
Congenital lues, 105
Congenital recessive atopic dermatitis triad, 548
Congenital rubella syndrome (CRS), 100, 101–102, 575
Congenital syphilis, 105–106, **540**, 576

Congenitally deaf children, babbling, abnormalities in, 130, 135, 137, 138
Congestive heart failure, 99
Conjugate procedure, 270
Connexin 26, 189–190
Connexin 26 (Cx26) hearing loss, 189–191
Connexin 26 mutations, 190
Consanguineous marriages, 65, 110
Conscious sedation, 366
Consensus Statement on Early Identification of Hearing Impairment in Infants and Young Children (National Institute on Deafness and Other Communication Disorders), 391
Consonants, 30
  fricative consonants, 32, 33
  infant's use of, 129
  occlusives, 32
  plosives, 32, 33
  stop consonants, 32
  voiced-unvoiced cognate pairs, 32
Continuous reinforcement, 267
Contralateral acoustic reflex pathway, 328, 329, **329**, 331
Contrecoup effect, 196
Conversational speech levels, **31**
Cooing, 147
Corneal dystrophy, 560
Cornelia de Lange syndrome, 69, **538**, 553
Cortical auditory evoked potential (CAEP), 358
Counseling
  for auditory neuropathy spectrum disorder, 594
  genetic counseling, 109–111
  hearing aid orientation and counseling, 449–451
  parental support groups, 237
  for parents of hearing-impaired children, 47, 229, 231–233, 237, 420, 497, 594
Count-the-dots audibility, 450–451, **451**
Coup injury, 196
CP. *See* Cerebral palsy
CPA. *See* Conditioned play audiometry
Craniofacial anomalies (CFAs), hearing loss and, 39, 41, 89–90, **260**, **538**, 548, 550, 553, 559, 572
Craniofacial dysostosis, 553

Crib-O-Gram, 389
Critical period, 143, 147
Cross-check protocol, 248–249, 276, 297
Cross-model regeneration, 117
Crossed acoustic reflex pathway, 328, 329, **330**
Crossing over (genetics), 58, 59
Crouzon disease, 169, 170
Crouzon's syndrome, 64, **538**, 553–554, **554**
CRS. *See* Congenital rubella syndrome
Cryptophthalmos, 554
CSOM. *See* Chronic suppurative otitis media
Cued speech, 519
Cultural needs, deaf culture, 497–499, 514
Cushing's symphalangism, 554
CVS. *See* Chorionic villus sampling
CX26 hearing loss. *See* Connexin 26 (Cx26)
        hearing loss
Cystic fibrosis, 65, **375**
Cytogenetics, 60–61, **61**, **62**
Cytomegalovirus (CMV) infection, congenital,
        102–104, **539**, 555
Cytosine, in DNA, 53, **54**

D

Day schools, 499, 501
db HL (hearing level), 11
db SL (sensation level), 11
db SPL (sound pressure level), 11
de Grouchy syndrome, 565
Deaf-blindness, 304–305
Deaf children. *See* Hearing-impaired children
Deaf culture, 497–499, 514
Deaf education programs, 492
"Deaf speech," 33, 38–39, 496
Deafness
    causes of, **396**
    congenital, 39, 89
    defined, 484
    economic burden of, 41–43
    genetic origins of, 52
    risk factors for, 390, 395–396
    use of term, 24
Decibels (dB), 10–11
Decision matrix analysis, 377–378, **377**
Deep sedation, 366
Deinstitutionalization movement, 499
Dekapascals (daPa), 323

Deletions (of chromosomes), 69
Denver system, 60
Deoxyribonucleic acid. *See* DNA
Descending pathway, 20
Desired Sensation Level (DSL) method, 447,
        453–454, **455**
Development delay, maturation index for, 265
Developmental theory, 265
DFMO. *See* Difluoromethylornithine
DFNB1 deafness, 190
Diabetes mellitus, hearing loss and, 202
Diagnostic genetic testing, 63, 110–111
Diastrophic dysplasia, 555–556
Diastrophic nanism syndrome, 555–556
Dibekacin, **541**
Dichotic speech tests, 157
Dieter's cells, 86
Difference theory, 265
Difficult-to-test children, 295–305, 309, 314,
        315, 316
    children with autism spectrum disorder
        (ASD), 302–304
    children with brain injury, 300–302
    children with deafness and blindness,
        304–305
    children with intellectual disability, 299–300
    children with multiple handicaps, 296–299,
        298
    children with pervasive developmental
        disorders (PDDs), 302–304
    developmentally delayed children, 418–419,
        591
    sedation for, 365–367
Difluoromethylornithine (DFMO), 193
Digital constrictions, **540**
Digital hearing aids, 430, 432
Digital signal processing (DSP), 430
Digitally programmable hearing aids, 430
DIP test. *See* Discrimination by Identification
        of Pictures (DIP) test
Diploid number, 56
Direct audio input (DAI), and hearing aids,
        431, 432
Directional microphones, in hearing aids,
        459–460
Discrimination, 155
Discrimination by Identification of Pictures
        (DIP) test, 288

Diseases
    congenital infections of newborns, 100–109
    inherited disorders, 63–64
    molecular genetic analysis, 62
    prenatal diagnostic tests, 62
    See also Infections
Distal 18q-, 565, **565**
Distortion product evoked otoacoustic
    emissions (DPEOAEs), 340, 343, **344**,
    345, 401, 408
DNA, 53, **54**
    base-pair arrangement, 53, **54**
    double-helix structure, 53, **54**
    function of, 56
    meiosis, 57, 58–59, **59**
    mitochondrial DNA, 69
    mitosis, 57–58, **58**
    molecular genetic analysis, 62
    polymerase chain reaction (PCR), 62
    protein synthesis, 56–57
Double-helix structure (DNA), 53, **54**
Down syndrome (trisomy 21), 100, 204–205,
    538, 556–557, **556**
    auditory screening of Down syndrome
        children, 300
    genetics of, 68, **68**
    prenatal blood test for, 63
DPEOAEs. *See* Distortion product evoked
    otoacoustic emissions
Drugs, ototoxic, 100, 192–193, 368, 397, **541**
DSL method. *See* Desired Sensation Level
    (DSL) method
DSP. *See* Digital signal processing
Duane syndrome, 550, 583
Ductus arteriosus, 80
Duplications (of chromosomes), 69
Dwarfism, 170, **538**
Dyschondrosteosis. *See* Madelung deformity

E

EAA. *See* Educational Audiology Association
EAHCA. *See* Education for All Handicapped
    Children Act of 1975
Ear
    anatomy and physiology of, **8**, 12, 14–16, **15**
    anomalies of, 89–90, 170, 258, 260
    auditory pathway, 7–8, **8**, **9**, 14–16

    developmental anomalies of, 89
    embryology of, 51, 72, **73**, 74, 75, 77, 80, 81,
        82, **83**, 84–86, **85**, **87**, **88–89**
    foreign bodies in, 171
    infections of, 4, 22, 174
    inner ear, 14
    medical examination by audiologist, 167,
        258, 260, **261**
    middle ear, 14
    otoscopy, 84, 260, **261**, 319
    outer ear, 12, 14
    speech and, 1
Ear canal
    anatomy of, 12, 14, 167
    atresia of external ear canal, 168–169, **168**,
        538
    bony growths of external ear canal, 171
    discharge from, 170
    embryology of, 80–82, **81**
    equivalent ear canal volume, 327
    malformations of, 167–170
    self-cleaning mechanism of, 167
Ear infections, 4, 22, 174
    See also Otitis media
Eardrum, 14
    perforated, 172–173, **173**, 178
Early Hearing Detection and Intervention
    (EHDI) programs, 214, 215, 393, 394, 395
Early intervention, 6, 211–245, 405
    2013 JCIH Supplement, 222–223
    about, 211–212
    for child with otitis media, 239–242
    Early Hearing Detection and Intervention
        (EHDI) programs, 214, 215, 393, 394, 395
    family-centered services, 223–228, **226**, 238,
        486
    hearing dogs, 244–245
    implementation of, 212–215
    Individualized Family Service Plan (IFSP),
        215
    language and literacy skills and, 493
    LENA system, 220–221
    optimal strategies for, 221–223
    reading to the child, 493
    research studies, 216–220
    telepractice, 242–244
    time between age of detection and age of
        intervention, 213–214

Early Language Milestone Scale, 241
Early Speech Perception (ESP) test, 292
Earmolds, 433, 462–464, **463**
Earphones, noise level in, 197
Ears. *See* Ear
Earwax (cerumen), 14, 21, 170–171
ECMO. *See* Extracorporeal membrane oxygenation
ECochG. *See* Electrocochleography
Ectoderm, 70, **71**, 81
EDN3 gene, 582
EDNRB gene, 582
EDR. *See* Electrodermal response
Education, 483–533
    advocates for hearing-impaired children, 506
    audiologist in educational setting, 484–487, 506, 522, **523–524**
    bilingual-bicultural education, 520
    challenges in teaching deaf and hearing-impaired students, 502–507
    of children with otitis media, 241–242
    classroom acoustics, 159, 522, 524–526
    classroom interpreters or note takers, 521, 522
    communication methods, 507–520
    communication with peers, 497–499
    cost of, 42, 43, 502, **502**
    current status of, 499–502
    day schools, 499, 501
    deaf education programs, 492
    deinstitutionalization movement, 499
    exclusion programs, 502
    Free Appropriate Public Education (FAPE), 488, 505
    goals for child with hearing loss, 490–499
    IEP for hearing-impaired students, 488, 500, 505–507
    itinerant programs, 501
    language goals in, 491
    Least Restrictive Environment (LRE), 488–489, 505, 522
    literacy and, 491–495
    mainstreaming, 506, 511–512, 520–522
    mental health goals, 495
    parents' role in, 530–533
    personal FM systems for children, 526, 527–530
    personalized instruction, 506
    public school education, 499–500
    reading level and comprehension, 491–492
    residential schools for deaf and hard-of-hearing children, 499, 500–501
    resource rooms, 501
    school environment, 500–502
    self-contained classrooms in schools, 501, 521
    special education, 43–44, 502
    special schools, 499, 501
    speech intelligibility as goal, 496–497
    supportive services, 506
    U.S. legislation for. *See* Legislation (U.S.)
    See also Schools
Education for All Handicapped Children Act of 1975 (EAHCA), 464, 483, 487, 489, 522
Educational audiologist, 484–487, 506, 522, **523–524**
Educational Audiology Association (EAA), 485, 502
Edwards syndrome, 578–579
Efferent pathway, 20
EHDI programs. *See* Early Hearing Detection and Intervention (EHDI) programs
18q deletion syndrome, 565
Eighth cranial nerve, 17
Electroacoustic hearing aid check, 447
Electrocochleography, 363–365, **363**
Electrodermal response (EDR), 386
Embryoblast, 70
Embryology, 70–90
    embryonic development, 72, 74–77, **74**, **75**
    fetal development, 70, 77–90
    pre-embryonic stage, 70–72, **71–73**
    teratogens and, 74, 80
Embryonic development, 72, 74–77, **74**, **75**
Embryonic disk, 70, 72, 74
Emotional content of speech, 33, 37
Encephalitis, **538**
Endoderm, 70, **71**, 81
Endolymph, 14, 16
Endolymphatic duct, 85
Engelmann's syndrome, **538**
Enlarged vestibular aqueduct (EVA), 193–194
EOAEs. *See* Evoked otoacoustic emissions
Equivalent ear canal volume (Veq), 326–327, **326**, **327**

ERCC6 gene, 553

ERCC8 gene, 553

ESP test. *See* Early Speech Perception (ESP) test

Ethacrynic acid, 193

Eustachian tube, 82, 84, 175, **175**

EVA. *See* Enlarged vestibular aqueduct

Evidence-based early intervention research studies, 216–217

Evoked auditory responses, 345–347, **345**, 369, **370**

Evoked otoacoustic emissions (EOAEs), 340, 399, 401–405, **402**, **404**, 408, 418

Exons, 56, 57

Exostoses, 171

Expressive language, 127

External auditory meatus, 80–82, **81**, 84

External ear
    anatomy of, 166–167
    embryology of, 75, 77, 82, **83**, **84**
    inflammatory conditions of, 172
    malformations of, 167–170
    medical conditions of, 166–173

External ear canal
    atresia and stenosis of, 168–169, **168**, **538**
    bony growths of, 171

External otitis, 170, 172

Extracorporeal membrane oxygenation (ECMO), 94, 98

EYA1 gene, 548

F

Face
    developmental anomalies of, 39, 41, 89–90
    fetal development of, 80–82, **81**, 86–87

Facial nerve, **81**

Facioscapulohumeral muscular dystrophy, 569

Familial, use of term, 52

Family
    communications in and childhood hearing loss, 43
    history of hearing loss, **538**
    mental health of hearing impaired child and, 495
    reading to the child, 493
    See also Parents

Family-centered early intervention services, 223–228, **226**, 238, 486

Family pedigree, 63, **66**

Fanconi's anemia syndrome, **538**, 557

FAPE. *See* Free Appropriate Public Education

FAS *See* Fetal alcohol syndrome

Father, academic and language outcomes and, 493

FDA *See* Food and Drug Administration

Federal programs for early intervention, 215–216

Feedback canceling algorithm, hearing aids, 431

Feigning hearing loss, 305–307

Female karyotype, 61, **61**

Fertilization, 70, 76

Fetal alcohol syndrome (FAS), **539**, 557–558

Fetal development, 70, 77–90
    auditory system, 118–119
    branchial structures, 81–82, **81**
    circulatory system, 79–80
    ear, 82, **83**, 84–86, **85**, **87**, **88–89**
    face, 80–82, **81**, 86–87
    maternal infections during pregnancy and, 100–109
    respiratory system, 76, 77, 78–79
    teratogens and, 74, 80

Fetus, 77
    growth of, 77–78, **78**
    intrauterine sound discrimination, 119–120
    prenatal diagnostic tests, 62
    prenatal hearing, 118–121
    ultrasonography, 62
    See also Fetal development; Prenatal development

FGFR2 gene, 554

Figure ground, 155

Fingerspelling, 512, 513, 514

First and second brachial arch syndrome, 560, 577

First arch syndrome, 89

First branchial arch, 75, **81**, 82, 84, 86, 87, 89

FISH (fluorescence in situ hybridization), 61

Fitting pediatric hearing aids, 426–428, 438–439, **439**, 446–447
    assessment, 443–445
    DSL method, 447, 453–454, **455**
    for infants, 440, 444, 455–456
    NAL approach, 453
    orientation and counseling, 449–451

prescriptive methods, 452–456, **455**
probe microphone measurements, 439–443, **439**, **441**, 447–448
protocol for, 443–452
validation, 451–452
verification, 447–448
5-minute Apgar evaluation, 164
FMR1 gene, 558
Food and Drug Administration (FDA), 426, 466
Foramen ovale, 80
Foregut, embryology of, 76
Formants, 30, 33
Fourth branchial arch, **81**, 82
Fragile X syndrome, 558
Fraser syndrome, **539**, 554
Free Appropriate Public Education (FAPE), 488, 505
Freidreich ataxia, **539**
Frequency, defined, 10
Frequency lowering, 459
Frequency response, 458–460
Frequency transposition, 459
Fricative consonants, 32, 33
Friedreich's ataxia, 558–559, 594
Frontonasal prominence, 86
Functional compensatory plasticity, 118
Functional gain, 449
Functional hearing loss, 305–307
Furosemide, 193, **541**
Furuncle, of the external ear canal, 172

G

GAEL-S. *See* Grammatical Analysis of Elicited Language-Simple Sentence Level
Gallaudet College, 514
Galvanic skin response, 386
Gametes, 66, 70, 76
Gametogenesis, 59
Gap-junction proteins, 190
Gargoylism, 170
Gas exchange, 77, 78–79
GASP. *See* Glendonald Auditory Screening Procedure
Gastrointestinal system, embryology of, 76
Gastrulation, 70
Gavage feeding, 94–95

GDF5 gene, 554
Gender, genetic basis for, 56, 76
General anesthesia, 366
Genes, 53, 55–57
See also Genetic disorders; Genetics; Mutations
Genetic counseling, 109–111
Genetic disorders
autosomal dominant disorders, 64–65, **66**
autosomal recessive disorders, 65, **66**
carriers, 65, **66**
chromosomal abnormalities, 67–69, **68**
Connexin 26 (Cx26) hearing loss, 189–191
consanguineous marriages, 65, 110
genetic counseling, 109–111
inheritance of, 63
single-gene defects, 64–65, **66**, 67, **67**
"skipped generation," 65
teratogens and, 80
X-linked disorders, 65, 67
Genetic screening, 382–385
Genetic testing, 63
for Connexin 26 mutations, 190–191
ethical dilemmas, 110–111
Genetics
basic principles of, 52–63
brain plasticity, 117
cell division, 55, **55**, 57–59
chromosomal abnormalities, 67–69, **68**
congenital anomalies, 67
congenital deafness, 39
diploid number, 56
fertilization, 70, 76
gametogenesis, 59
genetic disorders, inheritance of, 63
haploid number, 56, 57
of human pre-embryonic stage, 70–72, **71–73**
karyotype, 56
meiosis, 57, 58–59, **59**
mitochondrial inheritance, 69
mitosis, 57–58, **58**
protein synthesis, 56–57
recombination, 58, 59
single-gene defects, 64–67
See also Chromosomes; Cytogenetics; DNA; Genes; Genetic disorders; Molecular genetics; Mutations

Genome, 57

Gentamicin, 192, 368, **541**

Germ cell layers, 70

Germ layers, 69–70, **71**, 72, 76–77

Gestational age, estimating, 164–165

GJB2 gene, 190, 581

Glendonald Auditory Screening Procedure (GASP), 292

Glossopharyngeal nerve, **81**

Glottal sounds, 33

"Glue ear," 179

Goldenhar's syndrome, **539**, 559, **559**

Gonads, 76

Grammatical Analysis of Elicited Language-Simple Sentence Level (GAEL-S), 494

Grammatical rules, hearing loss and, 36, 38

Guanine, in DNA, 53, **54**

Guide for the Evaluation of Hearing Handicap (American Academy of Otolaryngology), percentage of hearing loss scale, 28–29

H

Haemophilus influenzae, 182, 200, 567

Hair cells, 15–16, **15**, 17, 86, 338, 340, 363

Hallgren syndrome, 560, 580

Hammer, anvil, and stirrup, 14

Hand-hearing syndrome, 560, **560**

Hands and Voices (support group), 237

Haploid number, 56, 57

Harboyan syndrome, 560

Hard-of-hearing, defined, 24, 483, 484

Hawaii, universal newborn hearing screening, 393

Head shadow (head diffraction), 457

Head Start Performance Standards, 405, 408, 409

Head-turn responses, 274

Hearing

auditory maturation, 121, **122**, 123–127, 250–252, 264–265

auditory pathway for, 7–8, **8**, **9**

bone conduction pathway, 8–9, **9**

brainstem auditory pathway, 17–20, **18–20**

damage to from hearing aids, 460–462

defined, 149

developmental questionnaire for parents, 132, **133–134**, 135–136, 253, **254**, **256–257**

fetal development of, 86

listening, 148–151, **150**

neonatal hearing development, 121, **122**, 123–127

neural activity involved in, 16–20, **17–20**

neuroelectrical signals of, 16–17

prenatal hearing, 118–121

speech and, 1

Hearing aid battery, as foreign object in ear, 171

Hearing aids, 423–481

about, 423–424, 428–432

acoustic coupling, 463

assessment for, 443–445

attractiveness to children, 431, 433

for auditory processing disorders, 160

behind-the-ear (BTE) models, 428, **429**, 434–435

binaural, 456–458

Bluetooth connectivity of, 434

bone anchored hearing aids (BAHA), 436–437, **437**

bone conduction hearing aids, 436

for children with otitis media, 241–242

completely in-the-canal (CIC) models, 436

components of, 429–430

count-the-dots audibility, 450–451, **451**

damage to hearing from, 460–462

digital models, 430, 432

digitally programmable models, 430

direct audio input (DAI) and, 431, 432

earmolds, 433, 462–464, **463**

feedback canceling algorithm, 431

frequency response, 458–460

functional gain, 449

in-the-canal (ITC) models, 429, 436

in-the-ear (ITE) models, 428–429, 435–436

for infants with ANSD, 590–591

insertion loss, 440

looking/listening check for, 464, **465**

operation of, 429

orientation and counseling, 449–450

output, 460–461, **461**

parental management of children's hearing aids, 424–425, 464–465

remote programming of, 430

replacement of, 42

selecting and fitting, 424, 426–428, 438–439, **439**, 446–447

sound channel, 462
telephone compatibility of, 434
types, 433–438
validation of, 451–452
verification of, 447–448
waterproof, 430, 434
Hearing dogs, 244–245
Hearing-impaired children
    advocacy for, 486, 506
    annual evaluation, 332–333
    assessment for hearing aids, 443–445
    babbling in, 139
    communication with peers, 497–499
    cost of education of, 42, 43, 502, **502**
    deaf culture, 497–499, 514
    early intervention, 6, 211–245
    educational goals for, 490–499
    functional hearing loss, 305–307
    High-Risk Register for Deafness, 387–388,
        390
    infant babbling in, 130, 135, 137, 138
    language deprivation, effect of on infant, 146
    language difficulties of, 494
    learning to listen, 148–151, **150**
    psychoeducational performance of, 507
    See also Auditory screening; Infants;
        Newborns; Toddlers
Hearing loss (general)
    about, 20–30
    age of identification of, 212–214
    ambient noise and, 36
    childhood infections and, 199–202
    in children. *See* Childhood hearing loss
    degree and severity of, 24–25
    diabetes mellitus and, 202
    economic burden of, 41–43
    educationally significant hearing loss,
        483–484, **484**
    effect on speech and language, 35–39, **40**, 41
    feigning, 305–307
    functional hearing loss, 305–307
    genetic counseling, 109
    genetic origins of, 52
    grammatical rules and, 36, 38
    hair cells and, 16
    from hearing aids, 460–462
    as hidden disability, 2–7
    High-Risk Register for Deafness, 387–388,
        390

language development and, 5–6, 44, 130
lifetime loss of income and, 42
medical disorders and, 163–209, **537–543**,
    543–583
noise and, 196–198
ototoxic medications, 100, 192–193, 368,
    397, **541**
problems in adulthood, 44
risk factors for, 390, 395–398
statistics, 394
suspicion of, 420
syndrome and condition list for, **537–543**,
    543–583
viral diseases and, 202
visual acuity and, 504–505
See also Central auditory processing
    disorder; Conductive hearing loss; Mixed
    hearing loss; Sensorineural hearing loss
Hearing loss in children. *See* Childhood
    hearing loss
Hearing screening. *See* Auditory screening
Hearing threshold level (HTL), 328
Hearing thresholds, 11–12
Heart
    embryology of, 76
    in fetus, 79
Heart. *See* Circulatory system
Heart rate response audiometry, 388
Hemifacial microsomia, **539**, 560–561
Hemoglobinopathy, **375**
Hemophilia, genetics of, 67
Hensen's cells, 86
Hereditary sensory and autonomic
    neuropathies (HSANs), 576
Heredity
    mitochondrial inheritance, 69
    use of term, 52
    See also Genetic disorders; Genetics
Herpes simplex virus (HSV), 200–201, **539**
Herrmann's syndrome, **539**, 561
Hertz (Hz), 10
HIB vaccine, 566
HIE. *See* Hypoxic ischaemic encephalopathy
High-Risk Register for Deafness, 387–388, 390
Hindgut, embryology of, 76
Hirschsprung disease, 582
Hispanic Health and Nutrition Examination
    Survey of 1990, 25
HIV, 106, 107

HIV infection, congenital, 106–108
HMD. *See* Hyaline membrane disease
Hospital-based hearing screening protocols, 403
Hospitals
    NICU (Neonatal/Newborn Intensive Care Unit), 90, 92–96, 163, 385, 397
    perinatal care, 90–93, **91**
HSANs. *See* Hereditary sensory and autonomic neuropathies
HSV. *See* Herpes simplex virus
HTL. *See* Hearing threshold level
Human vocal range, 34
Hunter-Hurler syndrome, 170, **539**, 561–562, **562**
Hunter's syndrome, **539**, 561–562, **562**
Huntington's disease, genetics of, 55
Hurler-Scheie syndrome, 561
Hurler's syndrome, 561
Hyaline membrane disease (HMD), 96–97
"Hybrid" cochlear implant, 469
Hydrocephalus, **539**, 562–563, **562**
Hyoid arch, **81**, 82
Hyperbilirubinemia, 95, 166, **539**
Hyperostosis corticalis generalisata, 581
Hypoxic ischaemic encephalopathy (HIE), **539**

I

IDEA. *See* Individuals with Disabilities Education Act
IDEIA. *See* Individuals with Disabilities Education Improvement Act of 2004
IEP. *See* Individualized Education Program
IFSP. *See* Individualized Family Service Plan
Illinois Test of Psycholinguistic Abilities (ITPA), 241
Immitance. *See* Acoustic immitance measures
Immitance meters, 328, 406
Immune system, of premature infants, 199
Impedance, 316
    See also Acoustic immitance measures
Impedance meters, 316, 328
Implantation (of embryo), 70, 72
In-the-canal (ITC) hearing aids, 429, 436
In-the-ear (ITE) hearing aids, 428–429, 435–436
Incidence, auditory screening, 379

Incidence rate, 379
Incidental learning, 150
Incus, 14, 81, **81**, 84, 170
Individualized Education Program (IEP), 488, 500
Individualized Family Service Plan (IFSP), 215
Individuals with Disabilities Education Act (IDEA), 215, 216, 483, 487–490, 522
    eligibility for services, 488
    Free Appropriate Public Education (FAPE), 488, 505
    history of, 487
    Individualized Education Program (IEP), 488, 500, 505–507
    Least Restrictive Environment (LRE), 488–489, 505, 522
    legislative growth of, 489–490
    procedural safeguards, 489
Individuals with Disabilities Education Improvement Act of 2004 (IDEIA), 490
Infant-Toddler Meaningful Auditory Integration Scale (IT-MAIS), 591
Infantile renal tubular acidosis, 557
Infants
    acoustic immitance measures in, 334–337
    acoustic stapedial reflex responses in, 335, 336
    auditory input given to, 130
    auditory maturation responses, 121, **122**, 123–127, 250–252, 264–265
    auditory neuropathy spectrum disorder in, 588
    babbling, 130, 132, 135, 137
    baby's first words, 129
    behavioral hearing tests on, **122**, 123–127, 271–277, **273**, **276**
    birth defects in, 51
    brain of, 115, 117
    cardiovascular system disorders, 99–100
    central nervous system disorders, 100
    congenital infections, 100–109
    development of oral communication, 127–132
    discrimination of speech sounds, 36
    ear anatomy in, 84
    early phonetic learning in, 121, **122**, 123–127
    equivalent ear canal volume in, 327

fetal development of, 70, 77–90
first vocal sounds, 113, 128–129, 137–138
fitting hearing aids for, 440, 444, 455–456
hearing loss statistics, 3–4, 394
hearing screening methods, 405–409
language acquisition by, 1–2
middle ear effusion (MEE) in, 188, **188**
monitoring infants with "transient" ANSD, 593–594
mother's voice, 113, 119, 120
multiple handicapping conditions of, 213, **213**
otoscopy in, 335–336
perception of speech signals by, 113
physiologic hearing tests on, 310–315, **312**
prelinguistic vocalizations, 138, 139
prenatal development, 70–77
prevalence of hearing loss in, 27
reflexive behaviors of, 251
respiratory system disorders, 96–99
response to sound, 121, **122**, 123–126, 250–252
risk factors for deafness, 390, 395–398
startle response, 121, 123, 124, 251, 268, 309
tympanometry in, 334–335, 336–337, 406–409, **407**
See also Hearing-impaired children; Newborns
Infections
congenital infections of newborns, 100–109
hearing loss and, 199–202
See also Diseases
Inferior colliculi, 19
Inferior vena cava, 79
Inheritance of genetic disorders, 63
Inherited disorders, 63–64
Inner ear
anatomy of, 14
congenital malformations of, 198–199
development anomalies of, 89–90
embryology of, 72, **73**, 74
fetal development of, 84–86, **85**, 89
Inner ear aplasia, 198–199
Inner hair cells, 15, **15**, 17, 86
Insert earphones, 249, **249**
Insertion loss, 440
Intensity, defined, 10
Intensive care nursery (ICN). See NICU

Intermittent reinforcement, 269
Internal auditory meatus, 17
Interphase, 57
Interpreters for the deaf, 515, 521, 522
Interstitial deletions, 69
Intervening sequences, 57
Intervention strategies. See Early intervention
Interweaving Staircase Procedure, 277
Intraventricular hemorrhage (IVH), **540**
Introns, 56–57
Inversions (of chromosomes), 69
Ipsilateral acoustic reflex pathway, 328–329, **329**
ITC hearing aids. See In-the-canal (ITC) hearing aids
ITE hearing aids. See In-the-ear (ITE) hearing aids
ITPA. See Illinois Test of Psycholinguistic Abilities
IVH. See Intraventricular hemorrhage
Ivory bone disease, 572

J

Jaundice, 95, 165, 166
Jervell and Lange-Nielsen syndrome (JLNS), 100, **540**, 563
JLNS. See Jervell and Lange-Nielsen syndrome
Joint Committee on Infant Hearing (JCIH), 394–395
2000 Position Statement, 396
2007 Position Statement, 222, 395, 397, 427, 443
2013 Early Intervention Supplement, 222–223
Early Hearing Detection and Intervention (EHDI), 395
history of, 390, 391, 392
on risk factors, 387

K

Kanamycin, 192, **541**
Karyotype, 56
female karyotype, 61, **61**
human karyotype, 68
male karyotype, **60**, 61
Karyotype layout, 60

KCNE1 gene, 563
KCNQ1 gene, 563
Keratoderm hereditaria mutilans, 581
Keratopachyderma, **540**
Kernicterus, 166
Klein-Waardenburg syndrome, 582
Klippel-Feil syndrome, 170, **540**, 550, 563–564, **563**, 583

L

Labiodental sounds, 33
Lack of penetrance, 64
Language
    defined, 139
    development of oral communication, 127–132
    prosody of, 30, 36
    structure of, 1
    See also Communication; Language development; Speech sounds
Language and speech screening
    for children with otitis media, 240–241
    speech awareness threshold (SAT), 274, 283
    speech detection threshold (SDT), 283
    speech perception testing, 286–293, **287**, **291**, **292**
    speech reception threshold (SRT), 283–286, **285**
    speech sample, 258, 279
Language association-element method, 510
Language development
    concept development and, 503–504
    critical period of, 144
    developmental questionnaire for parents, 132, **133–134**, 135–136, 253, **254**, **256–257**
    developmental speech milestones, 130–132, **131**, **259–260**
    discrimination of speech sounds and, 36, 120
    educational goals, 491–495
    family involvement in, 492–493
    hearing loss and, 5–6, 44, 130
    hereditary deafness and, 39, 41
    incidental learning, 150
    in infants, 1–2, 114–115
    listening, 148–151, **150**

    maternal communicative skills and, 493
    mild hearing loss and, 37
    moderate hearing loss and, 37–38
    in newborns, 113
    optimal periods for speech and language learning, 143–148
    overheard speech, 150, 151
    profound hearing loss and, 38–39
    sensory deprivation and, 145–148
    severe hearing loss and, 38
    stages in, 136–140, **140–142**, 142–143
    studies in, 136–140, **140–142**, 142–143
Language Environmental Analysis. *See* LENA system
Lanugo, 77, 165
Laryngotracheal tube, 76
Late auditory evoked potentials (AEPs), 357–359, **358**
Latency-intensity functions, 349–350, **350**
Lateral facial dysplasia, 560
Lateral olivocochlear neurons, 20
Laurence-Moon-Biedl-Bardet syndromes, **540**, 564
Laurence-Moon syndrome, 564
Least Restrictive Environment (LRE), 488–489, 505, 522
Legislation (U.S.)
    American Recovery and reinvestment Act of 2009 (ARRA), 290
    Education for All Handicapped Children Act of 1975 (EAHCA), 464, 483, 487, 489, 522
    Individuals with Disabilities Education Act (IDEA), 215, 216, 472, 487–490, 522
    Individuals with Disabilities Education Improvement Act of 2004 (IDEIA), 490
    No Child Left Behind Act of 2001, 490
LENA Digital Language Processor, 221
LENA Research Foundation, 220
LENA system, 220–221
LEOPARD syndrome, **540**, 564–565
Leri-Weill disease. *See* Madelung deformity
Lexical Neighborhood Test (LNT), 293
Lexington School for the Deaf, 510
Liability model with threshold effect, 67
LIFE. *See* Listening Inventory for Education
Lifetime prevalence, 379
Limb-girdle muscular dystrophy, 569

Linguadental sounds, 33

Lip reading, 513

Liquids (speech sounds), 33

LiSN & Learn auditory training software (NAL), 161

Listening, 148–151, **150**

Listening and Spoken Language, 511

Listening Inventory for Education (LIFE), 154

Literacy, audiologists and, 491–495

LNT. *See* Lexical Neighborhood Test

Localization, 143, 155, 267

Long arm 18 deletion syndrome, 565, **565**

Long QT syndrome, **540**

Looking/listening check, for hearing aids, 464, **465**

Loop diuretics, 192, 193

Loud music, 197

Loudness, defined, 10

Loudness summation, 457

Loudspeaker systems, classrooms, 159

LRE. *See* Least Restrictive Environment

Lumbar puncture, 199–200

M

MAC. *See* Minimal Auditory Capabilities Battery

Madelung deformity, 565–566

Mainstreaming, 506, 511–512, 520–522

Major organ systems, embryology of, 72, 74, 76–77

Male karyotype, **60**, 61

Malleus, 14, 81, **81**, 84

Malleus anomalies, 170

Mandibular arch, 75, **81**, 82

Mandibular dysostosis, 577

Mandibular prominence, 86

Mandibulofacial dysostosis, 89, **538**, 546

Manual communication, 508, 512

Manually coded English (MCE), 518–519

Mapping, 442, 470

Marble bone disease, 572

MarkeTrak VII study, 27

Marshall syndrome, **540**, 566

MAS. *See* Meconium aspiration syndrome

Mastoid antrum, fetal development of, 82, 84

Mastoid bone, 437

Mastoiditis, 180, 181, 186–188

Maternal infections, 100, 199, 201, **539–540**, 555

Maternal voice, 113, 119, 120

MaterniT21 test, 63

Maxillary prominences, 86, 87, 90

MCDI. *See* Minnesota Child Development Inventory

MCE. *See* Manually coded English

MD. *See* Muscular dystrophy

Meaningful Differences in the Everyday Experiences of Young American Children (Hart & Risley), 220

Measles, 566

Meatal plug, 84

Mecham Verbal Language Development Scale, 241

Meckel's cartilage, 81, 84

Meconium, 98

Meconium aspiration syndrome (MAS), 97, 98

Medial olivocochlear neurons, 20

Medial olivocochlear pathway, 20

Medical assessment of newborns, 164–166, **165**

Medical disorders

    childhood infections, 199–202

    of external ear, 166–173

    and hearing loss, 163–209

    medical assessment of neonates, 164–166

    otitis media, 173–189

    sensorineural hearing loss and, 189–199

    syndrome and condition list for hearing loss, **537–543**, 543–583

Medical examination

    by audiologist, 167, 258, 260, **261**

    otoscopy, 84, 260, **261**, 319

Medications, ototoxic, 100, 192–193, 368, 397, **541**

MEE. *See* Middle ear effusion

Meiosis, 57, 58–59, **59**

Melatonin, 365

Membranous cochlea, 86

Membranous labyrinth, 85

Memory, 155

Meningitis, 199–200, **540**, 566–567

Mental health, of hearing impaired child, 495

Mental retardation, 299

Mesoderm, 70, **71**, 81

Metaphyseal dysplasia, 574

Michel aplasia, 198, **537**

Microphones
   in hearing aids, 459–460
   probe microphone measurements, 439–443, **439**, **441**, 447–448
   remote microphone FM technology, 528
   remote microphone hearing aids (RMHAs), 160
Microtia, **168**, 169, 437, 574
Middle ear
   anatomy of, 14
   congenital malformations of, 169–170
   disorders of, 415–418
   fetal development of, 82, 84
   negative middle ear pressure, 323, **324**, 325, 331, **333**, 418
Middle ear anomalies, 170
Middle ear effusion (MEE), 188
Middle ear infections. *See* Otitis media
Middle ear ossicles, 14
Middle-latency evoked response (MLR), 355–357, **356**, **370**
Midgut, embryology of, 76
Mild hearing loss
   about, 24, 37
   handicapping effects of, 37, **40**
   language learning and, 37
   prevalence of, 26
Minimal Auditory Capabilities Battery (MAC), 293
Minimal hearing loss, 28–30
Minimum response level (MRL), 271, 276
Minnesota Child Development Inventory (MCDI), 219
MITF gene, 582
Mitochondria, 69
Mitochondrial disorders, **540**
Mitochondrial DNA, 69
Mitochondrial inheritance, 69
Mitosis, 57–58, **58**, 70
Mixed hearing loss, 22, **23**
MLNT. *See* Multisyllabic Lexical Neighborhood Test
MLR. *See* Middle-latency evoked response
MMR vaccine, 568
Mobius syndrome, 170, **540**, 567–568, **567**
Moderate hearing loss, 24
   handicapping effects of, 37–38, **40**
   language learning and, 37–38, **40**
   prevalence of, 26

Moebius syndrome, **540**, 567–568, **567**
Molecular cytogenetics, 61
Molecular genetic analysis, diseases, 62
Molecular genetics, 61–63
Monaural low-redundancy speech tests, 157
Mondini aplasia, 89–90, 198–199, **537**
Monosomy, 68
Monosomy 18q, 565
Monosyllabic, Trochee, Sondee (MTS) test, 292
Moraella catarrhalis, 182
Moro response, 121, 123, 124, 268, 309
Mother's voice, 113, 119, 120
Mouth
   cleft lip and palate, 90, 203–204, **538**, 551, **551**
   fetal development of, 86
MPS I. *See* Mucopolysaccharidosis Type I
MRL. *See* Minimum response level
MTS test. *See* Monosyllabic, Trochee, Sondee (MTS) test
Muckle-Wells syndrome, **540**, 546, 568
Mucopolysaccharidosis Type I (MPS I), 561
Multiple-frequency tympanometry, 325
Multiple handicapping conditions, 213, **213**
Multiple lentigines syndrome, **540**, 564–565
Multisensory/syllable unit method, 510
Multisyllabic Lexical Neighborhood Test (MLNT), 293
Mumps, 201–202, 568
Mumps vaccine, 202, 568
Mumps virus, 202
Muscular dystrophy (MD), 568–569
Music, loud music and hearing loss, 197
Musical toys, noise level of, 197
Mutations, 55
   CHD7 gene, 551
   COL4A5 gene, 546
   Connexin 26 mutations, 190
   EDN3 gene, 582
   EDNRB gene, 582
   ERCC6 gene, 553
   ERCC8 gene, 553
   EYA1 gene, 548
   FGFR2 gene, 554
   FMR1 gene, 558
   GDF5 gene, 554
   GJB2 gene, 581
   KCNE1 gene, 563

KCNQ1 gene, 563
MITF gene, 582
NDP gene, 570
NIPBL gene, 553
NLRP3 gene, 546
NOG gene, 554
PAX3 gene, 582
SIX1 gene, 548
SIX5 gene, 548
SLC4A11 gene, 560
SLC26A2 gene, 556
SMC1A gene, 553
SMC3 gene, 553
SNAI2 gene, 582
SOX10 gene, 582
TGFB1 gene, 549
Usher's syndrome, 581
Mycoplasma pneumoniae, 178
Myotonic muscular dystrophy, 569
Myringotomy, **177**, 203, 320

N

Nanism syndrome, 555–556
Nasals (speech sounds), 33
National Acoustics Laboratories, 447, 453
National Center for Hearing Assessment and
    Management (NCHAM), 402, 405
National Consortium on Deaf-Blindness, 304
National Deaf-Blind Child Count, 304
National Health and Nutrition Examination
    Surveys. *See* NHANES II and III
National Institute for Occupational Safety and
    Health (NIOSH), 196
National Institute on Deafness and Other
    Communication Disorders, 391
National Institutes of Health, 391, 392,
    472–473, 474
National Registry of Interpreters for the Deaf,
    515
National Technical Institute for the Deaf, 514
Native Americans, otitis media in, 189
Natural language method, 510
NCHAM. *See* National Center for Hearing
    Assessment and Management
NDP gene, 570
Negative middle ear pressure, 323, **324**, 325,
    331, **333**, 418
Negative reinforcement, 269

Neomycin, 192, **541**
Neonatal hearing development, 121, **122**,
    123–127
Neonatal hyperthyroidism, **375**
Neonatal/Newborn Intensive Care Unit. *See*
    NICU
Neonatal ventilators, 93–94, 98
Nephrosis, **540**
Nervous system, embryology of, 71–72, **72**, 74,
    76
Neural folds, 71, 72, **72**
Neural groove, 71, 72
Neural plate, 71, 72
Neural tube, 72, 76
Neurofibromatosis type I, 569–570
Neurofibromatosis type II, 66, **540**, 569–570
Neurogenesis plasticity, 118
Neurons, 115, 117
Neuroplasticity, 114–118, 143–144
New York, hearing screening program in, 393,
    408
Newborn and Infant Hearing Screening and
    Intervention Act (1999), 393
Newborn hearing loss
    High-Risk Register for Deafness, 387–388,
        390
    prevalence of, 384–385
Newborn hearing screening, 3, 121–127, **122**
    auditory brainstem response (ABR)
        audiometry, 266, 392, 587–588, 592
    for auditory neuropathy spectrum disorder,
        594
    Auditory Response Cradle, 389
    automated ABR (A-ABR), 399–401, **400**,
        404–405
    behavioral hearing tests, 247–307
    Crib-O-Gram, 389
    developmental milestones, **122**
    evoked otoacoustic emissions (EOAEs), 340,
        399, 401–405, **402**, **404**
    heart rate response audiometry, 388
    history of, 373–374, 385–387
    hospital-based hearing screening protocols,
        403
    methods, 399–405
    operant reinforcement audiometry, 270
    respiration audiometry, 388–389
    startle response, 121, 123, 124, 251, 268, 309
    universal screening, 390–399, 403, **404**

Newborns
  Apgar evaluation, 164, **165**
  auditory maturation responses, 121, **122**,
    123–127, 250–252, 264–265
  behavioral hearing tests, 266–268
  cardiovascular system disorders, 99–100
  central nervous system disorders, 100
  congenital infections, 100–109
  estimating gestational age of, 164–165
  genetic screening, 382–385
  hearing development in, 121, **122**, 123–127
  incidence of single-gene disorders, 53
  jaundice in, 95, 165, 166
  medical assessment of, 164–166
  middle ear effusion (MEE) in, 188, **188**
  mother's voice, 113, 119, 120
  NICU care for, 90, 92–96, 163, 385, 397
  nutritional assistance for, 94–95
  perception of speech signals by, 113
  prenatal development, 70–77
  prevalence of hearing loss in, 27
  respiratory system disorders, 96–99
  response to sound, 121, **122**, 123–126,
    250–252, 264–265
  Rh incompatibility and, 165–166
  sound discrimination in, 120, 131
  speech sounds in, 131
  startle response, 121, 123, 124, 251, 268, 309
  See also Infants; Newborn hearing loss;
    Newborn hearing screening
NHANES II and III (National Health and
  Nutrition Examination Surveys), 26, 414
NICU (Neonatal/Newborn Intensive Care
  Unit), 90
  hearing impairment incidence in, 163, 385, 397
  noise level in, 95–96
  technology in, 93–96
NIHL. *See* Noise-induced hearing loss
NIOSH. *See* National Institute for
  Occupational Safety and Health
NIPBL gene, 553
Nitrogen mustard, 193
NLRP3 gene, 546
No Child Left Behind Act of 2001, 490
NOG gene, 554
Noise
  classroom acoustics, 159, 522, 524–526
  hearing loss and, 196–198

Noise-induced hearing loss (NIHL), 414
Noise level, in the NICU, 95–96
Nondisjunctions, 68
Nonorganic hearing loss, 305–307
Nonsyndromic hearing loss, 55, 63
Nontraditional inheritance, 69
Noonan's syndrome, **541**
Norrie's disease, 570
Norries syndrome, **541**
North Carolina, hearing screening program in,
  408
Northwestern University Children's Perception
  of Speech (NU-CHIPS) test, **287**, 289, 290
Notochord, 71, 72
NU-CHIPS test. *See* Northwestern University
  Children's Perception of Speech
  (NU-CHIPS) test
Nutrition, in the NICU, 94–95

O

OAEs. *See* Otoacoustic emissions
OAV. *See* Oculo-auriculo-vertebralia spectrum
Obama, Barack, 490
Objective hearing tests, 309, 310
  See also Physiologic hearing tests
Occlusives, 32
Oculo-auriculo-vertebralia spectrum (OAV),
  541
Oculocutaneous albinism, 545
Olivocochlear neurons, 20
1-minute Apgar evaluation, 164
Oocyte, 59
OPD I and, II, 572
Operant behavior, 269
Operant discrimination, 270
Operant reinforcement, 270
Operant reinforcement audiometry, 270
Ophthalmologist, as treatment partner, 45–46,
  398
Optic atrophy, **541**, 570
Optico-cochleo-dentate degeneration, 570–571
Optimized Hearing Test Algorithm, 277
Oral-aural teaching programs, 508
Oral clefts, 90, 203–204, **538**, 551, **551**
Oral communication, 2
  adequate hearing for development of, 130
  development of, 127–132

developmental questionnaire for parents, 132, **133**–**134**, 135–136, 253, **254**, **256**–**257**

developmental speech milestones, 130–132, **131**, **259**–**260**

listening, 148–151, **150**

See also Language

Oral-mandibular-auricular syndrome, 560

Organ of Corti, 14, 15, 86, 338

Ossicles, 14, 81, 84

Osteodental dysplasia, 552

Osteogenesis imperfecta, **541**, 571, **571**

Osteomas, 171

Osteopetrosis, **537**, 544, 571–572

Otic capsule, 170

Otic pits, 74, 84

Otic placodes, 84

Otic vesicle, 84–85

Otitis externa, 170, 172

Otitis media (middle ear infections), 173–189

acute otitis media, 177–178

adhesive otitis media, 179–180, **180**

bullous myringitis, 178–179

cholesteatoma following, 180, 181, 185–186, 187, **187**

chronic suppurative otitis media (CSOM), 180, 186

classification of, 177–180

complications of, 184

diagnosis of, 176

Down syndrome associated with, 204

early intervention for children with, 239–242

etiology of, 175–176, **175**

external otitis, 170, 172

hearing loss and, 406, 416–418

mastoiditis following, 180, 186–188

in Native Americans, 189

neonates and infants prone to, 188, **188**

nonresponsive otitis media, 184

as public health issue, 174

risk factors for, 176–177

serous otitis media, 179, **179**, 406

statistics for, 4

symptoms of, 176

treatment of, 180–185

tympanometry, 332, **334**

tympanosclerosis following, 184–185

Oto-facio-cervical dysmorphia, 582

Otoacoustic emissions (OAEs), 193, 337–345, **339**, 412–413, 587, 593

Otocysts, 84, 85

OTOF gene, 586

Otoferlin (OTOF) gene, 586

Otomandibular dysostosis, 560

Otopalatodigital syndrome, 572

Otoplasty, 167

Otorrhea, 184, 189

Otoscopy, 84, 260, **261**, 319, 335–336

Ototoxic medications, 100, 192–193, 368, 397, **541**

Outer ear, anatomy of, 12, 14

Outer hair cells, 15–16, **15**, 17, 338, 340

Output, hearing aids, 460–461, **461**

Overheard speech, 150, 151

Ovum, 59

P

p arms, 56

Paget's disease, 170, **541**

Palatal sounds, 33

Palate

cleft palate, 90, 203–204, **538**, 551, **551**

developmental anomalies of, 90

fetal development of, 80, 87

Parents

case history from, 255, **256**–**257**, 257–258, **259**–**260**

children's development and, 123–132, 531

counseling for, 47, 229, 231–233, 237, 420, 497, 594

developmental screening questionnaire for, 132, **133**–**134**, 135–136, 253, **254**, **256**–**257**

educational assistance for children, 530–533

emotional needs of, 237

family-centered early intervention services, 223–228, **226**, 238, 486

family history, 257

father and academic and language outcomes, 493

getting diagnosis of hearing loss from audiologist, 212, 227–233, 234–237, 414–415

hearing aid orientation and counseling, 449–451

Parents *(continued)*
  involvement in education, 506
  maternal communicative skills and language development, 493
  mental health of hearing impaired child and, 495
  monitoring children's hearing aids, 464, **465**
  reading to the child, 493
  stages of adjustment to child's hearing loss, 230
  support groups for, 237
  See also Family
Partial 18q deletion, 565
Pascal (unit), 11
PAX3 gene, 582
PBK-50 word lists, 288, 290, 293
PCR (polymerase chain reaction), 62
PCV3. *See* Pneumococcal conjugate vaccine
PDDs. *See* Pervasive developmental disorders
Peabody Picture Vocabulary Test, 241
Pediatric audiologists. *See* Audiologists
Pediatric hearing aids. *See* Hearing aids
Pediatric hearing loss. *See* Childhood hearing loss
Pediatric speech audiometry, 283–286
Pediatric Speech Intelligibility (PSI) test, **287,** 289–290, **291**
Pena-Shokeir syndrome Type, II, 553
Pendred's syndrome, 194, **541**, 572–573
Perforated eardrum, 172–173, **173**, 178
Periauricular abnormalities, **541**
Perichondritis, 172
Perilinguistically deafened children, 472
Perilymph, 14, 16
Perilymph fistula (PLF), 194–195
Perinatal care, 90–93, **91**
Period prevalence, 379
Peripheral nervous system, embryology of, 76
Periventricular leukomalacia (PVL), **541**
Persistent fetal circulation (PFC), 97
Persistent pulmonary hypertension of the newborn (PPHN), 97–98, **541**
Personal FM systems
  for auditory processing disorders, 160, 209
  in school setting, 526, 527–530
Personal music players, noise level in, 197
Pervasive developmental disorders (PDDs), 205, 302–304

PFC. *See* Persistent fetal circulation
Pharyngeal arches, 74
Pharyngeal pouches, 81, 82, 84
Pharynx, 82, 129
Phenylketonuria (PKU), 65, **375**, 382
Phonetically Balanced Kindergarten word lists. *See* PBK-50 word lists
Phototherapy, for jaundice, 95, 166
Phylogeny, 51
Physiologic hearing tests, 309–371
  acoustic immitance measures, 315–337
  audiometric assistant in, 310
  auditory brainstem evoked responses (ABR), 205, 266, 347–355, 392, 418–419, 444, 587–588, 592
  auditory middle-latency evoked response (MLR), 355–357, **356**
  auditory steady-state response (ASSR), 359–363, **360**, **361**, 444
  distortion product evoked otoacoustic emissions (DPEOAEs), 340, 343, **344**, 345, 401, 408
  electrocochleography, 363–365, **363**
  evoked auditory responses, 345–347, **345**, 369, **370**
  evoked otoacoustic emissions (EOAEs), 340, 399, 401–405, **402**, **404**, 408, 418
  late auditory evoked potentials (AEPs), 357–359, **358**
  otoacoustic emissions (OAEs), 337–345, **339**
  sedation for, 365–367
  toddlers and, 310–315, **312**
  transient evoked otoacoustic emissions (TEOAEs), 340, 341, **342**, 343, 392, 401, 408
  vestibular evaluation, 367–368
Piebaldness, **541**
Pierre Robin syndrome, 89, 170, **541**, 573
Pili torti, 548
Pimple, of the external ear canal, 172
Pinna
  anatomy of, 12, 14, 166–167, **167**, 463
  malformation of, 52, **538**
  microtia, **168**, 169, 437, 574
  shape of, 167, 463
Pitch, defined, 10
PKU. *See* Phenylketonuria
Placenta, 70, 78

Plasticity. *See* Neuroplasticity
Play conditioning audiometry, 277–283, **280**
PLF. *See* Perilymph fistula
Plosives, 32, 33
Pneumatic otoscopy, 319
Pneumococcal conjugate vaccine (PCV3), 182
Pneumococcal infections, 182
Pneumothorax, 97
Point prevalence, 379
Polar body, 59
Polymerase chain reaction. *See* PCR
Polyneuropathy, **541**, 570
Portable stereos, noise level in, 197
Positive reinforcement, 269
Postlinguistically deafened children, 472
PPD. *See* Pervasive developmental disorders
PPHN. *See* Persistent pulmonary hypertension
    of the newborn
Preauricular appendages, 168, **168**, 573–574,
    574
Pregnancy
    fertilization, 70, 76
    implantation, 70, 72
    length of normal pregnancy, 70
    placenta, 70, 78
    prenatal diagnostic tests, 62
    quickening, 77
    Rh incompatibility, 165–166
    teratogens and, 74, 80
    term pregnancy, 70
    See also Fetal development; Prenatal
        development
Preimplantation diagnosis, 110
Prelinguistically deafened children, 472
Premature birth, 70
Premature infants, infections associated with
    hearing loss, 199
Prenatal development, 70–77
    embryonic development, 72, 74–77, **74, 75**
    pre-embryonic stage, 70–72, **71–73**
    stages of, 70
Prenatal diagnostic tests, 62
Prenatal hearing, 118–121
Preschool children, hearing screening,
    409–410, **410**
Prescriptive fitting methods, 452–456, **455**
Prevalence, auditory screening, 378–379
Prevalence rate, 379

Probe microphone measurements, 439–443,
    439, **441**, 447–448
Profound hearing loss, 24
    babbling and, 130, 135, 137
    handicapping effects of, 38–39, **40**
    language learning and, 38–39, **40**
    prevalence of, 26
Progressive diaphyseal dysplasia, 548
Prosody, 30, 36
Protein synthesis, genetics, 56–57
Proximal symphalangism, 554
Pseudoconductive hearing loss, 249
Pseudohypertrophic muscular dystrophy, 569
PSI test. *See* Pediatric Speech Intelligibility
    (PSI) test
Pulse oximetry, 93
"Punctured" eardrum, 172–173, **173**, 178
Pure oralism/auditory stimulation, 510
Pure tone audiometry, 332, 406, 411
Pure tones, 10, 11, 19
PVL. *See* Periventricular leukomalacia
Pyle's syndrome, **542**, 572, 574

Q

q arms, 56
Q-tips, 171
Quickening, 77
Quinine, 193, **541**

R

Rattles, noise level of, 197
RDS. *See* Respiratory distress syndrome
Reading comprehension, 492
Reading level, 491–495
Real-ear amplified response (REAR), 442, 447
Real-ear to coupler difference (RECD), 442,
    448, 454, 460
Real-ear unaided gain (REUG), 440
REAR. *See* Real-ear amplified response
Rearrangement (chromosomal), 68, 69
RECD. *See* Real-ear to coupler difference
Receptive language, 127
Recombination, 58, 59
Rectum, embryology of, 76
Refsum's syndrome, **542**, 574
Registry of Interpreters for the Deaf (RID), 515

Reichert's cartilage, 81

Remote microphone FM technology, 528

Remote microphone hearing aids (RMHAs), for auditory processing disorders, 160

Renal tubular acidosis, 557

Residential schools for deaf and hard-of-hearing children, 499, 500–501

Resource rooms, in schools, 501

Respiration, in fetus, 77, 78

Respiration audiometry, 388–389

Respiratory distress syndrome (RDS), 96–97

Respiratory system, 77–79, 96

Respiratory system disorders, in newborns, 96–99

Response decrement, 127

Reticular formation, 19

Retinitis pigmentosa-dysacusis syndrome, 580

Retraction pocket, 185

REUG. *See* Real-ear unaided gain

Reverberation time (RT), 525

Rh incompatibility, 165–166

Rhode Island Hearing Assessment Project, 391–392

Ribonuclear acid. *See* RNA

Ribosomal RNA, 57

Ribosomes, 56

Richards-Rundle syndrome, **542**, 574–575

RID. *See* Registry of Interpreters for the Deaf

Risk factors, for deafness, 390, 395–398

RMHAs. *See* Remote microphone hearing aids

RNA, 56

Rochester method, 515, 517

Rock concerts, loud music and hearing loss, 197

Rosenthal's canal, 17

RT. *See* Reverberation time

Rubella, 100, 101–102, **539**, 575

Ruptured eardrum, 172–173, **173**, 178

S

S/N. *See* Signal-to-noise ratio

Saccule, 86

Salicylates, 193

SAT. *See* Speech awareness threshold

Scala media, 15, 16

Scala tympani, 16

Scala vestibuli, 16

SCAN–3:C Tests for Auditory Processing Disorders for Children, 157–158

Scheibe aplasia, 198, 199, **537**

Scheie syndrome, 561

Schools

    challenges in teaching deaf and hearing-impaired students, 502–507

    classroom acoustics, 159, 522, 524–526

    deinstitutionalization movement, 499

    educational audiologist, 484–487, 506, 522, **523–524**

    exclusion from, 502

    hearing screening programs in, 408, 410–411, **415**

    Individualized Education Program (IEP) for hearing-impaired students, 488, 500, 505–507

    public school education for hearing-impaired children, 499–500

    resource rooms, 501

    self-contained classrooms in, 501, 521

    See also Education

Schwann syndrome, 575–576

Screening

    developmental screening questionnaire for parents, 132, **133–134**, 135–136, 253, **254**, **256–257**

    See also Auditory screening; Behavioral hearing tests; Difficult-to-test children; Language and speech screening; Newborn hearing screening; Physiologic hearing tests

Screening Instrument for Targeting Educational Risk (SIFTER), 154

SDT. *See* Speech detection threshold

Secobarbital, 366

Second branchial arch, 75, **81**, 82

Secretory otitis media, 179

Sedation, for physiologic hearing tests, 365–367

SEE. *See* Signing Exact English

Segmentation, 34, 36

Self-contained classrooms, in schools, 501, 521

Semicircular canals, fetal development of, 86

Sensitive time periods, 143

Sensitivity, of auditory screening, 378

Sensitivity prediction with the acoustic reflex (SPAR) test, 297–298, 337

Sensitized speech tests, 154
Sensorineural hearing loss, 22, **23**, 384
  bilateral, **375**
  child assessment questionnaire, **256–257**
  Connexin 26 (Cx26) hearing loss, 189–191
  meningitis and, 200
  from ototoxic drugs, 192
  perilymph fistula and, 194–195
  unilateral, 191–192
Sensory deprivation, and language
    development, 145–148
Sensory radicular neuropathy, 576
Sepsis, 201
Sequence, 535
Serous otitis media, 179, **179**, 406
SERT. *See* Sound Effects Recognition Test
Severe hearing loss, 26, 38, **40**
Sex cells, 56, 57, 58–59, **59**
Sex chromosomes, 56
Sexual maturity, 59
SIFTER. *See* Screening Instrument for
    Targeting Educational Risk
Signal-to-noise ratio (S/N), 34
Signing, 496, 512–513, 518–522
Signing Exact English (SEE), 519–522
Silent otitis media, 179
Single-gene defects, 64–67
  autosomal dominant disorders, 64–65, **66**
  autosomal recessive disorders, 65, **66**
  incidence of, 53
  X-linked disorders, 65, 67
Single probe tone tympanometry, 325
Single-sided deafness. *See* Unilateral hearing
    loss
Sisomicin, **541**
SIX1 gene, 548
SIX5 gene, 548
SLC4A11 gene, 560
SLC26A2 gene, 556
Slight hearing loss, handicapping effects of, **40**
SMC1A gene, 553
SMC3 gene, 553
SNAI2 gene, 582
SOAEs. *See* Spontaneous otoacoustic
    emissions
Sound
  binaural summation, 456
  head shadow effect, 457

infant's response to, 121, **122**, 123–126,
    250–252
  of mother's voice, 113, 119, 120
  nature of, 9–12
Sound Auditory Training (Plural Publishing),
    161
Sound Effects Recognition Test (SERT), **287**,
    289
Sound-field distribution, 525
Sound pressure, 11
Sound pressure level (SPL), 11
SOX10 gene, 582
SP. *See* Summating potential
SPAR test. *See* Sensitivity Prediction with the
    Acoustic Reflex (SPAR) test
Special care baby unit (SBCU). *See* NICU
Special education, 43–44, 502
Specificity, of auditory screening, 378
Speech
  acoustic features of, 126
  acoustics of, 30–35
  of autistic individuals, 206
  cochlear implants and, 474
  connected speech, 35
  conversational speech levels, **31**
  "deaf speech," 33, 38–39, 496
  developmental questionnaire for parents,
    132, **133–134**, 135–136, 253, **254**,
    256–257
  developmental speech milestones, 130–132,
    131, **259–260**
  emotional content of, 33, 37
  infant's first vocal sounds, 113, 128–129
  infant's response to, 125
  intensity of, 34
  nasals, 33
  optimal periods for speech and language
    learning, 143–148
  of profoundly deaf children, 33, 38–39
  referral guidelines for children with speech
    delay, 136, **136**
  segmental aspects of, 125
  supersegmental patterns, 33
  suprasegmental information, 35, 125
Speech awareness threshold (SAT), 274, 283
"Speech banana," **13**
Speech delay, referral guidelines for children
    with, 136, **136**

Speech detection threshold (SDT), 283
Speech intelligibility
    and cochlear implants, 478
    of "deaf speech," 39
    as educational goal, 496–497
    speech bands for, **32**
Speech intensity, 34
Speech-language pathologist, as treatment
    team partner, 45, 398
Speech mapping, 442, 470
Speech perception testing, 286–290, **287**, **291**,
    292–293, **292**, 452
Speech reception threshold (SRT), 252,
    283–286, **285**
Speech sample, 258, 279
Speech screening. *See* Language and speech
    screening
Speech sounds
    about, 11, 12, **13**, 30
    acoustic cues, 34, 35
    acoustics of, 30–35, **31**, **32**
    affricatives, 33
    auditory input given to infants, 130
    classification of, 33, 36
    consonants, 30
    discrimination of and language
        development, 36, 120
    formants, 30, 33
    fricative consonants, 32, 33
    hereditary deafness and, 39, 41
    infant's discrimination of, 129
    infant's response to, 125
    liquids, 33
    mild hearing loss and, 37, **40**
    moderate hearing loss and, 37–38, **40**
    in newborns, 131
    occlusives, 32
    place of production of, 33
    plosives, 32, 33
    profound hearing loss and, 38–39, **40**
    segmentation, 34, 36
    severe hearing loss and, 38, **40**
    slight hearing loss and, **40**
    "speech banana," **13**
    stop consonants, 32
    stressed speech sounds/words, 35
    variation in acoustic parameters of, 33–35, **34**
    voiced-unvoiced cognate pairs, 32
    vowels, 30–31

Speechreading, 513
Spermatononia, 59
Spinal ganglia, 72
Spoken language, prosody, 30, 36
Spontaneous otoacoustic emissions (SOAEs),
    340
Squeaky toys, noise level of, 197
SRT. *See* Speech reception threshold
Stapedial artery, 84
Stapedial muscle, 14, 327, 328
Stapedius reflex, 328
Stapes, 14, **81**, 84, 170, 328
Stapes anomalies, 170
Startle response, 121, 123, 124, 251, 268, 309
State programs, for early intervention, 215–216
Static admittance, 325–326
Stenger test, 306
Stenosis, 168
Stereocilia, 15, 16
Stickler syndrome, **542**, 566
Stimulus-response-reinforcement paradigm,
    269–270
Stomodeum, 86
Stop consonants, 32
Streptococcus pneumoniae, 182
Streptomycin, 192, 368, **541**
Stressed speech sounds/words, 35
Submucous cleft palate, 203
Summating potential (SP), 363
Superior laryngeal nerve, **81**
Superior olivary body, 19
Superior vena cava, 79
Supernumerary hillocks, 168, **168**
Supersegmental patterns, 33
Suprasegmental information, 35
Surfactant, 77, 96
Swimmer's ear, 172
Synaptic plasticity, 118
Synaptic pruning, 116
Syndactyly, 546, 554
Syndrome, 535
Syndromic hearing loss, 55
Syphilis, congenital, 105–106, **540**, 576

T

T-levels, 471
Tangible reinforcement operant conditioning
    audiometry (TROCA), 282–283

Tay-Sachs disease, genetics of, 65
TC. *See* Total communication
Technology, in the NICU, 93–96
Tectorial membrane, 16
Teenagers, prevalence of hearing loss in, 27
Teleaudiology, 242
Telepractice, 242–244
Templin-Darley Tests of Articulation, 241
Temporal bone fracture, 195–196
Tensor tympani, 14
TEOAEs. *See* Transient evoked otoacoustic emissions
Teratogens, 74, 80
Term pregnancy, 70
Test of Auditory Comprehension, 293
Testing. *See* Auditory screening; Behavioral hearing tests; Difficult-to-test children; Language and speech screening; Physiologic hearing tests
Texas, universal newborn hearing screening, 393
TGFB1 gene, 549
Therapeutic abortion, ethical dilemma of, 110
Third branchial arch, **81**, 82
Thymine, in DNA, 53, **54**
Tietz-Smith syndrome, 545
Tobramycin, 192, **541**
Toddlers
    behavioral hearing tests for, 277–283, **280**
    hearing screening methods, 405–409
    physiologic hearing tests for, 310–315, **312**
Tonsillectomy, 181
Tonsillitis, 181
Tonsils, 181
Top-down treatments, 159
TORCH infections, 108–109
Total communication (TC), 508, 517–518
Toxoplasmosis, congenital, 104–105, **540**
Toxoplasmosis gondii, 104–105
Toys, noise level of, 197
TPP. *See* Tympanogram peak pressure
Tracheoesophageal fistula, 76
Transfer RNA, 57
Transient evoked otoacoustic emissions (TEOAEs), 340, 341, **342**, 343, 392, 401, 408
Translocations (of chromosomes), 69
Traumatic brain injury (TBI), 300
Treacher Collins syndrome, 64, 89, 169, 170, 437, **542**, 577, **577**

Treatment plan, 45–47, 398
    audiologists with specialty training, 47–49
    counseling in, 47, 229, 231–233, 237, 420, 497, 594
    hearing aids, 445–446
    See also Hearing aids
Treponema pallidum, 106, 576
Trigeminal nerve, **81**
Triplet, 56
Trisomy 13–15 syndrome, 90, **542**, 578, **578**
Trisomy 18 syndrome, **542**, 578–579, **579**
Trisomy 21. *See* Down syndrome
TROCA. *See* Tangible reinforcement operant conditioning audiometry
True babbling, 132
Tube feeding, 95
Tubes in the ears, 182–184, **183**, 203
Turner mosaicism, 579
Turner's syndrome, 68, **542**, 579–580
Tympanic cavity, 84
Tympanic membrane, 14, 16, 84
    about, 173
    myringotomy, **177**, 203, 320
    perforation of, 172–173, **173**, 178
    tubes in the ears, 182–184, **183**, 203
    views of, **177**, **178**, **179**, **180**, **185**, **188**
Tympanic membrane ventilation tubes, 182–184, **183**, 203
Tympanogram peak pressure (TPP), 318, 418
Tympanograms, 319, 321, **322**, 323, **324**, 325, 331, 407
Tympanometric curve width, 407
Tympanometry, **318**, 319–321, **320**, **322**, 323, **324**, 325
    in infants, 334–335, 336–337, 406–409, **407**
    middle ear effusion and, 416–417
    for school-age children, 412
Tympanoplasty, 173
Tympanosclerosis, 184–185
Tympanostomy tubes, 182–184, **183**, 203
Tympanotomy, 176, **177**
Type I Cockayne syndrome, 553
Type II Cockayne syndrome, 553
Type III Cockayne syndrome, 553

U

Ultrasonography, of fetus, 62
Unbalanced translocations, 69

Uncrossed acoustic reflex pathway, 328, 329, **330**
Unilateral hearing loss, 24–25, 26, 37, 191
Unilateral microtia, 169
Unisensory approach, 511
Universal newborn hearing screening, 390–399, 403, **404**
Unvoiced stop consonants, 32
Urinary system, embryology of, 76
U.S. Food and Drug Administration (FDA), 426, 466
U.S. government
Early Hearing Detection and Intervention Department, 393
federal programs for early intervention, 215–216
Usher-Hallgren syndrome, 580
Usher's syndrome, 46, **542**, 580–581
Utricle, 86

V

Vaccination, 100
Validation, of hearing aids, 451–452
Van Buchem syndrome, 581
van der Hoeve's syndrome, 170, **542**, 571, **571**
Vancomycin, 192
Variability in expression, 65
Velar sounds, 33
Ventilators, neonatal, 93–94, 98, **542**
Veq. *See* Equivalent ear canal volume
Verification, of hearing aids, 447–448
Vernix caseosa, 77, 401
Vestibular aqueduct, 193–194
Vestibular evaluation, 367–368
Videoconferencing technology, 244
Videonystagmography, 368
Viral diseases, hearing loss and, 202
Viral infections, congenital, 100
Viral meningitis, 200, 567
Visual acuity, and deafness, 504–505
Visual reinforcement audiometry (VRA), 252, 266, 271–277, **273**, **276**, 444–445, 449
Visual reinforcement operant conditioning audiometry (VROCA), 277

Visually reinforced infant speech discrimination (VRISD), 275
Vocal range, 34
Vohwinkel-Nockemann syndrome, **542**
Vohwinkel syndrome, 581
Voice, vocal range, 34
Voice-onset time (VOT), 136
Voiced stop consonants, 32
Voiced-unvoiced cognate pairs, 32
Volunteers, for auditory screening, 398–399
Von Recklinghausen's syndrome, **542**, 544
Vowel Perception Test, 293
Vowels
acoustics of, 30–31
infant's use of, 129
VRA. *See* Visual reinforcement audiometry
VRISD. *See* Visually reinforced infant speech discrimination
VROCA. *See* Visual reinforcement operant conditioning audiometry

W

Waardenburg-Shah syndrome, 582
Waardenburg's syndrome, 55, 65, 194, **542**, 545, 581–582, **582**
Western Electric 4-A audiometer, 410
Western Electric Fading Numbers test, 410–411
WHO. *See* World Health Organization
Wildervanck's syndrome, **543**, 550, 582–583
Winter syndrome, **543**
Word Intelligibility by Picture Identification (WIPI) test, 288
World Health Organization (WHO), 196

X

X-linked disorders, 65, 67

Z

Zygotes, 56, 70